DISEASES OF THE EYE AND SKIN

A COLOR ATLAS

DISEASES OF THE EYE AND SKIN

A COLOR ATLAS

H. BRUCE OSTLER, M.D. (DECEASED)

Clinical Professor and Research Ophthalmologist
Department of Ophthalmology
Francis I. Proctor Foundation
University of California
San Francisco, California

HOWARD I. MAIBACH, M.D.

Professor
Department of Dermatology
University of California
San Francisco, California

AXEL W. HOKE, M.D.

Clinical Professor
Department of Dermatology
University of California
San Francisco, California

IVAN R. SCHWAB, M.D., F.A.C.S.

Professor of Clinical Ophthalmology
Department of Ophthalmology
University of California, Davis
Sacramento, California

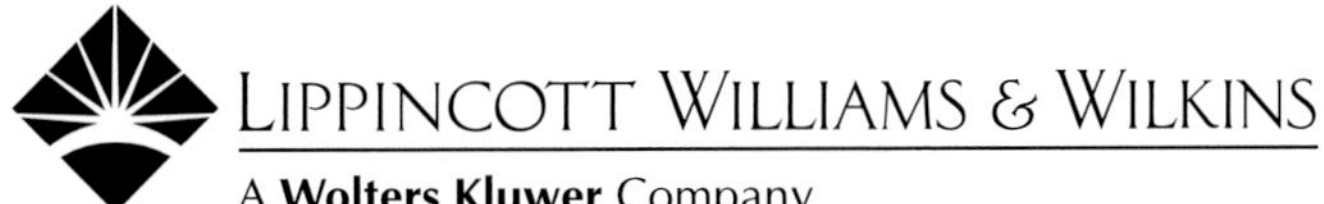

LIPPINCOTT WILLIAMS & WILKINS
A **Wolters Kluwer** Company
Philadelphia · Baltimore · New York · London
Buenos Aires · Hong Kong · Sydney · Tokyo

Acquisitions Editor: Jonathan Pine
Developmental Editor: Michael Standen
Production Editor: Sheila Higgins
Manufacturing Manager: Colin Warnock
Cover Designer: Christine Jenny
Compositor: Lippincott Williams & Wilkins Desktop Division
Printer: Walsworth Publishing

© **2004 by LIPPINCOTT WILLIAMS & WILKINS**
530 Walnut Street
Philadelphia, PA 19106 USA
LWW.com

Printed in the USA

Library of Congress Cataloging-in-Publication Data

Diseases of the eye and skin: a color atlas / H. Bruce Ostler ... [et al.].
    p. ; cm.
  Includes bibliographical references and index.
  ISBN 0-7817-4999-9
    1. Skin—Diseases—Atlases. 2. Eye—Diseases—Atlases. I. Title: Diseases of the eye and skin. II. Ostler, H. Bruce.
    [DNLM: 1. Eye Diseases—Atlases. 2. Skin Diseases—Atlases. WW 17 O852 2003]
RL81.O885 2003
616.5′0022′2—dc22

                                                                2003056498

10 9 8 7 6 5 4 3 2 1

To my wife Marian, my son Bruce Ostler II, my daughter Teresa Jacobson, and my grandchildren Geff, Pete, Johanna, Tom, Matt, Gabe, Jake, Jessica, Sam, Alex, Shannon, and Bruce, with special thanks to the fellows at the Francis I. Proctor Foundation for their continuing questions.

H.B.O.

To my wife Adriene and my daughters Marisa and Diana without whose encouragement and support this project would not have been completed.

A.W.H.

To my wife Nora and my son Nathan who have sustained me; my patients who have taught me; and the medical students, residents, and especially my fellows who have stimulated me to keep up with them.

I.R.S.

CONTENTS

PREFACE

Bruce Ostler had an interest in dermatology, and, of course in his specialty, ophthalmology for as long as I knew him. For example, I remember his spontaneous discussion about temperature—induced dermatoses, among other external diseases, and I marveled at his knowledge of the topic that might otherwise be considered out of his immediate field. He was a consummate physician; he was interested in the diseases of the anterior segment and external eye, and his depth of understanding included a comprehensive knowledge of dermatologic diseases. For him, understanding the external diseases of the eye to his satisfaction meant understanding diseases of the skin as well. He satisfied that need and then managed to stimulate a generation of fellows at the Francis I. Proctor Foundation in San Francisco to be similarly interested in diseases of the eye and skin. He succeeded more than he will ever know. As a former fellow of Dr. Ostler, I am a witness to his enthusiasm in teaching the skill of diagnosis. He was able to acquire the historical and physical findings of a patient's problem and, with the help of an almost photographic memory, he could quickly recite the differential list and synthesize the diagnosis. But surprisingly, this was not his greatest skill. That lay in his ability to stimulate medical students, ophthalmology residents, and especially clinical fellows to think, ask the right questions of the patient and the patient's examination, create the differential diagnosis, and establish the diagnosis. The process is called synthesis and is the single most important skill for a physician. It is a difficult one to teach. His professional endeavor was to teach, and his humble nature and subtle style will be remembered by all those he taught. His success in this quest is echoed in generations of students represented by former Proctor fellows and those we teach.

External diseases of the eye are rarely confined to the ocular surface. These diseases often cross the ocular mucous membrane surface to the skin surface directly or indirectly, or may be manifested by cutaneous disease at a remote cutaneous site. The skin and the eye share many common tissues, and an immune system as the first line of defense for the body against external insults and diseases. These myriad diseases are common and represent a large proportion of patient complaints for an ophthalmologist and certainly for a dermatologist.

Dr. Ostler had a dream to create an encyclopedia of diseases of the eye and skin in a text that is well illustrated with a comprehensive differential diagnostic list. This book began with the initiation of his career in 1956 after his completion of his fellowship at the University of Iowa, where he had been an intern, resident, and fellow in external diseases of the eye. He began writing in the mid-1990s and asked two experienced, knowledgeable, and renowned dermatologists, Drs. Hoke and Maibach, to help him create such a text. Unfortunately, Dr. Ostler died before this text could be completed.

I was honored when asked to complete this text, and I knew I would not be able to match his skill and understanding of this field. Nevertheless, I wanted to see his dream realized. This book represents that realization. If the reader is stimulated by reading this comprehensive text, the success should be credited to Drs. Hoke, Maibach, and especially Dr. Ostler.

There are several who should be recognized in this text. Dr. Ostler's children, Bruce Ostler II and Teresa Jacobsen were instrumental in keeping this project alive. Their heartfelt love for their father came through as they provided stewardship to assure completion and publication of this text. Charley Mitchell, as well as others who knew Dr. Ostler at Lippincott Williams & Wilkins also deserve credit for maintaining faith in the book and nurturing it to publication. Special thanks go to Donna Dator who gave so generously of her evenings and weekends to help meet transcription deadlines.

At least one other individual deserves mention. Dr. Ostler made innumerable trips to a variety of countries in the developing world, and on arriving in the clinic he was to visit, he would simply say "How can I help?" This work further broadened his encyclopedic knowledge of ophthalmic and dermatologic conditions and introduced him to others who shared his same interests. Through this work, he met and worked tirelessly with Yasin Al Quibati at the leprosarium in Yemen. Dr. Ostler and Dr. Al Quibati, a dedicated dermatologist in Taiz, Yemen, were working toward building an improved hospital for their patients when civil war erupted in Yemen. Unfortunately, this project was never completed.

Especially, Dr. Ostler would also have expressed his heartfelt thanks to the fellows who worked with him for more than a quarter of a century, for as those of you who teach know, students always stimulate with their insistent questions and wide-eyed curiosity. The greatest paean of thanks goes to the patients. Dr. Ostler's patients recognized that he cared greatly for their welfare. Our patients provide us the opportunity to learn more about each disease process, if we only take the time to listen, watch, and provide a helping hand when we are able. Dr. Ostler did all of that. It is from our patients and those we teach that we received the inspiration to produce this text.

This book offers extensive clinical photographs and explanatory text to document the disease presentations that include differential diagnoses. These photographs are provided in an effort to expand the understanding and "pattern recognition" of these diseases. The detailed descriptions of the anatomy and physiology of the epithelial manifestations of these diseases should assist the reader in their recognition. Our goal is to be as comprehensive as possible and to include an expanded differential for the ophthalmologist and the dermatologist, assisting in the management of their patients.

This book is a tribute to Dr. Ostler and his interest in the fields of dermatology and ophthalmology, but it should also be seen as his educational dream. We hope it will stimulate and teach.

Ivan R. Schwab, M.D., F.A.C.S.

1

INTRODUCTION

The layman, the medical neophyte, and the average physician are often amazed at the ability of an experienced dermatologist or ophthalmologist to make a lightninglike diagnosis following an almost casual glance at a cutaneous eruption or a keratitis. Yet both disciplines of medicine are based on the visual image conveyed. Colors, hues, configurations, shapes, distribution, and arrangement of lesions are emblems of various diseases, just as alphabetical letters or musical notes are emblems for words or songs.

Ophthalmology and dermatology have many things in common. Both are highly specialized disciplines that rely heavily on visual inspection and history for diagnosis. Both use meaningful descriptions that are readily understood by members of their own discipline but that often cause frowns and puzzlement to members of other medical disciplines because of the unusual terminology. Both have diseases in common, especially those that involve the skin, lid, conjunctiva, cornea, lens, and retina because of their contiguity and their embryologic derivation. The skin and the eye are highly specialized organs and often reflect pathology in other areas of the body. Both are sensitive to ultraviolet and x-ray irradiation, and the skin and ocular structures are often highly sensitive to topical and parenteral medications used both by ophthalmologists and dermatologists and by members of the medical profession in general.

ANATOMY AND ORGANIZATION OF THE SKIN

The skin is composed of the epidermis, the underlying dermis, and the subcutaneous fatty tissue lying directly beneath the dermis (Fig. 1-1).

The epidermis is a superficial, stratified, cellular structure composed of stratified epithelium that is produced in the basal layer at the dermoepidermal junction, then progressively differentiates as it moves toward the skin surface. The epidermal layers can be differentiated into basal cell, prickle cell, granular, and horny layers. Other cells in the epidermis include melanocytes, Langerhans' cells, and Merkel cells.

The dermis is made up of connective tissue composed of collagen and elastin. It contains fibroblasts, histiocytes, mast cells, blood vessels, and autonomic and sensory nerves in great abundance. The sweat glands are also located in the dermis, but their ducts and openings extend through the epidermis to the skin surface.

The dermoepidermal junction separates the dermis and epidermis, lends mechanical support to the skin, and serves as a protective barrier against large molecules gaining access to the subcutaneous tissue. It has an undulating shape called the *rete ridge* that projects into the dermis. The hair follicles and pilosebaceous units also project into the dermis, which further accentuates the undulating shape.

All skin areas contain eccrine glands, but various regions are notable for the presence or absence of terminal or vellus hair follicles, sebaceous glands, and apocrine glands. The glabrous, or nonhairy, skin (skin of the palms and soles) possesses sebaceous glands, encapsulated sense organs, and ridges (fingerprints or dermatoglyphics), but no hair follicles. The hair-bearing skin has both vellus and terminal hair-bearing follicles, sebaceous glands, and, in some areas, such as the axilla, apocrine glands.

Vellus hair represents soft, unmedullated hair less than 2 cm long. Terminal hair represents the long, strong hair of the adult and is found in the scalp, brows, lashes, male beard, axilla, and pubic regions.

ANATOMY AND ORGANIZATION OF THE EYE

Eyebrows

The eyebrows are the two raised arches of skin, containing multiple, short, thick hairs that overlie the supraorbital margins. The action of the frontalis muscle that is attached to the eyebrows gives much of the facial expression. The brow helps to warn of tactile danger to the eye and orbital rim and helps prevent perspiration from running into the eye. It is often involved in congenital and infectious diseases.

Eyelids

The lids are two movable folds of skin that serve to protect the eye (Fig. 1-2). Their layers include the following:

1. A very thin and easily irritated and inflamed skin.
2. A lax, nonfatty connective tissue that is wrinkled and becomes easily stretched (especially in the presence of edema).
3. Striated muscle that serves to open and close the lid.
4. Tarsus, composed of dense fibrillary connective tissue that contains the meibomian glands and gives support to the lid.
5. Tarsal or palpebral conjunctiva that lines and is firmly attached to the tarsus.

The free border of the lid is called the lid margin and is readily divided into an anterior and posterior border. The anterior border is rolled and contains several rows of lashes arranged one behind the other that serve to tactically warn of flying objects. Those in the upper lid are larger and more numerous. Modified sweat glands (glands of Moll) and Zeis glands (sebaceous glands) open onto the anterior lid margin and into the lash follicles.

The anterior border is separated from the posterior border by a fine gray line, which is more of a surgical than an anatomic line. The posterior border contains the orifices of the meibomian glands and ends with the conjunctiva.

The palpebral fissure represents the elliptical space between the lids. It is bordered laterally by the lateral canthus and medially by the medial canthus. Near the nasal extremity of the upper and lower lid margin is a small elevation of skin termed the *lacrimal papilla,* which contains the orifice (lacrimal puncta) of the lacrimal canaliculus.

The caruncle is derived from skin and is located at the medial angle of the eyelids. It contains sebaceous glands and sweat glands, and its surface is covered by fine, nonpigmented hair.

The lid participates in many infectious, as well as inflammatory, congenital, neoplastic, and dermatologic conditions.

The Lacrimal System

The lacrimal system is conveniently divided into secretory and excretory portions. The secretory portion produces the tears and contains the lacrimal gland (palpebral and orbital lobes), accessory lacrimal glands, lacrimal gland ductules, and goblet cells. The lacrimal gland is located in the orbital lacrimal fossa. The accessory lacrimal glands and goblet cells are found in the conjunctiva. The tears provide constant moisture for the eye and through their dilutional and slushing action serve to carry infectious particles and noxious substances away from the cornea and conjunctiva. The lacrimal glands participate in many of the same congenital, viral, granulomatous, and neoplastic diseases as the skin.

The excretory portion of the lacrimal system begins with the lacrimal puncta; extends into the lacrimal canaliculi, the common canaliculus, lacrimal sac, nasolacrimal duct; and finally ends under the inferior turbinate of the nose. Many of the congenital, inflammatory, infectious, and neoplastic disease processes that involve the nose or midfacial region also involve the excretory portion of the lacrimal system.

Conjunctiva

The conjunctiva is a thin, transparent membrane that lines and is firmly adherent to the inner surface of the eyelids (palpebral conjunctiva), then folds back on itself at the superior and inferior fornices to cover the anterior sclera. It has minimal connections to the inferior and superior fornices, fine connections to the sclera, and firm connections to the limbus and the palpebral surfaces. It participates in many infectious, immunologic, and allergic conditions, and is sensitive to ultraviolet irradiation.

Cornea

The cornea is the transparent fibrous coat of the eye. Seen from in front, it appears round. It is transparent in health but quickly becomes cloudy when diseased. It fuses with the sclera at the limbus and is normally avascular. It is readily infected once its surface epithelium is broken; it participates in many congenital, infectious, inflammatory, and allergic conditions; and it is sensitive to ultraviolet irradiation.

Sclera and Episclera

The sclera makes up about five-sixths of the fibrous coat of the eye. It is shaped like a sphere and fuses with the cornea at the limbus. It is white and is traversed by many vessels and nerves that pass into the interior of the eye. It can be conveniently divided into an anterior and posterior segment. Both segments participate in inflammatory disorders but are rarely involved in infectious processes.

The episclera is a loose connective tissue located external to and covering the sclera. It is traversed by many vessels and nerves, and readily participates in inflammatory disorders.

Uvea

The uvea represents the middle coat of the eye. It is dark brown because of the pigment-bearing cells that partially comprise it. The uvea is composed of the iris, ciliary body, and choroid. The iris is a disc-shaped membrane located anterior to the lens. In its center is a large opening, the pupil. The iris arises from the ciliary body. The ciliary body lies between the iris anteriorly and the choroid posteriorly. It is composed of the ciliary muscles and ciliary processes. The choroid is that part of the uvea that lies posterior to the ciliary body and is composed of blood vessels and nerves that serve to provide nourishment for the retina and sensory and motor nerves for the iris and ciliary muscles. The uvea participates in many inflammatory and infectious diseases.

Retina

The retina represents the innermost coat of the eye. It is perfectly transparent and is composed of supporting tissue and nervous tissue for the reception and transmission of visual impulses. It participates in many systemic, inflammatory, and infectious diseases.

Lens

The lens lies between the iris and the vitreous. It is colorless, is transparent, and has a lenticular shape. It gradually becomes opaque with aging, and the process is often speeded up by inflammation or infection of the uvea or other ocular structure.

Vitreous

The vitreous is a colorless, gelatinous mass that fills the posterior portion of the eye. It lies between the retina posteriorly and the lens anteriorly, and it participates in many inflammatory conditions of the uvea and retina.

EXAMINATION OF THE SKIN AND EYE

An accurate history is essential and should include the following:

1. The major complaints and their duration, the mode of onset, the location of any lesions, the course of the disease with and without treatment, and the associated symptoms, especially those of itch and pain.
2. A history of allergy or untoward reactions to drugs or chemicals.
3. A history of present medication, and present and past illnesses.
4. The presence of similar complaints in family members or those living in close proximity.

5. These and other questions should be elaborated upon, and will be suggested, as the patient is questioned and examined.

The skin of the lid and the skin in general must be examined in a good light, preferably daylight. Ophthalmologists, who choose to have easily controlled artificial light so that they can use ancillary optical instruments, may find this difficult. However, subtleties of change in skin and mucous membrane color are often missed in artificial light, and it is good to take a moment to at least open the drape to look at some lesions.

Often mistakes are made because the entire skin surface is not examined. To be sure, ophthalmologists are not equipped to examine the skin extensively. However, it is wise for both ophthalmologists and dermatologists to remember that the patient is not just made of skin or of the eye. He or she is a whole, living subject, and much information can be gleaned from looking at that subject from other aspects than just with the slit-lamp, a penlight, or the naked eye.

Physical touch and palpation of the hands, face, and especially the lids can be important even to the ophthalmologist. Lichenification, papules, dryness of the skin, subcutaneous nodules, lymph nodes, and other changes are best appreciated when felt. One of my favorite memories is that of watching my old professor (an ophthalmologist at that) tenderly palpate a skin lesion so that he could properly assess its character.

At this point, ophthalmologists then turn their attention to evaluation of the visual acuity, visual fields, pupils and pupillary reactions, extraocular movements, corneal sensation, intraocular pressure, and slit-lamp examination of the lid, lid margin, conjunctiva, cornea, anterior chamber, and lens. Following dilatation of pupils, the fundus is also evaluated.

Dermatologists, on the other hand, turn their attention to examination of skin under magnification, evaluate the hair where indicated, and often resort to biopsies for histologic studies or patch testing for determination of hypersensitivity.

The clinical findings are recorded with specific attention to location, morphology of individual lesions, grouping of the lesions, and presence of other factors. Following this, the diagnostic possibilities are considered, as well as the need for further study.

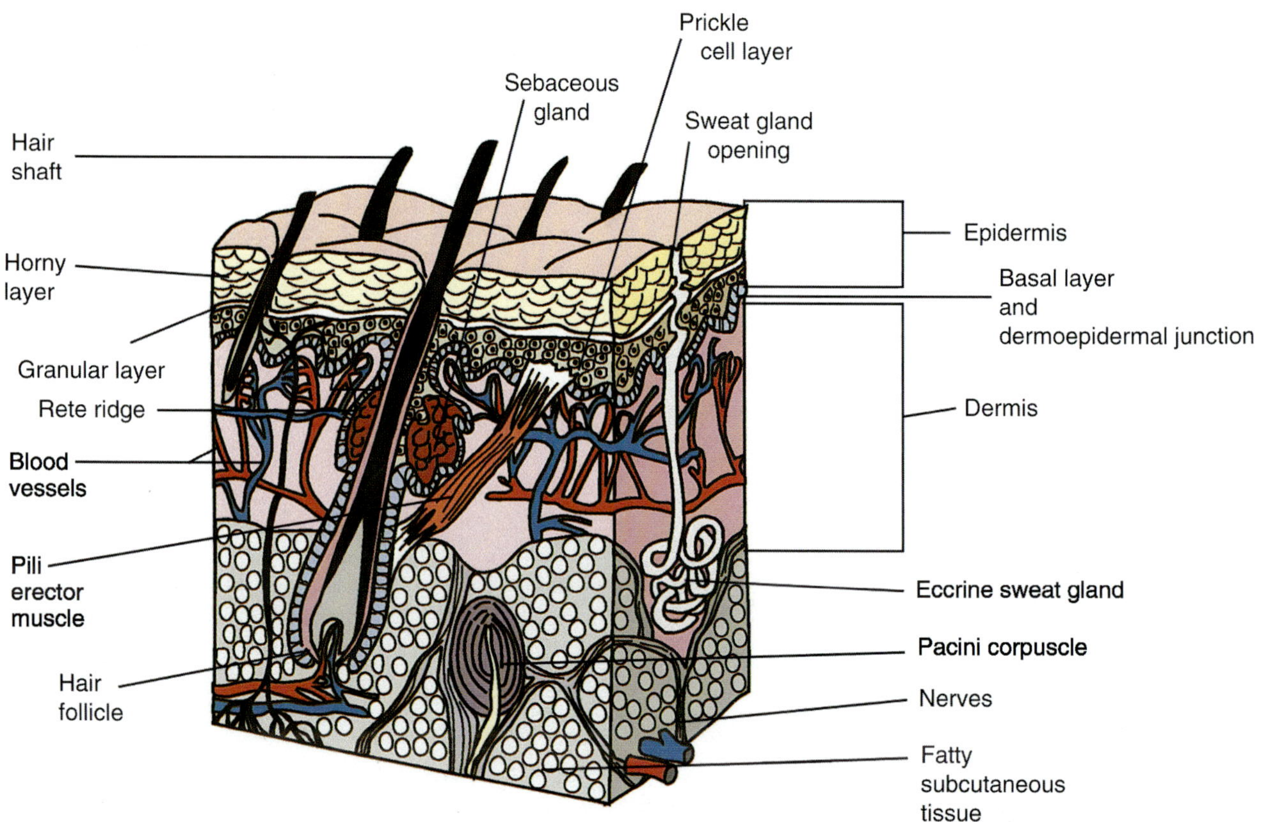

FIGURE 1-1. Schematic drawing of the histology of the skin. (Image courtesy of LifeART. Copyright © 2002 Lippincott Williams & Wilkins. All rights reserved.)

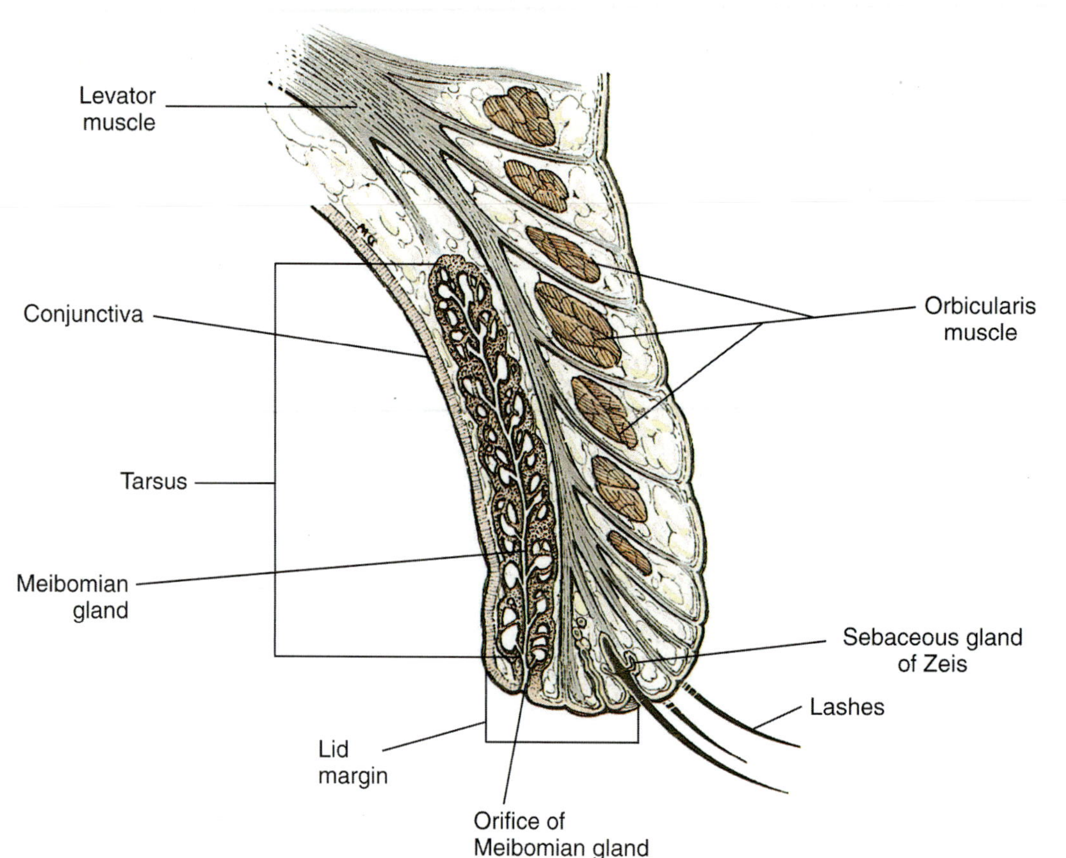

FIGURE 1-2. Schematic drawing of the histology of the eyelid. (Reprinted from Agur AMR, Lee MJ. *Grant's atlas of anatomy,* 10th ed. Philadelphia: Lippincott Williams & Wilkins, 1999, with permission.)

2

ALLERGIC DISORDERS

ATOPIC DERMATITIS

Atopic dermatitis is characterized by an eczematoid eruption that usually involves the forehead, neck, cheeks, and flexor surfaces of the arms and legs. It is often associated with a personal or family history of allergy, xerosis, immunologic peculiarities, and abnormal cutaneous vascular function. The symptoms are often exacerbated during the spring and fall, and may be associated with elevated serum IgE and peripheral eosinophilia.

Atopy usually begins in infancy and continues for many years, with periods of remission and exacerbation. It often improves during puberty and recurs during the third decade of life. Spontaneous remissions often occur after many years, and, with advancing age, the eruption may completely disappear; but atopic disease may last a lifetime.

Skin Features

Atopic dermatitis is characterized by acute, subacute, or chronic itch, superficial symmetric inflammation, weeping, crusting, and lichenification. The area of involvement varies for infants (Figs. 2-1 and 2-2), children (Figs. 2-3 and 2-4), and adults (Fig. 2-5). Occasionally, it involves the entire body.

The type of rash varies with age. In infants, the lesions are usually exudative and have a prominent picture of vesicles and crusting, and usually involve the forehead, cheeks, and extensor surfaces of the forearms and legs. In children 18 months to 12 years of age, dryness and lichenification involving the sides of the neck and flexural creases of the elbows, knees, wrists, and ankles are commonly seen. A mild periocular pigmentation may be seen, and a reticulated pigmentation often occurs on the sides of the neck. Pityriasis alba, characterized by branny desquamation of the skin followed by atrophy, may involve the lids and other facial areas (Fig 2-6). In adults, the lesions are thickened and lichenified, and usually involve the skin of the face, neck, palms, soles, flexural creases, and genitalia. Dryness (a minor degree of ichthyosis) is characteristic, and there is an increased transdermal loss of water in all age groups.

Associated stigmata include ridging and pitting of the nails; itchy skin; proclivity for the flexural creases to lichenify (Figs. 2- 4 and 2-7); abnormal vascular response to cold or trauma (constriction of the small vessels); increase in the fine palmar creases; abnormal sweat response (rash aggravated by sweating); alopecia areata; and Dennie line (Fig. 2-3). The Dennie-Morgan fold, or Dennie line, is present at or soon after birth and may be a harbinger of future allergy. It represents a crease of the lower lid similar to that seen in Down syndrome. The fold begins immediately below the medial margin of the lower lid and extends obliquely laterally and downward.

Ocular Features

Atopic patients often complain of ocular itching and burning. The atopic lid lesions are similar to skin lesions elsewhere, often are secondarily infected with staphylococci, and may include superantigen-producing bacteria, especially with increased severity of the skin lesions. These may persist for years even after the general eruption has subsided; infrequently, they persist for life. Other lid features include Dennie line (Fig. 2-3); thinning or loss of the brow or lateral aspect of the brow (Fig. 2-7) (madarosis), believed to be caused by rubbing; and a marginal blepharitis similar to staphylococcal blepharitis (Figs. 2-8 to 2-10).

Madarosis is common and often develops in the late stages of atopy; the lashes of the lower lid usually disappear first (Fig. 2-11). Atopic keratoconjunctivitis (Figs. 2-9, 2-12, and 2-13), Trantas dots (Fig. 2-14), and conjunctival scarring are common (Figs. 2-15 and 2-16). Limbal papillae are occasionally evident (Fig. 2-17). In some instances, limbal cysts develop (Fig. 2-18). They develop at the upper limbus in atopic keratoconjunctivitis and serve as evidence of previous disease. About a third of atopic patients develop a conjunctivitis characterized by itch, tearing, redness, edema, papillary hypertrophy, Trantas dots, stringy mucoid discharge, and conjunctival scarring. Trantas dots (focal, chalky-appearing concretions, composed of eosinophils) are often found near giant limbal papillae in atopic keratoconjunctivitis and may cause a foreign-body sensation. The edema, hyperemia, and fine papillary hypertrophy cause the upper and lower tarsal conjunctiva to appear milky and velvety. The milky appearance and fine papillary hypertrophy are readily apparent, while the conjunctival scarring is less apparent and appears as fine white lines against the reddish milky background. Fine stellate or linear conjunctival scars may occur in the inferior cul-de-sac and on the tarsal conjunctiva along with mild shrinkage of the inferior fornix. Occasionally, giant papillae resembling flat-topped polygonal cobblestones develop on the inferior and superior tarsal conjunctiva, at the upper limbus, and in the interpalpebral fissure area. The stringy mucoid discharge often causes blurred vision and irritation that results in rubbing, further irritation, and production of more mucus.

Corneal findings include an epithelial keratitis, frequently seen on the superior cornea, (Fig. 2-19). Corneal epithelial loss is often preceded by a syncytial epithelial keratitis (a fine, white haze that simulates flour dusted on the superior cornea) in the mid to superior cornea, quickly followed by slight staining of the epithelium with fluorescein. Eventually, the epithelium exfoliates, leaving an oval superficial ulcer (Fig. 2-20). Mucus, cellular debris, leukocytes, and epithelial cells then fill and adhere to the ulcer bed. Occasionally, a fine epithelial keratitis of the inferior cornea occurs as another form of syncytial epithelial keratitis leading to superficial ulceration. Central bacterial or viral corneal ulcers are common complications of atopic keratoconjunctivitis and reflect the increased incidence of staphylococcal organisms on the eyelids together with reduced cell-mediated immunity in such patients (Figs. 2-21 and 2-22). Superficial and deep corneal neovascularization often occur in response to a corneal ulcer, although neovascularization (superficial corneal vascularization in the form of a micropannus, gross peripheral vascularization, or, rarely, complete vascularization) often occurs in atopic keratoconjunctivitis without evidence of corneal suppuration. The vascularized area is usually hazy, and the vessels may be quite prominent. Keratoconus, characterized by a central, symmetric, conelike protrusion; pellucid marginal degeneration, characterized by a thin and ectatic inferior part of the cornea; and keratoglobus, characterized by diffuse corneal thinning most marked in the periphery may all occur in atopic dermatitis.

Other ocular features include punctal stenosis and tearing or keratoconjunctivitis sicca (dry eye), retinal detachment, and an allergic shiner characterized by bluish discoloration surrounding the orbit. A shieldlike or star-shaped anterior subcapsular cataract (Fig. 2-23) may be seen but is believed to be less common than the same opacity seen as a posterior subcapsular cataract. The posterior subcapsular cataract, however, may be a consequence of long-term treatment with corticosteroids.

URTICARIA

Urticaria is a common complaint and represents a transient erythematous or edematous swelling (wheal) of the dermis (Fig. 2-24). Acute urticaria is the most common. It persists less than 2 to 3 months and is usually associated with a familial or personal history of atopy. Chronic urticaria per-

TABLE 2-1. KNOWN TRIGGERS FOR URTICARIA AND ANGIOEDEMA

Major Nonallergic Causes
  Physical factors (cholinergic form of urticaria)
    Heat, cold, sunlight, pressure, injury, physical exercise, hot showers, excitement
  Arthropod bites and bee stings
  Food additives
    Cinnamic acid or aldehyde, sorbic acid, sodium benzoate
  Medications
    Atropine, pilocarpine codeine, morphine
  Neurogenic factors
    Tension
  General medical illnesses (acquired C1 esterase inhibitor deficiency)
    Lupus erythematosus
    Lymphoma and carcinoma
Major Allergic Causes
  Medications
    Penicillin, sulfonamides, aspirin, nonsteroidal antiinflammatory drugs, ACE inhibitors, streptomycin
    Sera and vaccines
  Inhalants
    Feathers; animal dander, hair, and saliva; grass pollen, mold spores, house dust, tobacco smoke
  Foods
    Shell fish, fish (especially old fish), strawberries, tomatoes, nuts, pork, eggs, mushrooms, fruit, chocolate, milk and cheese, spices, yeast, flour
  External contactants
    Cosmetics and chemicals
    Textiles
    Latex

sists longer than 2 to 3 months, and although individual lesions may last only a day or so, new lesions appear at irregular intervals. It is usually nonallergic but may be familial. Table 2-1 lists some urticarial triggers.

Contact Urticaria, or Immediate Reaction Syndrome

Contact urticaria, or immediate reaction syndrome, may be nonimmunologic (NICO) or immunologic (ICO). It usually occurs on the hands or around the mouth, and arises from direct contact with an allergen such as food additives, drugs, grass pollen, algae, lichens, animal saliva or dander, rubber gloves, and industrial substances. The reaction often extends beyond the area of direct contact. Sometimes simultaneous symptoms develop from other organ involvement. Not infrequently, there is a generalized urticaria; rarely, an anaphylactic reaction occurs.

Nonimmunologic contact urticaria occurs without previous sensitization and is caused by the offending agent (e.g., a chemical released from an arthropod or from a plant) directly influencing the dermal blood vessel wall, through nonimmunologic release of histamine or SRS-A (slow-reacting substance A), or by way of the alternate pathway that includes properdin.

Immune complex urticaria is acute (e.g., serum sickness), persisting several weeks, or chronic, and may last many months or years. Acute forms are often caused by parenteral serum or drugs (e.g., penicillin), and occasionally foods. In the chronic forms, the antigenic trigger is often not identified, and the picture suggests an urticarial vasculitis.

Skin Features

Urticarial lesions usually involve only the dermis, whereas angioedema usually involves both skin and subcutaneous tissue, and, when acquired, may be associated with a lymphoproliferative disorder. Urticaria occurs on any area of the body surface, including the palms, soles, lips, tongue, larynx, and genitalia. At onset there is intense itch, quickly followed by the sudden eruption of evanescent wheals (hives) with pseudopods and intense swelling surrounded by an erythematous halo. As the wheal subsides, the central area flattens, giving an annular appearance. Linear urticarial lesions are characteristic of acute allergic reactions to poisonous plants such as poison oak or poison ivy. Papular urticaria is often caused by insect bites and may persist for many days. A central pit is found in flea or gnat bite forms of urticaria.

The immediate type of reaction in other organs includes asthma–tracheal or pulmonary involvement; rhinitis–nasal mucous membrane involvement; conjunctivitis–conjunctival involvement; dysphagia and oral swelling-oropharyngeal involvement; and nausea, vomiting, and diarrhea–gastrointestinal involvement. Fever, flushing, headaches, joint pains, hematuria, anuria, hypotension, and shock may also occur.

Immune complex urticaria causes persistent, painful, tender urticaria that tends toward bruising. Constitutional symptoms (fever, arthropathy, and an elevated sedimentation rate) may also occur. In chronic immune complex urticaria, the symptoms last 24 hours or longer.

Physical urticaria is in the form of dermatographism, literally "writing on the skin" (whealing and itch) at sites of trauma, friction, or scratching (Fig. 2-25). Sometimes the cause is inapparent. Pressure urticaria (a form of physical urticaria) comes on only after several hours of prolonged pressure but may persist longer than 48 hours.

Cholinergic urticaria, sometimes called *micropapular urticaria,* is distinctive. Small wheals persisting several minutes or longer usually develop on the trunk in association with sweating induced by any cause. Occasionally, there is itch without whealing.

Ocular Features

Itch and lid edema and erythema are common. The typical wheal develops rapidly and progresses to a more generalized edema, which then spontaneously disappears after a few hours. Tearing and conjunctival chemosis are common.

ANGIOEDEMA

Angioedema (angioneurotic edema, Quincke edema, giant urticaria) is similar to urticaria, except the lesions are larger, involve the subcutaneous tissue, and usually do not itch. The two are often associated, and both may be caused by the same factors. Angioedema may occur suddenly and cyclically or intermittently. It usually lasts only a few hours, occasionally days or weeks, and usually involves the lids, lips, genitalia, and, less commonly, the tongue and larynx.

Recurrent angioedema may cause permanent hypertrophic tissue changes (redundant skin and subcutaneous tissue) that hangs loosely between attacks, whereas during attacks it is filled with edema fluid.

HEREDITARY ANGIOEDEMA

Hereditary angioedema is autosomal dominant and may begin in early childhood. It is manifested by recurrent skin and mucous membrane swelling, which are often associated with a reticulated erythema. Nausea, vomiting, colic, and urinary symptoms may accompany the attacks. Trauma (especially dental trauma) may induce the attacks.

Skin Features

Hereditary angioedema usually begins in infancy and is often associated with massive urticarial lesions. Often there is a history of repeated attacks of edema of the skin, respiratory tract, and gastrointestinal tract. The swelling begins suddenly and persists 1 to 2 days. Gastrointestinal involvement causes recurrent episodes of colicky abdominal pain and vomiting. Death may occur from laryngeal obstruction.

Ocular Features

Itch, lid edema, and erythema, and conjunctival chemosis are common in angioedema (Fig. 2-26). Infrequently, chronic angioedema presents as a cellulitis. Other ocular findings include corneal edema; orbital angioedema with itch, pain, extreme lid swelling, chemosis, and proptosis; and occasionally, optic neuritis and blindness. Occasionally, the orbital angioedema is recurrent.

In the exceptional case, iridocyclitis, anterior chamber hemorrhage, vitreous opacities, and secondary glaucoma develop in acute angioedema, and several cases of central serous retinopathy (edema of the macular region) have been observed.

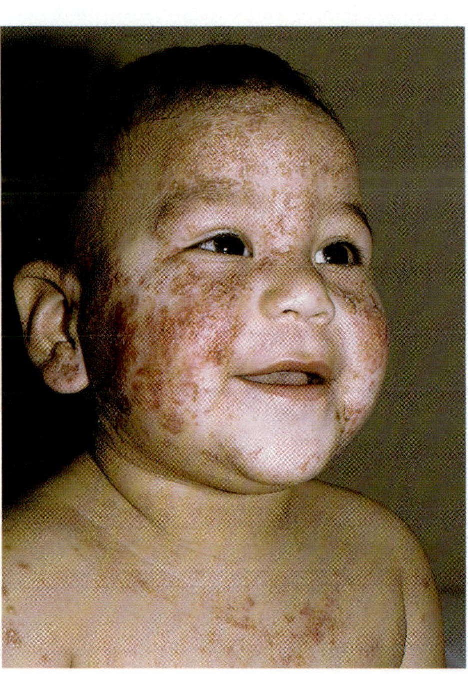

FIGURE 2-1. Severe atopic eczema of cheeks, forehead, external ears, and chest. Edema and erythema of upper eyelids is evident.

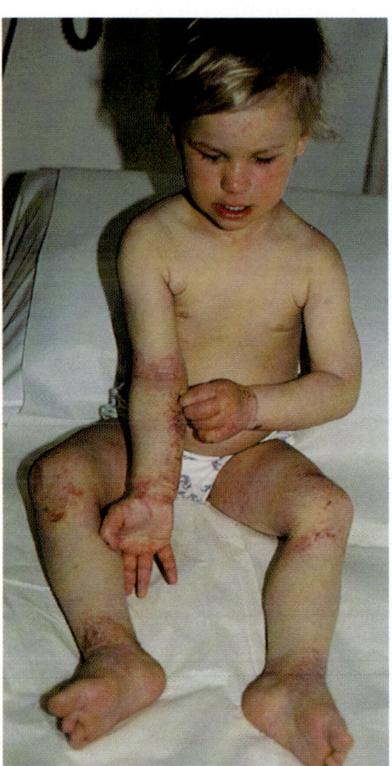

FIGURE 2-2. Subacute dermatitis of the antecubital fossae, knees, and ankles in a child with atopic eczema. Constant itching robbed the child of sleep and made him irritable and tearful.

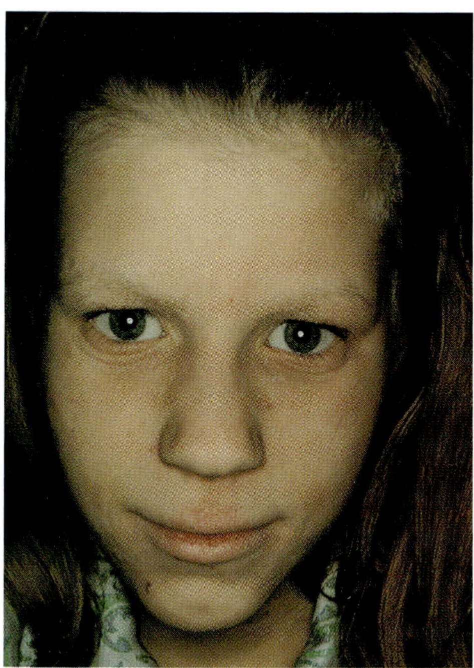

FIGURE 2-3. Young girl with atopic eczema since infancy demonstrating Dennie lines (also called *atopic pleats*) on lower eyelids as well as thinning of the lateral brows.

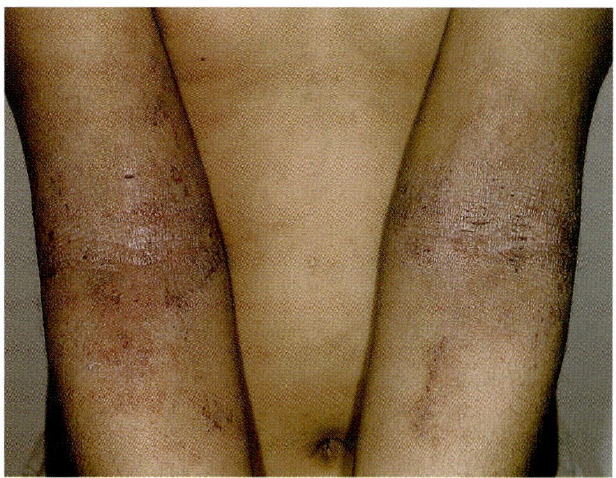

FIGURE 2-4. Subacute eczema with mild lichenification of antecubital fossae. Heavy colonization with *Staphylococcus aureus* is common.

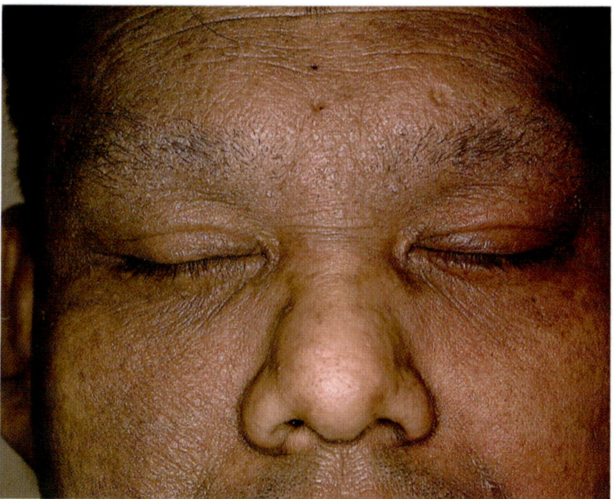

FIGURE 2-5. Lichenification, increased skin pigmentation, and lid thickening in an adult with chronic severe atopic eczema.

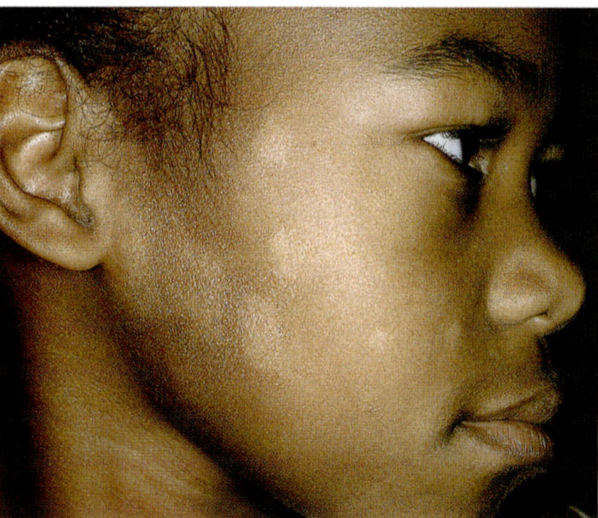

FIGURE 2-6. Pityriasis alba manifest by hypopigmented, slightly scaly maculae on cheeks and eyelid. This common finding in patients with atopic eczema is often misdiagnosed and treated as fungal infection (Tinea faciale).

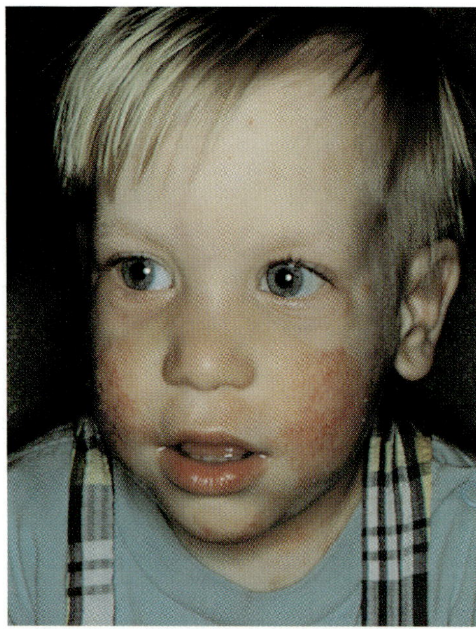

FIGURE 2-7. Atopic eczema in a sibling of patient shown in Fig. 2-3. Note thinning of lateral brows due to frequent rubbing, as well as Dennie lines of folds. Eczema of cheeks, chin, and neck is frequent at this age.

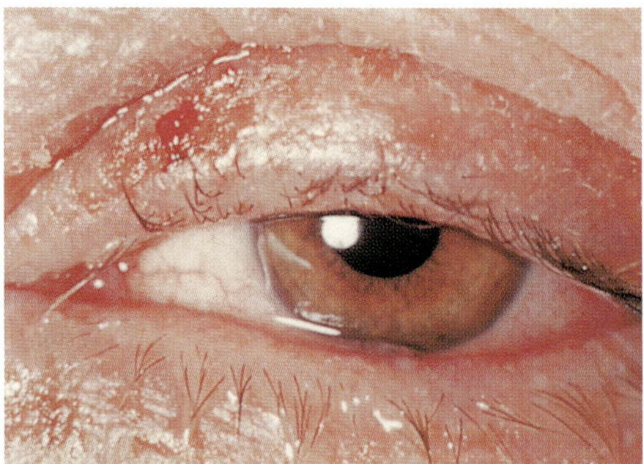

FIGURE 2-8. Eczematoid lid reaction in atopy. This patient with atopy and secondary staphylococcal infection demonstrates marked lid edema, erythema, and crusting; increased tear meniscus; conjunctival hyperemia; and a mild mucoid discharge that is evident in the central tear film.

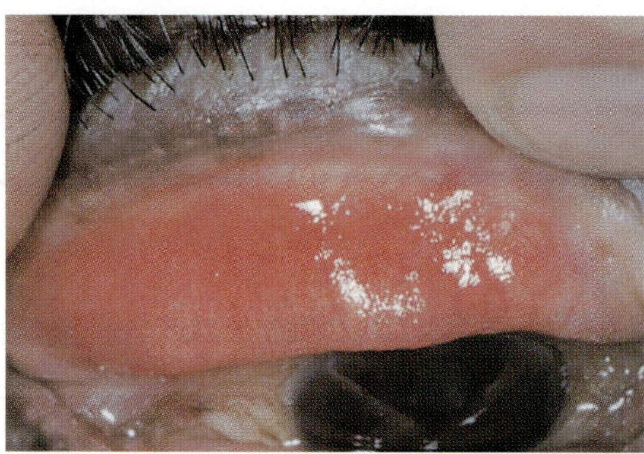

FIGURE 2-9. Conjunctival papillary hypertrophy and severe blepharitis in atopy. Lid margin discoloration, a fine papillary conjunctival hypertrophy, and some mucus are evident in this 49-year-old male. Each fine red point in the tarsal conjunctiva represents a papilla.

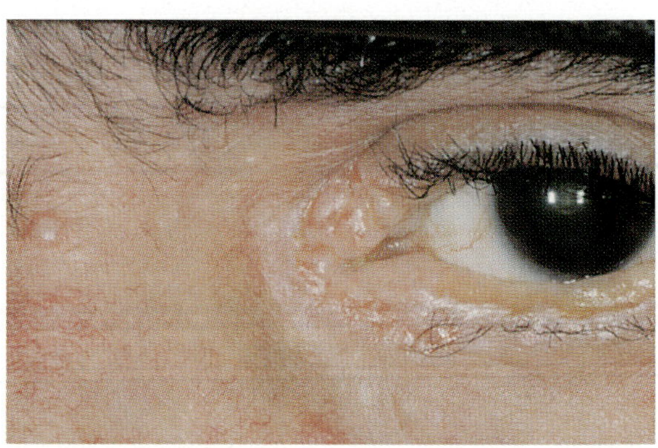

FIGURE 2-10. Severe lid thickening and lichenification of the medial canthal region atopic keratoconjunctivitis. A pustule can be seen on the bridge of the nose.

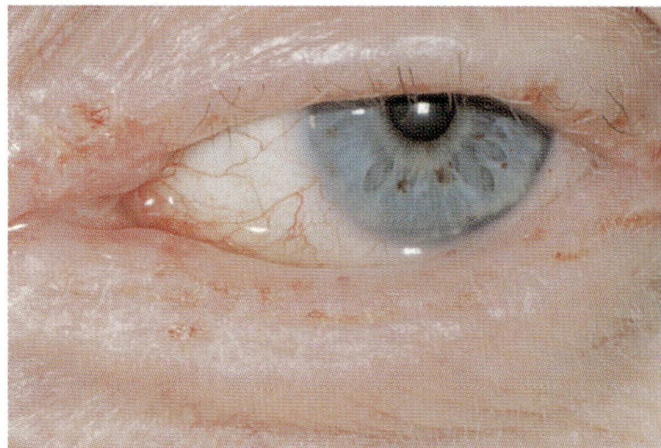

FIGURE 2-11. Lower lid lash loss and thinning of lashes in the upper lid, lid thickening, excoriation, crusting, and lichenification in atopy.

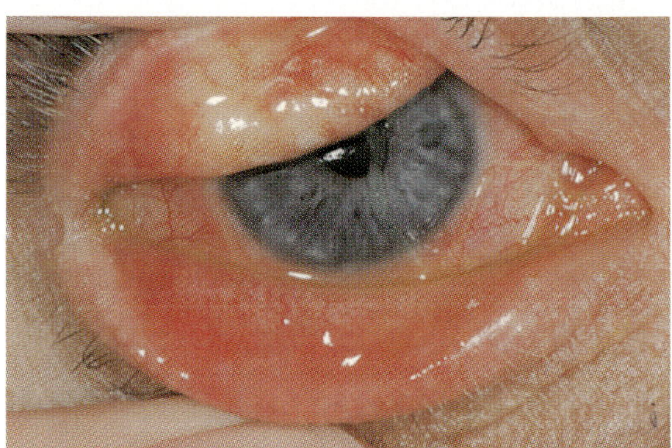

FIGURE 2-12. Atopic conjunctivitis. Increased skin folds and hyperemia, a mucous strand (crossing the cornea), a milky velvety appearance of the inferior conjunctiva, and a few giant papillae of the upper tarsus are seen in this patient.

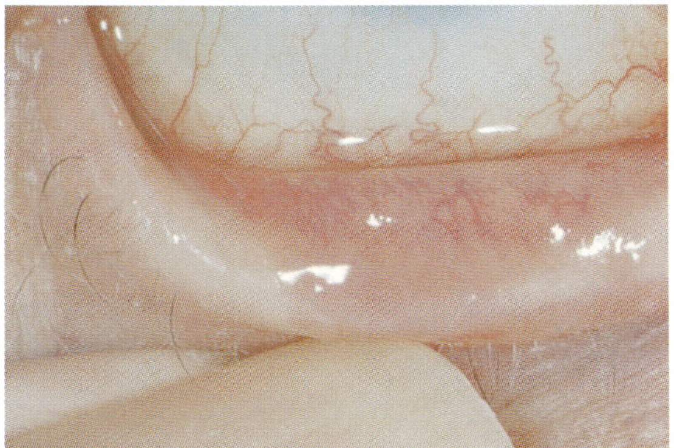

FIGURE 2-13. Milky appearance of the conjunctiva in atopic keratoconjunctivitis. Lash thinning, individual lash poliosis, and a milky appearance of the conjunctiva are all evident.

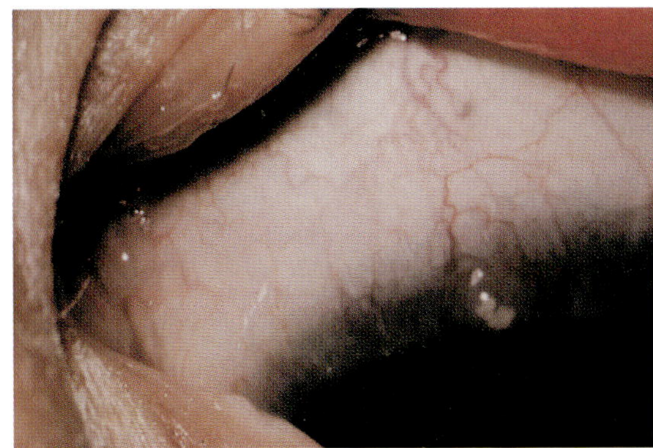

FIGURE 2-14. Trantas dots. A large Trantas dot surrounded by mucus and two smaller ones are evident to the left of the large one.

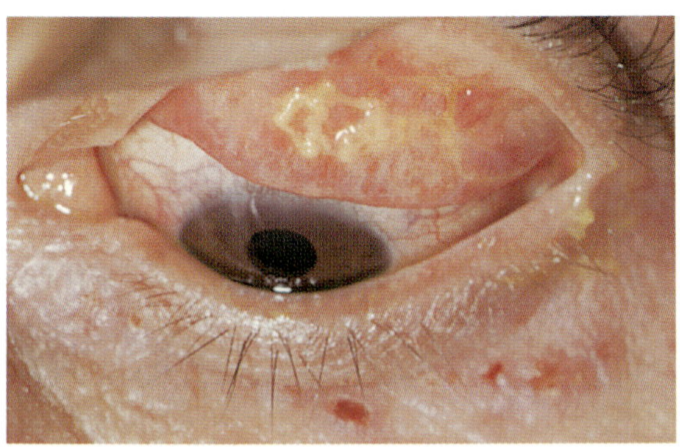

FIGURE 2-15. Excoriation of the lids, stringy mucoid discharge, papillary hypertrophy, and conjunctival scarring.

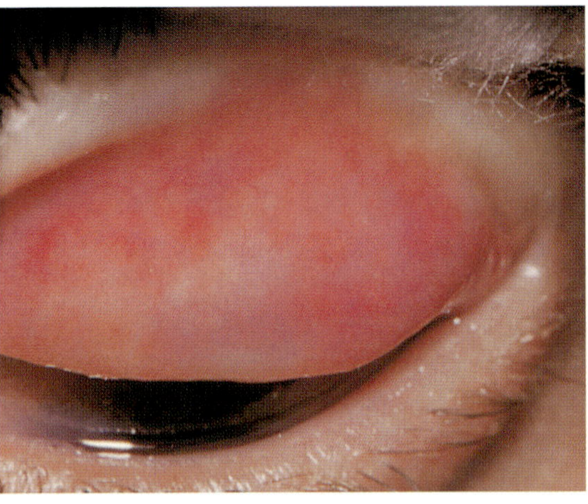

FIGURE 2-16. Milky-appearing conjunctiva, fine papillary hypertrophy, and conjunctival scarring.

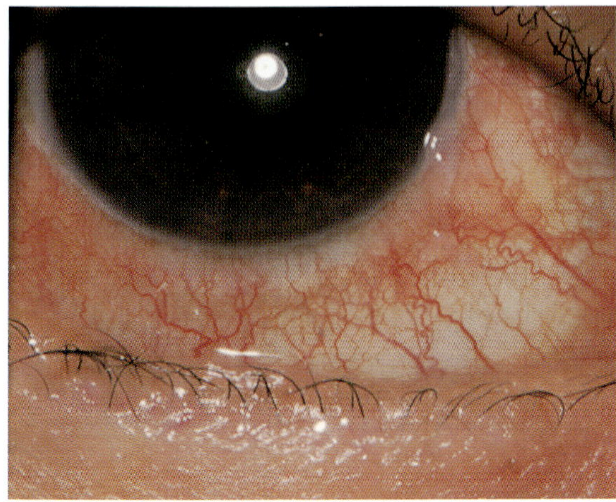

FIGURE 2-17. Limbal papillae, moderate increased redness, and mild conjunctival edema. The limbal papillae are located at the 4 to 6 o'clock limbus.

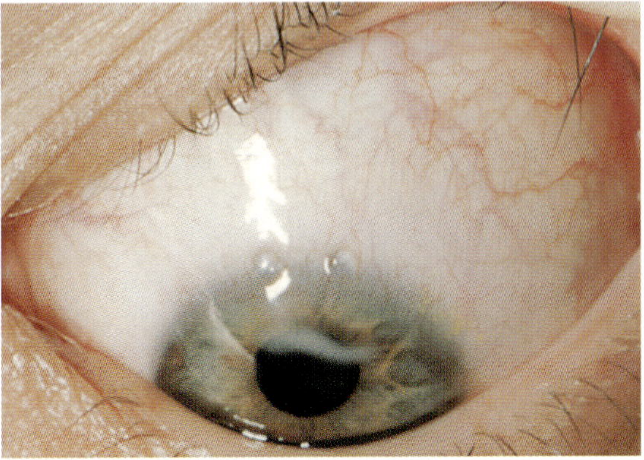

FIGURE 2-18. Misdirection of several lashes, two clear limbal cysts, and a linear corneal scar are evident in this patient with a history of atopic keratoconjunctivitis and herpes simplex keratitis.

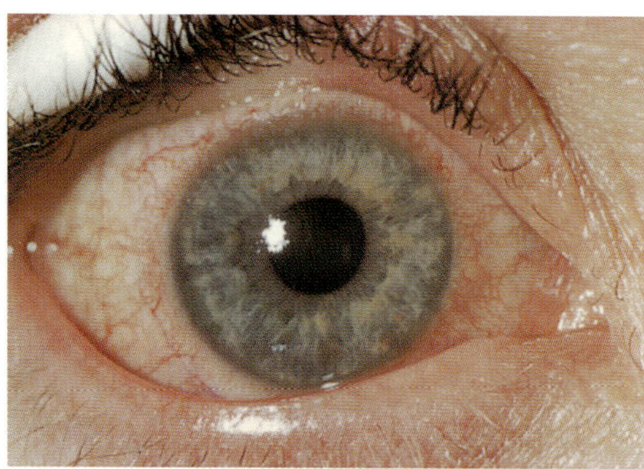

FIGURE 2-19. Lid margin hyperemia, reduced tear film, and a fine epithelial keratitis in atopy. The fine epithelial keratitis is manifested by the irregular light reflex.

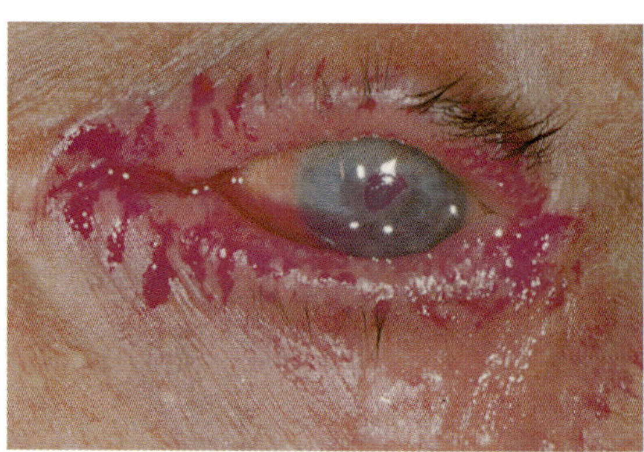

FIGURE 2-20. Oval superficial corneal ulcer stained with Bengal rose. Excess Bengal rose is evident on the lid margin and in the tear film. The lower lid is thickened from edema.

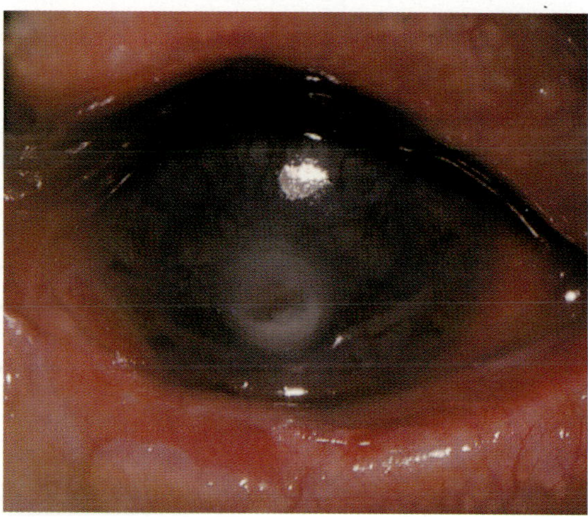

FIGURE 2-21. Severe lid margin irregularity, lash loss, marked conjunctival papillary hypertrophy, almost total superficial corneal vascularization, and a central corneal infiltrate with marked corneal thinning in atopic keratoconjunctivitis.

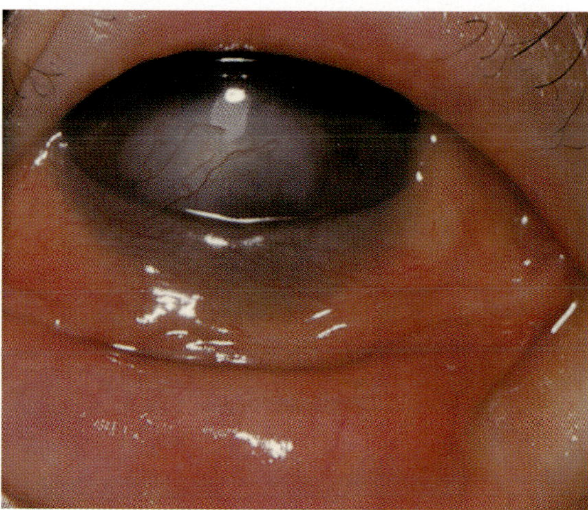

FIGURE 2-22. Severe milky-appearing papillary hypertrophy of the inferior tarsal conjunctiva, moderate bulbar chemosis, and paracentral corneal scar in atopic keratoconjunctivitis. This patient has had atopic keratoconjunctivitis for more than 35 years.

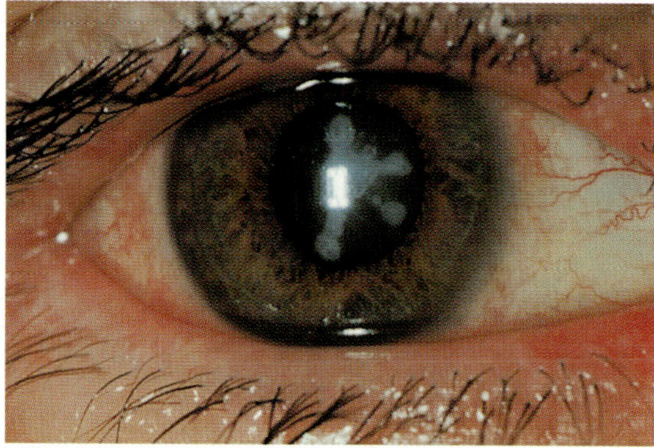

FIGURE 2-23. Anterior subcapsular shieldlike cataract in atopy. Moderate lid margin injection, increased tear meniscus, and moderate mucoid discharge are all evident.

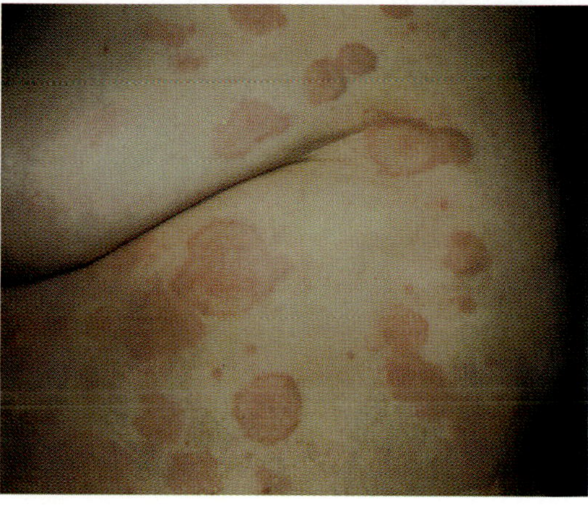

FIGURE 2-24. Urticaria of the chest and trunk. Urticaria lesions have a sharply demarcated border such as is illustrated in this patient.

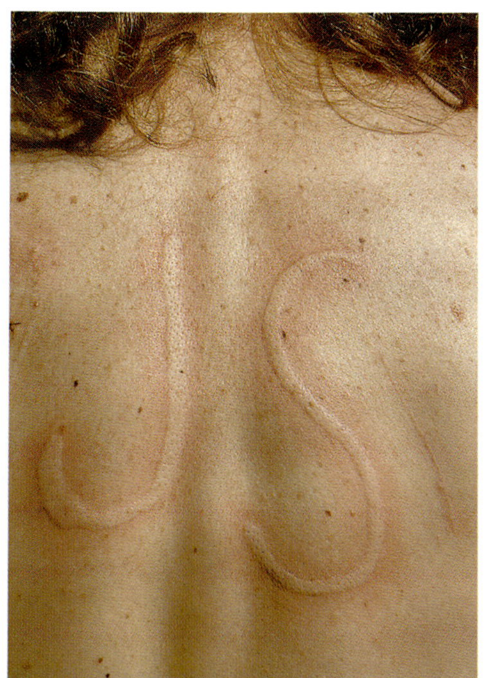

FIGURE 2-25. Dermatographism ("writing on the skin").

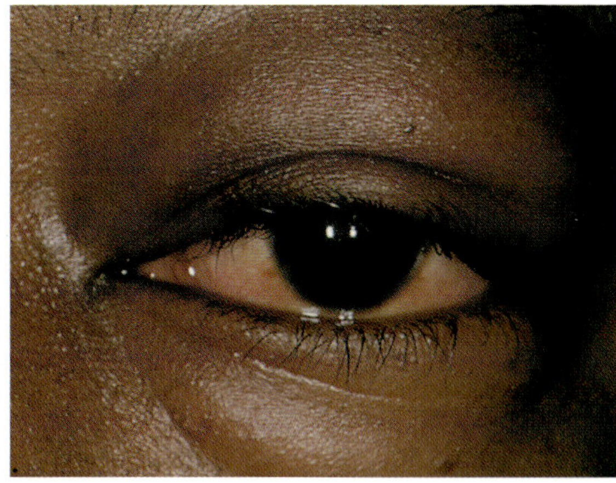

FIGURE 2-26. Lid and conjunctival angioedema following a diagnostic test with diethyl carbamazepine for onchocerciasis about 1 hour previously.

3

CONTACT DERMATITIS

Contact dermatitis represents a reaction to environmental substances such as drugs, cosmetics, preservatives, dyes, plant resins, and heavy metals, and usually involves exposed body areas, with approximately 85% of cases occurring in women. Most cases are nonimmunologic, being caused by irritants (irritant dermatitis). Allergic contact dermatitis, or contact hypersensitivity, is immunologic and usually represents a form of delayed hypersensitivity, induced either by a specific substance, a hapten that complexes to a self-component (skin protein), or a photoallergic reaction to a topically applied agent such as soap containing tribromosalicylanilide.

Irritant contact dermatitis develops within minutes of exposure to the offending substance. Allergic contact dermatitis, once the hypersensitivity has developed, occurs 8 to 120 hours (average, 24 to 48 hours) after contact with the substance. In both forms of contact dermatitis, the offending substance often acts in concert with a defatting agent (e.g., excessive moisture and alkalies), which damages the surface film and stratum corneum, allowing the irritant or allergen to reach the dermis. Sometimes the offending substance serves as both an irritant and an allergen.

Irritant dermatitis may develop without previous exposure to the offending agent, whereas, at other times, repeated exposure is necessary before the cumulative effect overcomes the recuperative processes of the skin to induce inflammation.

The offending agents can usually be identified from location of the dermatitis and by obtaining a history of the use of agents known to cause hypersensitivity, by testing the skin for possible agents, by eliminating all possible contactants, and by returning gradually to the various substances, one at a time.

In allergic contact dermatitis, the cell-mediated immune mechanisms are called forth only after the patient becomes sensitized to the substance or closely related substances, and, not infrequently, the patient has been exposed to the substance for many months before sensitization occurs. The allergens are usually small haptens that act as antigens by binding to dermal proteins.

In photoallergic contact dermatitis, the offending substances are activated by UV light before the reaction develops. The substance sometimes causes both photoallergic and allergic contact dermatitis.

Irritants and contact allergens may act in concert. The irritant breaks down the skin barrier, allowing the allergen to readily reach the dermis and to trigger the immune response sequence. Physical factors (e.g., microtrauma, friction, low humidity, heat, or cold) may also help break down the skin barrier.

The initial contact dermatitis episode is usually mild, whereas repeated exposure may result in a more widespread and severe eruption. Occasionally, local exposure to a substance induces general hypersensitivity, and, conversely, systemic exposure causes a severe local reaction.

CLINICAL MANIFESTATIONS

Contact dermatitis mimics almost any form of eczema. It often causes intense itch, burn, and sting.

Irritant Contact Dermatitis

Irritant contact dermatitis is often superimposed on other skin conditions (e.g., atopic dermatitis, psoriasis, and even allergic contact dermatitis). It usually begins with a few patches of dry, red, or chapped skin. The skin then becomes dry, scaly, and thickened; later, fissures and lichenification develop. In cumulative irritant contact dermatitis, the thin, exposed skin (e.g., finger webs, face, and eyelids) is involved first. In irritant contact dermatitis induced by volatile chemicals [e.g. Mace (chloracetophenone)] (Fig. 3-1), the face, eyelids, conjunctiva, and respiratory tract are often involved first.

Allergic Contact Dermatitis

Allergic contact dermatitis usually causes erythema, edema, papules, and papulovesicles, which progress to vesicles and blisters and finally to a weeping dermatitis with exudation and crusting (Figs. 3-2 and 3-3). The skin often becomes secondarily infected. The chronic phase is characterized by a dry, scaly, thickened skin with fissures and lichenification. A contact dermatitis arising from exposure to the plastic and/or nickel in the temple of the frame of spectacles often causes a reaction behind the ear (Fig. 3-4).

Allergic contact dermatitis caused by plants (e.g., *Rhus* genus—poison ivy, oak, and sumac) is often characterized by linear streaking (Fig. 3-5), irregular spotting, and more striking vesiculation; the vesicular fluid is cloudy and yellowish. Lesions may be found on the sides of the fingers, as well as on the genitalia in males; in some instances, the dermatitis becomes generalized.

OCULAR FEATURES OF CONTACT HYPERSENSITIVITY

The lid, especially the upper lid, is commonly affected by a contact dermatitis and may be the first or the only area involved. Mascara, eyeshadow, hair dye, or other hair products (Fig. 3-10), or the plastic or nickel in spectacles are common causes (Fig. 3-4). The lower lid is usually the major area involved when the substance is contained in eye medications (Figs. 3-6 to 3-8). Findings include erythema, acute edema, crusting, tearing, an eczematoid reaction, and lichenification. Often the reaction causes edema of both lids and extends onto the cheek. Nail polish sometimes causes a contact dermatitis of the lid or of the sides of the neck (Figs. 3-9 and 3-11).

The conjunctiva is occasionally involved. The reaction is usually severe and is associated with tearing, redness, mucopurulent discharge, generalized hyperemia, chemosis, and a moderate to severe papillary reaction, especially of the lower fornix and tarsus (Figs. 3-7 and 3-9). When the conjunctiva is involved secondarily, the reaction may be overlooked because of the severe lid reaction. Infrequently, the conjunctiva is affected following use of systemic medication.

Contact reactions of the cornea occasionally occur from topical eye medications. The reaction is characterized by a fine epithelial keratitis, loss of large areas of the corneal epithelium, or, more frequently, small, yellow necrotic opacities near the limbus. The latter usually occur in response to thimerosal used for the care of soft contact lenses.

Phototoxic Contact Dermatitis

Phototoxic contact dermatitis resembles a severe sunburn. It is usually limited to areas of exposure but may be diffuse (Fig. 3-12). Hyperpigmented areas often develop and persist for long periods of time.

Photoallergic Contact Dermatitis

Photoallergic reactions are similar to allergic contact dermatitis, with erythema, papules, vesicles, and blisters. Initially, these lesions are usually limited to exposure areas, sparing areas just below the brows, under the chin, and behind the ears. Later, more distant sites may be involved; the reaction then resembles a sunburn.

Since photoallergic contact dermatitis is immune mediated, there is a delay of several days after the sun exposure before the skin reacts. On the other hand, phototoxic dermatitis is seen within hours after exposure, is sharply limited to the sun-exposed sites, and appears very much like a severe acute sunburn.

Infectious Eczematoid Dermatitis (Infective Dermatitis, Microbial Eczema)

Infectious eczematoid dermatitis (infective dermatitis, microbial eczema) represents an eczematous skin reaction induced by a hypersensitivity reaction to microorganisms (bacteria, fungi, or viruses) or their products. The condition differs from infected atopic dermatitis or contact dermatitis.

Bacterial hypersensitivity reactions may occur to staphylococci, less commonly to beta-hemolytic streptococci or to *Mycobacterium tuberculosis.* Fungal hypersensitivity occurs to *Candida* spp., the dermatophytes, and probably *Pityrosporum* yeasts. Eczematization from viral hypersensitivity occurs in molluscum contagiosum infections (Fig. 3-13). The eczematoid reaction is probably a cell-mediated immune reaction to bacterial, fungal, or viral antigens acting as haptens; is often aggravated by scratching and rubbing; and may persist for years because of the rubbing. The initiating infection may be local or at another location, such as the conjunctiva, skin of the feet, scalp, or anterior nares. The lesions display an ill-defined area of advancing erythema that is often associated with microvesicles and have a tendency to oozing, thick lamellar scaling, and crusting. They often occur around discharging sinuses, around the ear in cases of chronic otitis media, and in areas that are moist.

The eczematoid reaction in molluscum contagiosum occurs near the nodules and clears as the nodules disappear. It usually begins as a small erythematous fissure at the inner or outer canthus or in the fold of the upper eyelid and is then followed by vesiculation, pustulation, crusting, and lichenification. The conjunctivitis and keratitis that usually accompanies the dermatitis helps to differentiate this condition from contact dermatitis.

Id Reactions

Id reactions are pruritic, eczematoid, lichenoid, or vesicular in character. They develop as a reaction to tuberculoprotein in tuberculosis (tuberculid), as a hypersensitivity reaction to *Candida albicans* (candidid), or as a distant focus of a dermatophyte infection, especially one that causes a large amount of inflammation (a dermatophytid). The id itself should not be thought of as a focus of infection.

Tuberculids are usually disseminated and are arranged symmetrically. They are classified as papulonecrotic (Fig. 3-14), lichen scrofulosorum, acne scrofulosorum, lichenoid, and nodular. Tuberculids of the lid present as chronic, multiple, small, papular, or papulonecrotic skin lesions. Conjunctival tuberculids are small, evanescent conjunctival nodules, which arise and fade spontaneously. They represent miliary tubercles that arise from small foci of tubercle organisms, which, upon reaching the area, cause a significant hypersensitivity reaction. Papulonecrotic tuberculids of the bulbar conjunctiva are usually associated with an interstitial keratitis. Corneal tuberculids are similar to those of the conjunctiva. They cause corneal scarring and usually vascularize.

Candidids usually occur on the hands or in the groin and are eczematoid in character. Dermatophytids are eczematous, lichenoid, vesicular, macular, papular, or similar to erysipelas. Infrequently, they present as erythema nodosum, erythema multiforme, or erythema annulare gyratum.

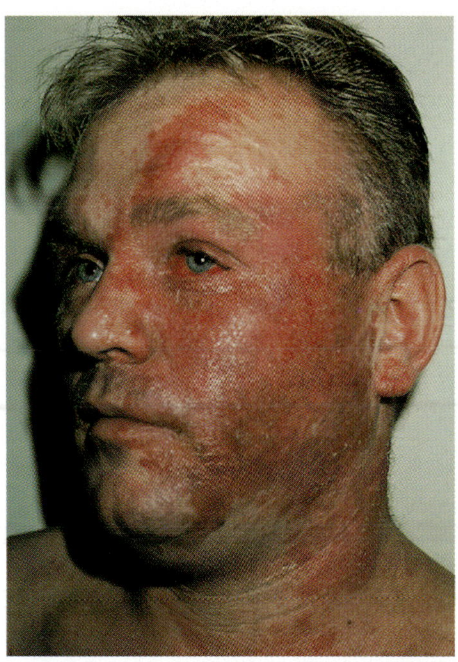

FIGURE 3-1. Irritant contact dermatitis of the face and neck caused by Mace. This man was sprayed in the face at close contact with Mace. The resulting changes represent an irritant form of contact dermatitis. The ocular erythema represents both a conjunctival reaction and subconjunctival hemorrhages. Note the mild amount of mucus in the tear film at the inferior border of the cornea.

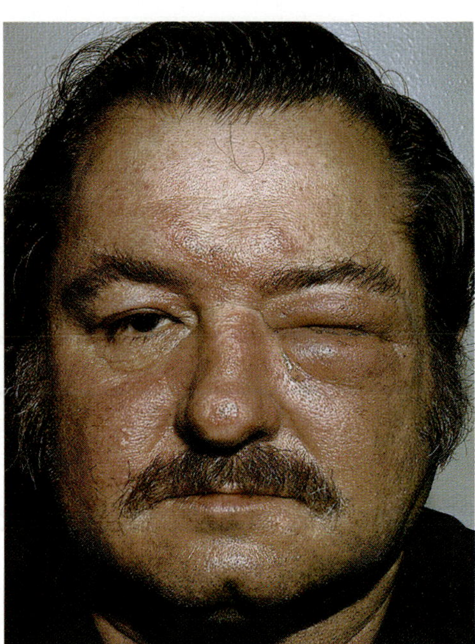

FIGURE 3-2. Contact dermatitis from poison oak with marked lid edema.

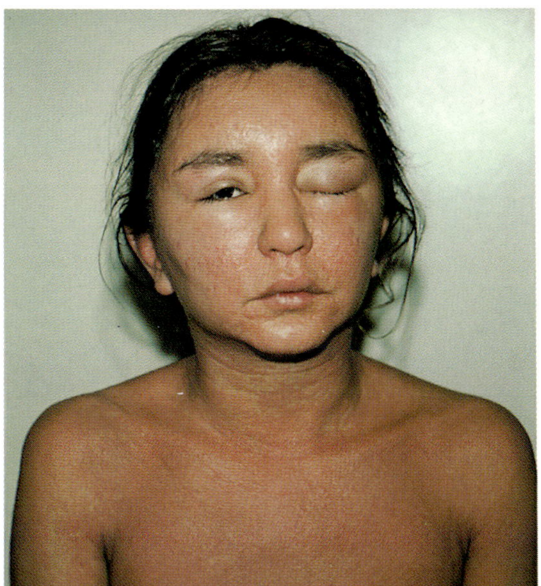

FIGURE 3-3. Acute contact dermatitis following use of a sulfacetamide eyedrop. Note edema of forehead and eyelids. The rash has spread to involve not only the face but also the trunk and arms.

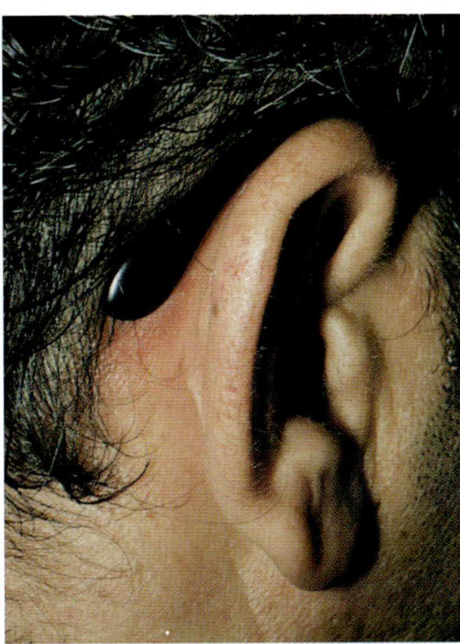

FIGURE 3-4. Contact dermatitis to the plastic in the frames of a pair of glasses. (The patient reacted to both the plastic in the frame as well as to nickel.)

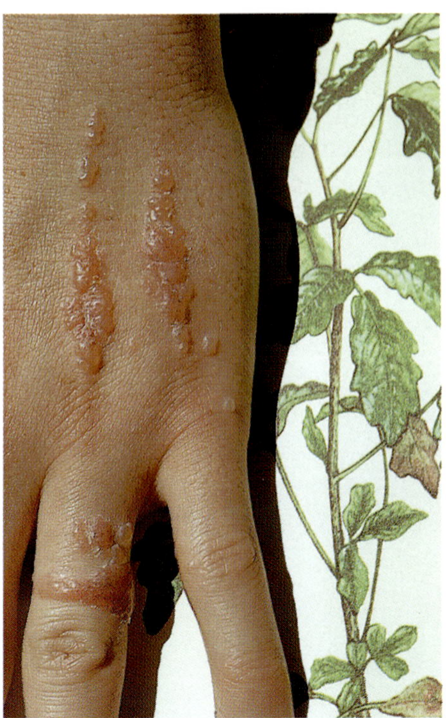

FIGURE 3-5. Allergic contact dermatitis to poison oak. Note characteristic linear pattern of vesicles from exposure to plant.

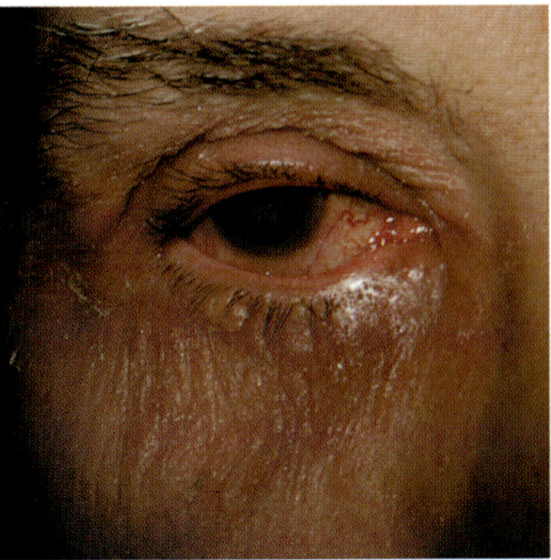

FIGURE 3-6. Contact dermatitis with increased pigmentation, thickening of the lower and upper lids, and conjunctival hyperemia from use of neomycin eye drops.

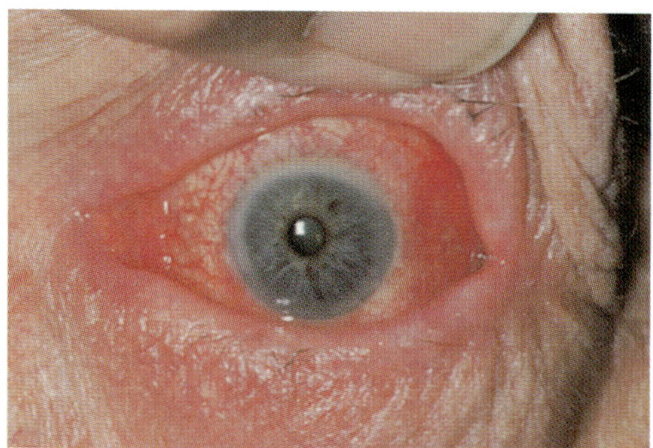

FIGURE 3-7. Contact dermatitis of both lids and the conjunctiva secondary to the use of boric acid.

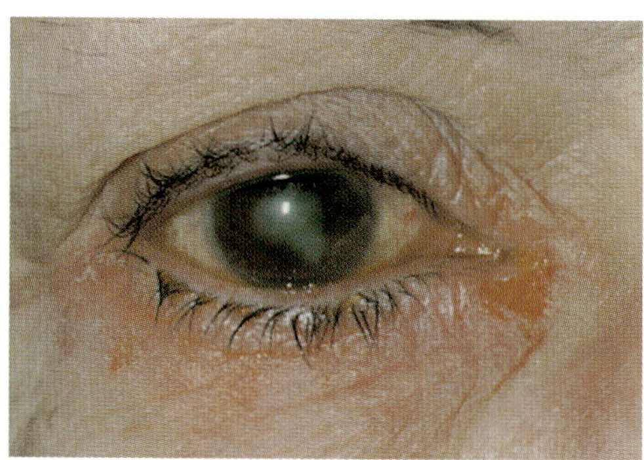

FIGURE 3-8. Contact dermatitis with lichenification and moderate tearing from homatropine used for corneal infection. The central corneal scar was caused by the central corneal infection.

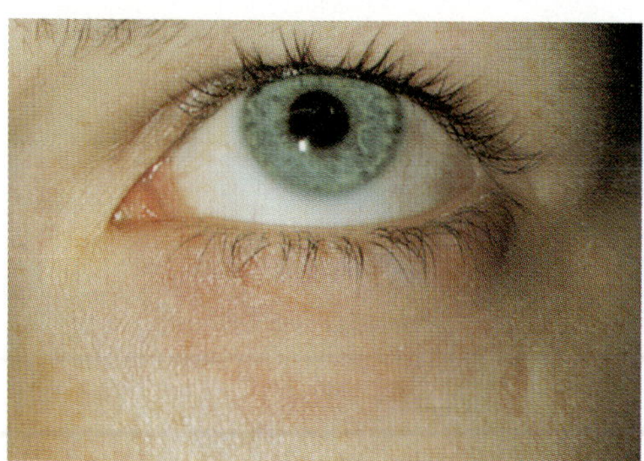

FIGURE 3-9. Contact dermatitis of the eyelid from use of nail polish. Allowing the polish to dry completely before touching face may prevent this problem.

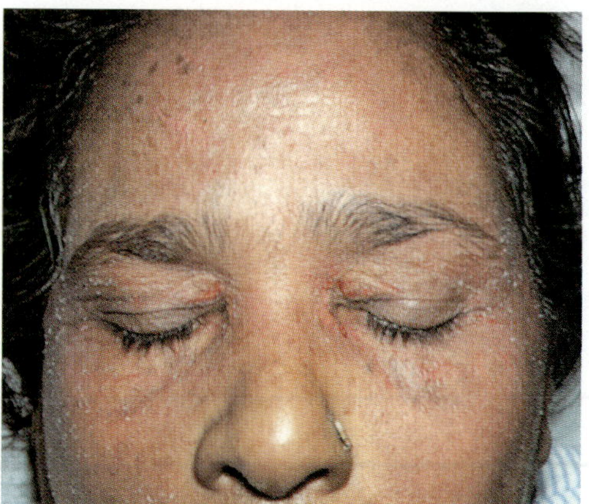

FIGURE 3-10. Acute allergic contact dermatitis from exposure to hair dye.

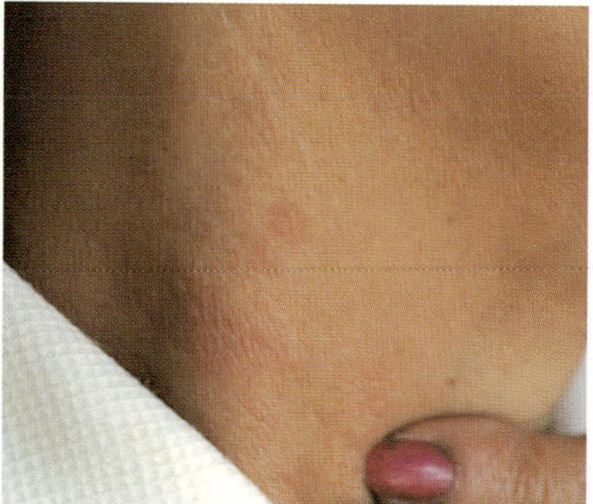

FIGURE 3-11. Contact dermatitis of the neck from nail polish. A common site for this problem.

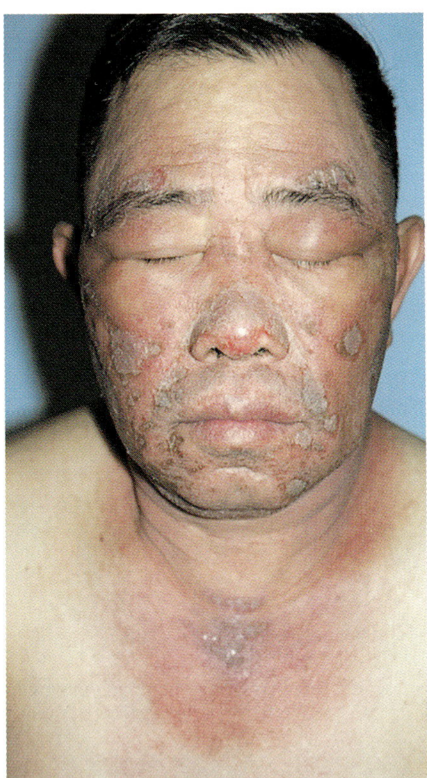

FIGURE 3-12. Severe phototoxic dermatitis. Note the relative sparing of the forehead (shielded by a cap he was wearing) and the mid anterior neck.

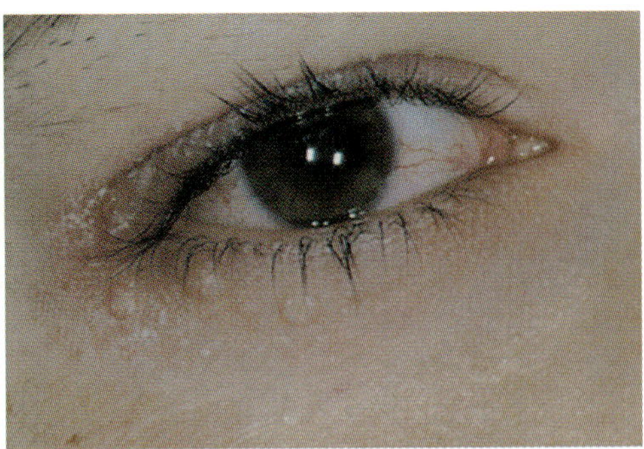

FIGURE 3-13. Eczematoid reaction of the lateral canthal region and lower eyelid associated with molluscum contagiosum nodules. The eczematoid reaction disappeared following removal of the molluscum nodules.

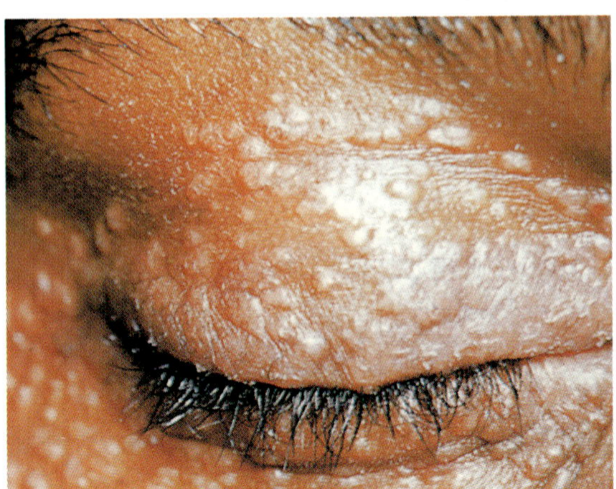

FIGURE 3-14. Papulonecrotic tuberculids of the lid. (Photograph courtesy of Dr. Phillips Thygeson.)

4

THE PHOTODERMATOSES

The photodermatoses are probably acquired, immunologic disorders; they must be differentiated from other light-exacerbated dermatoses, such as lupus erythematosus and chemical photosensitivities.

POLYMORPHOUS LIGHT ERUPTION

Polymorphous light eruption (PLE) usually affects women (the ratio of women to men is 3:1) who live in temperate climates. It is believed to have a familial transmission pattern, although the evidence is variable. It is probably the most common photodermatosis and usually begins in the first two decades of life. It affects all races and is usually provoked by sunlight (especially bright summer sunlight), but it may be provoked by ultraviolet A (UVA) and sometimes by broad-band ultraviolet B (UVB) exposure. Polymorphous light eruption is induced by sun exposure of more than 15 minutes. The lesions develop within hours and last several hours or days, but with continued sun exposure they may persist for weeks. They typically involve those areas receiving the greatest sun exposure (nasal bridge, cheeks, front of the chin, sides and back of the neck (Fig. 4-1), V area of the upper chest, dorsolateral aspects of the arms, and dorsum of the hands and feet). (Other areas, although light-exposed, are sometimes unaffected.)

The eruption varies from person to person and includes the following:

1. Eczematous lesions associated with lichenification and residual hypo- and/or hyperpigmentation.
2. Symmetric, erythematous, or skin-colored papular eruptions. The papules are usually pruritic, are grouped, and can be large or small; in some instances they coalesce to form smooth or irregular confluent plaques.
3. Vesicles, papulovesicles, or generalized facial edema.
4. Pruritic erythema and vesicles (juvenile spring eruption) in young boys, which preferentially involve the helix of the ears.

The lesions usually recur indefinitely during the summer months, then gradually remit in the fall without scarring. Occasionally, fever, chills, headaches, and nausea are associated with the skin eruption.

Conjunctival Changes

Increased conjunctival pigmentation and limbal papillae are often associated with the skin eruption of polymorphous light eruption (Fig. 4-2).

ACTINIC PRURIGO AND HEREDITARY POLYMORPHOUS LIGHT ERUPTION OF NATIVE AMERICANS

Actinic prurigo has many characteristics of PLE. It is familial in about 50% of cases, usually occurs in children under the age of 10 (especially young girls), and tends to clear in puberty. Sensitivity to UVA is probably more common and more important than that to UVB. A similar eruption (familial polymorphous light eruption) occurs in Native Americans of North and South America of any age group (Fig. 4-3). Hereditary PLE of Native Americans is autosomal dominant, is more common during summer, and frequently is induced by UVA and sometimes UVB exposure. It is often associated with atopy and remits during adolescence. There is often associated chronic papillary conjunctivitis.

Both actinic prurigo and hereditary PLE of Native Americans are characterized by an itchy, symmetric, erythematous, papular, or nodular eruption of skin areas (such as the face and lower lip) that are exposed to light (recurrent chilitis, especially in Native Americans), and of distal areas of the extremities. It usually spares the forehead, especially near the hairline, and the proximal areas of the extremities. Other findings include excoriation, eczematization, crusting, and lichenification. The facial lesions often heal with minute, linear, or pitted scars.

HYDROA VACCINIFORME (HUTCHINSON SUMMER ERUPTION, HYDROA AESTIVALIS)

Hydroa vacciniforme usually begins before the age of 4, then remits in the late teens. It is more frequent in males and represents a severe, recurrent vesicular skin eruption of sun-exposed skin areas that usually occur during the spring and summer months. The cause is unknown, but this disorder must be distinguished from erythropoietic protoporphyria. Prurigo aestivalis (Hutchinson summer prurigo) is a mild variant of hydroa vacciniforme that leads to less severe scarring.

Mild stinging, burning, or pain of the exposed skin areas (face, ears, neck, arms, and hands) usually develops 1 to 2 hours following sun exposure. Soon thereafter, scattered or confluent, symmetric, erythematous, and sometimes hemorrhagic vesicles and bullae develop, which are filled at first with a clear, then cloudy, fluid. Umbilication and crusting develop within days, and healing occurs with hypopigmented, pocklike, or occasionally, telangiectatic scars within weeks. Rarely, it causes constitutional symptoms of fever, headache, and malaise.

In hydroa aestivalis, the primary lesions are pruritic edematous papules that tend to become confluent.

Ocular Features of Hydroa Aestavilis

Tearing and photophobia are common in hydroa aestivalis. Lid scarring may occur, leading to conjunctival and corneal changes from secondary exposure. Other conjunctival changes, although rare, include limbal chemosis, gelatinous granulations, vesiculation, and scarring (Fig. 4-4).

Corneal involvement includes epithelial vesiculation, ulceration, band-shaped keratopathy, stromal infiltration, and dense stromal opacities leading to corneal neovascularization and blurred vision.

SOLAR URTICARIA (URTICARIA PHOTOGENICA)

Solar urticaria (urticaria photogenica) may be primary, occur secondary to use of drugs or chemicals, or arise from exogenous photosensitization.

Primary solar urticaria probably represents a type I hypersensitivity from a fixed cutaneous or circulating antigen that is induced by UV or visible radiation. Infrequently, it occurs in lupus erythematosus, lymphocytoma cutis, polymorphous light eruption, or other urticaria. It is usually recurrent, occurring between the ages of 10 and 50 and more frequently in females.

Secondary solar urticaria is probably nonimmunologic, arising from exposure to chemicals such as tar, pitch, and dyes; from use of drugs such as benoxaprofen; and in patients with erythropoietic protoporphyria.

The skin features usually begin within minutes of sun exposure and include tingling, irritation, and erythema followed by edema without whealing or by raised, multiple or confluent, whitish, well-demarcated wheals. The lesions then fade after 1 or 2 hours, leaving only minimal redness. Usually, it involves all the sun-exposed skin areas, but it occasionally spares the face and dorsum of the hands. Following the eruption, the exposed areas are insensitive to further sun exposure for hours to days.

Headache, nausea, faintness, bronchospasm, or syncope may develop if the whealing is widespread and severe.

CHRONIC ACTINIC DERMATITIS (PHOTOSENSITIVITY DERMATITIS AND ACTINIC RETICULOID SYNDROME)

Actinic reticuloid syndrome is probably the most severe variant of the chronic actinic dermatitis group of diseases. It usually occurs in elderly males and is characterized by severe photosensitivity to all wavelengths of visible light with clinical features suggestive of lymphoma.

The photosensitivity is persistent and begins with erythema and edema in light-exposed areas. Later, there is scaling, pigmentation, and severe leonine thickening. In some instances, papules, nodules, and plaques develop, and the lesions may be excoriated and lichenified because of itch. Other skin features include vitiligo-like depigmentation, a pseudolymphomatous eruption, or an eczematoid eruption. The lesions occur on sun-exposed areas such as the scalp, face, sides and back of the neck, upper chest, and dorsal surfaces of the forearms and hands. Protected areas—including the area behind the ears, upper eyelids, finger webs, and skin creases—are spared, although in long-standing cases, the protected areas become involved. In many instances, there are coexistent contact dermatitis, endogenous eczema, and airborne allergies; occasionally, mycosis fungoides is associated.

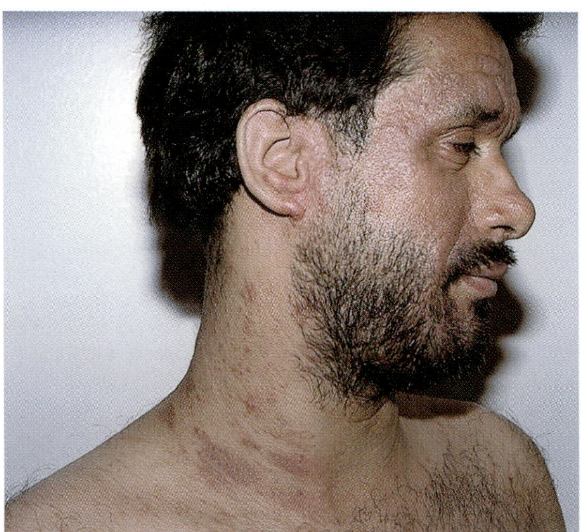

FIGURE 4-1. Patient with chronic polymorphous light eruption showing papules, plaques, and edema, especially of forehead and eyelids. Note resemblance to lesions seen in lepromatous leprosy.

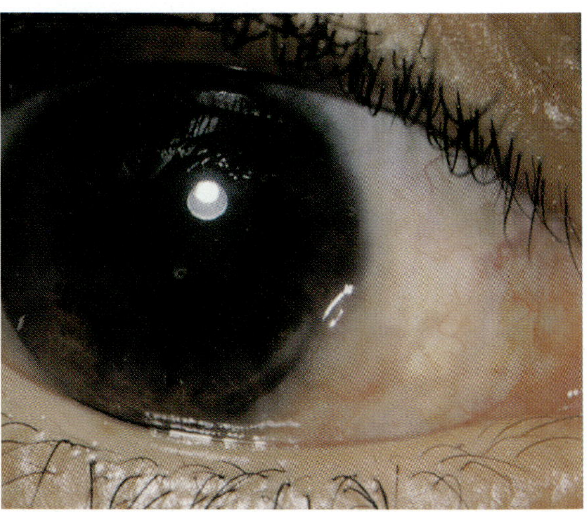

FIGURE 4-2. Limbal involvement with conjunctival pigmentation and papillary hypertrophy in polymorphous light eruption. The arcuslike corneal opacity central to the giant papillae represents a pseudogerontoxon that arises from prolonged hyperemia of the limbus in that area.

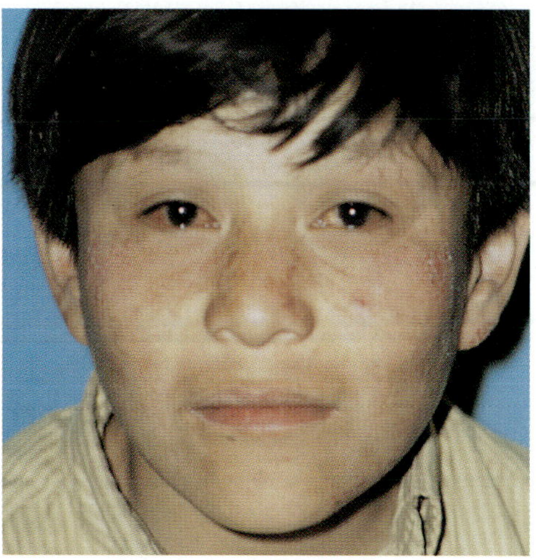

FIGURE 4-3. Familial polymorphous light eruption in a Native American. Eczematoid lesions of the malar eminences, conjunctival hyperemia, and limbal swelling are evident in this 12-year-old Navajo Indian.

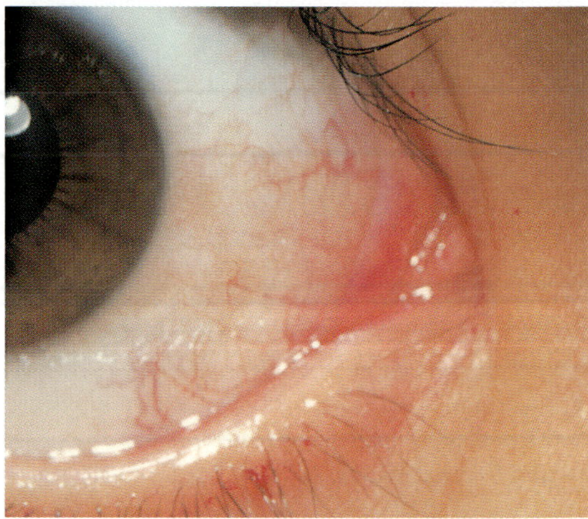

FIGURE 4-4. Hydroa aestivalis of the conjunctiva with bulbar conjunctival hyperemia, chemosis, and a mild, fine, punctate conjunctival staining near the limbus, evident with Bengal rose stain.

5

DISORDERS OF KERATINIZATION

Keratin disorders are characterized by an abnormal and usually thicker than normal stratum corneum, caused by increased cellular production, failure of desquamation, and abnormalities in cellular adhesions or by changes in the cellular junction complexes.

ICHTHYOSIS

Ichthyosis is characterized by excessive generalized, noninflammatory scaling. It is usually present at birth or develops in the first year of life. There are four major hereditary forms:

1. Ichthyosis vulgaris.
2. Lamellar ichthyosis (nonbullous congenital ichthyosiform erythroderma).
3. Epidermolytic hyperkeratosis (bullous congenital ichthyosiform erythroderma).
4. X-linked ichthyosis.

Two other skin conditions (the collodion baby and harlequin fetus) are often classified as ichthyosis; ichthyosis is also a constant feature of several syndromes. Occasionally, it occurs secondary to systemic diseases or metabolic abnormalities.

Ichthyosis Vulgaris (Ichthyosis Simplex, Autosomal Dominant Ichthyosis)

Ichthyosis vulgaris (ichthyosis simplex, autosomal dominant ichthyosis) is autosomal dominant and has a high penetrance. It usually develops after the age of 3 months, progressively gets worse for a period of time, and then improves as the patient gets older.

Skin Features

Ichthyosis vulgaris is characterized by a fine, branny, white desquamation, which has a predilection for the trunk and extensor surfaces of the extremities (especially the legs) (Figs. 5-1 and 5-2), but also occurs on the face (forehead and cheeks). It does not involve the flexor surfaces of the joints. A discrete, shiny hyperkeratosis of the elbows, knees, and ankles may be evident, and the palms and soles have mild keratoderma and evidence of splitting. The follicular orifices, especially over the upper arms and thighs, may be plugged (keratosis pilaris). Occasionally, the skin is only dry and rough.

Ocular Features

Ichthyotic scales may develop on the lid and lashes. Corneal changes include punctate corneal epithelial erosions, stromal opacities, and, later in life, a band-shaped keratopathy (Fig. 5-3). A central retinal dystrophy has been reported, although it is not well understood.

Lamellar Ichthyosis (Nonbullous Congenital Ichthyosiform Erythroderma, Ichthyosis Congenita)

Classic lamellar ichthyosis (nonbullous congenital ichthyosiform erythroderma, ichthyosis congenita) is autosomal recessive, although several reports also suggest autosomal dominant inheritance. The child is often premature. The skin may have thick, horny, polygonal, shieldlike plates or warty excrescences with minimal erythroderma. At other times the scales are thin and white, easily flake off, and are associated with marked erythroderma. Infrequently, the infant presents as a collodion baby with lamellar ichthyosis becoming manifest after shedding of the collodion membrane. Lamellar ichthyosis may be associated with small stature, mental retardation, and other developmental abnormalities.

Skin Features

The child is born with generalized erythroderma that is often especially prominent over the face, causing the skin to appear taut, red, and shiny (Fig. 5-4). In severe disease, white, brown, or black scales are uniformly distributed over the entire body, but usually the flexural areas (knees, elbows, and ankles) are the most severely involved. The pinna may be small, may be deformed, and may have a crumpled appearance. The palms and soles usually show some degree of keratoderma or at least increased skin markings. Itch may be present and in some instances is severe.

The nails are often stippled, ridged, and thickened. The hair is usually normal, but occasionally there is moderate scalp scaling. Sometimes the scalp and body hair are sparse and abnormally fine.

Ocular Features

Lid changes include lid scaling and mild to severe ectropion and lagophthalmos that may be cicatricial in nature. Conjunctival hyperemia, thickening, and keratinization, as well as corneal ulceration, scarring, and vascularization often occur from exposure. Band keratopathy sometimes develops in childhood or later life. Photophobia is often a constant companion.

Collodion Baby (Lamellar Exfoliation of the Newborn, Lamellar Ichthyosis)

At birth, the collodion baby (lamellar exfoliation of the newborn, lamellar ichthyosis) is encased in a smooth, thick, tough, inelastic, glistening, and translucent membrane that eventually fissures, peels, and sheds between 18 and 46 days. The membrane causes ectropion of all four lids, distortion of the pinna, effacement of the nose, and eversion of the lips (Fig. 5-5). The child is often premature. Death may occur in as many as 25% from dehydration or hypothermia. These infants have marked temperature instability, defective barrier function, cutaneous infections, hypernatremic dehydration, and septicemia. Following desquamation, the skin occasionally appears normal, but usually there are fine, white, branny scales, and in later infancy or childhood, the patient often develops lamellar ichthyosis.

Ocular Features

The ectropion that occurs at birth may lead to lagophthalmos because of cicatricial shortening of the upper lid (Fig. 5-5).

Harlequin Fetus (Ichthyosis Congenita, Keratosis Diffusa Foetalis)

The harlequin fetus (ichthyosis congenita, keratosis diffusa foetalis) is usually premature and has a low birth weight. The condition is probably autosomal recessive. The face, trunk, extremities, palms, and soles are encased in large, flat, platelike scales with deep crevices that run transversely and vertically, causing the skin to appear hard, fissured, and hyperkeratotic with a diamondlike pattern. The ears and nose are effaced and distorted. The lips are everted and often give the appearance of a "fish-mouth." The extremities are flexed. The hair and nails are absent or hypoplastic. Death often occurs within hours or weeks. Surviving babies may develop nonbullous ichthyosiform erythroderma.

Ocular Features

At birth there is a severe ectropion of the upper and lower eyelids; the chemotic, red conjunctiva often protrudes between the eyelids and covers the cornea.

Bullous Ichthyosiform Erythroderma (Epidermolytic Hyperkeratosis)

Bullous ichthyosiform erythroderma (epidermolytic hyperkeratosis) is autosomal dominant, although many cases are sporadic. It occurs with equal frequency in males and females and is characterized by hyperkeratosis and blistering of the skin.

Skin Features

The patient develops a generalized erythema and localized scaling and blistering soon after birth (Fig. 5-6). The blisters develop on the trunk and in areas of trauma, such as the knees and elbows. The scaling and blistering usually persist for 7 to 8 years (Fig. 5-7) and, occasionally, throughout life. The erythema usually disappears by middle age.

Hyperkeratotic areas with a rippled or beaded appearance develop in late infancy and persist for life. They are more prominent over the flexural surfaces and sometimes around the umbilicus. Occasionally, there is keratoderma of the palms and soles; sometimes the hyperkeratosis is generalized. The ears may have a crumpled appearance. Pruritus may be severe. The nails and hair are usually normal, although the scalp hair may be encased in the hyperkeratotic areas.

Ocular Features

Scaling of the lids and accumulation of scales on the lashes may be seen. Ectropion is unusual except in severely affected infants.

X-Linked Recessive Ichthyosis (Sex-Linked Ichthyosis)

X-linked recessive ichthyosis (XLI) (sex-linked ichthyosis) is uncommon and is characterized by large, dark scales on the neck, trunk, and extremities, usually developing within the first 3 months and persisting throughout life. The palms and soles are usually spared. Cryptorchidism, hypogonadism, and infertility have been observed.

Skin Features

The large, thick, dark-brown scales impart a "dirty appearance" to the scalp, sides of the face, neck, trunk, abdomen, and extensor and flexor surfaces of the extremities (Fig. 5-8). The scales also occur in the axillae and antecubital fossae in children and in the popliteal fossae in adults. Sometimes the skin of the palms and soles is slightly thickened.

Ocular Features

Ocular features include the following:

1. Scales on the lids and lashes.
2. Deep gray-white stromal corneal opacities distributed throughout the posterior cornea at the level of Descemet membrane. They are more pronounced in the adult. (Similar but less pronounced opacities may also be seen in clinically normal females.)
3. Punctate epithelial erosions and brushlike branching of the corneal nerves without diffuse thickening.
4. Peripheral granular retinal pigmentation.

MISCELLANEOUS ICHTHYOTIC DISORDERS

Anosmia, X-Linked Recessive Ichthyosis, Hypogonadism, and Various Neurologic Manifestations

This rare disorder is characterized by anosmia, X-linked recessive ichthyosis, hypogonadism, and various neurologic manifestations and includes mirror movement of the hands and feet, and ocular features of decreased visual acuity, iris hypopigmentation, strabismus, and nystagmus.

X-Linked Dominant Ichthyosis (XDI)

X-linked dominant ichthyosis (XDI) begins as a generalized erythroderma and scaling followed by a persistent linear and whorled pattern of hyperkeratosis, generalized follicular atrophoderma, and localized loss of scalp hair. Other features include chondrodysplasia punctata (stippled epiphyseal calcification), kyphoscoliosis, short stature, and cataracts.

Conradi–Hunermann Syndrome and Rhizomelic Chondrodysplasia (Chondrodysplasia Punctata, Congenital Stippled Epiphyses)

The Conradi–Hunermann (or Conradi–Hunermann–Happle) syndrome is a form of ichthyosiform erythroderma characterized by erythema, hyperkeratosis (linear ichthyosis), short stature, transient epiphyseal stippling of the long bones in infancy (epiphyseal stippling is seen by X-

ray, is nonspecific, and occurs in a wide variety of disorders; it is not a constant feature of the Conradi–Hunermann syndrome), and anterior cortical cataracts. It is X-linked dominant and occurs almost exclusively in females. It shows increased disease expression in successive generations (anticipation). The abnormalities are less severe and occur less frequently than in rhizomelic chondrodysplasia punctata; they are compatible with life.

Patients with rhizomelic chondrodysplasia punctata have severe abnormalities, including neuronal atrophy with psychomotor retardation, spasticity, and, sometimes, defective heart valves. This syndrome is autosomal recessive. Patients usually die before the age of 2.

Associated abnormalities include short stature, moderate to severe scoliosis, short asymmetric limbs, hexadactyly, frontal bossing, and dysmorphic facial features.

Skin Features

The shiny erythema is extensive. A whorl-and-swirl pattern of thick, yellow, adherent plaques occurs on the trunk and extremities at birth or within several months following birth. Within a few weeks, they lead to skin atrophy, a follicular atrophoderma (patulous hair follicles), and patchy cicatricial alopecia. The hair is coarse, irregularly twisted, and lusterless. The nails are flattened and often split into layers.

Ocular Features

Rhizomelic chondrodysplasia punctata is associated with hypertelorism; in the Conradi–Hunermann syndrome, the brows are usually sparse. Congenital, dense, anterior cortical cataracts occur in both forms. Optic nerve hypoplasia and atrophy may occur in the rhizomelic form, but their manifestations are variable.

Sjögren–Larsson Syndrome

The Sjögren–Larsson syndrome is autosomal recessive and is characterized by moderately severe lamellar ichthyosis, severe mental deficiency, spastic paresis, keratitis, cataracts, and maculopathy. There is some controversy as to whether some collodion babies have Sjögren–Larsson syndrome.

Neurologic abnormalities develop soon after birth and may progress until puberty. They include spastic diplegia or tetraplegia, mental retardation, epilepsy, speech defects, and occasionally, contractures of the hips and knees.

Skin Features

Patients with Sjögren–Larsson syndrome have an ichthyosis at birth, variable in appearance, that develops fully during infancy. It is characterized by scaling and patchy hyperkeratosis of the flexural surfaces; the face, palms, and soles are only mildly involved. A generalized mild erythroderma may be evident. Defective sweating and dermatoglyphic abnormalities (deviant finger and palm dermal-ridge patterns) may occur. Tooth enamel dysplasia and serrated teeth are also seen.

Ocular Features

Patients with Sjögren–Larsson syndrome have severe photophobia. Ichthyotic lid changes, blepharoconjunctivitis, and red lid margins are common. Corneal changes include punctate erosions, stromal opacities, and neovascularization.

Retinal changes described as glistening intraretinal dots are found in the macular region, along with retinal pigment epithelial changes (pale atrophic spots or gray to black circular pigmentary spots), and peripheral granular retinal pigmentation. Fluorescein angiography reveals transmission defects of the retinal pigment epithelium in the region of the macula. The fundus changes are independent of the cerebral symptoms.

Refsum Syndrome (Heredopathia Atactica Polyneuritiformis)

Refsum syndrome (heredopathia atactica polyneuritiformis) is autosomal recessive and is characterized by ichthyosis, cerebellar degeneration, progressive polyneuropathy, sensory deafness, and retinitis pigmentosa. The ichthyosis and degenerative changes usually begin during the second and third decades of life.

The neuromuscular features include a chronic progressive peripheral polyneuropathy, nerve deafness, anosmia, muscle atrophy, and elevated cerebrospinal fluid protein without pleocytosis. The cerebellar degenerative features include dysarthria, ataxia, scanning speech, and intention tremor. Skeletal abnormalities include kyphoscoliosis; pes cavus; epiphyseal dysplasia of the shoulders, elbows, and knees; and alteration in the size of the metacarpals, metatarsals, and phalanges. In later life, cardiac abnormalities (cardiomyopathy and arrhythmia) may be observed. Death may occur from cardiac failure.

Skin Features

Ichthyosis is not a constant feature but usually develops during the second decade of life. It is similar to ichthyosis vulgaris, with generalized branny desquamation of dirty-brown scales. The fingernails may short and broad.

Ocular Features

Night blindness, concentric visual field constriction, poor dark adaptation, and color vision defects develop before the third decade of life. Occasionally, there is photophobia. The pupils are miotic and dilate poorly. Nystagmus, poste-

rior subcapsular cataracts, and choroidal atrophy have been observed. The retinitis pigmentosa is progressive and results in narrowed retinal vessels, retinal pigmentation and depigmentation, intraretinal bone spicule pigmentation, a waxy optic nerve pallor, and vitreous degeneration.

Rud Syndrome

Rud syndrome is characterized by oligophrenia, epilepsy, hypogonadism, and ichthyosis. It is probably autosomal recessive with genetic heterogeneity. Neurologic abnormalities include moderate to severe oligophrenia and major or minor epilepsy. Nerve deafness and conduction deafness may also occur.

Sexual infantilism includes sparse pubic hair and hypoplastic genitalia. Males have sparse facial and axillary hair; females show lack of menstruation. Developmental anomalies include dwarfism, partial gigantism, arachnodactyly, and abnormal hands and feet.

The skin features vary from a mild, generalized branny desquamation to a severe ichthyosis of the extensor surfaces of the extremities or a severe generalized ichthyosis. Acanthosis nigricans of the flexures may be seen along with generalized skin thickening. Alopecia and absent or hypoplastic teeth are occasional abnormalities. Ocular features include cataract, retinitis pigmentosa, ptosis, strabismus, nystagmus, and blepharospasm.

Dorfman–Chanarin Syndrome

Dorfman–Chanarin syndrome is autosomal recessive and characterized by a disorder of the metabolism of neutral lipids with deposition of fat droplets in multiple tissues. It is manifested by lamellar ichthyosis, mental retardation, microcephaly, hepatosplenomegaly, myopathy, neurosensory deafness, cataracts, and/or impaired vision.

KID Syndrome (Keratitis, Ichthyosis, and Deafness Syndrome)

KID syndrome is probably autosomal dominant and is an acronym for *k*eratitis, *i*chthyosis, and *d*eafness. A nonprogressive neurosensory deafness develops at birth or within the first 2 years of life and is probably the result of cochlear–saccular abnormality. Patients often have recalcitrant cutaneous bacterial and fungal infections. Squamous cell skin carcinomas may also be found.

Skin Features

The skin is red, dry, and thickened at birth. Later keratodermal, rugose, well-marginated plaques with a serpiginous outline develop on the extremities, cheeks, and periocular skin. Perioral furrows become evident, and pronounced follicular plugging leading to follicular hyperkeratotic spines, and fine dry scales occur. Severe diffuse hyperkeratosis with a characteristic stippled or reticular surface pattern develops on the palms and soles. About half of the patients have scalp hypotrichosis. The nails are dystrophic, and there is diminished sweating. Oral mucosal leukoplakia is common.

Ocular Features

Photophobia is prominent in older children. The brows and lashes are sparse. The keratitis is characterized by epithelial irregularity and ulceration, corneal neovascularization, infiltration, and superficial pannus. It usually begins before adolescence and causes decreased vision (Fig. 5-9).

Ichthyosis–Cheek–Eyebrow Syndrome

The ichthyosis–cheek–eyebrow (ICE) syndrome is autosomal dominant and is characterized by ichthyosis vulgaris, prominent full cheeks, and sparse lateral eyebrows.

Acquired Ichthyosis

Acquired ichthyosis occasionally accompanies Hodgkin disease, lymphosarcoma, Kaposi sarcoma, mycosis fungoides, rhabdomyosarcoma, carcinomatosis (adenocarcinomas of the lung, colon, and breast), leprosy, systemic lupus erythematosus, hypothyroidism, hyperparathyroidism, AIDS, sarcoidosis, chronic renal failure, polycythemia rubra vera, and gross nutritional deficiencies.

Some medications also induce ichthyosis, including cholesterol-lowering drugs such as clofibrate and niacin. Dixyazine (a phenothiazine tranquilizer) has also been found to cause a reversible ichthyosis, depigmentation, hair loss, and cataracts.

ICHTHYOSIS WITH HAIR SHAFT ABNORMALITIES

The group of disorders that involves ichthyosis with hair shaft abnormalities includes Tay syndrome and PIBIDS (an acronym for *p*hotosensitivity, *i*chthyosis, *b*rittle hair, *i*mpaired intelligence, *d*ecreased fertility, and *s*hort stature). PIBIDS syndrome has ocular significance because of its association with cataracts and retinal dystrophy. The ichthyosis is a form of congenital ichthyosiform erythroderma.

XERODERMA (XEROSIS, ASTEATOSIS, WINTER ECZEMA, WINTER ITCH)

Xeroderma represents a milder form of abnormal keratinization than ichthyosis. It is characterized by persistent generalized noninflammatory scaliness, with the earliest changes being fine accentuation of skin markings followed by irregular reticulate red fissuring, pruritus, and lichenifi-

cation from scratching. It occurs in atopic dermatitis, "winter itch" (a condition arising in individuals who are exposed to low temperatures and made worse by frequent bathing), and wasting disorders such as nutritional deficiencies, malignant disease, and leprosy.

FOLLICULAR KERATOSES

The follicular keratoses comprise a number of conditions characterized by prominent plugs of keratin in the follicular orifices.

Keratosis Pilaris Atrophicans (Ulerythema Ophryogenes)

Keratosis pilaris atrophicans (ulerythema ophryogenes) begins at birth or soon thereafter and is autosomal dominant. Erythema and small keratotic papules develop in the lateral aspect of the eyebrows and then extend to the medial brow, sometimes to the forehead and scalp, leading to follicle destruction and cicatricial alopecia of the brows, sometimes of the scalp, along with pitted depressed scars. Similar changes may occur in the beard areas of young men, and in some patients the extremities are also involved. It may also occur in conjunction with hereditary woolly hair. The condition is symmetric and is usually found in blond individuals.

Keratosis Pilaris Decalvans (Keratosis Follicularis Spinulosa Decalvans)

In keratosis pilaris decalvans (keratosis follicularis spinulosa decalvans), an X-linked dominant condition, numerous milia of the face develop during infancy, followed by follicular plugging of the skin of the nose, cheeks, neck, and extensor surface of the extremities that may be quite prominent. Atrophoderma of the cheeks and cicatricial alopecia of the scalp and brows develop during childhood. Infrequently, there is complete regrowth of hair without scarring. Limited palmoplantar keratoderma may develop during childhood; hair abnormalities and reduced sweating may also be found. In heterozygous females, the alopecia and ocular findings are less severe.

Other associated abnormalities include physical and mental retardation, atopy, deafness, recurrent infections, and aminoaciduria. Ocular abnormalities include photophobia, corneal stromal opacities, and vascularization.

Pityriasis Rubra Pilaris (PRP, Pityriasis Pilaris)

Pityriasis rubra pilaris (PRP) comprises a group of conditions in which there are varying degrees of circumscribed follicular keratosis and erythema. Other potential findings include hypothyroidism, leukemia, and multiple seborrheic warts.

PRP involves both sexes with equal frequency and begins during adulthood or childhood. There are five types:

Type I—adult onset, classical.
Type II—adult onset, atypical.
Type III—juvenile onset, classical.
Type IV—juvenile onset, circumscribed.
Type V—juvenile onset, atypical.

Some childhood cases are autosomal dominant. Acquired cases occur at any age. The cause of acquired cases is unknown. The authors are concerned with the classical forms (type I and type III), and, except for age of onset, both are similar. Sometimes the juvenile form is precipitated by an acute infection.

Skin

PRP often involves the scalp first, and the lesions are indistinguishable from seborrheic dermatitis. Characteristic lesions are seen on the head, neck, or upper trunk, appearing as erythematous, slightly scaly macules that are soon followed by profuse numbers of follicular acuminate papules (erythematous perifollicular papules with central plugs). In some instances, the papules coalesce to form plaques. Adjacent areas become erythematous, and, over a 1- to 3-month period, the lesions spread from the face and scalp downward, leaving small areas of normal skin within the erythematous areas (Fig. 5-10). A diffuse, branlike scaling then occurs on the scalp; hyperkeratotic and yellow scaling occurs on the palms and soles, often with painful fissures; the dorsal aspects of the proximal phalanges often become involved; the nails become discolored and grossly thickened with subungual accumulations of keratinous debris. Oral lesions are uncommon but appear as a diffuse hyperkeratosis or resemble lichen planus. In most patients, the condition resolves spontaneously after 1 to 3 years.

Ocular Features

PRP may cause a mild to severe ectropion. Corneal changes are uncommon, although keratinization, peripheral keratitis, pannus, interstitial keratitis, and epithelial erosions may be seen (Fig. 5-11).

Darier Disease (Keratosis Follicularis, Darier–White Disease)

Darier disease (keratosis follicularis, Darier–White disease) is autosomal dominant, but many new cases arise as mutations. Characteristic skin lesions develop before the age of 30.

Skin Features

Symmetric skin-colored, yellow-brown, or brown; firm; rather greasy; crusted papules develop in the seborrheic areas of the skin (face, neck, shoulders, chest, and midline of the back) and legs (Figs. 5-12, 5-13, 5-14, and 5-15). The papules coalesce to form vegetating malodorous irregular warty plaques or papillomatous masses in the flexures of the trunk (groins and anogenital region) and on the face (especially the scalp, scalp margins, forehead, ears, and nasolabial folds), or small, leukodermatous macules develop on the trunk and extremities. Punctate keratoses, pathognomonic pits, or hyperkeratosis develops on the palms and soles. Infrequently, hemorrhagic macules are seen on the hands and feet. Nail findings include broad, white or red, slightly translucent, longitudinal bands. Subungual hyperkeratosis may also be present.

Mucous membrane lesions include white, umbilicated, or cobblestone papules of the tongue, buccal mucosa, palate, epiglottis, pharyngeal wall, esophagus, vulva, or rectum. Confluence of the papules may produce leukoplakia-like plaques. Occasionally, the salivary glands are blocked, and hypertrophy of the gums may occur.

Ocular Features

Irregular, peripheral, epithelial opacities and central cobweb-like linear opacities occur in the corneal epithelium, and are best seen with the pooling of topical fluorescein. These nebulous opacities are often associated with central irregularities in the corneal epithelium. The eyelid margin can be afflicted with hyperkeratotic plaques, and these may become secondarily infected during topical treatment with etretinate.

KERATINIZATION AND PIGMENTATION DISORDERS

Acanthosis Nigricans

Acanthosis nigricans is characterized by pigmentation and hyperkeratosis with papillomatous elevations and a velvety texture. There are five types:

Type 1. Hereditary benign acanthosis nigricans (autosomal dominant) is present at birth or develops during childhood or at puberty (Fig. 5-16).
Type 2. Benign acanthosis nigricans occurring as part of
  A. Endocrine disorders (Addison disease, Cushing disease, hypothyroidism, and insulin-resistant diabetes mellitus types A, B, and C).
  B. Various ovarian tumors (ovarian stromal luteomas, ovarian dermoid cysts, polycystic ovarian disease).
  C. Hypogonadal syndromes with insulin resistance (Prader–Willi syndrome, Alstrom syndrome, and others).
  D. Miscellaneous syndromes (ataxia telangiectasia, Bloom syndrome, Capozucca syndrome, Crouzon

disease, Lawrence–Seip syndrome, leprechaunism, Rud syndrome, Wilson disease, and the syndrome of acral hypertrophy and muscle cramps).

    E. The HAIR–AN syndrome (*h*yper *a*ndrogenis, *i*nsulin *r*esistances–*a*canthosis *n*igricans) indicates those females with evidence of increased androgen levels who develop acanthosis nigricans due to mutation in the insulin receptor gene.

Type 3. Pseudoacanthosis nigricans associated with obesity (Fig. 5-17). This form of acanthosis nigricans is benign and often reversible with weight reduction. Lesions usually develop in the body folds (axillae, groins, and natal cleft), the inner and upper thighs, and labia majora.

Type 4. Drug-induced acanthosis nigricans (Fig. 5-18). The condition arises in association with consumption of high doses of nicotinic acid, glucocorticoids, oral contraceptives, estrogens, and triazinate (a folic acid antagonist).

Type 5. Malignant acanthosis nigricans (associated with malignancies such as adenocarcinoma or, rarely, lymphoma). The lesions are extensive, and palmar hyperkeratosis is common. Irritation is a common complaint. Increased pigmentation is a prominent finding even in areas free of hyperkeratosis. The nails are often ridged or brittle; loss of scalp hair and eyebrows is common.

Acanthosis nigricans occurring in response to insulin or insulin-like growth factors is less severe than when associated with malignancies.

Clinical Features

The most common sites of involvement are the scruff and sides of the neck, axillae, groins, and anogenital region. Other flexural areas, the submammary region and the umbilicus, are occasionally involved. Infrequently it is generalized. A gray-brown or black thickened pigmented area develops that often feels dry and rough early in the disease process (Fig. 5-18). The area then becomes covered with small papillomatous elevations that give a velvety texture to the involved areas. The lesions progress to form rugose, nipplelike, or large warty excrescences. The benign forms of the disease regress or remain stationary following puberty.

Malignant forms of acanthosis nigricans sometimes arise a year or more before the symptoms of the underlying malignancy. In some instances, acanthosis nigricans regresses following tumor removal. The mucous membranes, including the esophageal mucosa and mucocutaneous areas, are involved in about half of the cases of the malignant variety. Warty papillomatous lesions are often seen about the lips.

Ocular Features

Acanthosis nigricans is characterized by pigmentation and hyperkeratosis with papillomatous elevations and a velvety texture. Warty, papillomatous thickening sometimes occurs in the periocular skin in the malignant form of acanthosis nigricans and may be the presenting complaint (Fig. 5-19).

Alstrom Syndrome

Alstrom syndrome is characterized by short stature, obesity, acanthosis nigricans, baldness, kyphoscoliosis, hypogonadism, renal dysfunction, hyperuricemia, hypertriglyceridemia, insulin-dependent diabetes mellitus, and sensorineural deafness. The mental development is normal. It is probably autosomal recessive.

Loss of vision develops in the first decade of life from retinitis pigmentosa (salt-and-pepper pigment abnormalities, marked vascular attenuation, and later diffuse chorioretinal atrophy with evidence of large clumps of retinal epithelial pigment).

POROKERATOSIS

Porokeratosis represents a keratotic lesion that develops from a clone of dysplastic cells. It is associated with increased incidence of carcinomas.

Porokeratosis of Mibelli

Porokeratosis of Mibelli represents a condition in which there are isolated lesions of porokeratosis. It is autosomal dominant but may occur sporadically or follow immunosuppression. Males are involved two to three times more frequently than females.

Skin Features

The eruption is characterized by annular or raised atrophic or hyperkeratotic dry plaques with horny concretions and plugs (Fig. 5-20). The plaques are surrounded by a keratotic, fine, raised or furrowlike border. The lesions may be single, few in number, or many and small. They usually develop on the extremities and often spread centrifugally, producing an annular or oval figure. Scalp involvement produces patchy alopecia. They have a potential for malignant change. Rarely, lesions develop on the face. They also occur in the genital area or, occasionally, on the buccal mucosa and undersurface of the tongue.

Ocular Features

Hyperkeratotic lesions similar to the skin lesions have been described on the cornea.

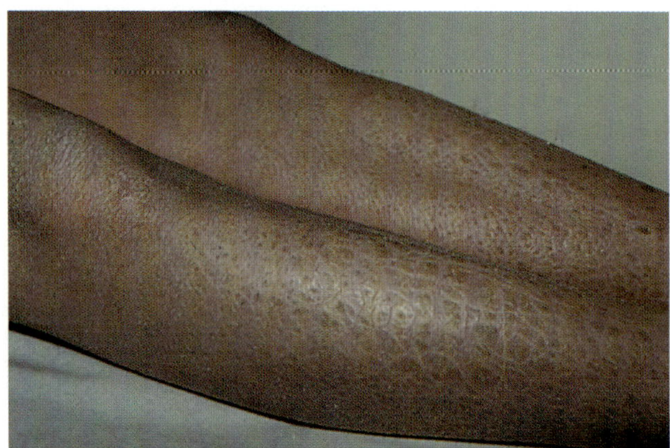

FIGURE 5-1. Ichthyosis of the legs.

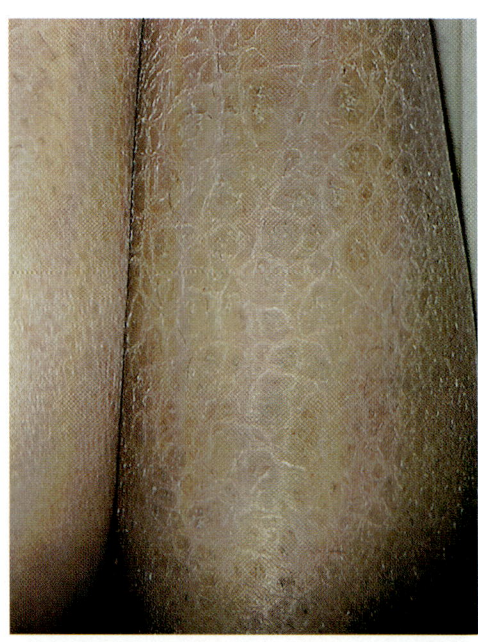

FIGURE 5-2. Ichthyosis vulgaris of the extensor surfaces of the arms.

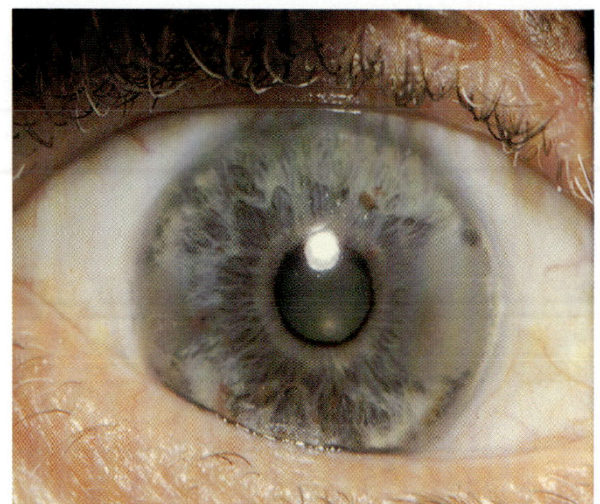

FIGURE 5-3. Band-shaped keratopathy in ichthyosis vulgaris. The keratopathy and slight visual loss had developed over 3 years. There is mild lid thickening but no ichthyotic scales. The band keratopathy is evident both medially and laterally.

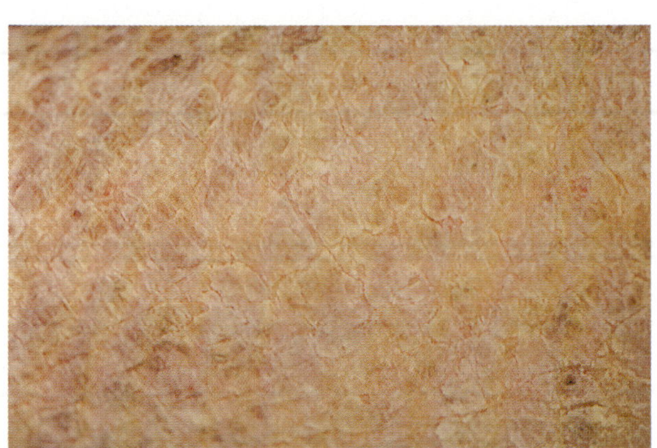

FIGURE 5-4. Lamellar ichthyosis of the extensor surface of the leg.

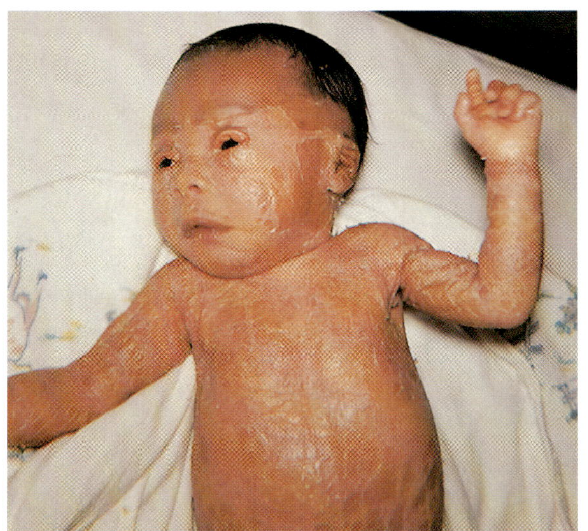

FIGURE 5-5. Collodion baby (lamellar exfoliation of the newborn, lamellar ichthyosis). Ectropion of both upper lids, distortion of the pinna, and the inelastic, thick, translucent membrane are evident.

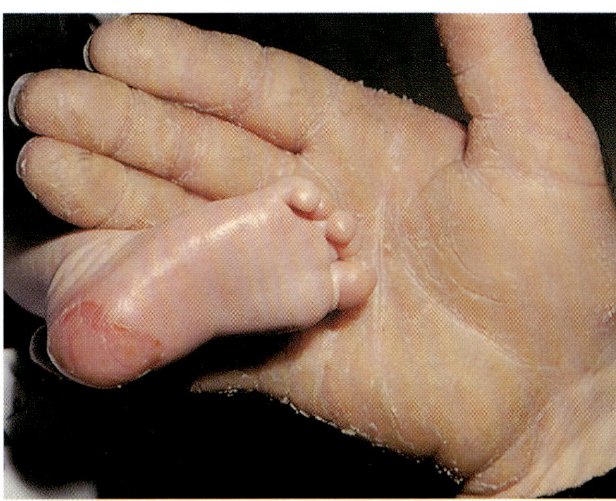

FIGURE 5-6. Bullous ichthyosiform erythroderma in father and infant. The father's hyperkeratotic hands and the infant's erythrodermatous hyperkeratotic soles are readily seen. The condition is present in four generations of this family.

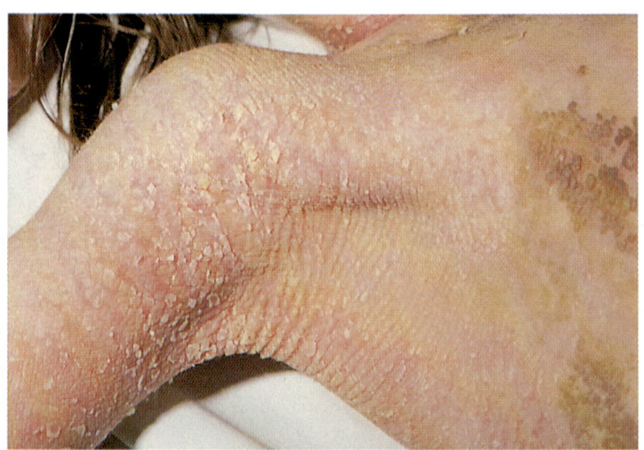

FIGURE 5-7. Bullous ichthyosiform erythroderma involving the axillae.

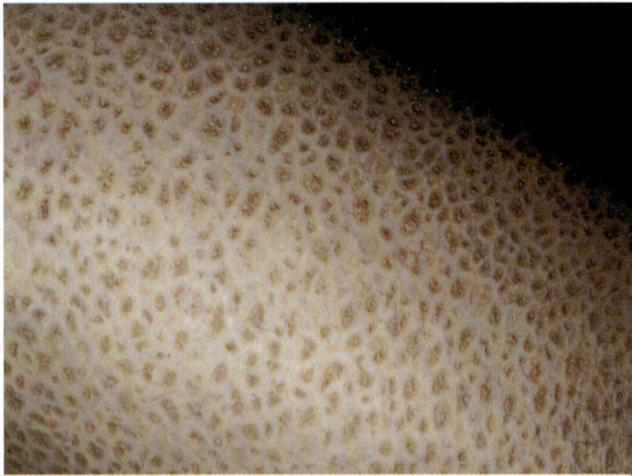

FIGURE 5-8. X-linked recessive ichthyosis with scaling of the extensor surfaces of the arm.

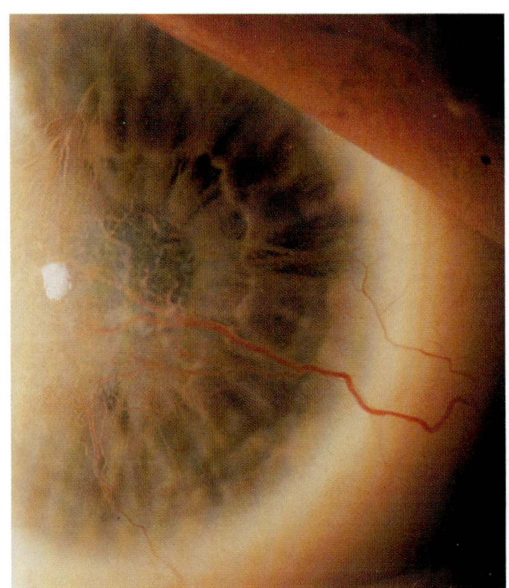

FIGURE 5-9. Epithelial irregularity and corneal neovascularization in the KID syndrome. (Photograph courtesy of Suzanne Banuvar.)

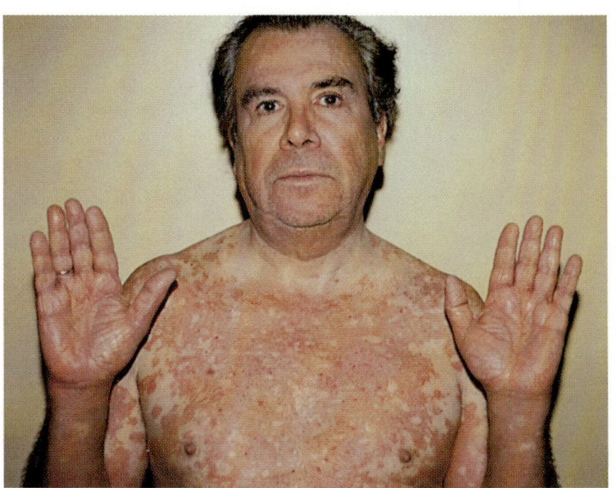

FIGURE 5-10. Pityriasis rubra pilaris (PRP).

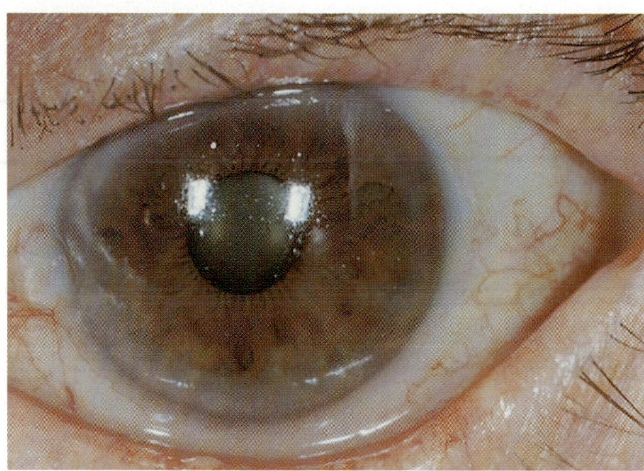

FIGURE 5-11. Keratinization of the lateral limbus and a peripheral keratitis in pityriasis rubra pilaris.

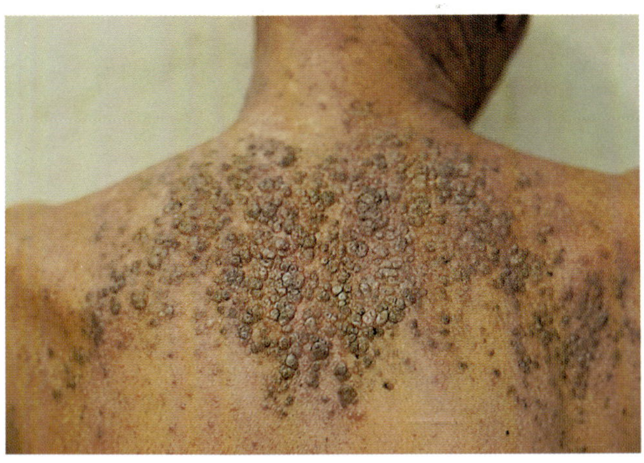

FIGURE 5-12. Darier disease showing the symmetric, greasy, crusted papules on the trunk, face, back, and legs.

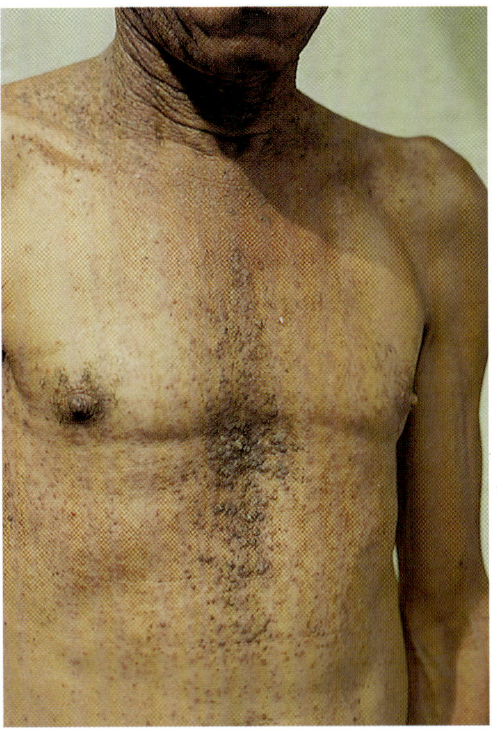

FIGURE 5-13. Darier disease.

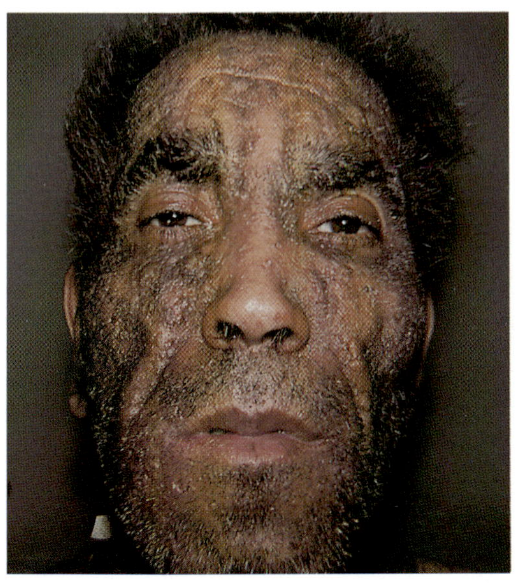

FIGURE 5-14. Darier disease.

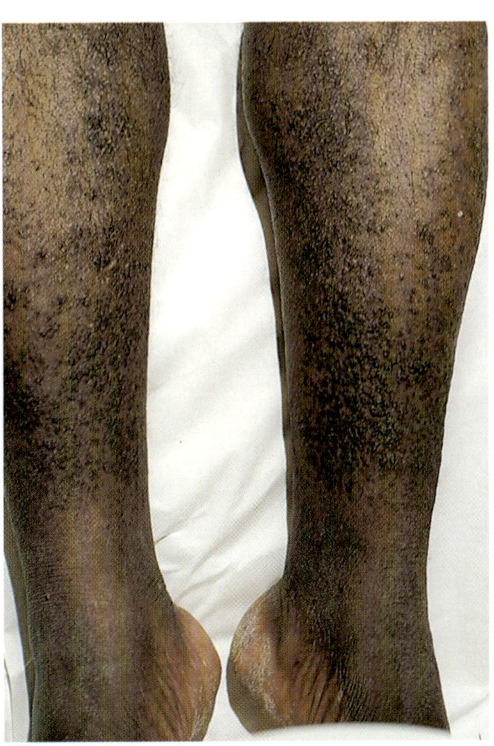

FIGURE 5-15. Darier disease.

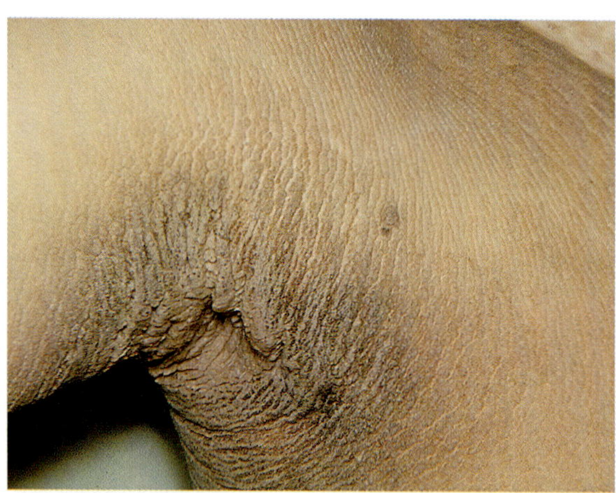

FIGURE 5-16. Hereditary benign acanthosis nigricans in a teenage boy. His severe lesions were malodorous, causing him significant social embarrassment. Treatment with dermabrasion resulted in only temporary improvement.

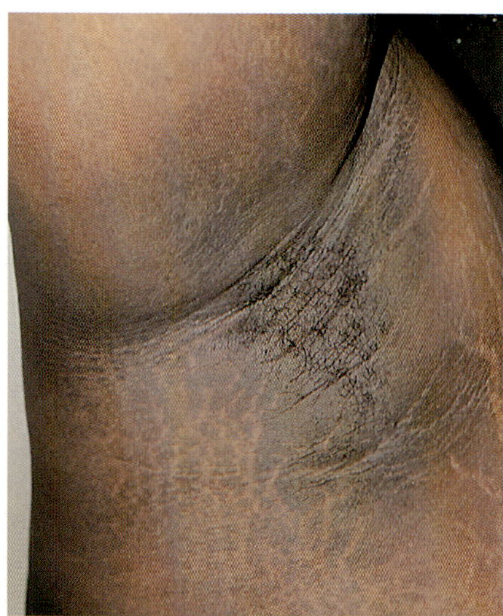

FIGURE 5-17. Pseudoacanthosis nigricans of the axilla. A commonly seen entity in dark-skinned, overweight young teenagers. These sites often are irritated from vigorous scrubbing in attempts to clean them.

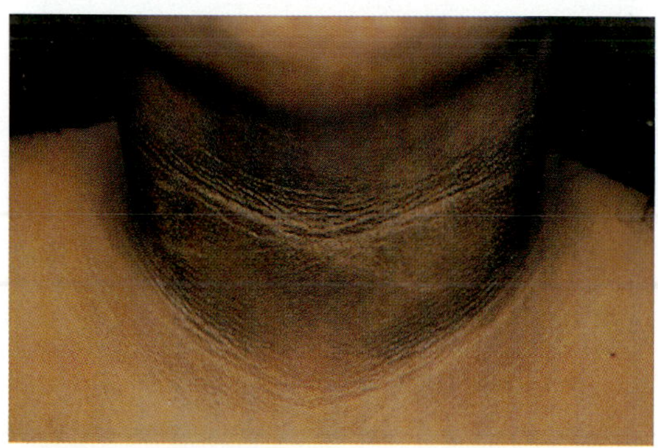

FIGURE 5-18. Acanthosis nigricans of the neck induced by high doses of nicotinic acid.

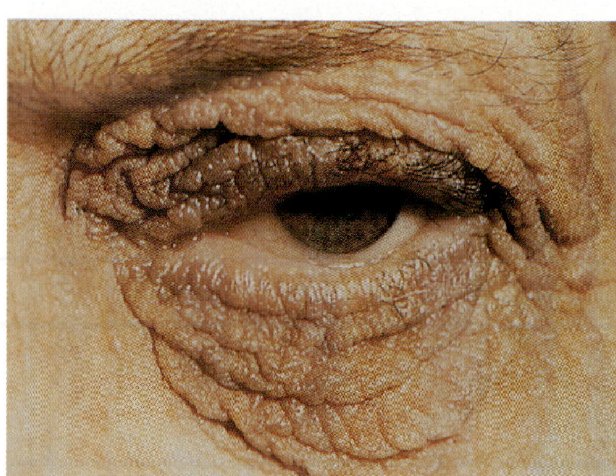

FIGURE 5-19. Acanthosis nigricans of the eyelids characterized by severe periocular thickening together with increased pigmentation. (Photograph courtesy of Dr. Alson E. Braley.)

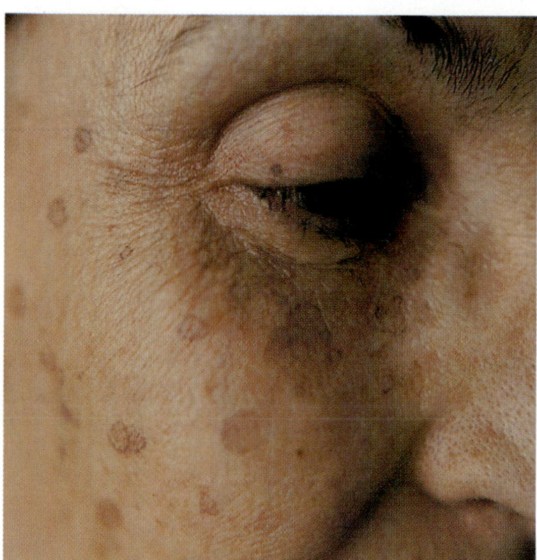

FIGURE 5-20. Porokeratosis of Mibelli involving the face. Note the subtle raised margins.

6

PIGMENTARY DISORDERS

Skin color is determined by the amount of melanin, the location of melanin and melanocytes, the state of the ratio between oxygenated and reduced hemoglobin, and the presence of carotenoids and other endogenous or exogenous pigments in the skin.

Melanin and the effect of sun exposure on melanin pigment are major determinants of skin color. Estrogen and pituitary hormones have some effect on melanin, as is seen in chloasma of pregnancy and increased pigmentation in Addison disease. Melanin pigment in the upper dermis causes a blue pigmentation (Riehl melanosis); melanocytes and melanin located in both the epidermis and dermis cause blue pigmentation as seen in the nevus of Ota and mongolian spot; a normal number of epidermal melanocytes with increased epidermal melanin pigment causes a brown pigmentation (melasma).

Carotenoids are yellow pigments, which are deposited in the epidermis and subcutaneous fat and, when present in excessive amounts, cause conspicuous yellowing, especially in areas of thick keratin layers and where there is a preponderance of subcutaneous fat. Carotinoids may be deposited in the peripheral cornea and may be mistaken for a Kayser–Fleischer ring. They are not deposited in the sclera. High serum levels of bilirubin cause scleral icterus, because it has a high affinity for elastic tissue and is deposited in the sclera. (Fig. 6-1). (Long-standing jaundice also causes the amount of skin melanin to be increased, which causes a bronze discoloration.)

About 75% of patients with ochronosis develop skin, sclera, and conjunctival darkening, and as early as the third decade, the cartilaginous tissue and many other body tissues become brownish-yellow in color. The pinna, concha, antihelix, and later, the tongue and antitragus become discolored; the darkened cartilage feels abnormally firm. Symmetric diffuse brown or black pigmentary deposits develop in the episclera and sclera near the insertion of the rectus muscles and appear like oil droplets in water on retroillumination (Fig. 6-1b). Sometimes the sclera has a blue-gray discoloration, especially laterally.

HYPERMELANOSIS

The hypermelanotic conditions associated with ocular disease, such as lentigines and lentiginosis, are discussed in Chapters 16 and 19; neurofibromatosis, in Chapter 11; xeroderma pigmentosum, in Chapter 10; and endocrine disorders, in Chapter 18. Facial hypopigmentation or hyperpigmentation in African patients is common, arising from exposure to agents such as skin-bleaching creams, mercury-containing skin-lightening soaps and creams, antimalarials, fixed drug reactions, and photosensitizing herbal concoctions.

Melanism

Melanism is autosomal dominant and is manifested by skin and sometimes meningeal hyperpigmentation, which is present at birth and increases in magnitude until about the age of 5 or 6. The iris may or may not be affected.

Periorbital Melanosis

Although some periorbital pigmentation is normal, it is usually an autosomal dominant trait. (The allergic shiner in atopic dermatitis is not due to melanosis but arises from venous stasis.)

Erythema Dyschromicum Perstans (Ashy Dermatosis of Ramirez)

Erythema dyschromicum perstans (ashy dermatosis of Ramirez) is an idiopathic dermatosis that is characterized by various shades of ashy gray macules, which have a red, slightly raised, infiltrated margin. The lesions vary in size and occur on the trunk (Fig. 6-1c), extremities, and face; they may coalesce to become quite extensive and may cause bilateral periorbital pigmentation.

Lentiginosis Profusa Syndrome (Multiple Lentigines Syndrome)

Lentiginosis profusa syndrome (multiple lentigines syndrome) carries the acronym LEOPARD syndrome (*l*entigines, *e*lectrocardiographic abnormalities, *o*cular hypertelorism, *p*ulmonary stenosis, *a*bnormalities of the genitalia, *r*etardation of growth, and *d*eafness). It is autosomal dominant, has a variable degree of expressivity, and probably arises as a defect in the neuroectodermal or neural crest stem cells. The lentigines are present at birth or develop soon thereafter and are most numerous on the neck and upper trunk. They increase in number until about puberty. Supernumerary teeth may also occur.

Cardiac abnormalities include conduction abnormalities and pulmonary and subaortic stenosis. Skeletal abnormalities include hypertelorism and mandibular prognathism. Sensorineural deafness is uncommon. Genital abnormalities include hypospadias, gonadal hypoplasia, and delayed puberty. Growth retardation may be seen.

Ocular Features

The ocular findings include hypertelorism, strabismus, nystagmus, ptosis, lagophthalmos, and corneal haze secondary to the lagophthalmos.

Peutz–Jeghers Syndrome (Period Lentiginosis)

Peutz–Jeghers syndrome (period lentiginosis) is autosomal dominant with variable degrees of expressivity. It is characterized by hamartoma polyps of the large and small intestine and pigmented skin, lip, and buccal mucosa lesions. It may be complicated by increased breast, reproductive organ, thyroid, and pancreatic malignancies.

Gastrointestinal polyposis, with a small increased incidence of malignancy, occurs with or without skin pigmentation, and, conversely, pigmentation occurs without gastrointestinal polyps. The polyps often lead to recurrent intussusception, spasm, irritability, ulceration, and rectal bleeding. Polyps may also occur in the upper respiratory tract, gallbladder, appendix, and ureter.

Skin Features

The pigmented macules occasionally involve the periorbital skin. Pigmented macules may be present at birth or, more usually, develop during infancy, but they may also develop later in life. Macules around the nose and mouth are smaller and darker than macules of the volar and dorsal aspects of the hands, feet, and terminal portion of the digits. The macules are lighter in color and less profuse in numbers in fair-skinned individuals.

Round or oval irregular pigmented patches occur on the lips (especially the lower lip) (Fig. 6-2), oral mucosa, and rarely, rectal mucosa. Infrequently, the nails are also pigmented. The pigmented skin and lip lesions may fade after puberty, whereas the buccal lesions do not fade.

Cronkhite–Canada Syndrome

Cronkhite–Canada syndrome is a nonfamilial, generalized gastrointestinal polyposis associated with skin pigmentation, alopecia, and onychodystrophy. The cause is unknown. The male-to-female ratio is 3 to 2. Patients develop diarrhea, abdominal discomfort, and anorexia, followed by weight loss, wasting, edema, and, sometimes, severe anemia from gastrointestinal bleeding. Multiple gastrointestinal hamartomatous polyps may develop, extending from the stomach to the rectum. Carcinoma occurs in about 15% of patients. Death is usually caused by gastrointestinal bleeding, protein deficiency, and wasting.

Skin Features

Pigmented macules occur on the face, trunk, extremities, palms and soles, and rarely, buccal mucosa. They are light to dark brown and vary from several millimeters to 10 cm in diameter. Skin edema is common. Alopecia of the scalp, brow, face, and body hair may develop over a period of weeks. Varying dystrophic nail changes (splitting, thinning, and partial onycholysis) or complete nail loss may develop rapidly. Cheilosis and papillary atrophy of the tongue may also be seen.

Following treatment or during remissions, the pigmentation and other ectodermal changes sometimes disappear.

Ocular Features

Brow alopecia, xanthelasma, skin pigmentation about the eyes, cataracts, and retinal pigmentary changes have been observed.

Incontinentia Pigmenti (Bloch–Sulzberger Syndrome)

Incontinentia pigmenti (Bloch–Sulzberger syndrome) is characterized by cutaneous, ocular, skeletal, dental, and central nervous system abnormalities. It is probably X-linked dominant and is lethal for males. Those cases that occur in males probably arise from mutation. The condition also occurs in the Klinefelter syndrome.

About one-third of patients develop central nervous system disorders that include psychomotor retardation, epilepsy, spastic di- or tetraplegia, hydrocephalus, and microcephaly. Skeletal abnormalities include spina bifida and skull and palatal defects.

Skin and Oral Features

Cicatricial alopecia, usually of the vertex, occurs in about 25% of patients, and dystrophic nail changes may be seen (Figs. 6-3 and 6-4). Incontinentia pigmenti has three distinct skin stages:

1. The inflammatory stage is present at birth or develops within the first few weeks of life and may be associated with pruritus. Recurrent crops of vesicles or small, tense bullae with surrounding erythema develop in a linear fashion on the extremities and with a less distinct linear arrangement on the trunk. Smooth, red nodules or plaques often accompany the vesicles or bullae, or they may precede the bullae. The lesions last several days or months and occasionally ulcerate.
2. The second stage, characterized by linear verrucous skin lesions of the dorsum of the hands and feet, begins 2 or more weeks after the inflammatory stage and persists for weeks or months; rarely, it occurs without the inflammatory stage.
3. The third stage is characterized by pigmented irregular streaks and whorls of blue-gray or slate-to-brown pigmentation of the trunk distributed along Blaschko lines (Fig. 6-3). They are more prominent during the first few years. Eventually, hypopigmented streaks and skin atrophy develop, especially on the lower extremities; these characteristics may be the only cutaneous abnormalities evident in the adult, although extensive and progressive hyperkeratotic lesions of the legs have been noted. Dental defects (delayed dentition, partial anodontia, and eruption of cone- or peg-shaped teeth) occur in about 60% of cases of incontinentia pigmenti (Fig. 6-4).

Ocular Features

Ocular abnormalities occur in about 30% of patients (Fig. 6-5). They are often unilateral and include microphthalmos, nystagmus, strabismus, myopia, focal conjunctival pigmentation, keratitis, cataracts, uveitis, retinal abnormalities, and blindness. The retinal abnormalities include arteriovenous (A-V) aneurysms, neovascularization, hemorrhage, exudative chorioretinitis with retinal detachment, retinal dysplasia, increased retinal pigmentation, and retrolental masses simulating retrolental fibroplasia.

Dyskeratosis Congenita (Zinsser–Cole–Engmann Syndrome)

Dyskeratosis congenita (Zinsser–Cole–Engmann syndrome) is X-linked recessive and, in affected females, may be autosomal dominant or recessive. It is manifested by skin atrophy and pigmentation, leukoplakia, nail dystrophy, predisposition to malignancy, and progressive bone marrow failure that leads to pancytopenia.

Gastrointestinal hemorrhage, malignancies, diarrhea, ascites, and noncirrhotic portal hypertension develop in a significant number of patients. Chronic respiratory tract involvement has also been observed. Physical and mental retardation occasionally occur. Impaired cell-mediated immunity may be seen. Minor skeletal anomalies, a small sella turcica, heart block, hypospadias, hypogonadism, and meatal stenosis are uncommon.

Skin Features

Poikiloderma, reticulated pigmentation, and atrophy with prominent telangiectasis develop in the sun-exposed areas of the neck, upper chest, arms, thighs, and greater part of the trunk during early childhood. Occasionally, it affects the entire skin. Occasionally, skin changes are delayed until the second or third decade, when fine, reticulate, gray-brown pigmentation develops. The skin atrophy usually involves the extremities, dorsum of the hands and feet, and genitalia. Malignant changes may occur in involved areas.

The soles and palms may be thickened, may be hyperhidrotic, and may blister with trauma. Sometimes the muscles and bones of the hands and feet also show atrophic changes. The hair of the scalp, brows, and lashes may be lusterless and sparse, and in some instances, the brows and lashes are absent. Almost all patients have progressive nail dystropy, with longitudinal ridging and splitting followed eventually by pterygium unguis and complete nail loss.

The buccal mucosa, the palate, and especially the lateral margins of the tongue sometimes develop bullae or painful ulcerations that may lead to hyperkeratosis, leukoplakia, and malignant changes during the third to fifth decade. Infrequently, similar lesions occur on the urethral meatus, vagina, glans penis, and anus. Nasopharyngeal atresia has been observed. Dysphagia may occur from esophageal involvement. Dental involvement includes increased caries, gingival recession and bleeding, short-blunted roots, tooth mobility, and severe alveolar bone loss.

Ocular Features

Blepharitis, ectropion, trichiasis, and loss of the lashes and brows, conjunctival bullae, and white plaques sometimes occur. In more than three-fourths of cases, epithelial hyperplasia causes punctal obliteration and epiphora. Congenital cataracts have been observed.

Hemochromatosis (Hanot–Chauffard Syndrome)

Hemochromatosis (Hanot–Chauffard syndrome) is characterized by hyperpigmentation, diabetes, cirrhosis, increased iron deposition in internal organs, cardiac disease, and occasionally, hypogonadism. It is more common in males and begins gradually, usually during the fourth to sixth decade. It is caused by chronic iron consumption, chronic liver disease in the face of iron consumption, congenital transferrin deficiency, and ineffective erythropoiesis in patients who are consuming iron. It is usually autosomal recessive, although many cases are idiopathic.

Other findings include anorexia and weight loss, testicular atrophy due to pituitary gland involvement, and arthropathy similar to rheumatoid arthritis but with a negative serology. Hepatomas are found in more than one-fourth of patients, especially elderly patients.

Skin Features

Cutaneous hyperpigmentation is the most common and often the earliest manifestation. The skin of the face, flexural creases, and exposed areas become metallic gray or gray-brown in color; occasionally, the buccal mucosa also becomes pigmented. The skin may be dry and atrophic, and palmar erythema and spider angiomas may develop. Occasionally, the skin around the nipple, genitalia, and exposure areas becomes depigmented. Scalp, axillary, and pubic hair alopecia may be found; sometimes koilonychia, onychia striata, and leukonychia occur.

Ocular Features

Limbal or diffuse conjunctival pigmentation develops in about 20% of patients.

Dermal Melanocytosis (Ceruloderma)

Dermal melanocytosis (ceruloderma) arises from failure of the dermal melanocytes to reach the basal layer of the epidermis during migration from the neural crest. The lesions are present at birth and are slate-brown or blue in color.

Oculodermal Melanocytosis (Nevus of Ota)

Oculodermal melanocytosis (nevus of Ota) involves the skin of the first and second division of the trigeminal nerve and often affects the sclera (Figs. 6-6 and 6-7). The lesions are usually congenital but may develop during childhood and often become progressively darker in childhood. Rarely, they develop during adulthood. They are more common in females and in Asians (Fig. 6-6). Associated skin, eye, and brain melanomas have been observed, but usually in whites.

Blue-gray macules and patches develop on the lids, cheeks, forehead, scalp, ala nasi, and pinna, and are sometimes confluent. Their edges gradually blend into normal skin. Infrequently, patients have similar pigmentation in the region supplied by the mandibular nerve with rare occurrence on the trunk. About 10% of patients have bilateral pigmentation. Melanosis may also occur in the oral and nasal mucosa. The upper and lower lids, the bulbar and palpebral conjunctiva, and the cornea may have various areas of brownish discoloration. Blue-gray scleral pigmentation (Fig. 6-7) occurs in more than 60% of patients and may be associated with heterochromia iridis.

Other ocular features include melanocytic infiltration and hyperpigmentation of the anterior chamber angle, iris, fundus, optic papilla, optic nerve, retrobulbar fat, orbital vessels, extraocular muscles, and periosteum of the orbital bone. Glaucoma and cataracts may also be seen. Malignant transformation may occur, especially in white patients, but usually there are no characteristic skin changes evident in those patients.

OTHER CAUSES OF HYPERPIGMENTATION
Riehl Melanosis

The cause of Riehl melanosis is unknown but probably represents a pigmented contact dermatitis related to use of tar derivatives, compounds in cosmetics, or nutritional or other factors. It is characterized by brownish-gray pigmentation involving most of the face, including the lids, and is especially intense over the forehead and temples. Sometimes it extends to the scalp, neck, and chest, and occasionally, to the forearms and hands. The pigmentation may develop quite rapidly. Small perifollicular macules may also occur in nonpigmented surrounding areas. The follicles are filled with horny plugs.

Drug-Induced Hyperpigmentation

Skin hyperpigmentation occurs as an adverse reaction to a variety of drugs. The phenothiazines react with melanin to form drug–pigment complexes. Heavy metals may be directly deposited in the skin, causing color changes. Some drugs induce pigmentation following inflammation, such as in fixed drug reactions and drug-induced lichenoid reactions, whereas other drugs act directly on chemical groups in cells to cause pigmentation (e.g., arsenic combines with sulfhydryl groups in the epidermal cells to cause pigmentation).

Phenothiazines

Discoloration can be seen on any sun-exposed area and can be evident on the lids, periocular region, forehead, cheeks, and nose (Figs. 6-8 and 6-9). Bluish-gray-to-purple skin discoloration develops as a phototoxic reaction in these skin areas in about 0.1% to 0.2% of patients taking phenothiazine. This is especially true for white females using high doses of chlorpromazine for prolonged periods. Sometimes it involves the nail beds. Paradoxically, lower doses of chlorpromazine over short periods of time may also cause purple discoloration in both sun-exposed and nonexposed skin areas.

The exposed bulbar conjunctiva often has a brownish discoloration, and brownish pigmentation may occur in the central corneal epithelium in a vortex pattern or, more diffusely, in the exposure area. Anterior lens capsule pigmentation may also occur.

Hydantoin

About 10% of patients taking hydantoin develop a chloasma-like bronze or fawn-colored, patchy pigmentation.

Arsenic

Inorganic arsenic administered over long periods of time may induce a diffuse or a "raindrop" pattern of pigmentation, especially on the trunk. Vitiligo is also increased. Arsenical keratosis may or may not be associated.

Antibiotics: Clofazimine and Minocycline

Clofazimine (Lamprene) used for leprosy causes redness of the cheeks, forehead, and other areas initially. Prolonged administration causes a violaceous-brown pigmentation (Fig. 6-10). Clofazimine in discoid lupus erythematosus causes dark reddish-blue pigmentation in the scarred areas induced by the disease.

Prolonged administration of high doses of minocycline may cause blue-brown pigmentation at inflammatory sites or a diffuse and generalized pigmentation in the sun-exposed areas of the body, including the sclera and nail beds, but sparing the palms and buttocks.

Antimalarial Drugs: Chloroquine and Hydroxychloroquine

Quinine and quinidine may cause generalized skin pigmentation (Fig. 6-11).

Mepacrine or quinacrine used as an antimalarial or anthelminthic may cause a greenish-yellow discoloration of the skin of the face, hands, and feet a few days after use. It does not affect the sclera. A slate-gray pigmentation similar to that seen in ochronosis and preferentially involving the cartilaginous structures such as the nose, epiglottis, and trachea may also occur in white patients receiving high doses of antimalarials. Sometimes the conjunctiva, palate, and nail beds are also involved.

In about 25% of patients, chloroquine or hydroxychloroquine administered over a period of several years causes blue-gray pigmentation of the face, neck, and less frequently, upper and lower extremities. Areas exposed to the sun and patches over the shins may become blue-black in appearance. The hard palate may appear blue-gray. There may also be diffuse nail pigmentation or pigmentation in transverse bands. The hair appears bleached. Ocular findings include a vortex keratopathy, macular changes, and severe reduction of vision (Fig. 6-11).

Amiodarone

Amiodarone infrequently causes photosensitivity, a gray-blue pigmentation of sun-exposed areas of the body, vortex epithelial opacity in the central cornea, decreased vision, photophobia, and halos around light (Fig. 6-12). Optic neuritis secondary to amiodarone can be a serious and unrecognized cause of visual loss.

Antitumor Drugs

Busulfan used for prolonged periods causes a diffuse brown pigmentation, which is more marked in non-whites with a dark complexion. Less frequently, it causes an addisonian pattern of pigmentation. Intravenous thiotepa may cause hyperpigmentation in skin areas occluded by adhesives, probably from accumulation of sweat in these areas. Topical use may cause depigmentation of the skin.

Oral Contraceptives

Brown hyperpigmentation of the forehead, malar eminences, and lower cheeks similar to chloasma of pregnancy occurs in about 30% of patients using oral contraceptives.

Heavy Metals

Gold may be deposited in the skin, conjunctiva, cornea, iris, ciliary body, choroid, and lens (Figs. 6-13 to 6-15). In sun-exposed skin, it produces a blue-gray-purplish tinge, probably through stimulation of melanin production in the dermis. It is diffusely deposited in the peripheral cornea and appears as dustlike or glittering granules (brownish, golden, or violet), whereas in the central corneal it is deposited anteriorly. In the lens, it is found in the anterior Y suture.

A gray-brown pigmentation of the conjunctiva or skin creases may occur from mercury deposition arising from repeated applications of ointments containing mercury.

Bismuth administration causes gray skin pigmentation similar to that seen in argyria. The conjunctiva, sclera, oral, vaginal, and colon mucosa may be involved.

Silver from medications or industrial sources may be deposited in the skin, causing a blue-gray color that is most intense on exposed skin; sometimes the discoloration is generalized, and the nails and mucous membranes may become pigmented.

Repeated topical instillation of argyrol often causes blue-gray discoloration of the conjunctiva, cornea, and skin of the eyelids. Corneal deposition of silver causes a peripheral yellow or brown ringlike opacity similar in many respects to a Kayser–Fleischer ring. Occasionally, the pigment involves all of Descemet membrane and, at the slit-lamp, resembles a sheet of fine, dustlike granules.

HYPOMELANOSIS

Hypomelanosis represents partial or complete absence of melanin in the skin and often the eyes. It is usually hereditary but may be acquired.

Albinism

Albinism represents an inherited congenital dilution of pigment that arises from disturbance in melanin synthesis. The degree of hypopigmentation varies from white to chocolate brown, but the dilution of pigment is always more than in unaffected relatives. It involves the skin, hair, and eyes (oculocutaneous albinism) or is confined to the eye (ocular albinism).

Oculocutaneous Albinism (OCA)

Oculocutaneous albinism (OCA) is uncommon. Except for autosomal dominant OCA, all variants are autosomal recessive. There are two major forms, tyrosinase-negative OCA characterized by total failure of melanin formation (demonstrated by plucked hair bulbs failing to darken when incubated with tyrosine), and tyrosinase-positive OCA, in which some pigmentation develops as the patient ages and in which the hair bulbs darken in the presence of tyrosine. Tyrosinase-positive OCA is more common and embraces various syndromes, including Prader–Willi, Hermansky–Pudlak, Chediak–Higashi, and Cross–McKusick syndromes.

Clinical Manifestations

In tyrosinase-negative OCA the skin is pink, the hair is white, and the irides are translucent, giving a prominent red reflex. In tyrosinase-positive OCA, the skin, hair, and eyes develop some pigment as the patient ages. Light tanning may occur, the hair becomes flaxen-yellow or red; in blacks, the skin becomes yellowish-brown with dark freckles sometimes developing in sun-exposed areas.

Ocular Features

Photophobia, decreased vision, and horizontal or rotary nystagmus, sometimes with head-nodding, are found in both forms of OCA but are more severe in tyrosinase-negative OCA. The patients also have misrouting of the optic fibers at the chiasm. The irides in tyrosinase-positive black patients may appear brown or tan, otherwise, in both tyrosinase-positive and tyrosinase-negative OCA, they are blue and transilluminate readily. Sometimes in albinoidism (hypopigmentation of the hair and skin and a positive hair bulb test), the irides transilluminate in a punctate pattern.

Increased visibility of the choroidal vessels, due to decreased amounts of retinal pigment epithelium, is found, and macular hypoplasia may occur, characterized by a normal perifoveal vasculature with absence of the foveal pit and the pigment of the macula lutea. Optic nerve hypoplasia is also common. OCA patients have an increased incidence of strabismus and refractive errors.

Hermansky–Pudlak Syndrome

Hermansky–Pudlak syndrome is a rare autosomal recessive form of tyrosinase-positive OCA. It is associated with a bleeding abnormality that arises from a storage-pool platelet defect. There is generally only mild pigmentary dilution of the skin and hair, and the melanin pigment abnormality is more marked in the eye. Inflammatory bowel disease, renal failure, and cardiomyopathy may be associated with this syndrome.

Cross Syndrome (Oculocerebral Syndrome with Hypopigmentation)

Cross syndrome (oculocerebral syndrome with hypopigmentation) is probably autosomal recessive. Patients have light-colored skin and hair from birth, and the albinism is weakly tyrosinase-positive. The patient is physically and mentally retarded, and progressive neurologic deterioration and athetoid movements with spasticity soon develop. Ocular features include coarse nystagmus, microphthalmos, a small opaque cornea, iris atrophy, cataracts, and bilateral optic atrophy.

Prader–Willi Syndrome

Prader–Willi syndrome arises from deletion of the long arm of chromosome 15 (15q-) and is characterized by early childhood obesity, mental retardation, emotional lability, hypotonia, hypogonadism, short stature, and often small hands and feet. Obstructive sleep apnea may be present, and the child often suddenly falls asleep during the daytime. Many patients are insensitive to pain and are prone to self-injury.

Skin and Ocular Findings

The facies is characteristic, with slit-eyes and down-turned nose (Fig. 6-16). Although subtle, about half of the patients have skin hypopigmentation. Tooth hypoplasia and caries may also occur.

About half of the patients have ocular pigmentary dilution that is sometimes quite subtle; radial translucent peripheral iris defects are more common. Strabismus nystagmus, foveal hypoplasia, field defects, and cataracts may also occur. Unlike in albinism, the chiasmal optic fibers are not aberrantly misrouted.

Ziprkowski–Margolis Syndrome

Ziprkowski–Margolis syndrome is a rare X-linked recessive condition characterized by white-pink hypopigmented skin that is sometimes associated with hyperpigmentation of the gluteal and scrotal skin and development at a later date of hyperpigmented areas on the extremities, trunk, and scalp. The patient has congenital sensorineural deafness, white hair, and sometimes heterochromia irides.

Ocular Albinism (OA)

Usually in ocular albinism (OA), only the eyes are clinically involved, although occasionally there is a mild skin hypopigmentation.

Ocular albinism encompasses the following:

1. The Nettleship–Falls type, which is X-linked recessive and is characterized by generalized uveal pigment dilution, photophobia, nystagmus, severe decrease in visual acuity, nystagmus, and foveal hypoplasia. The skin usually appears normal, but occasionally hypomelanotic macules are found, or, in some male patients, mild skin hypopigmentation is evident. In female carriers, the iris may transilluminate, and the fundus may have patchy or striated hypopigmentation.
2. The Witkop form, which is autosomal recessive.
3. The Forsius–Eriksson type, which is X-linked recessive and is associated with color blindness and axial myopia. The skin, hair, and eye color are normal.
4. The Winship type, which is X-linked recessive and is associated with a sensorineural deafness that develops at a later date.
5. The Lewis form, which is autosomal dominant and is associated with multiple lentigines and congenital neurosensory deafness.

Ocular Features of Ocular Albinism

Pigment hypoplasia is less evident in OA than in OCA, and sometimes the iris does not transilluminate; however, focal pigment hypoplasia often occurs as manifested by peripheral radial transillumination iris defects.

Piebaldism (White Spotting)

Piebaldism (white spotting) is an autosomal dominant condition characterized by a congenital patch of amelanotic skin. It probably represents several different genetic disorders and may not be a distinct entity. The amelanotic skin patches are present at birth and are usually located on the forehead, anterior trunk, flanks, and/or the mid-portion of the extremities. Islands of normal or hypermelanotic skin may be found inside of the amelanotic areas. Usually there is a diamond- or triangular-shaped, central white forelock. Heterochromia irides also occurs.

Waardenburg syndrome, Klein–Waardenburg syndrome, and BADS syndrome have many features of piebaldism.

Waardenburg syndrome Types I and II

In Waardenburg syndrome, the patient has a white forelock and congenital amelanotic skin areas of the forehead, which often contain normally colored or hyperpigmented macules. The anterior chest, abdomen, and extremities may also have areas of hypopigmentation. The lesions do not change over time, but premature graying of other areas of the scalp, brows, and lashes may occur.

Congenital, bilateral, symmetric sensorineural deafness occurs in both types but is more common in Waardenburg's type II syndrome. In both forms, the patient has a broad nasal root, closely set nares, small alar wings, a broad mandible, and an arched upper lip. Hirschsprung's megacolon occurs in both types but is more common in type II.

Ocular Features

Ocular features of both forms include synophrys (confluence) or hyperplasia of the eyebrows, heterochromia or hypopigmented irides, and fundus hypopigmentation. Lateral displacement of the inferior punctum and inner canthus (dystopia canthorum) is characteristically seen in Waardenburg type I syndrome. Occasional Waardenburg type I syndrome displays blepharophimosis. Marcus Gunn ptosis (jaw-winking) may occur in Waardenburg syndrome type II.

Klein–Waardenburg Syndrome

Klein–Waardenburg syndrome has all the features of Waardenburg type I syndrome plus congenital anomalies of the upper extremities (fusion of the carpal bones, syndactyly, absence of the upper limb and pectoral muscles, and flexion contractures and rigidity of joints). It is autosomal dominant.

BADS Syndrome

*B*lack locks, *a*lbinism, and sensorineural *d*eafness comprise BADS syndrome. Locks or clusters of black hair are found together with areas of white hair. Patients have marked sensorineural deafness. Ocular involvement includes photophobia, nystagmus, severe decrease in vision, translucent irides, and foveal hypoplasia.

Hypomelanosis of Ito (Incontinentia Pigmenti Achromians)

Hypomelanosis of Ito (incontinentia pigmenti achromians) is autosomal dominant and is more common in females. It is manifested by whorls and splashes of hypopigmentation that occur along Blaschko lines. The hypopigmentation appears as linear, mottled, or whorled streaks and splashes. It is either present at birth or develops within the first year of life. There are no preceding inflammatory signs. The hypomelanotic areas sometimes increase with time and later may repigment. About 75% of the patients have abnormal teeth. Many patients have musculoskeletal disorders and a length discrepancy of the extremities. Mental retardation and seizures are found in about 40% of patients.

Ocular Features

Ocular abnormalities occur in about 75% of patients and include epicanthal folds, hypertelorism, corneal opacities, heterochromia irides, pupillary dislocation and irregular margins, choroidal atrophy, retinal pigment abnormalities with patchy mottled hypopigmentation and increased striation in the periphery, strabismus, microphthalmos, small optic nerve, nystagmus, and myopia.

Vitiligo

Vitiligo affects all races and involves about 1% of the population (Figs. 6-17 and 6-18). About 30% of patients have a family history of vitiligo, and there is clustering of affected relatives. It usually occurs before the age of 20. There is often an associated autoimmune or endocrine disorder (Hashimoto thyroiditis, Grave disease, adrenal insufficiency, pernicious anemia, diabetes, hypoparathyroidism, or myasthenia gravis).

Initially, hypomelanotic macules develop in sun-exposed areas, (dorsum of the hands and face), especially around the eyes and mouth. Other frequently involved areas include areas that are normally hyperpigmented (axilla, groin, areolae, and genitalia) and areas subjected to trauma or repeated friction (e.g., feet, elbows, knees, and ankles). The lesions are usually symmetric but occasionally are unilateral or follow a dermatomal distribution. Sometimes there is trichrome vitiligo (partial hypomelanosis, complete melanosis, and normal skin located in the same area). The white patch is often surrounded by a hyperpigmented border.

The vitiliginous patches are usually convex; they irregularly increase in size. Smaller patches may fuse to form larger patches. Graying of the hair in older lesions may occur. Vitiligo gradually progresses over a period of months, then may remain quiescent. In some cases, especially in children, the areas partially repigment.

Discrete focal areas of choroidal and retinal depigmentation with some retinal pigment hypertrophy occur in about 40% of vitiligo patients. The changes sometimes represent inactive choroidal scars, other times retinal pigment degeneration. Usually there are no associated symptoms. About 8% of patients with vitiligo have an active uveitis (iridocyclitis or choroiditis).

Alezzandrini Syndrome

Alezzandrini syndrome is characterized by unilateral retinal degeneration followed after a few months or years by ipsi-lateral vitiligo, poliosis, and sometimes neurosensory deafness (Fig. 6-19).

Vogt–Koyanagi–Harada Syndrome

Vogt–Koyanagi–Harada syndrome occurs more frequently in Asians than in whites and is found more frequently during the third and fourth decade of life (Figs. 6-20 to 6-23). Initially, patients develop a trivial illness or a prolonged meningeal episode with nausea, severe headache, deep orbital pain, drowsiness, vertigo, pleocytosis, and occasionally, other neurologic signs (nuchal rigidity, papilledema, palsies of cranial nerves (III, IV, V, and VI), nystagmus, hemiparesis, and dysphasia). Many of these findings are transitory.

The second phase develops several months later and is characterized by iridocyclitis, scleritis, vitreitis, diffuse choroidal swelling, serous (exudative) retinal detachment, optic disc hyperemia, and dysacusis. The iridocyclitis is chronic and is often associated with the sudden onset of blurred vision; circumscribed retinal edema, usually of the posterior pole; and papilledema.

More than 50% of patients develop deafness or tinnitus from labyrinth involvement about 1 week after onset of the bilateral uveitis. Recovery of hearing is usually complete.

Vitiligo, alopecia, and poliosis occur late in the course of the illness, usually as the eye manifestations begin to resolve. The poliosis is usually limited to the brows and lashes but occasionally involves the scalp and body hair. The vitiligo is usually quite extensive. Alopecia occurs as a subtle diffuse loss of hair or as alopecia areata with patches of hair loss or sometimes diffuse hair loss. Alopecia totalis is uncommon.

Perilimbal depigmentation (Sugiura sign) may be the earliest sign of vitiligo. The poliosis and vitiligo are usually permanent.

The inflammation in Vogt–Koyanagi–Harada syndrome leads to an exudative retinal detachment, which is usually located in the inferior quadrants. Late in the course of the disease, the fundus may appear mottled and tessellated from loss of pigment (sunset-glow fundus). Blindness may occur.

Pityriasis Alba

Pityriasis alba represents a nonspecific dermatitis of unknown etiology (Fig. 6-24). It is characterized by multiple erythematous scaly patches, which, upon healing, leave areas of depigmentation. It usually affects children between the ages of 3 to 16, is more common in white patients, and often involves atopic diathesis.

The lesions affect the face, neck, arms, shoulders, trunk, and extremities, and occasionally are associated with mild pruritus. They appear as oval or round, erythematous, irregular plaques covered with fine scales. The margins are usually sharp and may be elevated. As the erythema subsides, the area becomes depigmented, although the fine scaling may persist. The leukoderma may persist for more than a year.

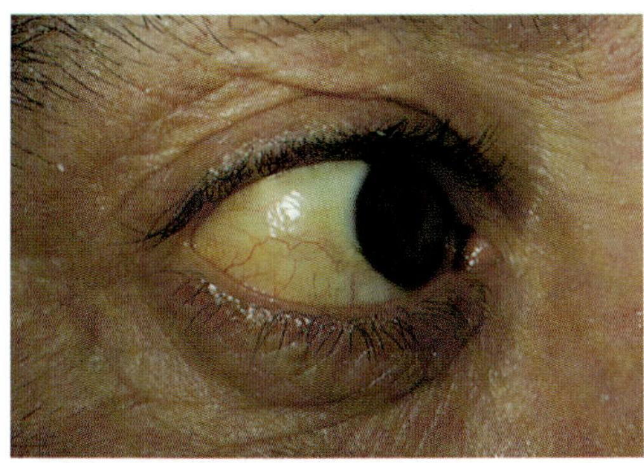

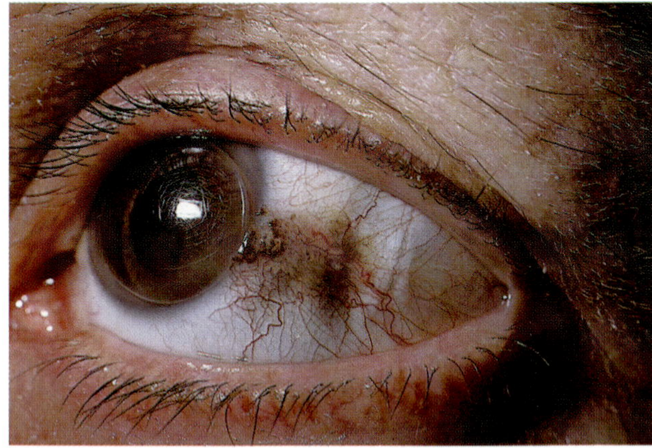

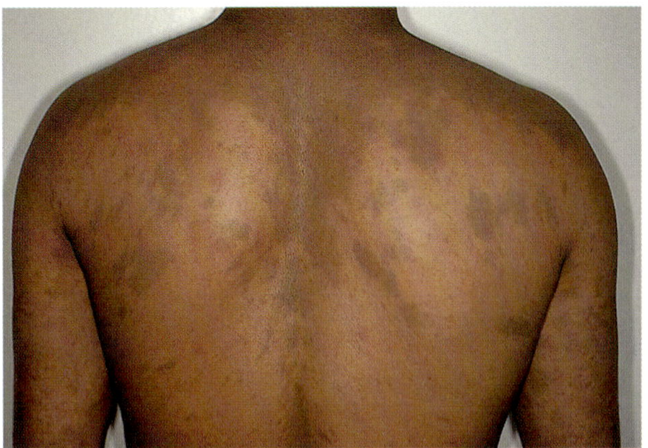

FIGURE 6-1. A: Scleral icterus in patient with hepatitis B. **B:** Scleral pigmentation near the insertion of the rectus muscle (Osler's sign) in Ochronosis. **C:** Erythema dyschromicum perstans (ashy dermatosis).

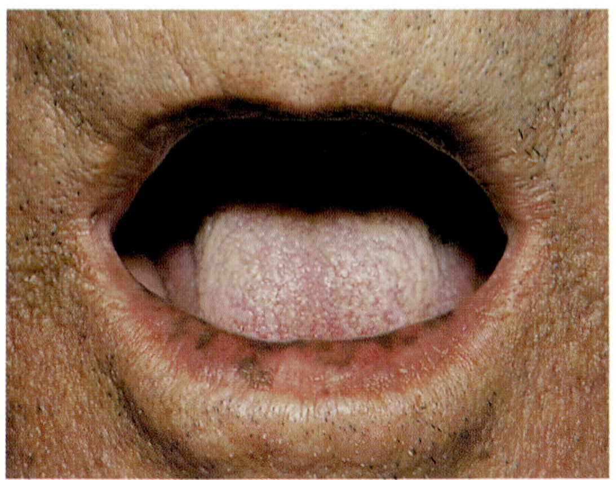

FIGURE 6-2. Pigmented patches of the lips in Peutz-Jegher syndrome. This patient had intestinal polyposis.

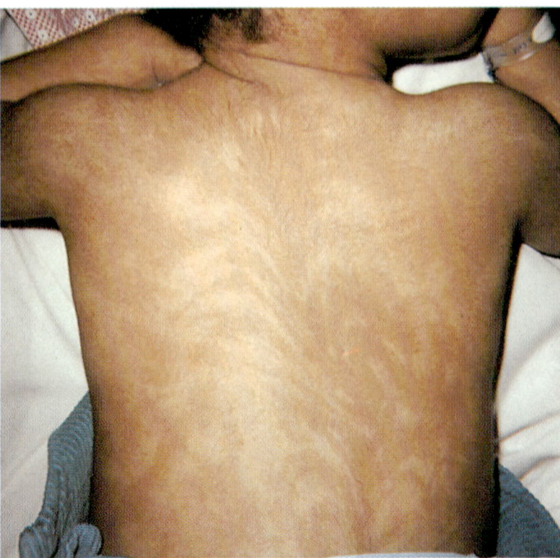

FIGURE 6-3. Pigmentation of the trunk following Blaschko lines in incontinentia pigmentosa.

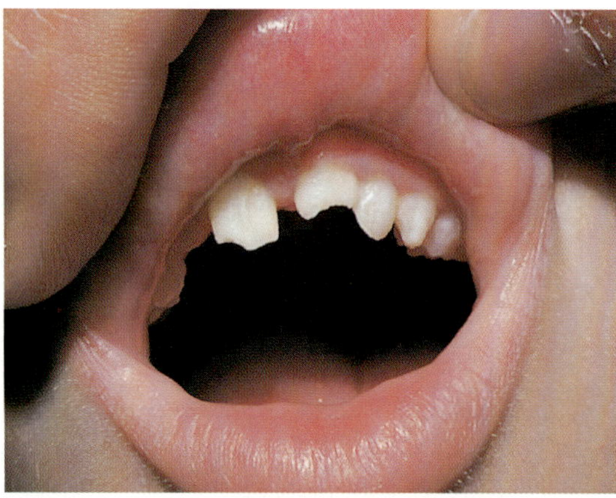

FIGURE 6-4. Cone- and peg-shaped teeth in incontinentia pigmenti.

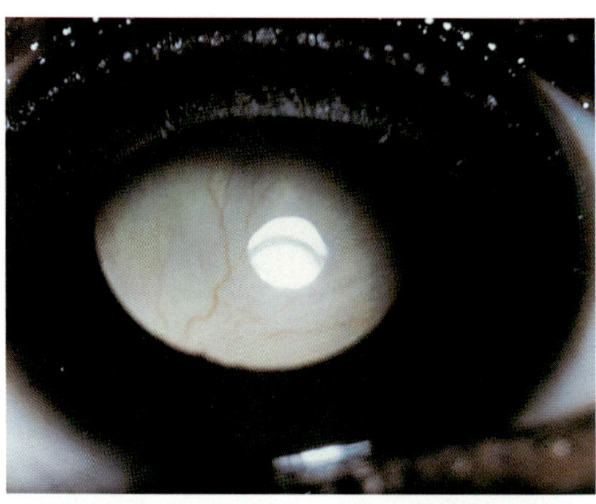

FIGURE 6-5. Pseudoglioma in incontinentia pigmenti. The pseudoglioma can be seen in the pupillary area. Vessels course over the white gliotic membrane. (Photograph courtesy of Dr. Philips Thygeson.)

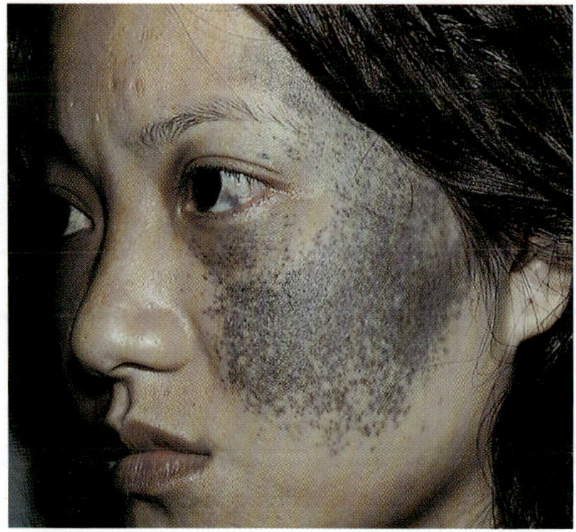

FIGURE 6-6. Nevus of Ota of the temple, cheek, and sclera in a young Asian female.

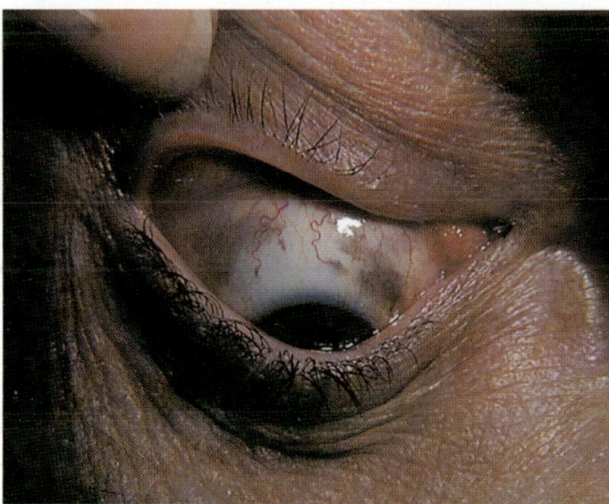

FIGURE 6-7. Nevus of Ota with slate-gray pigmentation of the sclera.

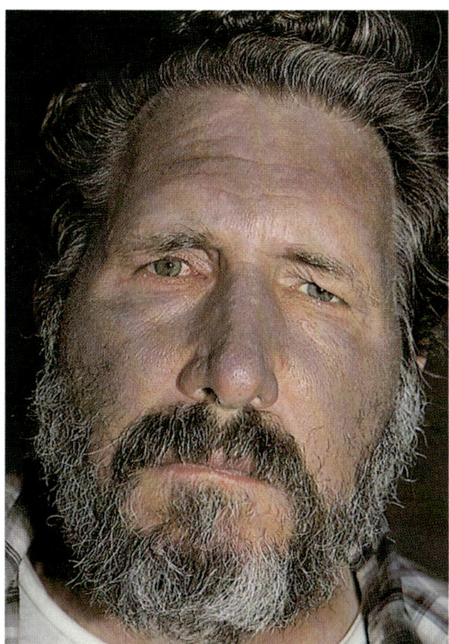

FIGURE 6-8. Skin pigmentation from phenothiazine use. This patient had used more than 1,200 mg of Thorazine daily for several years and during that time developed glaucoma thought to be related to use of the Thorazine.

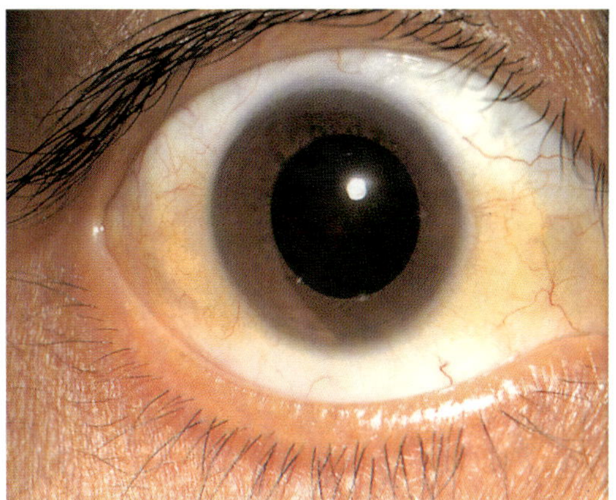

FIGURE 6-9. Conjunctival pigmentation caused by phenothiazine.

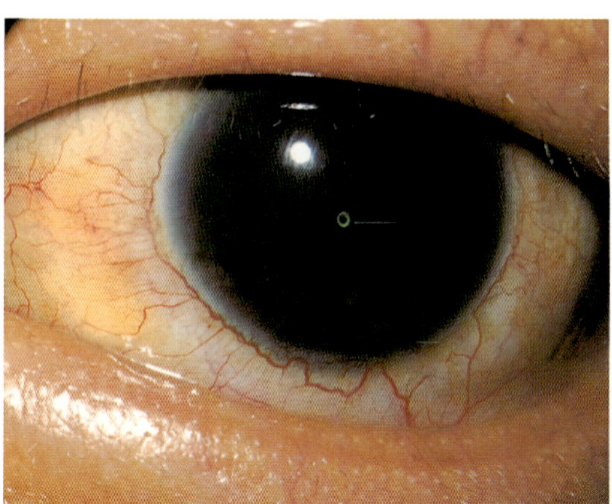

FIGURE 6-10. Yellow conjunctival pigmentation in the exposure area arising from use of clofazimine for leprosy. The lash loss is related to the disease process.

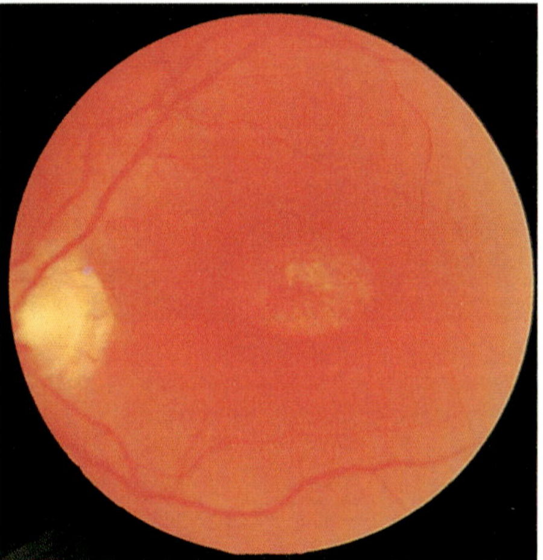

FIGURE 6-11. Chloroquine retinopathy. (Photograph courtesy of Dr. John Belmont.) Chloroquine retinopathy (often appearing as a bull's eye) may be induced by the prolonged administration of antimalarial drugs.

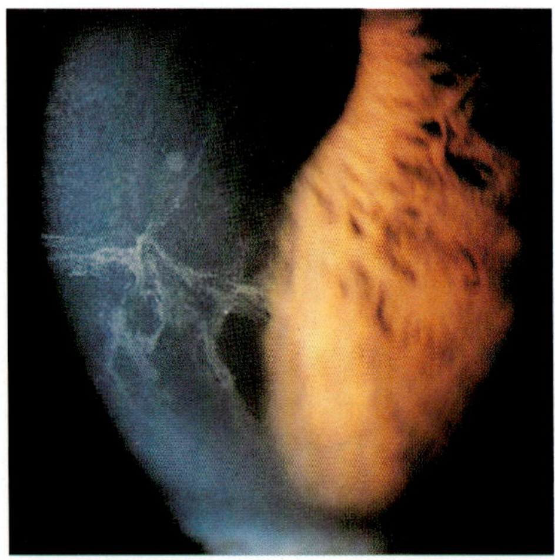

FIGURE 6-12. Amiodarone toxicity characterized as a vortex opacity of the corneal epithelium.

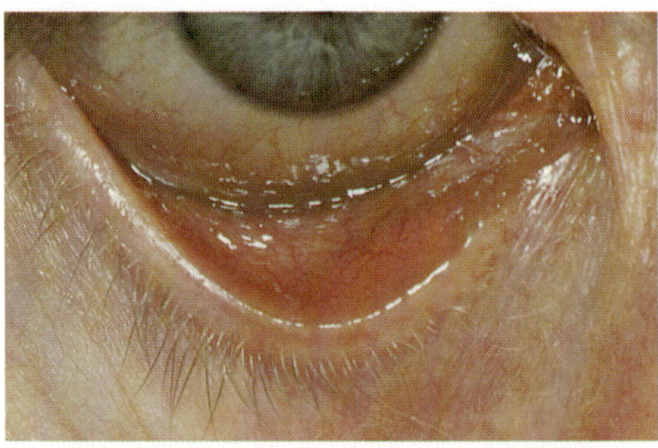

FIGURE 6-13. Argyria. Scleral and conjunctival pigmentation caused by prolonged use of Argyrol, a silver-containing compound used as an eye wash.

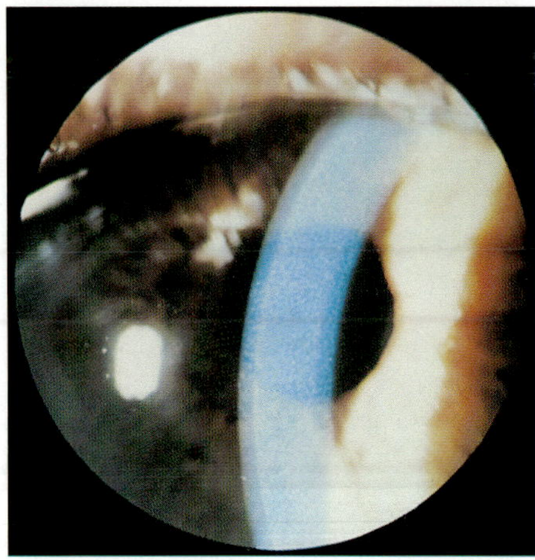

FIGURE 6-14. Silver deposition in the cornea. (Photograph courtesy of Dr. John Belmont.) A sheet of fine, dustlike granules is evident in the parallelepiped of the cornea.

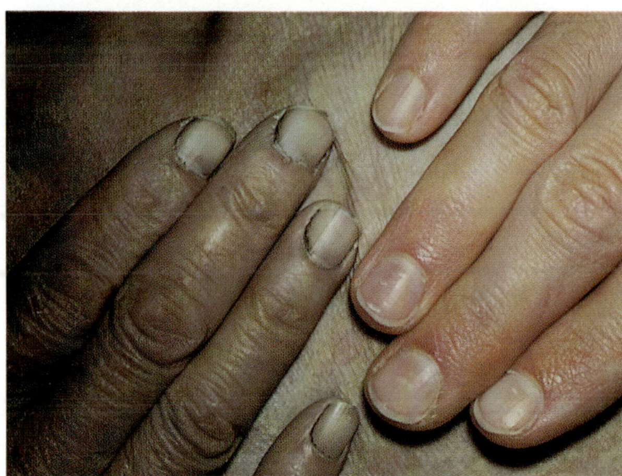

FIGURE 6-15. Argyria. Slate-gray colored pigmentation of the hand and bluish discoloration of fingernails (compared with a normal hand) in an elderly patient who had been using Argyrol as mouth wash and gargle for many years.

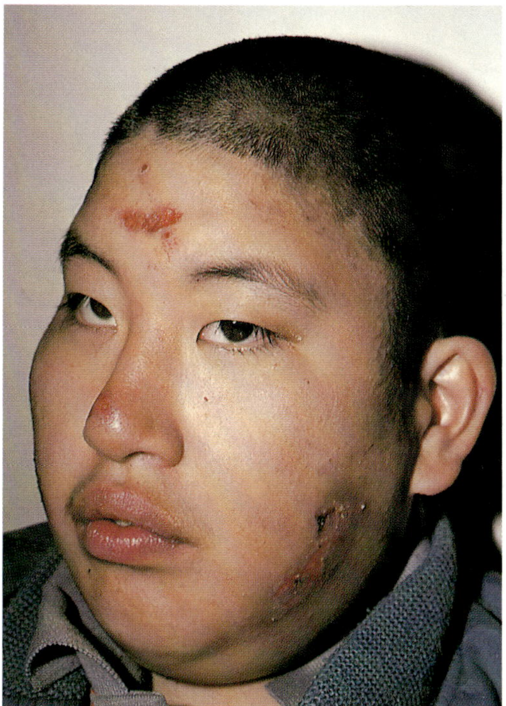

FIGURE 6-16. Mongolian slant to the eyes with Prader–Willi syndrome. The skin lesions were self-induced, which is not unusual because of insensitivity to pain.

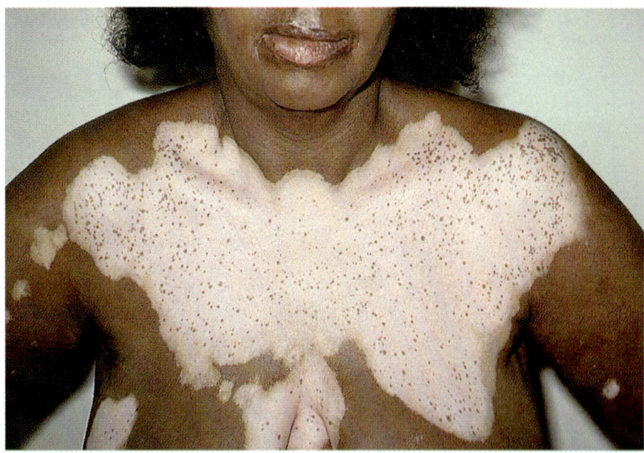

FIGURE 6-17. Vitiligo causing significant cosmetic concern in this dark-skinned female. Note small islands of repigmentation around hair follicles in response to treatment with ultraviolet A and psoralen.

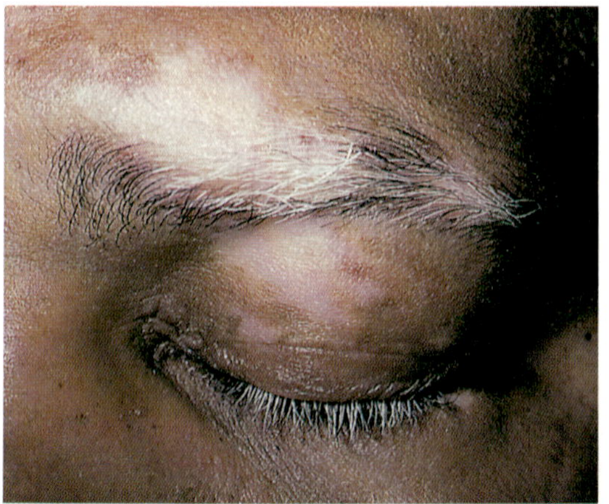

FIGURE 6-18. Vitiligo with poliosis of the lashes and brow.

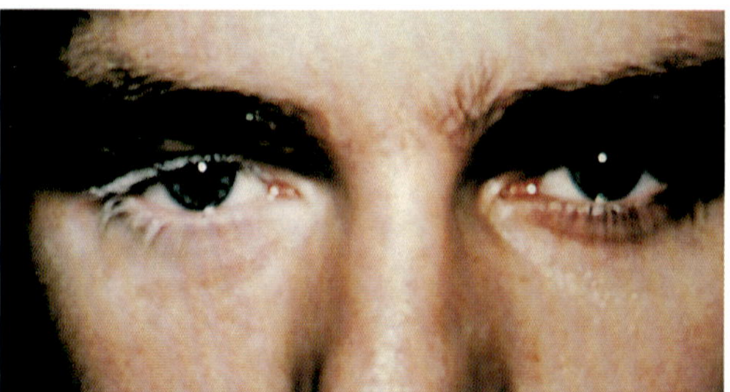

FIGURE 6-19. Periocular unilateral vitiligo and poliosis in Alezzandrini syndrome.

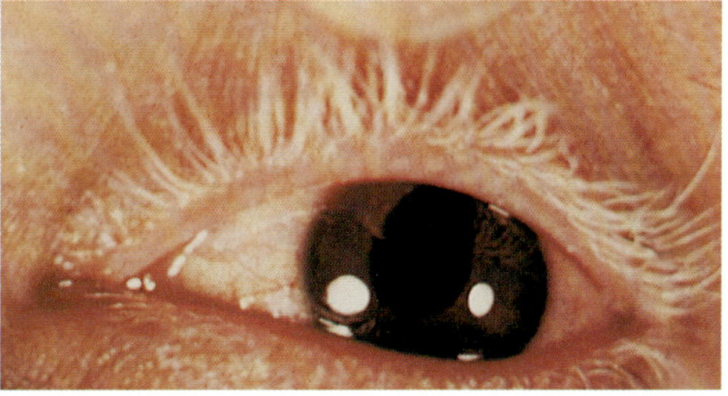

FIGURE 6-20. Poliosis in Vogt–Koyanagi–Harada syndrome. (Photograph courtesy of Dr. John Belmont.)

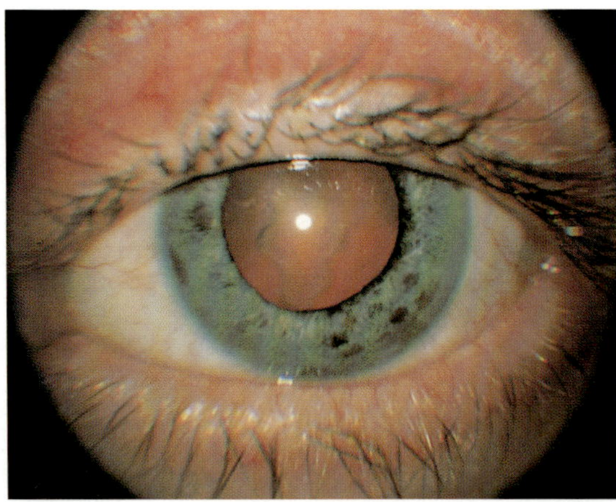

FIGURE 6-21. Vitreitis in Vogt–Koyanagi–Harada syndrome. In this patient with Vogt–Koyanagi–Harada syndrome, the exudative deposits are readily seen in the detached vitreous.

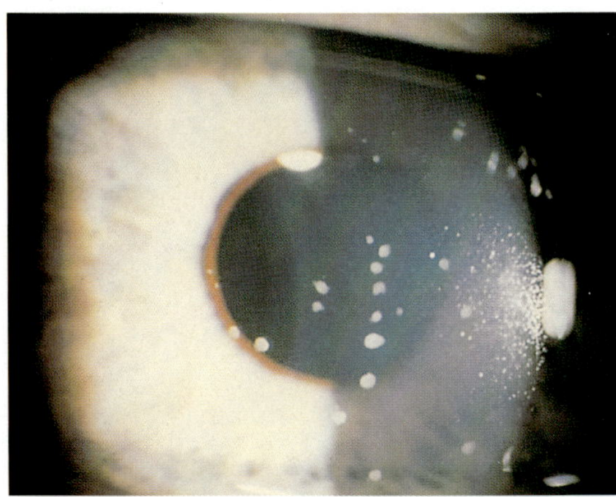

FIGURE 6-22. Keratic precipitates and anterior chamber flare in Vogt–Koyanagi–Harada syndrome.

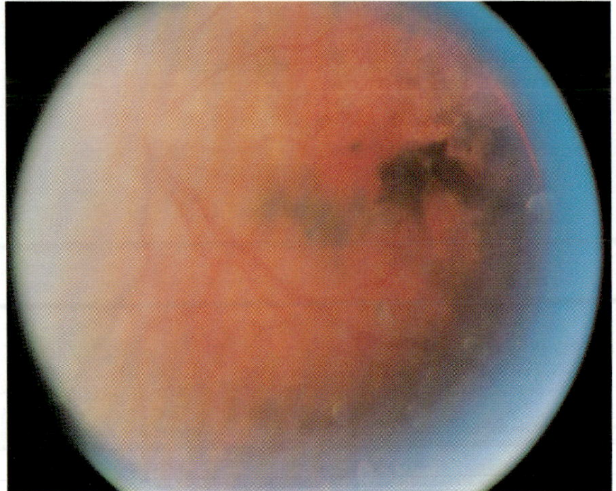

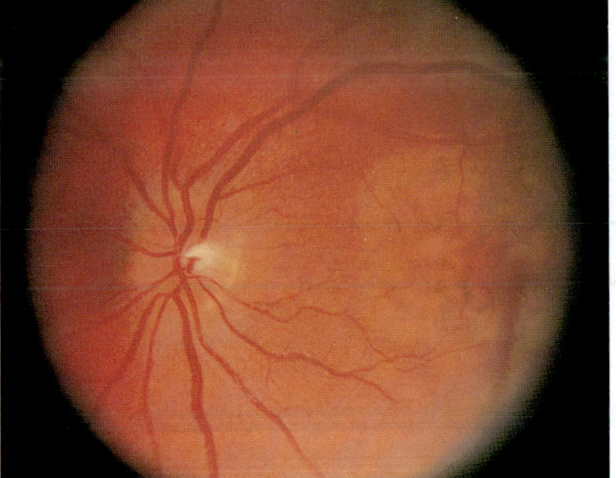

FIGURE 6-23. Fundus changes in Vogt–Koyanagi–Harada syndrome. Retinal pigment proliferation and atrophy are evident in this patient.

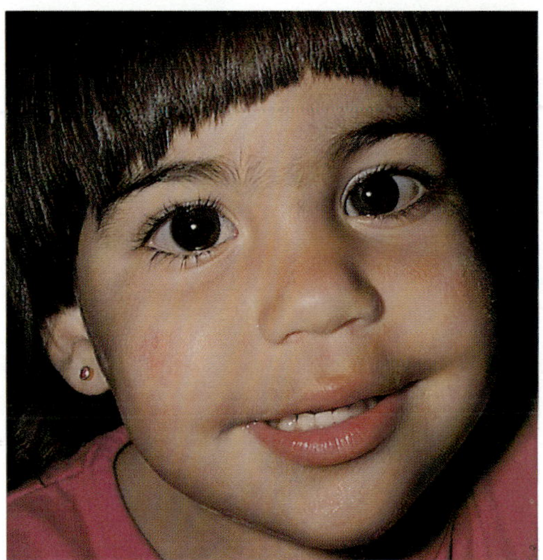

FIGURE 6-24. Pityriasis alba of the face in a 3-year-old child.

PAPULOSQUAMOUS DISORDERS

SEBORRHEIC DERMATITIS

Seborrheic dermatitis is a very common skin problem. Pityrosporum ovale, hormones, infection, nutrition, and emotional stress may play a role in its cause. It occurs during infancy and following puberty, persists into old age, and is more common in light-skinned males and in various disease states (e.g., Parkinson disease).

Infantile seborrheic dermatitis (Fig. 7-1) usually occurs only during the first few months of life. Its relationship to adult seborrheic dermatitis is unknown.

Skin Features

Seborrheic dermatitis usually involves the scalp, face, ears, and the postauricular (Figs. 7-2 and 7-3). presternal, and interscapular regions. In mild cases, there is erythema or mild scaling of the scalp, brow, and malar region or sometimes only dryness or oiliness of the skin folds. The medial aspect of the eyebrows, postauricular area, external auditory canals, and nasolabial folds are common areas of facial involvement. In more severe cases, oily yellowish scurf or dry scales of the scalp, face, chest, back, umbilicus, and body folds occurs. The disease is chronic with recurrent flare-ups. Redness, fissuring, and secondary infection are common.

Seborrhea begins perfidiously on the scalp with only a few scales; later, sharply marginated dry, scaly, or oily patches develop that have a yellow center and a reddish periphery. Occasionally, it causes itching. The lesions often extend beyond the hairline, forming a seborrheic corona. Chronic seborrhea may be associated with hair loss, but the mechanism(s) remains covert.

Anterior chest involvement is manifested by follicular papules covered with greasy crusts. Sometimes the intrascapular region and anterior chest in men are involved in a petaloid or a figured eruption with circinate patterns and fine brawny scales. Lesions of the flexural creases (axilla, groins, anogenital, submammary, and umbilical regions) present as diffuse erythema and greasy crusting. Seborrheic dermatitis in AIDS is often more severe and resistant to treatment.

Ocular Features

Lid margin seborrhea causes irritation, itch, lid edema, and lid margin hyperemia (Figs. 7-4 to 7-8). The posterior edge of the lid margin is red and irregular. Pityriasis sicca (scurf—dry, flaky, branlike scales) or pityriasis steatoides (yellow, greasy scales) is usually found on the lid margin. Often the scale adheres to the lash. Permanent lid margin irregularity and madarosis may occur in long-standing, neglected seborrheic blepharitis with secondary infection. Secondary staphylococcal infections are common.

Meibomian gland involvement causes burning, a feeling of heaviness, or a "tired feeling" in excess of the findings of a papillary conjunctivitis (chronic conjunctivitis meibomiana). The lids are swollen and thickened, the meibomian glands are markedly inspissated, large quantities of oil (often with a purulent character) can be expressed from the gland's orifices, and meibomian froth is evident on the lid margin. Eventually, chalazia may occur. Keratoconjunctivitis sicca develops in about 25% of patients.

Seborrheic keratitis is characterized by photophobia; a mild, fine to medium, or, occasionally, blotchy epithelial keratitis; and fine epithelial erosions of the lower one-third of the cornea or recurrent marginal corneal ulcers.

PERIORAL DERMATITIS

Perioral dermatitis most often occurs in young women (Fig. 7-9). Use of greasy lotions and topical glucocorticoids probably contributes to the development of this condition. It is characterized by a circumoral papular, pustular, or papulopustular flesh-colored eruption on an erythematous or scaly base. Sometimes the lesions involve the ala nasi, glabella, and eyelids. Healing may lead to scarring.

ROSACEA (ACNE ROSACEA)

Rosacea is a chronic, facial, inflammatory skin disorder characterized by symmetric flushing that leads to dilated telangiectatic vessels of the malar eminences, acneform lesions, and rhinophyma (Figs. 7-10 to 7-17). It often fluctuates in intensity. It is more common in light-skinned, blue-eyed patients between the ages of 30 and 50, and is about three times more common in women. Its cause is unknown, but it appears to be a vascular and immunologic disorder (increased vascular dilatation of the papillary dermal vasculature and inflammation) exacerbated by use of alcohol, hot drinks, spicy foods, sun exposure, menopause, and emotional disturbances. Chronic application of corticosteroids may lead to a steroid-induced rosacea.

It begins with transient episodes of periodic blotchy or diffuse hyperemia of the nasal area, adjacent forehead, cheeks, and chin. When fully developed, there are erythema, telangiectasis, swelling, and acneform lesions of the midfacial region; occasionally, there is only erythema and telangiectasis. The acneform lesions are both papular and pustular, and are similar to acne vulgaris except that there are no comedones and no scarring. Occasionally, granulomatous plaques form. Sometimes there is marked swelling during an exacerbation, and lymphedema may persist in one or more facial areas during remission. The involved areas feel cool to the touch, and the vessels blanch on diascopy. The skin is oily in appearance. Months or years after onset, the skin becomes thickened, telangiectatic, and red or purplish.

Rhinophyma (lymphedema, a bulbous hyperplasia of the soft tissue of the nasal sebaceous tissue, and connective tissue with a purplish-red color) frequently develops in rosacea, especially in males.

Ocular Features

Rosacea involves the lids and conjunctiva in more than 50% of cases, and, about 20% of the time the eye is involved first. Often the ocular and facial activity is not related, and the two progress independently. Rosacea causes burning, discomfort, and foreign-body sensation. It is frequently associated with staphylococcal blepharitis. Meibomian gland inspissation and oversecretion, seborrhea, collarettes, ulcerative lesions, and chalazia may be observed. The posterior lamella is preferentially involved.

Conjunctival involvement causes irritation, photophobia; tearing; watery, mucoid or, occasionally, mucopurulent discharge; diffuse conjunctival redness; and edema. Infrequently, small gray nodules develop in the interpalpebral fissure near the limbus and may ulcerate and then resolve. The conjunctival vessels are dilated, and garlandlike permanent dilatation of the limbal vessels may be seen.

About one-third of patients have corneal involvement that causes pain, redness, tearing, and photophobia. The keratitis may be limited to an epithelial keratitis, although a peripheral keratitis with superficial and deep corneal infiltrates is often the first sign of rosacea keratitis. The peripheral spadelike corneal opacities are very characteristic. The base of the opacity (the edge nearest the limbus) is narrower than the more central part and simulates in many respects the spade on a playing card. In some instances, sectorial scarring and vascularization occur in the inferior quadrants; infrequently, the entire cornea is involved. A fascicular lesion is common. It begins as a corneal subepithelial infiltrate just central to corneal vessels, which causes the vessels to gradually encroach further and further into the cornea. The infiltrates lead to progressive scarring central to the leash of vessels.

LEWANDOWSKY ROSACEA-LIKE ERUPTION

Lewandowsky rosacea-like eruption affects women in the third to sixth decades of life. It is characterized by pinhead-sized, reddish-blue or brownish micropapules of the cheeks, forehead, or, occasionally, most of the face. The papules are slightly indurated, are flattened, and have an erythematous base. They are self-limited and heal with small, pitted scars.

LUPUS MILIARIS DISSEMINATUS FACIEI, ACNITIS (ACNE AGMINATA)

Lupus miliaris disseminatus faciei, acnitis (acne agminata) is occasionally seen in young adults. It is characterized by discrete, dull brown papules with a yellow center that usually involve the eyebrows but may also involve the chin, temples, cheeks, and sometimes the limbs, trunk, or axilla. The papules usually pustulate, crust, and heal by scarring after several months. This disease is considered a variant of rosacea, and in spite of its name, has nothing to do with cutaneous tuberculosis.

PSORIASIS (PSORIASIS VULGARIS)

Psoriasis (psoriasis vulgaris) is a common, chronic, recurrent inherited skin disease, which is at times associated with arthritis and keratitis. The skin lesions are characterized by rounded, erythematous, dry patches or plaques covered by micaceous scales. Sites of predilection include the scalp, elbows, knees, sacral areas, and penis. Flexural sites such as the axilla, groin, and toe webs may also be affected.

Small, erythematous macules or maculopapules initially develop, then gradually enlarge and coalesce peripherally to form plaques of various shapes. The lesions are sharply delineated from the surrounding skin, have a salmon-pink color, and are covered with silver-white scales that are attached to the center of the lesion. Frequently, the central area of the scale, especially in long-standing lesions, piles up into layers, and the epidermis feels thickened to palpation. Removal of the scales reveals minute bleeding points (Auspitz sign). About 15% of patients have severe generalized psoriasis. Environmental factors play a role in expression of the disease. It usually begins during the second to fourth decade, but may start in infancy or old age. There is no sex predilection.

Known triggers include skin trauma (e.g., scratching— Koebner phenomenon), infections (e.g., streptococcal throat infections, AIDS), emotional stress drug ingestion (e.g., beta adrenergic blockers, lithium, and antimalarials), decrease or discontinuation of glucocorticoids, and endocrine factors (psoriasis may worsen postpartum).

Sunlight and relaxation usually improve the problem, though excessive sun or ultraviolet lamp exposure may cause psoriasis to appear at all burn sites (Koebner phenomenon). Itching or burning can cause much discomfort, but usually improves with ultraviolet light exposure.

Psoriatic arthritis is seen in 25% of patients. Asymmetric distal interphalangeal joints are often involved when significant psoriatic lesions are present. Oligoarthritis of hand joints and rheumatoid arthritis-like changes may occur. Ankylosing spondylitis is occasionally seen.

Skin Features

Pustular psoriasis is characterized by small pustules of the hands or feet or generalized pustules (Figs. 7-19 to 7-23). Inveterate psoriasis is manifested by thick, fissured patches covered with heavy scales in the lumbosacral region and buttocks. A clear peripheral zone (halo or ring of Woronoff) surrounds the plaques.

When lesions primarily involve the flexural areas, the condition is called inverse psoriasis, and here scaling is markedly reduced or absent. Psoriatic lesions that occur primarily in the distribution of seborrheic dermatitis (scalp and intertriginous areas) are referred to as seborrheic psoriasis or "seborrhiasis."

Psoriatic palmar and plantar eruptions are characterized by small, raised, hard, horny, keratotic thenar, and hypothenar lesions, sharply circumscribed lesions of the palms, and tips of the fingers and toes that may fissure and cause severe pain, or by poorly defined linear lesions with thick laminated scales. Occasionally, psoriasis presents as small white patches on the glans penis, buccal mucosa, and tongue. On the buccal mucosa and tongue, the plaques are gray, yellowish, or white, and are well demarcated. Sometimes in generalized psoriasis the lips have silvery scales.

Nail Changes

Nail changes (Fig. 7-24) occur in more than 50% of patients, but the severity varies from person to person and even from finger to finger. The changes include pitting, onycholysis (uplifting of distal portion from the nail bed), pale brownish discolorations ("oil spots"), and onychodystrophy. Extensive nail involvement is usually associated with psoriatic arthropathy.

Ocular Features

About 10% of patients develop ocular disease (Fig. 7-12, Figs. 7-25 to 7-29). Psoriatic lid involvement usually presents as a nonspecific blepharitis or blepharoconjunctivitis. Sometimes there is just redness and lid edema. Uncommonly, psoriatic patches develop on the lid and may involve the lid margin and eyebrows. Occasionally, there is lash loss, loss of the lid substance proper, ectropion, or trichiasis.

Psoriasis may cause a nonspecific conjunctivitis or small white or yellow patches or plaques with signs of chronic inflammation and discharge. The plaques usually arise from the lid margin; occasionally, they occur without lid involvement. Rarely, phlyctenular-like lesions develop at the limbus. Infrequently, conjunctival psoriasis leads to symblepharon formation.

Psoriatic corneal changes include a superficial punctate keratitis; epithelial thickening associated with multiple erosions, filaments, and patchy epithelial and anterior stromal infiltrates; superficial vascularized opacities overlying a deep, nonvascularized opacity; discrete subepithelial infiltrates; and indolent chronic corneal ulcers. A peripheral ulcerative keratitis resembling Mooren ulcer may be seen. Iridocyclitis may accompany the arthrotic form.

LICHEN PLANUS

Lichen planus (LP) is probably immunologically mediated and, in some patients, is associated with hepatitis C. It affects the skin and mucous membranes in about 2% of patients. Most cases occur during the fourth to sixth decade.

Skin Features

A mild or severe itch is a constant complaint of patients with lichen planus and is especially severe in hypertrophic lesions. The skin lesions begin insidiously and are characterized by symmetric, shiny, violaceous, polygonal, angulated, flat-topped papules that usually occur on the wrists, ankles, and lumbosacral areas (Figs. 7-30 and 7-31). The papules have a tendency to clear while others are forming. They usually occur in groups or are arranged in rings. Sometimes they become confluent, forming a single, large papule. Fine, white striae (Wickham striae) (Fig. 7-32) may be observed on the papule's surface, or sometimes there is a delicate scale on the surface or central umbilication. Other features include spiny lesions near hair follicles (lichen planopilaris) and erosions (bullous lichen planus) that involve the palms, soles, and mucous membranes. The lesions eventually flatten and heal, leaving areas of hyper- or hypopigmentation and occasionally atrophy. Hypertrophic lesions tend to occur on the shins and ankles, and are violaceous to reddish-brown verrucous plaques, which have a tendency to heal with scarring and atrophy. Scalp involvement may lead to atrophic, cicatricial patches of hair loss.

Oral Features

About 70% to 80% of patients with skin lesions have mucous membrane involvement, and mucous membrane involvement may occur without skin lesions (Figs. 7-33 and 7-34). Oral lesions cause discomfort, stinging, or pain. White papules with reticulated or lacy, white streaks develop on the vermilion border of the lips, buccal mucosa, tongue, and gingiva. Tongue lesions appear as fixed, white, slightly depressed plaques and sometimes as erosions (erosive lichen planus). The oral lesions are potentially malignant. LP occasionally involves the mucous membranes of the larynx, esophagus, stomach, bladder, genitalia, anus, and, very rarely, tympanic membrane.

About 10% of patients develop nail involvement, with thinning of the nail plate, exaggeration of the longitudinal lines, linear depressions of the nail plate, and pterygium unguis.

Ocular Features

Lichen planus rarely involves the lid, but can involve the conjunctiva (Fig. 7-35). Conjunctival lichen planus causes a foreign-body sensation and is characterized by a fine, white, lacy pattern in the tarsal conjunctiva reminiscent of Wickham's striae and, occasionally, of keratoconjunctivitis sicca.

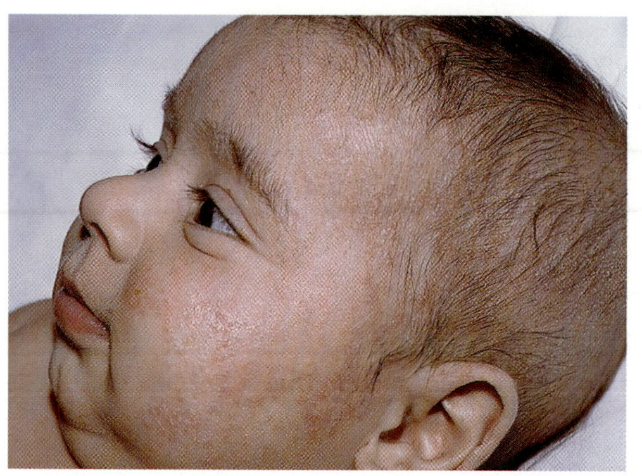

FIGURE 7-1. Seborrheic dermatitis in infancy. Note greasy erythematous scales of cheeks, brows, forehead, and scalp.

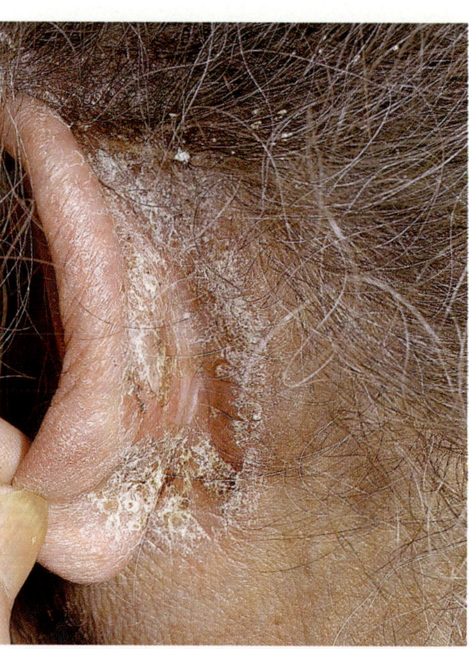

FIGURE 7-2. Retroauricular seborrheic dermatitis. It is sometimes difficult to differentiate seborrheic dermatitis from psoriasis, leading to the term *seborrhiasis.*

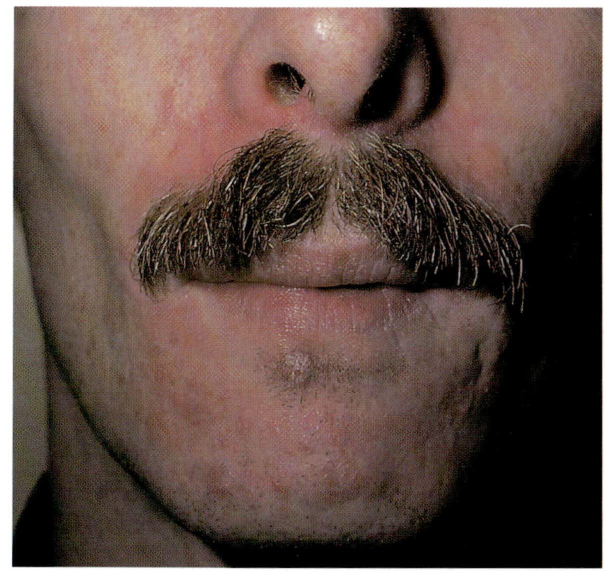

FIGURE 7-3. Seborrheic dermatitis in a patient with AIDS. This is often an early cutaneous sign of reduced immunity. Seborrheic dermatitis tends to be more severe and resistant to therapy in AIDS.

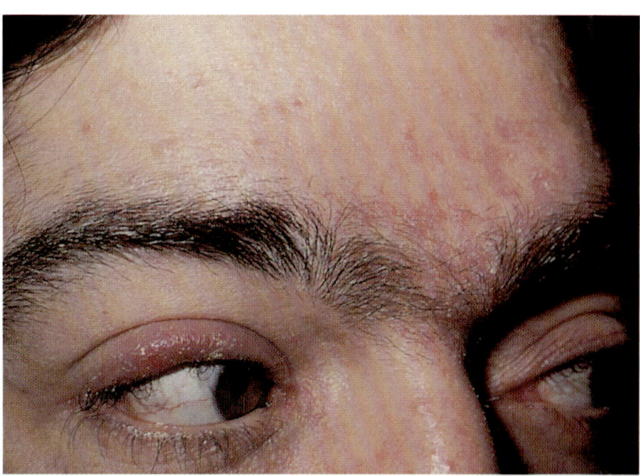

FIGURE 7-4. Seborrheic dermatitis and blepharitis in a patient with AIDS.

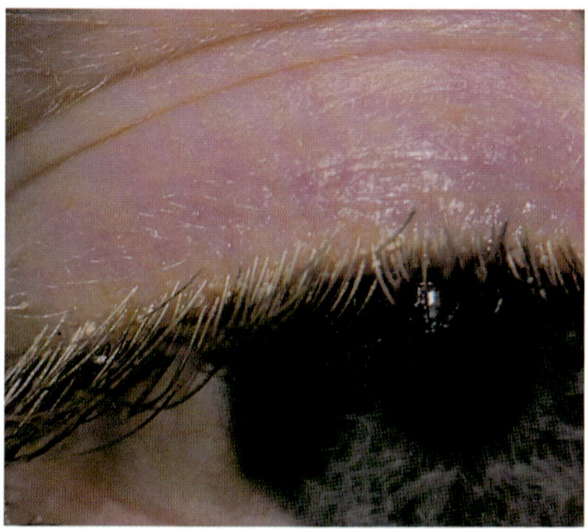

FIGURE 7-5. Seborrheic blepharitis. Pediculosis palpebrarum can be mistaken for seborrheic blepharitis.

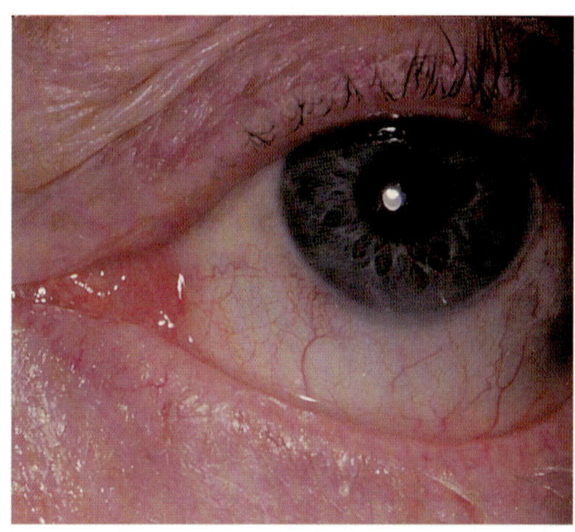

FIGURE 7-6. Seborrheic blepharitis and conjunctivitis.

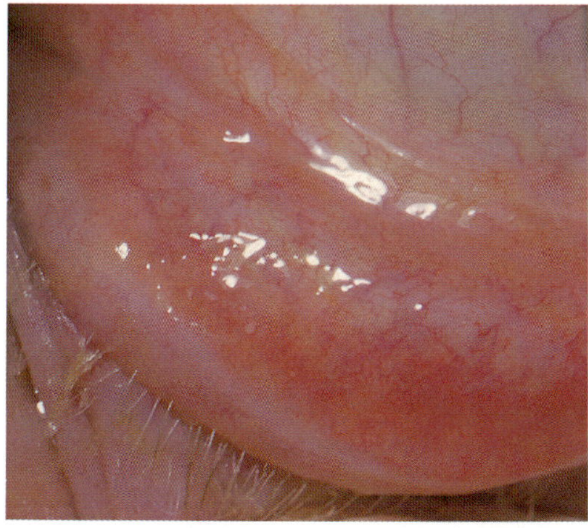

FIGURE 7-7. Seborrheic dermatitis. Papillary hypertrophy is evident on the inferior tarsus.

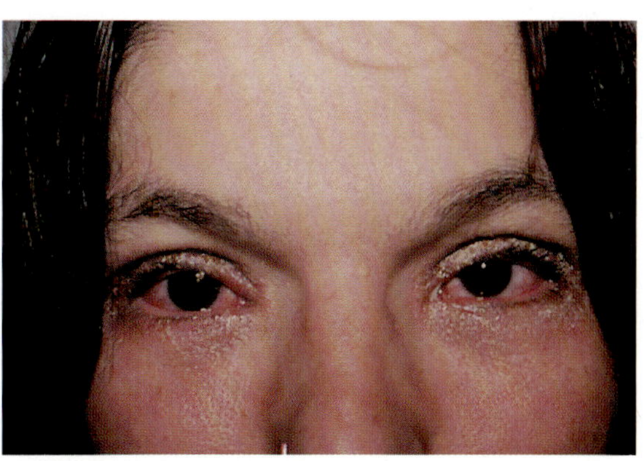

FIGURE 7-8. Severe blepharitis and conjunctivitis in seborrhea.

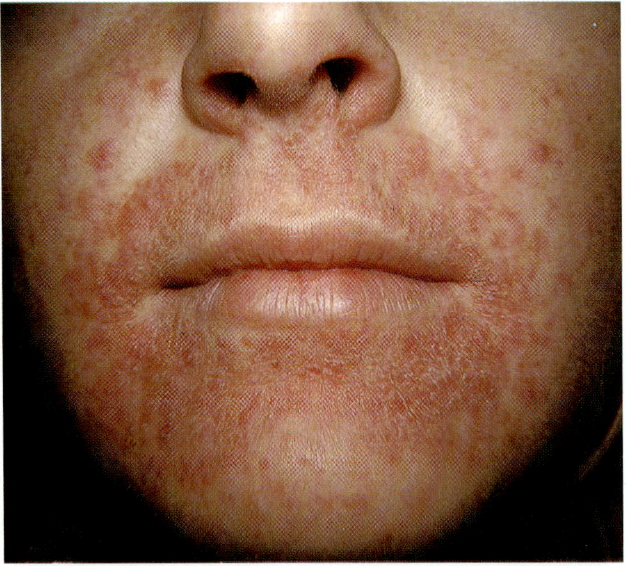

FIGURE 7-9. Perioral dermatitis in a young woman.

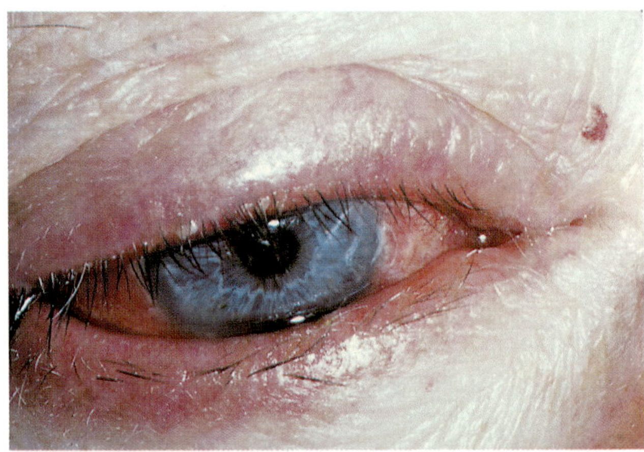

FIGURE 7-10. Acne rosacea of the lid. Severe lid erythema together with collarettes and conjunctival erythema are evident in this 28-year-old woman with acne rosacea.

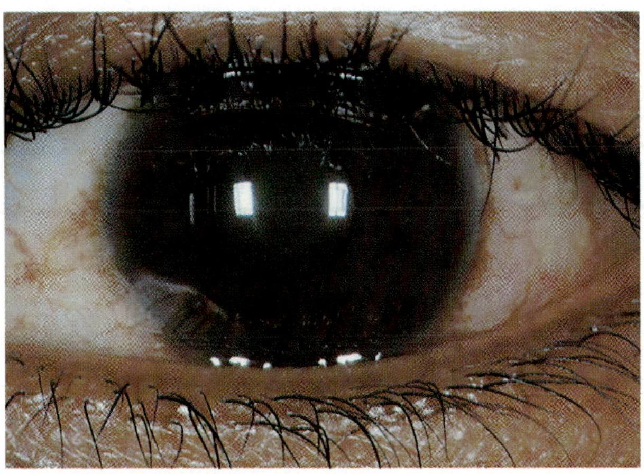

FIGURE 7-11. Spadelike corneal lesion in acne rosacea.

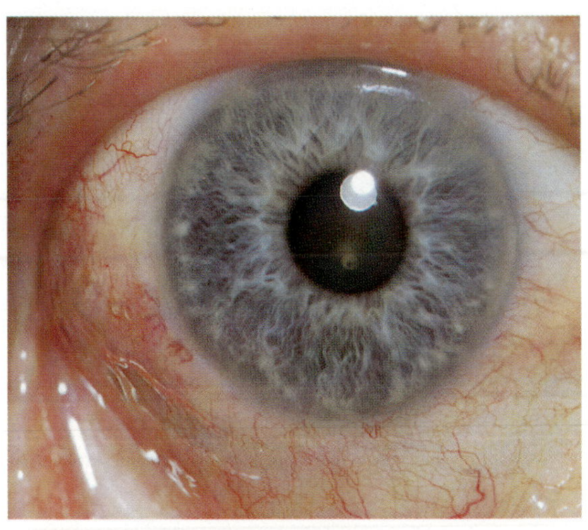

FIGURE 7-12. Dilated conjunctival vessels in acne rosacea.

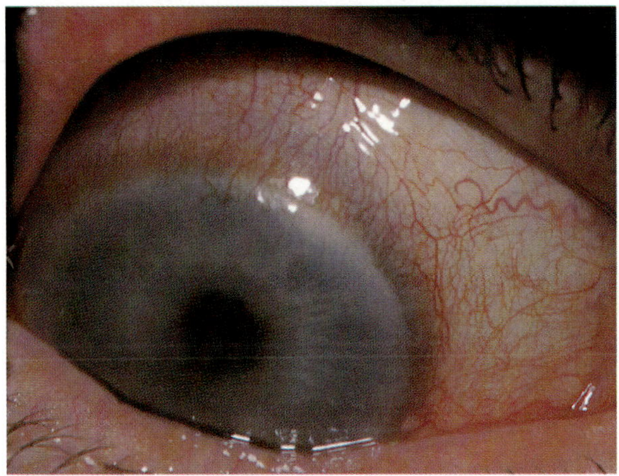

FIGURE 7-13. Early superficial corneal vascularization in acne rosacea. Small vessels can be seen at the one o'clock position, encroaching on the cornea together with some scleral thinning.

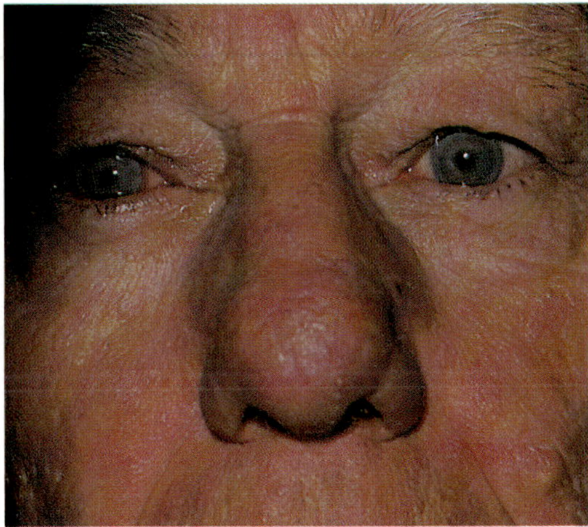

FIGURE 7-14. Moderate rhinophyma with mild, midfacial vascular dilatation. Tearing is caused by a peripheral keratitis.

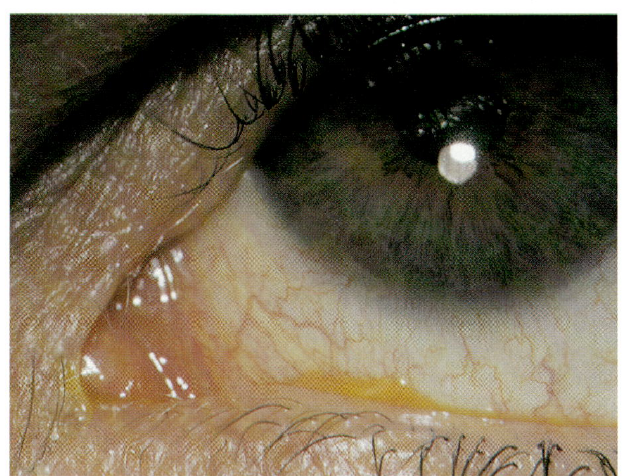

FIGURE 7-15. Spadelike corneal lesion located at the seven o'clock position in a patient with rosacea.

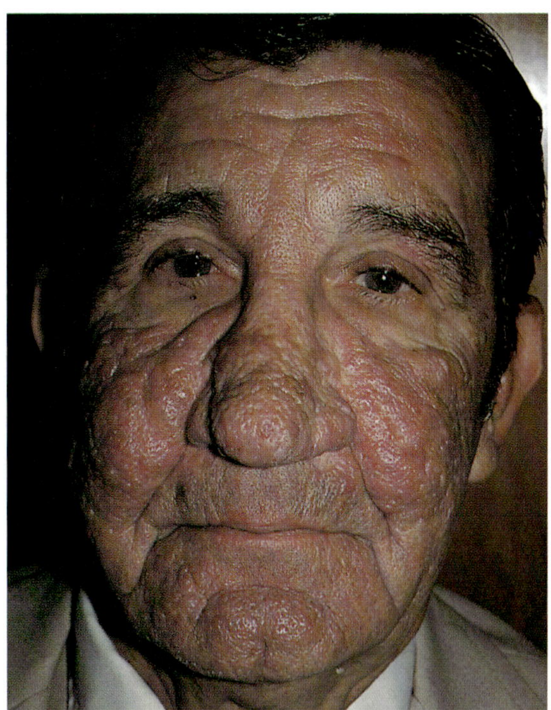

FIGURE 7-16. Severe acne rosacea with rhinophyma, and chronic conjunctivitis of the right eye.

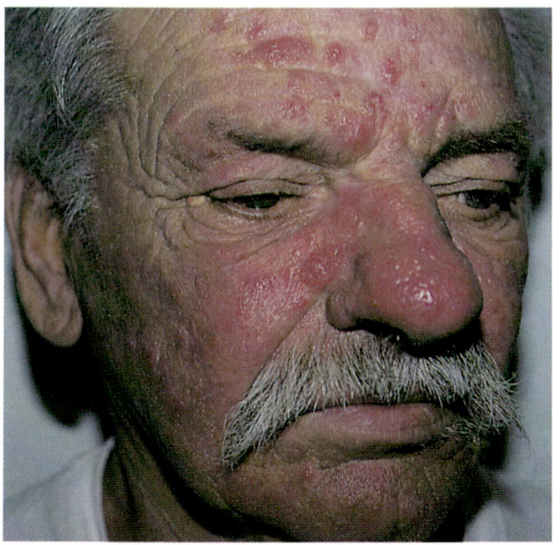

FIGURE 7-17. Rhinophyma and severe acne rosacea.

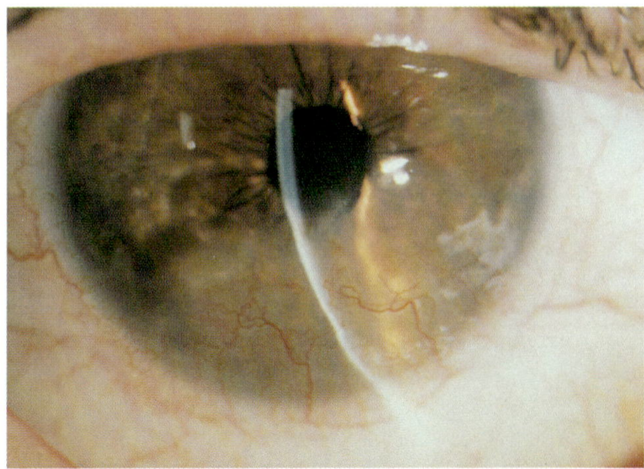

FIGURE 7-18. Sector vascularization of the inferior cornea in rosacea keratitis. There is a small corneal infiltrate at the margin of the pupil at six o'clock and in the mid cornea at seven o'clock.

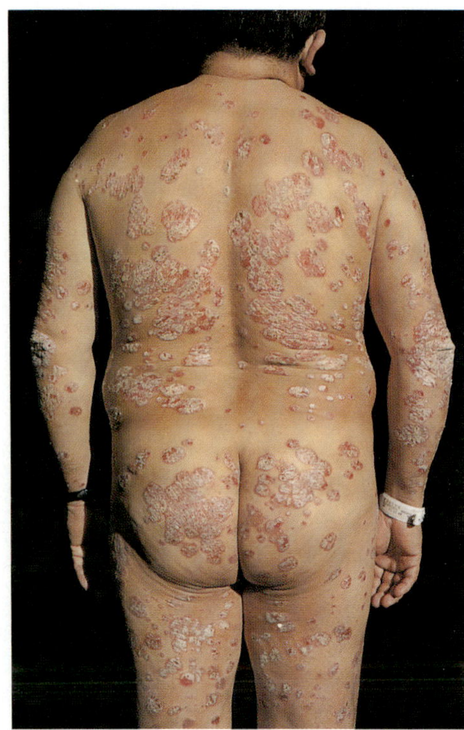

FIGURE 7-19. Widespread psoriasis. Note thick patches (plaques) over elbows.

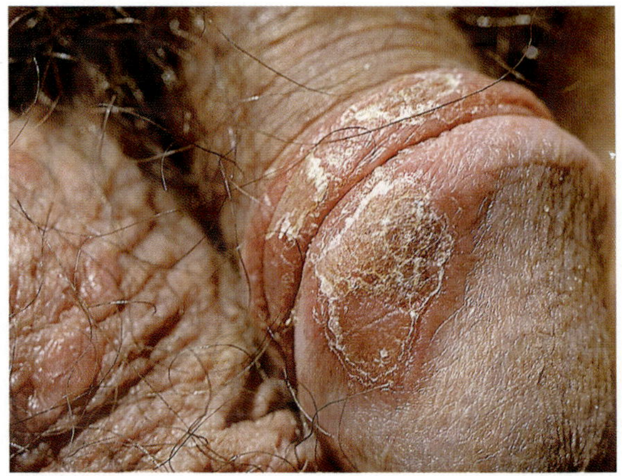

FIGURE 7-20. Psoriatic patches of penis resembling lesions in Reiter syndrome.

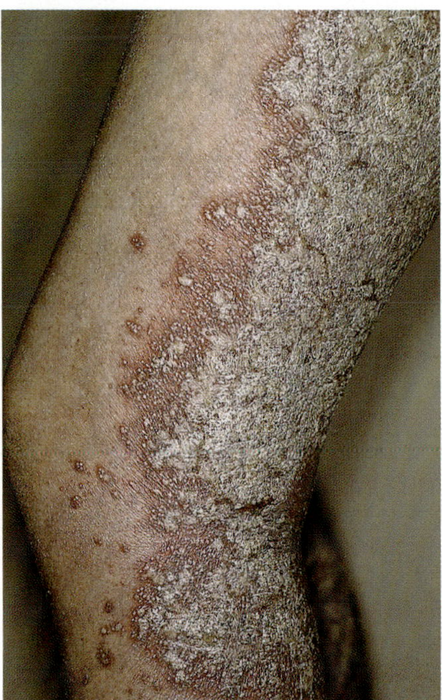

FIGURE 7-21. Pustular psoriasis. Note the multiple tiny pustules forming "lakes of pus." The patient had abused alcohol. She could not walk without severe pain and had to be hospitalized.

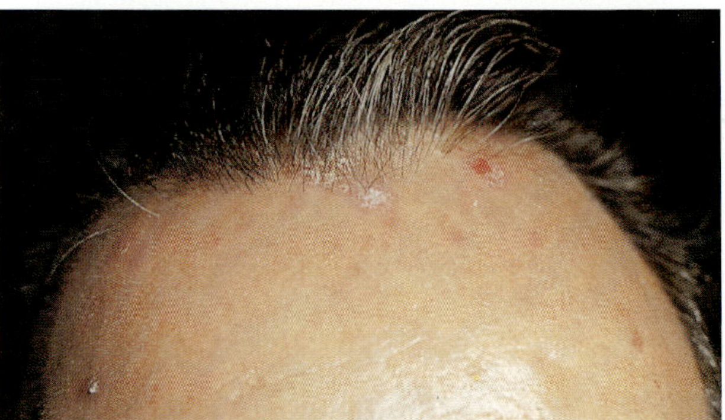

FIGURE 7-22. Psoriasis of the scalp. Note extension of psoriatic patches to the forehead in contrast to seborrhea, which on the scalp is usually confined to hair-bearing areas.

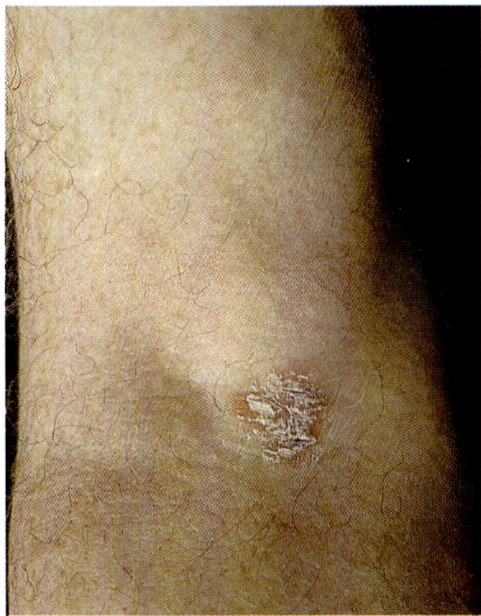

FIGURE 7-23. Psoriasis appearing at site of needle stick in the antecubital fossa (Koebner phenomenon).

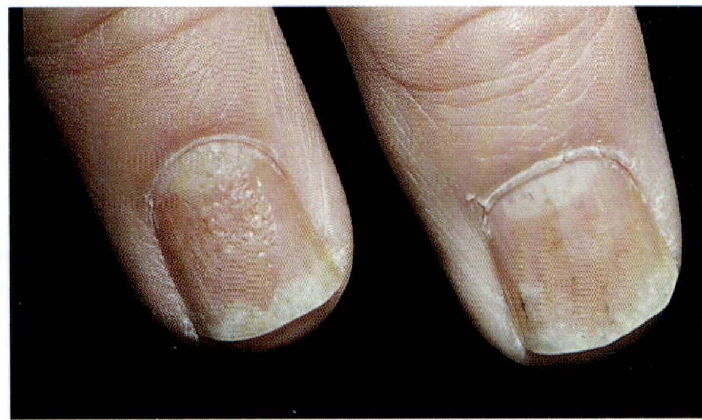

FIGURE 7-24. Nail involvement in psoriasis. Note characteristic pitting, distal onycholysis, and brown discoloration or "oil spots."

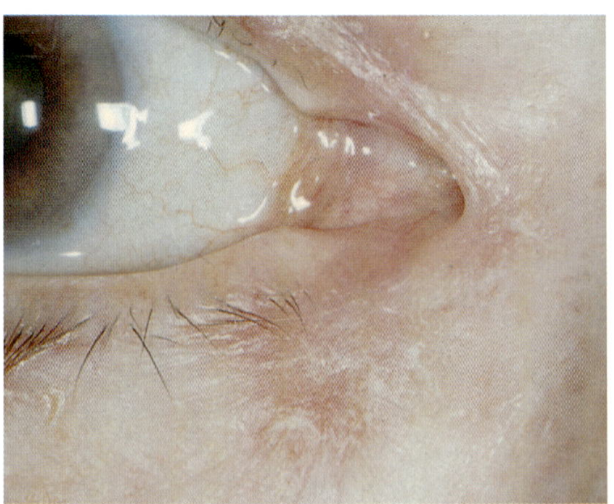

FIGURE 7-25. Nonspecific blepharitis in psoriasis with mild scaling.

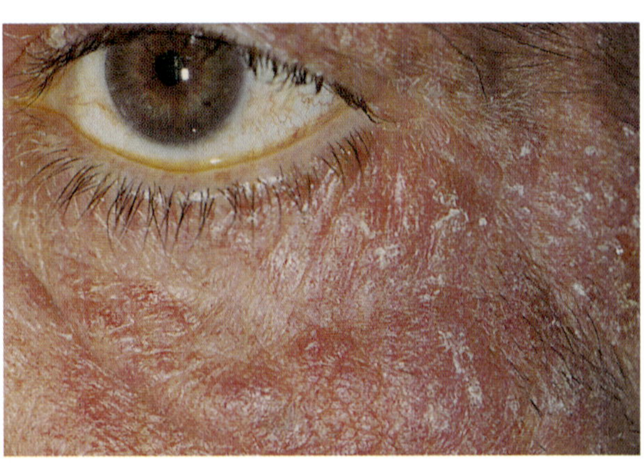

FIGURE 7-26. Thickening and silver scales of lid in psoriasis.

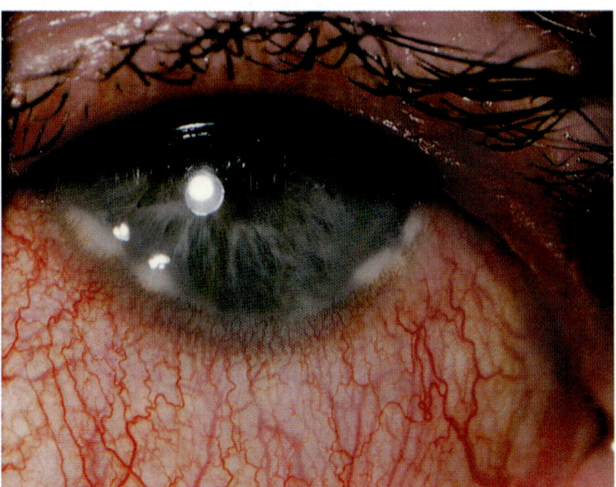

FIGURE 7-27. Marginal, anterior, stromal corneal infiltrates in psoriasis. (Photograph courtesy of Dr. Philips Thygeson.)

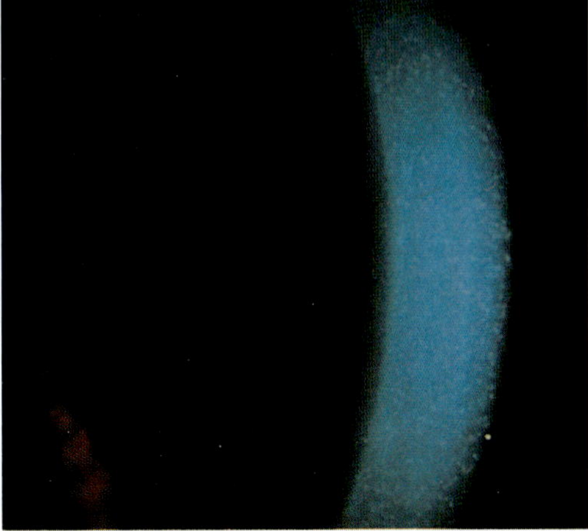

FIGURE 7-28. Superficial punctate keratitis associated with psoriasis. (Photograph courtesy of Dr. John Belmont.)

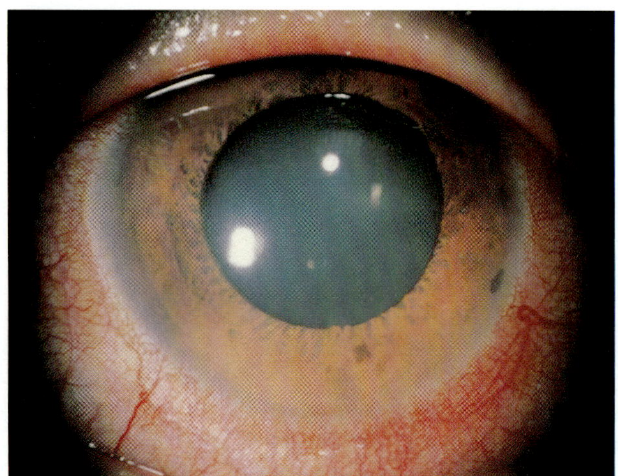

FIGURE 7-29. Diffuse episcleritis in psoriasis.

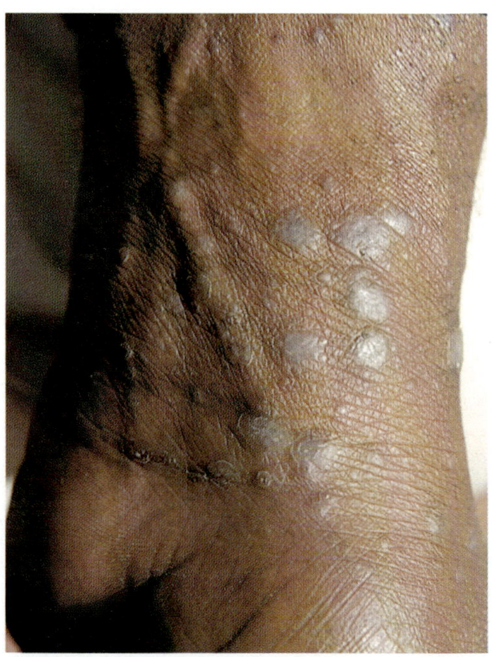

FIGURE 7-30. Lichen planus of the wrist in an African American. Note that in dark skin the lesions assume a more violaceous appearance.

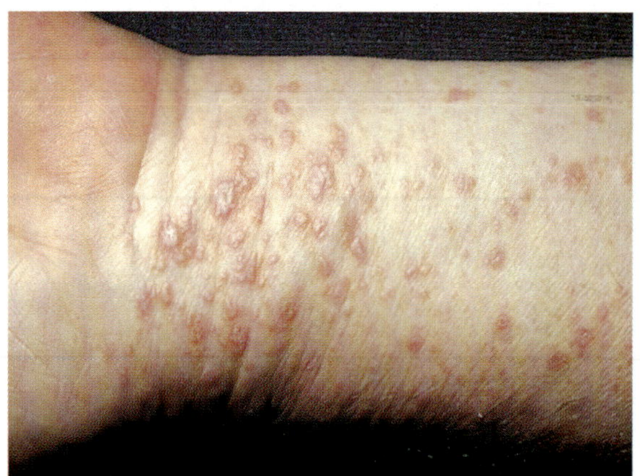

FIGURE 7-31. Lichen planus of the wrist in a Caucasian. Here the lesions look more erythematous.

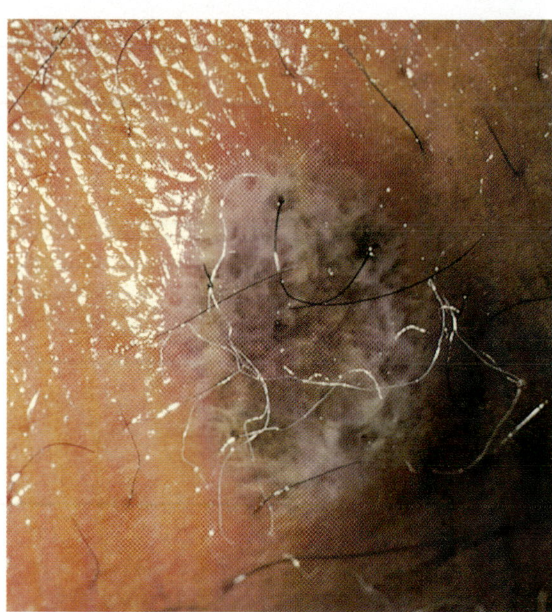

FIGURE 7-32. Wickham's striae in lichen planus.

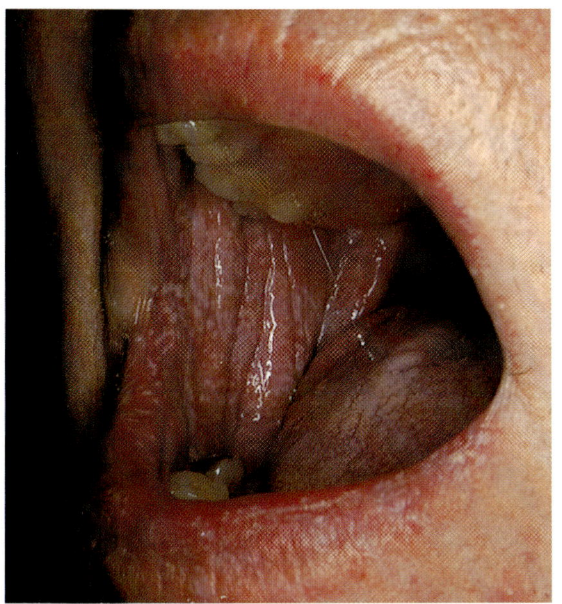

FIGURE 7-33. Oral involvement in lichen planus. The buccal mucosa, tongue, and lips are affected in this patient.

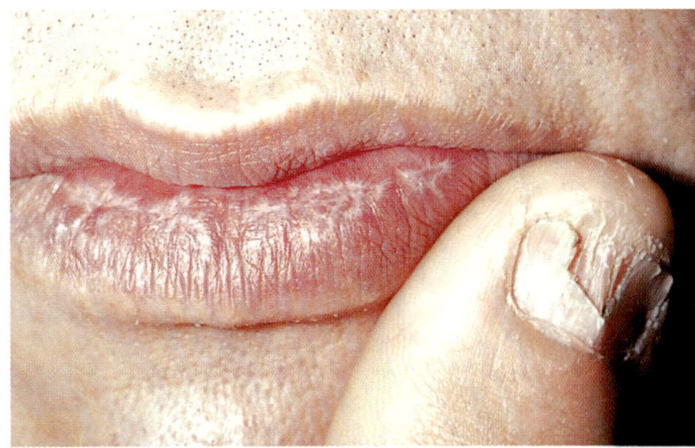

FIGURE 7-34. Lip and nail involvement in lichen planus. Note the centrally tented or pterygeal lesion of the nail that is characteristic of lichen planus.

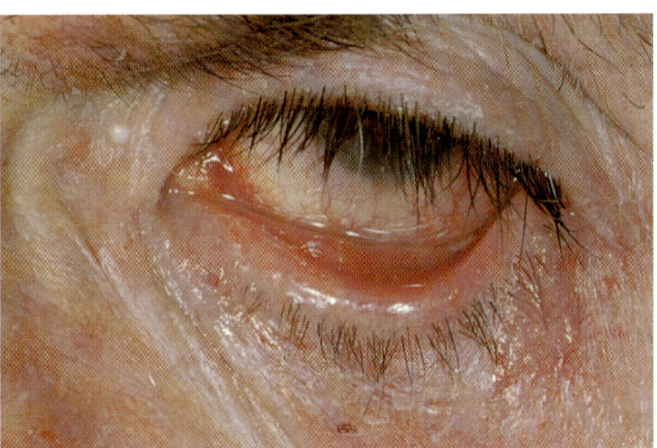

FIGURE 7-35. Lichen planus of the conjunctiva and skin. The excoriation and thickening of the skin of the eyelid are readily seen in this patient together with edema of the palpebral conjunctiva.

8

BULLOUS ERUPTIONS

Hereditary, immunologic, and acquired bullous eruptions often involve both skin and eye.

HEREDITARY BULLOUS ERUPTIONS

Epidermolysis Bullosa

Epidermolysis bullosa (EB) comprises a number of skin and mucous membrane diseases characterized by blisters, erosions, and, occasionally, scarring that develop following minor and often insignificant trauma. The various diseases are clearly distinct and are mediated by different mechanisms. All forms involve both skin and eye, but significant ocular involvement usually occurs in the hereditary autosomal recessive junctional and autosomal recessive dystrophic EB. Nonhereditary acquired EB also causes skin and eye changes.

EB is classified according to whether it causes nondystrophic, dystrophic, or atrophic skin, and mucous membrane changes or according to the anatomic location of the bullae.

Epidermolysis Bullosa Simplex (Simple Epidermolysis Bullosa)

In epidermolysis bullosa simplex (simple epidermolysis bullosa) the bullae are intraepidermal. Except for EB simplex lethalis and generalized EB simplex, which are autosomal recessive, all others are autosomal dominant. In each subset, blistering is usually present at birth or develops within the first 2 years of life, and only in the exceptional case are milia, scarring, or hair and nail involvement found. The subsets include the following:

1. EB simplex of the leg, feet, and hands (Weber–Cockayne). The Weber–Cockayne subset is the most common and usually affects the palms and soles and, occasionally, other skin areas that are subjected to mechanical trauma. As the patient gets older, thick, loose calluses develop on the soles and sometimes the palms. Focal oral erosions may occur in early infancy and are usually associated with bottle and breast feeding.

2. Generalized or Koebner form of EB simplex. The lesions are more widespread but are otherwise similar to the Weber–Cockayne variety. Recurrent esophageal blistering, erosions, and eventual strictures may be observed.
3. EB herpetiformis (Dowling–Meara). Here there are widespread, grouped (herpetiform) skin blisters, and, in some, nail dystrophy, milia, and scarring. Extensive and sometimes confluent calluses of the palms and soles and progressive hoarseness may develop.
4. Ogura (Gedde–Dahl) variant. This form is characterized by generalized blistering, deep hemorrhagic bruising, and onychogryphosis.
5. Mottled or reticular pigmented variant with atrophic scarring and nail dystrophy.
6. EB simplex superficialis characterized by subcorneal instead of intraepidermal cleavage, generalized blistering, striking mechanical skin fragility, development of milia and scarring, and often, postinflammatory hypo- or hyperpigmentation (Fig. 8-1).
7. EB simplex lethalis with or without myasthenia gravis and muscular dystrophy, characterized by increased infant death, generalized blistering, atrophic scarring, milia, nail dystrophy, and partial alopecia.

Ocular Features

Ocular involvement in EB simplex is uncommon and usually only mild. It includes a refractory blepharoconjunctivitis and a bilateral ringlike configuration of fine subepithelial cystic blebs in deep corneal epithelium. The latter leads to fine epithelial defects.

Junctional Epidermolysis Bullosa

Junctional epidermolysis bullosa is autosomal recessive and is characterized by blister formation in the lamina lucida of the basement membrane. The Herlitz and non-Herlitz subsets are the most common. Only the Herlitz subset has ocular features.

The Herlitz (junctional EB gravis, EB lethalis) subset frequently causes early death and is characterized by generalized blistering, striking mechanical skin fragility, milia, atrophic scarring, and absence of nail dystrophy. At about the age of 1 or 2, symmetrically exuberant granulation tissue develops in the periorificial region, nape of the neck, and upper and mid-trunk, which heals with atrophic scarring. Squamous cell carcinomas may develop in areas of chronic dermatitis. The nails are often discolored, thickened, and dystrophic.

Sometimes upper respiratory tract involvement (especially laryngeal involvement) leads to the necessity for a tracheostomy in early life. Oral blistering, erosions, ankyloglossia, and microstomia; enamel hypoplasia; recurrent esophageal erosions, blisters, and strictures; pyloric atresia and chronic malabsorption; and progressive scarring of any portion of the genitourinary tract may occur.

Ocular Features

Corneal epithelial bullae, recurrent epithelial erosions, and fine superficial corneal opacities may occur in the Herlitz variety of junctional EB.

Dystrophic Epidermolysis Bullosa

Dystrophic EB is autosomal dominant or recessive. The recessive form is associated with more severe skin and extracutaneous manifestations. Both forms have an increased incidence of aggressive squamous cell carcinomas, especially in areas of chronic blistering and scarring, which may lead to metastasis and death.

Autosomal dominant dystrophic EB is composed of:

1. The Pasini and the Cockayne–Touraine variants, characterized by generalized blistering, atrophic scarring, milia formation, and absence of nail dystrophy. The Pasini variant also has small, firm, white papules (albopapuloid lesions) on the trunk.
2. Transient bullous dermolysis of the newborn, which is less common and is characterized by generalized or localized blistering, scarring, milia, and nail dystrophy in early infancy (Fig. 8-2). The blistering disappears after the first year of life.

Autosomal recessive dystrophic EB is composed of:

1. The Hallopeau–Siemens variant, characterized by large, flaccid bullae, which involve all areas of the body at birth or during early infancy. Healing occurs with scarring, and by middle or late childhood, there is web formation of the digits (pseudosyndactyly) and later "mitten or glove deformity" due to complete encasement of the hands and feet by scar tissue (Figs. 8-3 and 8-4).
2. A mitis variant, characterized by generalized blistering and healing by scar formation. Pseudosyndactyly and "mitten deformity" do not occur in this form.
3. A localized form of recessive dystrophic EB, which also occurs and is primarily acral.

4. A recessive inverse dystrophic (dermolytic) EB variant begins with bullae and scarring at an early age, which then becomes less severe during adulthood. Areas of involvement include the inguinal folds, perineum, axilla, submammary area, neck, and lumbar regions. The proximal extremities may be involved, but the hands, feet, knees, and elbows are usually not involved, and acral webbing usually does not occur. The toenails are dystrophic or atrophic; the fingernails are minimally involved.

Mucous Membrane Features

Oral mucous membrane involvement and severe caries occur in all dystrophic forms of EB. Ankyloglossia, microstomia, and widespread scarring are found in the Hallopeau–Siemens variant. Severe esophageal involvement occurs in the generalized recessive dystrophic and recessive inverse dystrophic forms of epidermolysis bullosa. Chronic malabsorption and genitourinary system involvement with organ dysfunction also occur in generalized recessive dystrophic EB.

Ocular Features

Ocular findings include photophobia, lid ulceration, cicatricial entropion/trichiasis, and ectropion. The recessive form of epidermolysis bullosa dystrophica often causes a chronic conjunctivitis, scarring, and symblepharon. Recurrent corneal erosions, avascular widening of the limbus, and opacities at the level of Bowman's layer have all been observed.

Epidermolysis Bullosa Acquisita

Acquired epidermolysis bullosa is a chronic, blistering, immunologic disease that occurs in both noninflammatory and inflammatory forms. It involves all age groups (median age, 45 to 50 years). The noninflammatory form resembles hereditary epidermolysis bullosa and may lead to milia and atrophic scarring in areas of trauma and areas overlying bone. The inflammatory form causes widespread disease and is clinically similar to bullous pemphigoid.

Skin Features

Recurrent localized serous or hemorrhagic blisters develop in areas of trauma on the extensor surfaces of the extremities. The lesions heal with atrophic scars, milia, and hyperpigmentation. Infrequently, it causes cicatricial alopecia. Severe mucous membrane involvement is usually associated with severe skin disease. Erosions and intact blisters develop in the mouth, genitalia, esophagus, and larynx, and may lead to functional disability from scarring and stenosis.

Ocular Features

Lid skin involvement may lead to milia and conjunctival involvement to conjunctival scarring and symblepharon. Bilateral, small, subepithelial vesicles have been observed in the cornea, and peripheral corneal ulceration and scarring are a primary manifestation of the disease. Corneal perforation is uncommon.

Benign Familial Chronic Pemphigus (Hailey–Hailey Disease)

Benign familial chronic pemphigus (Hailey–Hailey disease) represents a recurrent vesicular and scaly skin eruption, which primarily involves the neck, axilla, and intertriginous regions. It is autosomal dominant with incomplete penetrance. Risk factors include humidity, heat, local friction, and mechanical trauma; viral (herpes simplex), bacterial (staphylococcal, streptococcal), and yeast (candida) infections; and ultraviolet irradiation.

Skin Features

The initial lesions develop about the age of puberty and are often associated with pruritus and burning. They consist of small, flaccid vesicles filled with clear then turbid fluid on a normal or erythematous base. The vesicles quickly erode and crust, and may form sharply demarcated erythematous plaques (Fig. 8-5). Occasionally, the central area resolves, producing a circinate border. The lesions involve the nape of the neck, axilla, and groin; less commonly, the periumbilical, perigenital, and perianal areas; infrequently, the scalp and glabrous regions; and rarely, the anterior chest, lateral arms, or vulva. Uncommonly, the disease presents as a generalized erythroderma, verrucous, or lichenified plaques; pruritic papules; or bullous lesions. In the perianal area, the lesions present as condyloma acuminata. The involved areas may develop basal cell epitheliomas or squamous cell carcinomas. Papular oral lesions have been described. Esophageal involvement leads to epigastric pain and distress.

Ocular Features

A keratoconjunctivitis may occur but is unusual.

IMMUNOLOGIC BULLOUS DISORDERS

The immunologically mediated bullous skin and/or mucous membranes disorders are those that can be evidenced by demonstration of *in vivo* bound (direct immunofluorescence) and circulating (indirect immunofluorescence) immunoglobulins directed against the epithelial intracellular substance and the basement membrane zone of the skin and/or mucous membranes (Fig. 8-6). Characteristically, direct immunofluorescence staining can be demonstrated using immunoglobulins directed against the basement membrane or the epithelial intercellular substances in these diseases.

Cicatricial Pemphigoid (Benign Mucous Membrane Pemphigoid)

Cicatricial pemphigoid (benign mucous membrane pemphigoid) is a variant of pemphigoid and represents a chronic subepithelial bullous disease. It causes mucous membrane scarring, especially of the oral mucosa (gingiva) and conjunctiva. Occasionally, it involves the skin. It is more common in women and usually occurs after the age of 45. It usually leads to significant morbidity within 2 years.

Skin Features

A generalized bullous eruption of short duration occurs in about one-third of patients. The bullae are localized on the scalp, on the face, or in the inguinal areas. The lesions develop in normal skin, are tense and dome-shaped, and usually recur in the same place at a later time. Less commonly, scaly, erythematous plaques with recurring peripheral bullae develop on the scalp and adjacent to affected mucous membranes. These lesions heal by scarring and sometimes produce cicatricial alopecia. Uncommonly, hyperkeratotic plaques develop on the distal extremities.

Mucous Membrane

About 85% of patients develop a persistent desquamative gingivitis of the labial and buccal gingiva of the tooth-bearing portion of the alveolar processes and sides of the tongue (Figs. 8-7 and 8-8). Later, vesicles and thick-walled bullae develop in other oral mucosal areas, such as the posterior fauces, pharynx, palate, and area under the tongue. The vesicles rapidly disintegrate to form eroded red areas covered with fine white lacy scars. Oral lesions cause little discomfort but occasionally bleed. Healing occurs by scarring, which may lead to contractions, strictures, and distortion of surrounding tissue.

Nasal mucous membrane involvement causes local discomfort, rhinitis, and nasal discharge. Laryngeal and esophageal involvement may cause hoarseness and, occasionally, strictures. Gastrointestinal tract involvement is manifested by diarrhea and rectal strictures. Genitourinary involvement may lead to bladder, urethral, and vaginal adhesions, and adhesions between the glans penis and prepuce.

Ocular Features

About 65% of patients develop irritation, pain, photophobia, tearing, and some discharge (Fig. 8-9). Lid involvement causes trichiasis, cicatricial entropion or ectropion, poliosis, and vitiligo, all of which occur late in the disease process.

The conjunctiva is involved early, and the process begins as a chronic catarrhal conjunctivitis with moderate papillary hypertrophy most marked in the inferior nasal or middle portion of the lower tarsus. Vesicles and small bullae then form that quickly break down, leading to punched-out ulcers covered by a thin, gray membrane. The surrounding conjunctiva appears hyperemic, and there is moderate to marked papillary hypertrophy and subepithelial fibrosis manifested by a fine, white membrane.

The scarring is progressive and eventually leads to symblepharon (Fig. 8-10), obliteration of the fornix, and ankyloblepharon (Fig. 8-11). The eyes are often dry from constant exposure, obliteration of the lacrimal gland orifices, and loss of the accessory lacrimal glands and goblet cells. The superior fornix and tarsal conjunctiva are generally less affected, although there is a moderate papillary hypertrophy of the upper tarsal conjunctiva during the active process and the subepithelial fibrosis may be seen on the upper tarsus (Fig. 8-12).

Corneal irregularity, opacification, neovascularization, and pannus develop as a result of improper lid surfacing, trauma, and drying. Recurrent corneal ulceration, thinning, and perforation may be seen. Eventually, the corneal surface becomes keratinized (Fig. 8-11).

Bullous Pemphigoid

Bullous pemphigoid usually develops after the age of 60. It is characterized by a prodromal nonspecific urticarial or eczematoid rash of the legs, followed after several weeks or months by large, tense, thick-walled bullae on a normal or erythematous base. These bullae usually involve the extremities and central abdomen but may involve most of the body (Fig. 8-13). The bullae usually contain clear fluid, occasionally blood-tinged or turbid fluid, and may reach a diameter of more than 6 cm. Some bullae rupture, leaving erosions that heal rapidly with mild postinflammatory changes, while others gradually flatten out and heal without rupturing.

Mucous membrane lesions are usually confined to the mouth and are less severe than those seen in pemphigus vulgaris. They heal without scarring.

Ocular involvement is uncommon, although symblepharon and obliteration of the inferior fornix have been observed.

Pemphigus Vulgaris

Pemphigus vulgaris represents an immunologically mediated disease characterized by intraepidermal bullae. It is more common in Ashkenazi Jews and generally begins between the ages of 40 to 60. The cause is unknown.

Skin Features

Skin blisters or bullae filled with clear fluid or, occasionally, pus develop on normal-appearing skin of the scalp, face, trunk, groin, axillae, and other pressure points. The blisters are often chronic, are readily unroofed, and produce painful denuded surfaces (Fig. 8-14). Both involved and normal skin have a positive Nikolsky sign (spreading a blister by lateral pressure on the skin). Occasionally, the denuded intertriginous areas develop vegetations with crusting and heaped-up epidermis, and the lesions often leave areas of hyperpigmentation with slight atrophy.

Mucous membrane lesions are common and are characterized by erosions and ulcerations that extend peripherally and heal only slowly. The gingiva, tongue, oral floor, and retromolar trigone are frequently involved; less commonly, the mucous membranes of the pharynx, esophagus, rectum, vulva, and cervix are involved.

Ocular Features

In some instances, ocular irritation, foreign-body sensation, and tearing precede the oral or skin lesions. Symmetric erosions of the lids, lid margins, and adjacent skin have been observed from transient vesicle formation (Fig. 8-15), and may lead to exposure or trichiasis from lid distortion by the crusted lesion. Conjunctival hyperemia, mucoid discharge, and pseudomembranes may occur. Rarely, conjunctival involvement leads to symblepharon and obliteration of the lower fornix.

Pemphigus Foliaceus and Pemphigus Erythematosus (Senear–Usher Syndrome)

Pemphigus foliaceus may represent the benign end of the spectrum of pemphigus vulgaris. The course is benign but prolonged. The skin lesions are characterized by small, superficial, flaccid blisters on an erythematous base, which are easily ruptured, leaving erosions that heal with crusting and scaling. The margins are usually sharply defined. The eruption is at first localized to the face, scalp, chest, and back; later it becomes more generalized. Sometimes the generalized lesions simulate exfoliative dermatitis with erythema, scaling, and crusting.

In pemphigus erythematosus the facial skin lesions often have a butterfly distribution simulating discoid lupus erythematosus and are erythematous, scaly, and hyperkeratotic. Sometimes the lesions occur in a distribution that suggests seborrheic dermatitis. Lesions on the trunk are similar to those seen in pemphigus foliaceus. Oral erosions and ulcerations are less common and less severe than in pemphigus vulgaris. Occasionally, the genital mucous membranes are involved. Conjunctival involvement is uncommon but is usually manifested as a purulent or pseudomembranous conjunctivitis.

Dermatitis Herpetiformis (During–Brocq Disease)

Dermatitis herpetiformis (DH) (During–Brocq disease) (Figs. 8-16 to 8-18) usually develops during the second to sixth decade and is more common in males. The etiology is unknown.

Skin Features

DH is characterized by a chronic, symmetric, intensely pruritic papulovesicular eruption of the extensor surfaces. Some patients complain of malaise during the acute disease. Many patients have an asymptomatic gluten-sensitive enteropathy, and many have steatorrhea and abnormal D-xylose absorption.

The skin eruption begins abruptly with intense pruritus, which is followed by recurrent groups of erythematous papules, urticarial wheals, or small vesicles. Occasionally, small bullae or eczematous changes develop that may become lichenified, but often the lesions are excoriated so rapidly that their character cannot be properly identified. Skin lesions develop on the extensor surfaces of the extremities (especially the knees and below the point of the elbow), sacral area (Fig. 8-16A), and natal cleft; less commonly, in the axillary folds, shoulders, trunk, scalp, and face. In about 50% of cases, the lesions lead to progressive pigmentation. The oral mucous membranes and occasionally the larynx are involved, but often there are no symptoms.

Ocular Features

Periocular skin lesions are often associated with burning, itching, and severe swelling around the eyes. Conjunctival involvement may lead to severe conjunctival scarring, obliteration of the fornix, and corneal scarring (Figs. 8-16 to 8-18).

Linear IGA Disease (Linear IGA Dermatitis Herpetiformis)

Linear IGA disease (linear IGA dermatitis herpetiformis) is differentiated from DH by the presence of linear IgA deposits in the lamina lucida or subbasal lamina zone.

Skin Features

The clinical manifestations are similar to those of DH, with development of pruritic, large or small, tense bullae in an annular or arciform grouping on normal or urticarial skin. The bullae heal without scarring. Occasionally, the lesions resemble erythema multiforme with targetlike lesions. Oral blisters and erosions often occur. There is no gluten-sensitive enteropathy.

Ocular Features

Moderate conjunctival chemosis is quite common, and the patients complain of ocular discomfort and hyperemia. Infrequently, it causes cicatricial entropion and trichiasis. Fine conjunctival scarring, shrinkage, and symblepharon may occur with secondary corneal ulceration in the presence of conjunctival involvement.

Chronic Bullous Dermatosis of Childhood (Juvenile Pemphigoid, Juvenile Dermatitis Herpetiformis)

Chronic bullous dermatosis of childhood (juvenile pemphigoid, juvenile DH) is a rare, self-limited disease that occurs only during childhood. It is probably a variant of linear IgA disease and cicatricial pemphigoid. The cause is unknown.

It begins acutely around the age of 4 or 5 and persists 2 to 4 years; then it spontaneously subsides. There are usually no symptoms. The initial attack is most severe and begins with large, clear, or, occasionally, hemorrhagic bullae on normal or erythematous skin of the inner thighs, genitalia, and buttocks. The scalp and perioral area may also be involved. Recurrent clusters of new bullae develop around old bullae during recurrent attacks. The lesions heal rapidly, causing hyperpigmentation.

Ocular Features

Ocular involvement may lead to irritation, redness, conjunctival scarring, and blindness.

Paraneoplastic Bullous Diseases

Bullous skin eruptions are sometimes associated with tumors such as malignant lymphomas, benign thymomas, retroperitoneal sarcomas, and chronic lymphocytic leukemia.

Skin Features

The eruption is polymorphous and has skin features of both pemphigus vulgaris and erythema multiforme. Occasionally, there are tense blisters as well as violaceous papules. The eruption has a propensity to involve the acral areas of the body. A severe stomatitis that involves the lips (similar to that seen in Stevens–Johnson syndrome) is commonly found.

Ocular Features

The disease may lead to severe shrinkage of the fornix and decreased tearing (Fig. 8-19).

ACQUIRED BULLOUS DISEASE

Toxic Epidermal Necrolysis (Scalded Skin Syndrome)

Toxic epidermal necrolysis (TEN) (scalded skin syndrome) is an acute blistering skin disease, characterized by skin tenderness and erythema followed by flaccid blistering and loss of full-thickness epidermis, which gives the appearance of scalded skin. It occurs in any age group but is more common in adults and affects females more frequently than males.

There are three groups of triggers, namely: drug exposure (e.g., sulfonamides, barbiturates), septicemia or administration of vaccines, and an idiopathic group in which no precipitating factor is identifiable.

Skin Features

The skin eruption begins with discrete erythematous macules or a morbilliform rash that quickly coalesces to form a diffuse erythroderma. A positive Nikolsky sign occurs in areas of erythema, and epidermolysis develops within hours producing flaccid bullae, which may rupture, leaving sheets of exfoliated skin that may extend over large areas of the skin surface (Fig. 8-20). Petechiae and hemorrhagic bullae may be a prominent part of the process. The epidermolysis reaches its maximum within 48 hours, following which unimpeded healing begins and continues for the next 2 to 4 weeks. Hair and nail loss may occur. There is minimal or no scarring unless there is secondary infection.

Often the skin of the hands and fingers peals off like a glove (Fig. 8-21). Erosive lesions of the mouth, esophagus, trachea, and genitourinary tract often occur during the first 24 to 48 hours. Stomatitis may be a prominent feature of the disease.

Ocular Features

Erosive corneal lesions occur in about 50% of patients. Corneal perforation and neovascularization have been observed. Lid edema is common during the acute phase, and the eruption often involves the lid. Meibomian gland metaplasia, trichiasis, and eyelid deformity may develop. Conjunctival hyperemia and infiltration, mucopurulent discharge, erosive lesions, and pseudomembrane formation frequently occur (Fig. 8-22). Upon healing, scarring, and symblepharon may be seen. The conjunctival scarring may cause keratoconjunctivitis sicca, punctal stenosis, and canalicular obliteration.

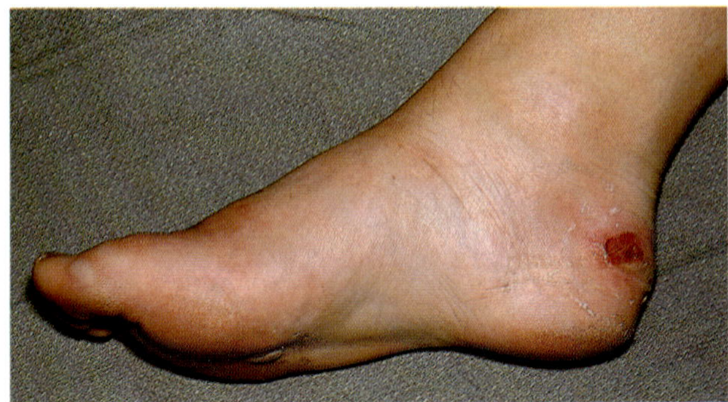

FIGURE 8-1. Epidermolysis bullosa simplex (Weber–Cockayne). Note erosions and bullae at sites of friction on heal, toe, and sole. This patient first became aware of this problem after prolonged hiking and sweating.

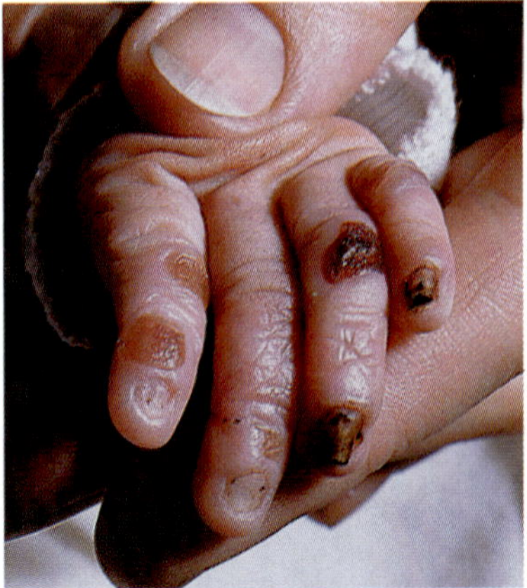

FIGURE 8-2. Dystrophic epidermolysis bullosa. Transient bullous dermolysis of the newborn. Note erosions, crusts, and nail dystrophy. (Photo courtesy of Dr. Paul Fasal.)

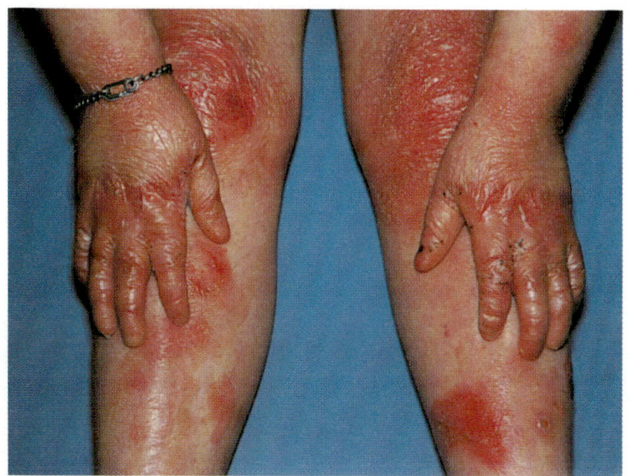

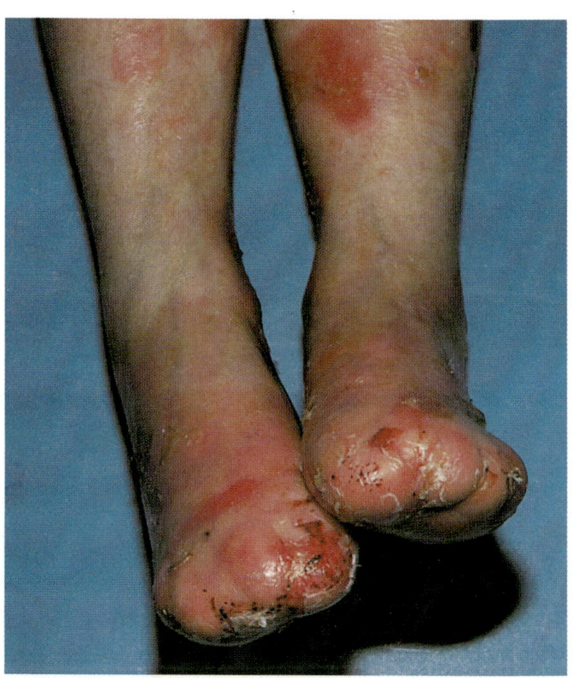

FIGURE 8-3. Dystrophic epidermolysis bullosa showing parchment-like scarring and beginning web formation of fingers, which is more apparent in this young child's feet in Fig. 8-4.

FIGURE 8-4. Dystrophic epidermolysis bullosa with severe pseudosyndactyly of toes.

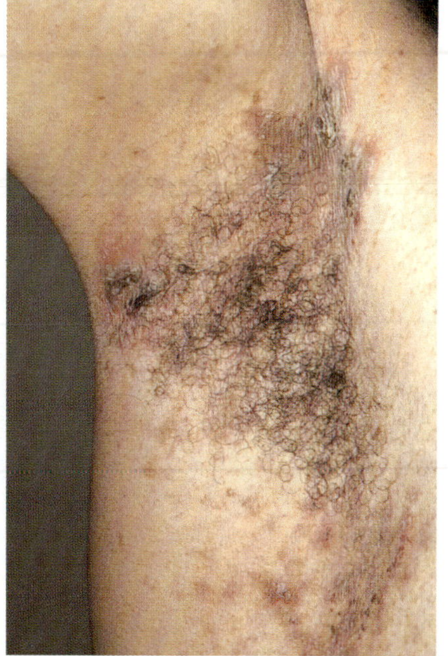

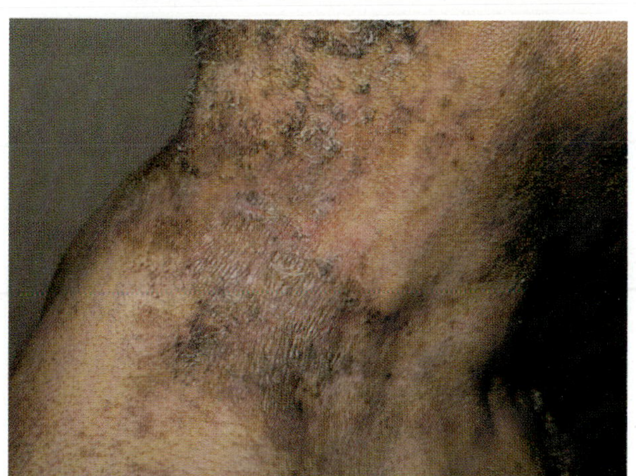

FIGURE 8-5. Hailey–Hailey disease involving the axilla (**A**) and neck (**B**). Note grouped vesiculopustules and crusts.

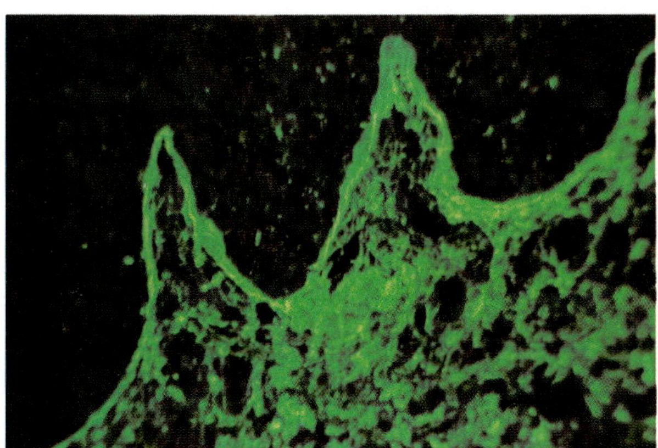

FIGURE 8-6. Indirect IgG staining of the basement membrane of the soft palate in cicatricial pemphigoid. (Photograph courtesy of Dr. Troy Daniels.)

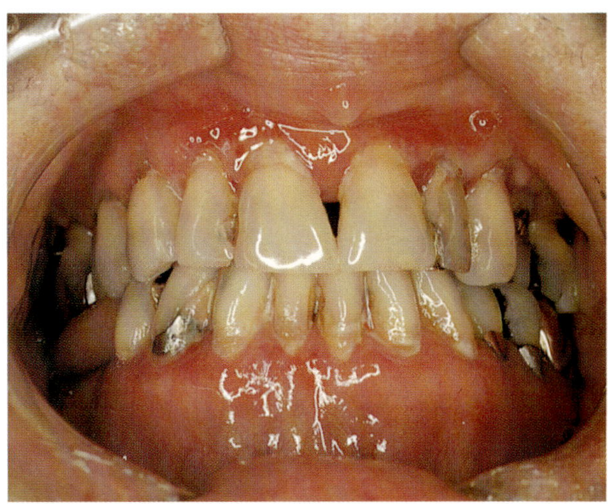

FIGURE 8-7. Desquamative gingivitis in the tooth-bearing portion of the alveolar processes in cicatricial pemphigoid. (Photograph courtesy of Dr. Troy Daniels.)

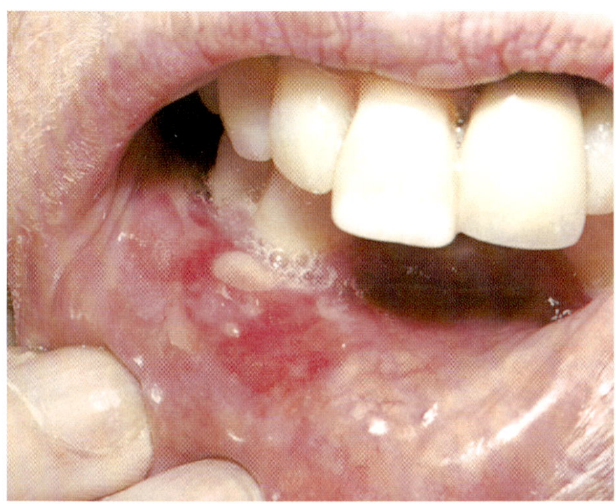

FIGURE 8-8. Cicatricial pemphigoid of the mouth. Differential diagnosis includes aphthae, traumatic lesions, and pemphigus.

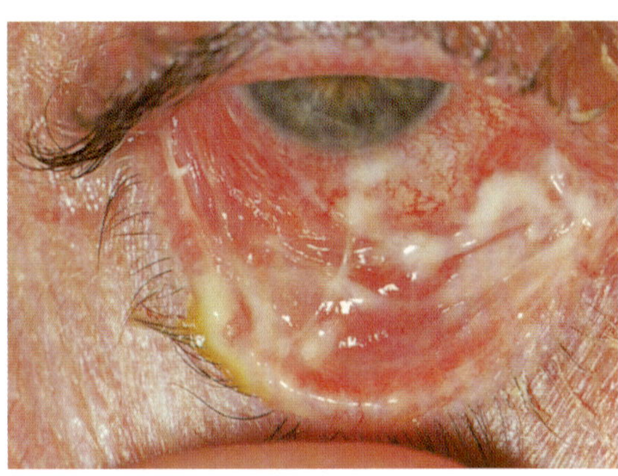

FIGURE 8-9. Severe mucoid discharge in cicatricial pemphigoid. The stringy mucoid discharge may be severe, as in this patient.

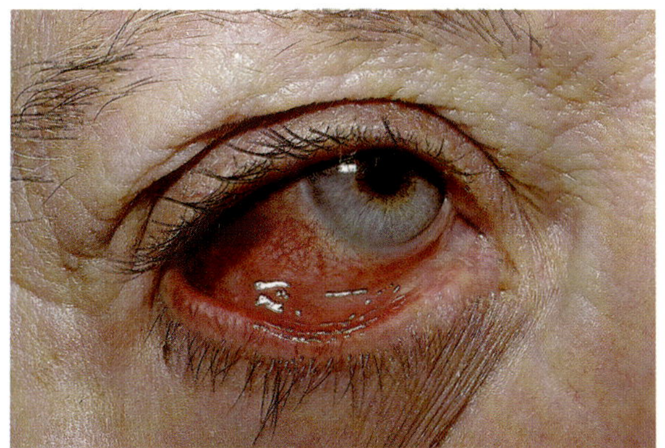

FIGURE 8-10. Early symblepharon formation in cicatricial pemphigoid.

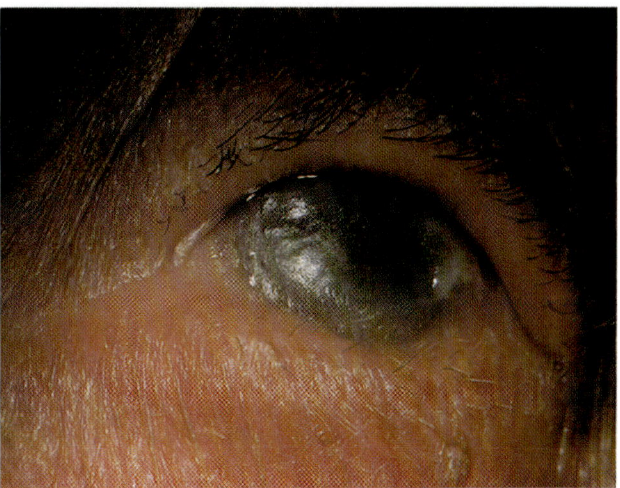

FIGURE 8-11. Final stage of conjunctival scarring with ankyloblepharon in cicatricial pemphigoid. Note keratinization of cornea.

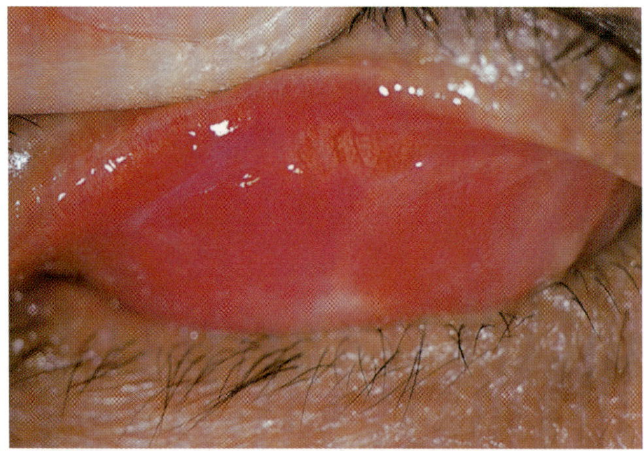

FIGURE 8-12. Superior tarsal conjunctiva during active cicatricial pemphigoid. Note the marked papillary hypertrophy, moderate mucoid discharge, and superficial flat scarring.

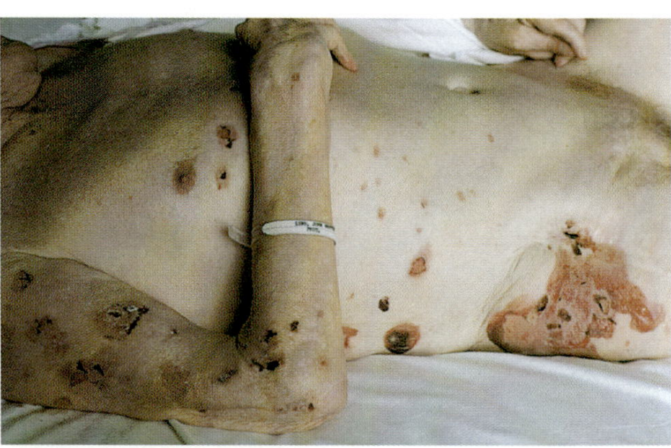

FIGURE 8-13. Bullous pemphigoid skin lesions. Note flaccid bullae and erosions.

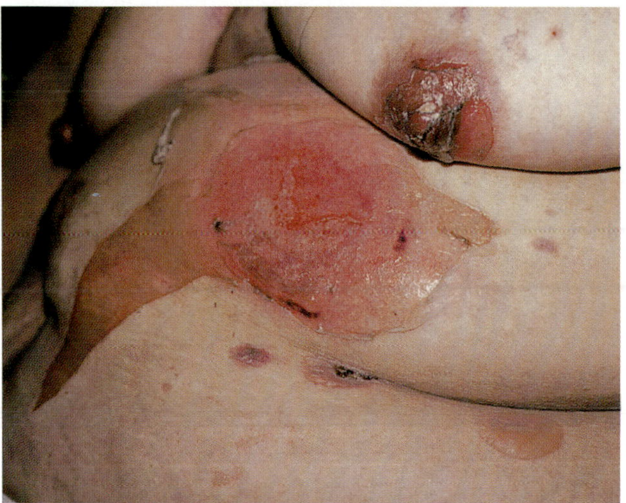

FIGURE 8-14. Pemphigus vulgaris in an elderly female with large bullae and painful erosions.

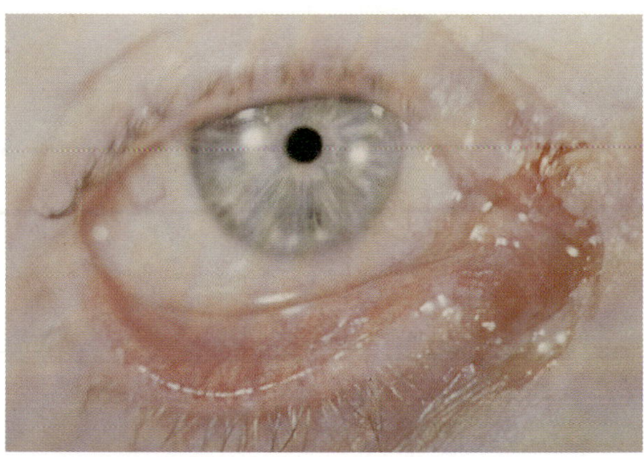

FIGURE 8-15. Superficial ulceration of the medial portion of the lower eyelid is evident in this patient with pemphigus vulgaris. Probably vesicles preceded the skin lesions.

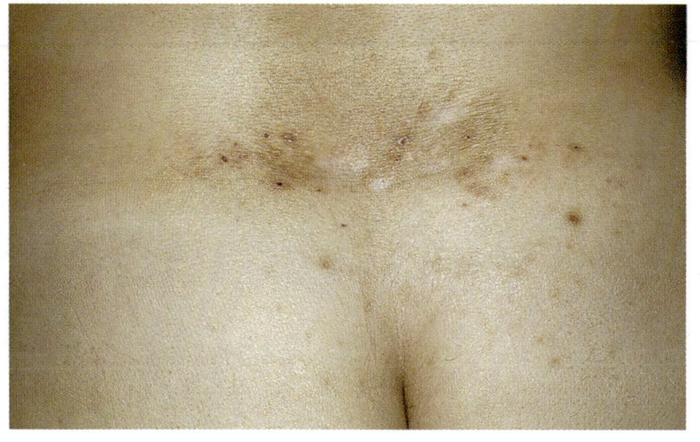

A

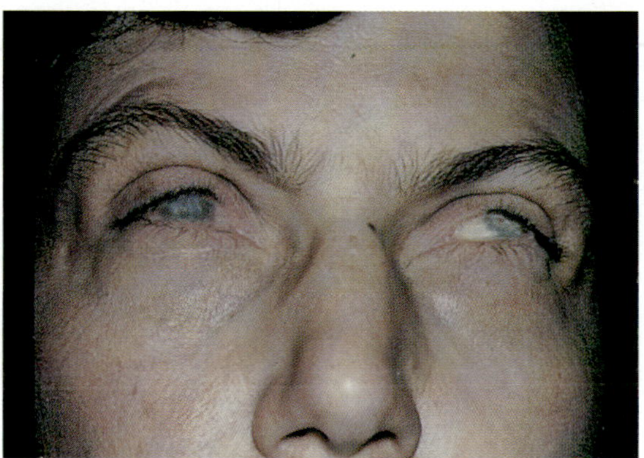

B

FIGURE 8-16. A: Dermatitis herpetiformis showing excoriated papulo-vesicles and scarring of sacral area in a patient with long-standing lesions. Considerable improvement was obtained by following a gluten-free diet and using dapsone. **B:** Late stages of dermatitis herpetiformis with severe conjunctival cicatrization.

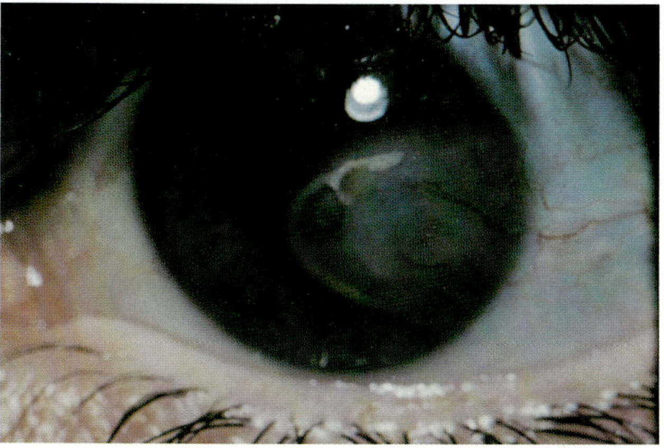

FIGURE 8-17. Peripheral corneal scarring with neovascularization in long-standing dermatitis herpetiformis.

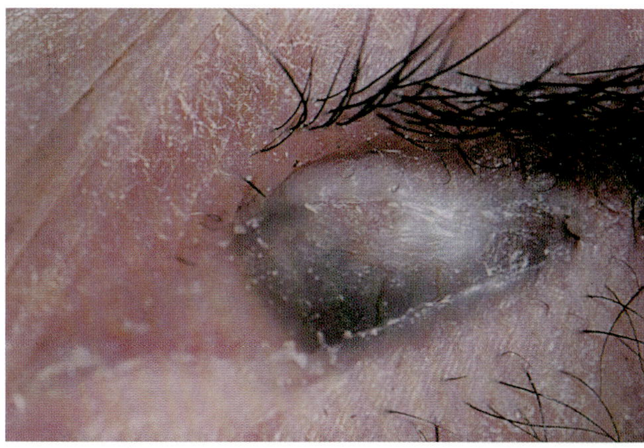

FIGURE 8-18. Obliteration of fornix and extensive conjunctival cicatrization in dermatitis herpetiformis. This is the same patient as the one depicted in Fig. 8-16B.

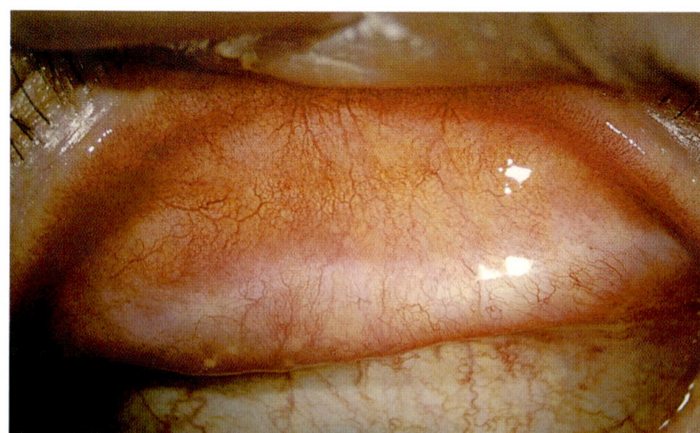

FIGURE 8-19. Foreshortening of the fornix and typical subepithelial fibrosis in paraneoplastic bullous disease.

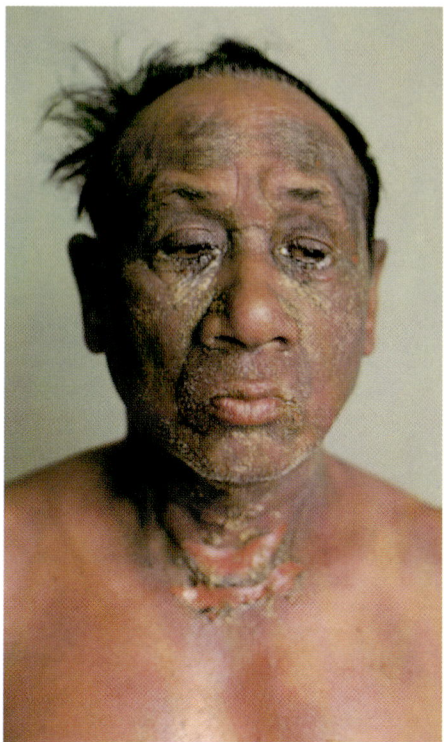

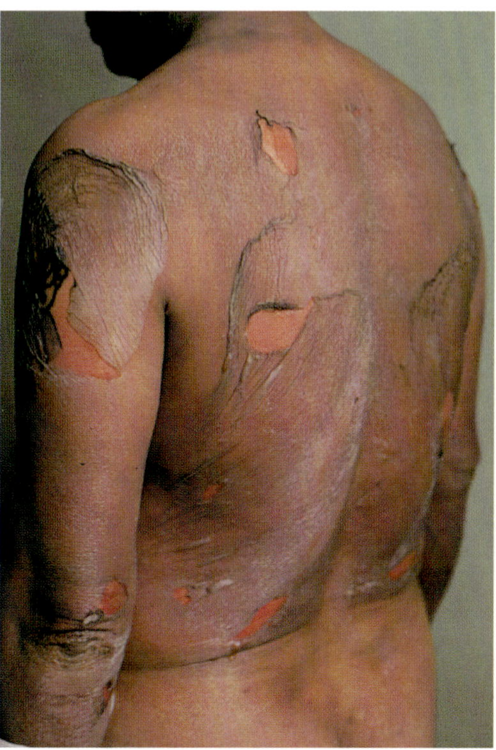

FIGURE 8-20. Toxic epidermal necrolysis caused by a sulfonamide diuretic showing classic flaccid bullae and denuded skin. Several years after this photograph was taken, the patient was unfortunately reexposed to a sulfonamide medication and despite treatment in a burn unit, died within a week.

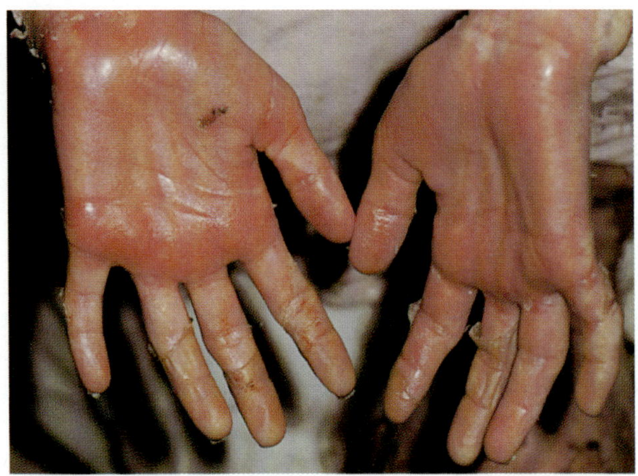

FIGURE 8-21. Denuded palms in toxic epidermal necrolysis.

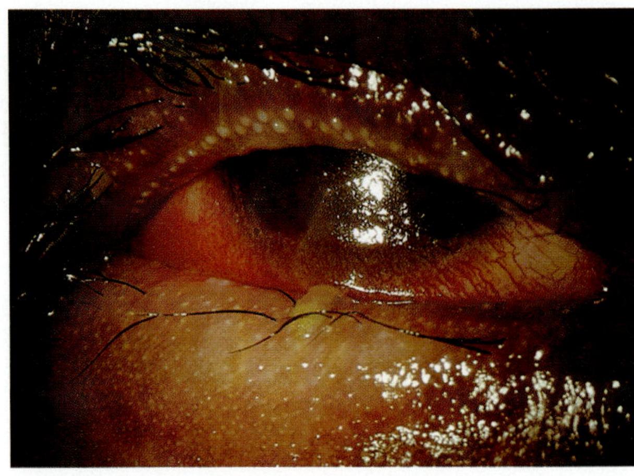

FIGURE 8-22. Conjunctival scarring secondary to toxic epidermal necrolysis. Acute phase shows conjunctival hyperemia, lash loss, and mucopurulent discharge.

CHROMOSOMAL DISORDERS AND DEVELOPMENTAL DEFECTS

Chromosomal disorders are caused by abnormalities in the structure or number of chromosomes. Usually, multiple malformations occur. As a general rule, any child born with more than one malformation should have chromosomal analysis. The chromosomal disorders represent deletions, inversions, duplications, ring formations, and translocations.

Deletion syndromes usually have one normal and one partially deleted chromosome. The terminology used for deletion syndromes includes the chromosome number, with the letter q standing for the long arm and the letter p for the short arm of the chromosome combined with a minus sign (e.g., deletion of the long arm of chromosome 13 is termed $13q^-$ syndrome; deletion of the short arm of chromosome 18 is termed $18p^-$ syndrome).

Ring forms arise from breakage of both arms of a chromosome followed by loss of the terminal end, which results in a ring form when the chromosome reunites at the break point. The terminology used for ring chromosome formation includes the letter r and the number of the chromosome (e.g., ring chromosome 18 is termed r18).

Trisomy represents an extra chromosome as exemplified in Down syndrome, in which there are three of chromosome 21 instead of the normal two chromosomes.

Mosaicism usually occurs following fertilization and results in the abnormal chromosomes being present in only a fraction of the body cells.

AUTOSOMAL CHROMOSOMAL DEFECTS

Chromosome 4 Abnormalities

Deletion of the Short Arm of Chromosome 4 (4p⁻ Syndrome)

Deletion of the short arm of chromosome 4 ($4p^-$ syndrome) causes the Wolf–Hirschhorn syndrome, characterized by retarded pre- and postnatal physical and mental development, characteristic facies, congenital heart disease, hypospadias, arthrogryposis, hypotonia, and seizures. The characteristic facial features include microcephaly, a long nasal root with prominent glabella, hypertelorism, ear anomalies, cleft lip and/or palate, and micrognathia.

Skin and Ocular Features

The skin features are limited to hemangiomas; the ocular features, to microphthalmia, strabismus, nystagmus, epicanthal folds, ptosis, iris coloboma, and cataracts.

Chromosome 5 Abnormalities

Deletion of the Short Arm of Chromosome 5 (5p⁻ Syndrome)

Deletion of the short arm of chromosome 5 ($5p^-$ syndrome) causes the cri-du-chat syndrome, so named because of the catlike mewing of the infant when crying. It is characterized by mental retardation, a round face during infancy, facial asymmetry, congenital heart disease, and transverse simian creases.

Skin and Ocular Features

The skin features are limited to hemangiomas; the ocular features, to epicanthal folds in infancy, squint, refractive errors, occasional congenital cataracts, optic nerve atrophy, and tortuous retinal arterioles.

Chromosome 11 Anomalies

Deletion of the Short Arm of Chromosome 11 (11p⁻ Syndrome)

Deletion of the short arm of chromosome 11 ($11p^-$ syndrome) results in aniridia and development of Wilms tumors.

Chromosome 13 Abnormalities

Some genes on chromosome 13 regulate development of the thumbs, fingers, and midfacial region. Diseases associated with chromosome 13 abnormalities include Wilson disease (Chapter 33), retinoblastoma, and osteosarcoma.

Deletion of Part of the Long Arm of Chromosome 13 (13q⁻ Syndrome)

The major characteristics of 13q⁻ syndrome are absence of the thumbs, a broad nasal bridge, forward-slanting incisors, microcephaly, and increased risk for developing osteosarcoma.

Ocular Features

The major ocular feature is development of retinoblastoma, which may then be transmitted to the patient's offspring in an autosomal dominant fashion. Other ocular features include microphthalmia, hypertelorism, ptosis, and epicanthus.

Chromosome 13 Ring Formation (R13)

Chromosome 13 ring formation (R13) is characterized by severe mental retardation, microcephaly, craniofacial dysmorphism with hypertelorism, epicanthic folds, a broad nasal bridge, triangular cranium, and large ears.

Trisomy 13 (Patau Syndrome)

Trisomy 13 (Patau syndrome) is usually lethal. It is characterized by a sloping forehead, low-set ears, a cleft lip and palate, and rocker-bottom feet. Cardiac defects and a variety of other visceral defects may be found. Characteristically, there is holoprosencephaly, arrhinencephaly or microcephaly, and mental retardation.

Skin Features

The skin features include localized scalp defect; capillary hemangiomas, especially of the forehead; cutis laxa of the neck; distal palmar axial triradii of the palm print; and hyperconvex nails.

Ocular Features

The abnormal ocular features include microphthalmos, anophthalmos, synophthalmus, and cyclops; hypertelorism, epicanthus, and absence of eyebrows; corneal opacities (Peters anomaly); anterior chamber angle anomalies; colobomas, sometimes associated with cartilaginous metaplasia of fibrovascular tissues; cataract; persistence of the hyaloid artery, tunica vasculosa lentis, and persistence and hyperplasia of the primary vitreous; and hypoplasia of the optic nerve.

Chromosome 14 Abnormalities

Ring Formation Chromosome 14 (R14 Syndrome)

Ring formation of chromosome 14 consistently results in both psychomotor and growth retardation, seizures, microcephaly, dolichocephaly, a high forehead, downward-slanting palpebral fissures and epicanthal folds, and a short neck. The central nervous system features include hypo- or hypertonia, tremor, and athetosis.

Skin and Ocular Features

Café-au-lait spots may involve the skin.

The ocular features include nystagmus, hypertelorism, and downward-slanting palpebral fissures. Isolated cases of Brushfield's spots, pigmentary mottling in the peripheral retina, and pinpoint white opacities of the macula have been described.

Chromosome 15 Abnormalities

Deletion of the Long Arm of Chromosome 15 (15q⁻ Syndrome)

Deletion of the long arm of chromosome 15 (15q⁻ syndrome) results in the Prader–Willi syndrome (Chapter 6).

Ring Formation of Chromosome 15 (R15 Syndrome)

Ring formation of chromosome 15 (R15 syndrome) often shows only mild phenotypic abnormalities. They include prenatal and postnatal growth retardation, mild mental retardation, microcephaly, micrognathia, anomalies of the radial axis, and a bird-headed profile. Ocular features are limited to hypertelorism and narrow palpebral fissures.

Chromosome 18 Anomalies

Deletion of the Short Arm of Chromosome 18 (18p⁻ Syndrome)

The abnormalities seen in this deletion syndrome usually occur in children born to mothers over the age of 30. There is no specific clinical syndrome, but abnormalities include prenatal and postnatal growth failure, mild to severe mental retardation, brachycephaly or microcephaly, muscle hypotonia, seizures, and dysmorphic features, including a broad nasal bridge; floppy, large, low-set ears; high-arched palate; receding chin; webbed-neck; a deep nuchal hairline; and a cleft palate.

Scalp alopecia and delayed tooth eruption often occur with the dysmorphic features. The dermatoglyphics may show an abundance of whorls and a distal palmar triradius.

Ocular Features

About half of the patients have hypertelorism, epicanthal folds, ptosis, and strabismus. Microphthalmia, cyclopia, coloboma, corneal leukoma, keratoconus, and glaucoma are less common.

Deletion of the Long Arm of Chromosome 18 (18q⁻ Syndrome)

Deletion of the long arm of chromosome 18 (18q⁻ syndrome) is more common in females. The patients have midfacial hypoplasia, deep-set eyes, large ears, a very prominent antihelix and antitragus, cleft palate and cleft lip, and multiple skeletal anomalies, including proximally inserted thumbs and second toes, clubfeet, and supernumerary ribs. The patients are usually quite short, and about 70% have microcephaly. They have retarded psychomotor and mental development, and muscle hypotonia. Eczema occurs in about 25% of patients.

Ocular Features

The ocular anomalies include microphthalmia, hypertelorism, and epicanthal folds; ptosis; nystagmus and strabismus; microcornea, corneal opacities, and corneal staphyloma; absence of the anterior chamber angle; coloboma of the iris, choroid, and retina; pale optic discs; glaucoma; and refractive errors.

Ring Chromosome 18 Syndrome (R18 Syndrome)

Ring chromosome 18 syndrome (R18 syndrome) is uncommon and generally presents with characteristics of both 18p⁻ and 18q⁻ syndromes (see earlier). Sometimes the patient is phenotypically normal.

Trisomy 18 (Edward Syndrome)

Trisomy 18 (Edward syndrome) occurs more often in children born to older women and usually causes spontaneous abortion or early neonatal death. It is characterized by polyhydramnios and prenatal growth retardation. Surviving children have severe postnatal growth and mental retardation. The clinical findings of a prominent occiput and narrow bifrontal diameter of the head along with small palpebral fissures and low-set and malformed ears are characteristic. Central nervous system abnormalities include hydrocephalus, cerebellar hypoplasia, corpus callosum defects, microgyria, deficiency of myelination, and meningomyeloceles. Many pulmonary, cardiac, and great vessel abnormalities have been described.

Skin Features

Skin features are limited to excess skin.

Ocular Features

The ocular features include orbital ridge hypoplasia, short palpebral fissures, inner epicanthal folds, ptosis, and corneal opacities. Less common findings are microphthalmos, hypertelorism, slanting of the palpebral fissures, iris coloboma, and cataract with persistent hyperplastic primary vitreous.

Chromosome 21 Abnormalities

Abnormalities of several genes in chromosome 21 help to explain the abnormalities in Down syndrome, namely:

1. A gene that codes for two enzymes important in purine metabolism and thus proper mental development.
2. The oncogene Ets-2, which is related to development of leukemia in Down patients.
3. A gene important in the aging process, which helps to explain the premature aging of Down patients.
4. The gene for amyloid beta protein, which comprises a major portion of the material that accumulates in Alzheimer disease and helps explain the Alzheimer-like brain changes that occur.
5. The gene for a structural component of the lens, which may explain the cataracts in Down syndrome.

Down Syndrome (Trisomy 21)

Down syndrome (trisomy 21) arises from nondisjunction of chromosome 21. The characteristic facial features include a small head; flat face; a short, broad nose; small, low-set, misshapen ears; a small, round mouth that is usually partly open; epicanthal folds; and slanting palpebral fissures.

The extremities are usually short and stumpy; the joint ligaments, lax; the hands, broad; and the fingers, short, cone-shaped, often webbed, and the little finger curved. The palms have a simian crease (a midpalmar transverse crease). The peripheral circulation is poor and often results in acrocyanosis. About 40% of patients have congenital heart defects. Recurrent respiratory infections are common, and the patients usually have delayed puberty.

Most are severely mentally retarded, with an IQ of less than 50. Epilepsy occurs in about 10% of patients, and after the age of 35, the patients often develop changes reminiscent of Alzheimer disease.

Skin Features

In early childhood, the skin is soft and velvety, but at about age 15, it becomes dry and loses its elasticity; later, there is mild to moderate xerosis. After the age of 20, many patients develop patchy lichenification on the upper arms, wrists, fronts of the thighs, and backs of the neck and ankles, which is probably a manifestation of atopic dermatitis. Livido reticularis occurs on the thighs, buttocks, and trunk.

In adult males, a chronic follicular papular eruption may be seen in the presternal and interscapular region. Other findings include elastosis perforans, syringomata, vitiligo, keratosis pilaris, and increased numbers of skin infections. Fissuring and thickening of the lips; angular chilitis; a thick, geographically fissured tongue; and purulent nasal discharge are common. The hair is fine and may be hypopigmented; alopecia may be quite extensive. The teeth are hypoplastic and slow to erupt.

Ocular Features

The upward-slanting palpebral fissures give the patient a mongoloid appearance and are usually associated with epicanthic folds that are more prominent in early childhood. The eyelids are thickened; the lashes, short and sparse. Syringomas of the eyelids are common, and chronic blepharitis may be seen. Keratoconus occurs in 15% to 30% of Down patients, and acute hydrops is not uncommon (Fig. 9-1). Other ocular features include cataracts (cortical flake opacities or arcuate opacities), seen in 10% to 50% of patients; a hypoplastic iris; and Brushfield spots (the latter being seen in about 75% to 85% of patients); strabismus; nystagmus; refractive errors; and occasionally, retinal detachment.

Chromosome 22 Anomalies

Chromosome 22 Trisomy

Chromosome 22 trisomy, also known as the cat eye syndrome because of the prominent iris colobomas, is characterized by microcephaly (45%), mild to moderate mental retardation (80%), preauricular tags or fistulas (90%), cardiovascular anomalies, renal and urinary tract anomalies, anal atresia, and musculoskeletal deformities.

Ocular Features

The ocular features include microphthalmia (25%), strabismus, inferonasal colobomas of the iris, choroid and optic nerve (65%), hypertelorism (50%), antimongoloid palpebral slant (40%), and congenital cataracts.

Derivative Chromosome 22

Patients with derivative chromosome 22 have a balanced translocation of the long arms of chromosome 11 and chromosome 22. The patients have mental retardation, preauricular skin tags or pits, low-set or large ears, a high-arched or cleft palate, micrognathia, septal heart defects with a patent ductus arteriosus, small penis, undescended testicles, and inguinal hernias.

Ocular Features

Ocular features include strabismus, hyper- or hypotelorism, and mongoloid or antimongoloid palpebral fissures.

SEX CHROMOSOMAL ANOMALIES

Klinefelter Syndrome

The Klinefelter syndrome represents trisomy of the sex chromosomes resulting in two X chromosomes and one Y. About 15% of patients have mosaicism with at least two distinct cell lines and a pattern of 46 XY/47 XXY. Phenotypically, the patients are males, but sperm cell and testosterone production are usually abnormal, and the patients are sterile. There is usually gynecomastia, and breast cancer is quite common. Some patients are moderately mentally retarded.

Skin and Ocular Features

Skin features include sparse facial and axillary hair. Ocular features include bilateral anophthalmos, strabismus, color vision abnormalities, hypertelorism, epicanthal folds, unilateral (or bilateral) radial, linear, corneal stromal opacities with focal posterior keratoconus, superior pseudopannus dislocated lens, uveal colobomas, a diffuse choroidal atrophy with mid-peripheral bone-spicule pigment clumps, retinitis pigmentosa, and optic atrophy.

Turner Syndrome

Turner syndrome is characterized by sexual infantilism, short stature, webbing of the neck (Fig. 9-2) and cubitus valgus. It is caused by a structurally defective X chromosome. (Most of the patients have 45 chromosomes with an XO sex chromosome complement in which the missing chromosome is lost before or at the time of fertilization. Others have 46 chromosomes with partial deletion of one of the X chromosomes.) Mosaicism is common. About 95% of fetuses are spontaneously aborted.

General Features

Patients have a characteristic facies with low-set ears, narrow maxilla, small mandible, high-arched palate, and webbed neck. Intelligence is usually normal. About one-fourth of the patients have congenital heart disease. Almost all have short stature, and many have a shield chest and widely spaced nipples. The ovaries are absent or abnormal, and there is an increased risk of gonadal malignancy. The external genitalia are normal, but secondary sexual characteristics do not develop. Skeletal deformities and hearing loss are also found.

Skin Features

The skin features include redundant lax skin, especially of the neck and buttocks; cutaneous and subcutaneous lymphatic hypoplasia; low nuchal hairline; peripheral edema of the dorsal aspect of the hands and feet; abnormal dermatoglyphics; multiple pigmented melanocyte nevi, especially over the upper part of the body; pedal hemangiomas that tend to resolve in early life; and a propensity for keloid formation. The nails are hypoplastic and have an increased convexity.

Ocular Features

Ocular findings include hypertelorism, epicanthus blepharitis or inversus, antimongoloid palpebral fissures, ptosis; strabismus with 10% red–green color blindness even though the patients are females. Rare findings include conjunctival cysts, microcornea, corneal nebulae, blue sclerae, and cataracts.

Noonan Syndrome (Noonan–Ehmke Syndrome)

Noonan syndrome (Noonan–Ehmke syndrome) is clinically similar to Turner syndrome but occurs in both sexes. The number of chromosomes is normal. The syndrome is probably autosomal dominant, but most cases are sporadic and probably arise from spontaneous mutation. About one-third of cases are complicated by polyhydramnios.

Characteristically, the patients have short stature; broad, short, webbed neck; low posterior hairline; pectus excavatum; and a shieldlike chest. The facies is characterized by hypertelorism, epicanthal folds, ptosis, low-set ears, small chin, and malocclusion of the front teeth. Many patients are mildly mentally retarded.

Cardiac defects, pectus excavatum, and vertebral defects are common. Hepatosplenomegaly occurs in about 50% of patients. About 77% of males have cryptorchidism; testicular hypoplasia and a small penis are common. Females usually have functional ovaries and are able to bear children.

Skin Features

Ulerythema ophryogenes (keratosis atrophicans) is a cutaneous marker for Noonan syndrome. Lymphedema of the feet and legs is more common than in Turner syndrome and persists longer. Coarse, woolly, light-colored hair and downy hypertrichosis on the cheeks or shoulders may be observed. In males, the beard and pubic hair are scanty.

Ocular Features

The lid features include hypertelorism (74%), ptosis (48%), downward-sloping palpebral apertures (38%), and epicanthic folds (39%). Other features include prominent corneal nerves (46%), anterior corneal stromal dystrophy (4%), cataracts, and uveitis, retinal findings (20%), colobomas, drusen of the optic nerve head, and hypoplasia of the optic nerve.

Developmental Defects

Developmental defects include malformations, deformations, and disruptions. They represent flaws that arise during intrauterine life and are thus congenital.

Congenital Absence of Skin

Congenital absence of skin arises from genetic defects, trauma, and intrauterine infection (e.g., varicella and herpes simplex infections). Congenital absence of skin and ocular abnormalities are found in the epidermal nevus syndrome, oculo-cerebro-cutaneous syndrome, bitemporal aplasia cutis congenita, and focal facial dermal dysplasia.

Oculo-Cerebro-Cutaneous Syndrome (Delleman–Orthuys Syndrome)

The skin features in oculo-cerebro-cutaneous syndrome (Delleman–Orthuys syndrome) include multiple or punched-out-appearing focal areas of cutaneous hypoplasia of the scalp, neck, and lumbosacral area. Skin tags measuring up to 1 cm in diameter usually occur around the eyes and nose. Other abnormalities include skull defects, porencephaly, cerebral malformations, and agenesis of the corpus callosum.

Ocular Features

The ocular abnormalities include orbital cysts, microphthalmia, and lid colobomas.

Bitemporal Aplasia Cutis Congenita (Setleis Syndrome)

Bitemporal aplasia cutis congenita (Setleis syndrome) is probably autosomal dominant and has incomplete penetrance. The patients have a leonine, aged facies; the nose and chin feel rubbery to palpation. The skin findings include bitemporal scarlike defects resembling forceps marks.

Ocular Features

The ocular findings include puckered periorbital skin, laterally deficient eyebrows that angle outward and upward. There is distichiasis (double row of lashes) of the upper lids and astichiasis (lashes not arranged in rows) of the lower lids.

Focal Facial Dermal Dysplasia (Hereditary Symmetric Aplastic Nevi of the Temples)

The anomalies are similar to those described for bitemporal aplasia cutis congenita. The syndrome is autosomal dominant. The skin lesions occur near the brow and present as atrophic, pigmented, puckered, hairless areas above the eyebrow that extend upward and outward.

Developmental Defects of the First Branchial Arch

First branchial arch developmental defects arise from arrested development during various stages of gestation.

Mandibulofacial Dysostosis (Treacher–Collins Syndrome)

Mandibulofacial dysostosis (Treacher–Collins syndrome) is autosomal dominant with complete penetrance but variable expression. New mutations are common. The facial features include (Figs. 9-3 and 9-4):

1. Circumscribed cicatricial alopecia and extension of terminal scalp hair onto the cheeks.
2. Orbital distortion with antimongoloid palpebral fissures and ptosis.
3. Absence or hypoplasia of the zygomatic arches and paucity of muscular aponeurosis of the midface.
4. Small, malformed pinna with stenosis of the external auditory meatus and accessory tragi.
5. Choanal atresia, micrognathia, small lower jaw, malocclusion, high palate, occasional cleft palate, and sometimes a cleft alveolus.

Secondary conductive-type deafness may arise from middle ear hypoplasia and dysmorphia. A narrow airway may cause chronic respiratory insufficiency and sleep apnea.

Other ocular findings include deformity of the lower orbital rim with lower lid pseudocolobomas (partial thickness colobomas), partial or total lash alopecia of the lower lids, bilateral absence of inferior lacrimal puncta, triangular shape of the palpebral fissures, and, rarely, dermolipoma and lens subluxation.

Hallermann–Streiff Syndrome (Oculomandibulodyscephaly with Hypotrichosis)

The inheritance pattern for Hallermann–Streiff syndrome (oculomandibulodyscephaly with hypotrichosis) is unknown. The birdlike facial features are distinctive, with a short head, beaked nose, small mouth, high-arched palate, and hypoplastic mandible. The children are often dwarfed, and the head is often misshapen with frontal bossing and brachycephaly, scaphocephaly, or microcephaly. Delayed closure of the fontanels may also occur.

The facial skin, especially in the midfacial area, is atrophic, and telangiectasia may be prominent. The scalp hair, although often normal at birth, becomes sparse, hypopigmented, and brittle, and there is frequently alopecia of the cranial suture lines. Although teeth are often present at birth, partial anodontia, hypoplasia, caries, and malalignment are common.

Ocular Features

Ocular findings include bilateral microphthalmia, scanty brows and lashes, and total or partial cataracts. The cataracts may cause secondary glaucoma. Infrequently, the patients have blue sclerae, chorioretinal scars, retinal folds, optic nerve colobomas, and strabismus.

Goldenhar Syndrome (Oculo-Auriculo-Vertebral Dysplasia)

The Goldenhar syndrome is usually sporadic. Most patients have facial asymmetry that arises from soft-tissue displacement, hypoplasia, or malposition. The maxillary, malar, and temporal bones are often hypoplastic and flattened.

The most common findings are accessory auricles and pits, which occur along a line between the ear and angle of the mouth. The pinna is frequently deformed, and preauricular skin tags are frequently seen (Fig. 9-5A). Preauricular sinuses, hypoplasia of the ossicles, and sensorineural or conductive hearing loss may occur. Occasionally, there is a low hairline along the forehead and temples.

Up to 15% of patients have a cleft lip or palate. Mandibular ramus agenesis, lateral facial clefts, and hypoplasia of the palatal and tongue muscles and of the accessory salivary and parotid glands may also occur.

Skeletal and muscular abnormalities include cervical vertebral fusion, vertebral hypoplasia, and hemivertebrae.

About 10% of patients have mental retardation. Other central nervous system abnormalities include microcephaly, unilateral arhinencephaly, occipital encephalocele, Arnold–Chiari malformation, hydrocephalus, aqueductal stenosis, agenesis of the corpus callosum, and aplasia of the 5th and 7th cranial nerve nuclei.

Ocular Features

Ocular findings include the following:

1. Microphthalmia, anophthalmia.
2. Upper lid coloboma, ptosis.
3. Epibulbar dermoids in the lower outer quadrant at the limbus, sometimes involving the peripheral cornea (Fig. 9-5B). Lipodermoids in the upper outer quadrant.
4. Nasolacrimal duct and canalicular obstruction with or without fistulas and ectopic puncta.
5. Reduced corneal sensation.
6. Iris and retinal coloboma.
7. Peripapillary choroidal hyperpigmentation.

8. Macular hypoplasia, tortuous retinal vessels.
9. Optic nerve hypoplasia, tilted optic disc.
10. Strabismus.

Congenital Inclusion Dermoid Cysts (Dermoid Cyst)

Most congenital inclusion dermoid cysts (dermoid cysts) arise from entrapped epithelium along the lines of embryonic fusion. They are subcutaneous, usually measure 1 to 4 cm in diameter, and are soft and doughy to palpation. Hair can often be seen projecting from a sinus opening. The cysts are usually found in the following areas:

1. Head: outer one-third of brow, middle of bridge of nose, orbit. They may extend intracranially.
2. Scalp: along suture lines; occipital area. They may extend intracranially.
3. Submental area: floor of the mouth.
4. Anterior neck.
5. Anterior chest wall.
6. Inguinal area.

Epidermal Nevus (Linear Nevus)

An epidermal nevus (linear nevus) represents a hamartomatous lesion of epidermal tissue. Hamartomas arise from mature or nearly mature structures that are part of the normal skin structure. Most occur on the head and neck, and, in more than one-third of cases, there are other organ system abnormalities (see epidermal nevus syndrome below).

Verrucous Epidermal Nevus (Nevus Verrucosus)

Verrucous epidermal nevi (nevus verrucosus) are epidermal hamartomas that are usually congenital but sometimes develop in childhood or adulthood. These hamartomas begin as pink or slightly pigmented velvety streaks or plaques that are either continuous, interrupted, or sometimes isolated (Fig. 9-6). They later darken and become keratotic. The epidermolytic forms (those that involve the palms and soles) are usually more verrucous and have an erythematous base. Flexural lesions are usually more velvety and may become macerated and foul smelling.

During childhood, keratinocytic nevi continue to extend in size, and new lesions may appear. During puberty, those with abundant sebaceous or apocrine elements often enlarge rather dramatically. Head and face lesions are uncommon, but oral mucous membrane lesions may present as papillary projections on the lip or in the mouth. Trunk lesions run in transverse bands or in an S-shaped curve but do not cross the midline. Lesions near the midline of the trunk and on the extremities are usually arranged more vertically. The development of nodules or ulcers in the lesion suggests neoplastic changes.

The ocular and other features of verrucous epidermal nevi are considered under epidermal nevus syndrome.

Organoid Nevus (Nevus Sebaceus of Jadassohn, Sebaceous Nevus)

Organoid nevi (nevus sebaceus of Jadassohn, sebaceous nevus) are congenital hamartomatous lesions composed primarily of sebaceous glands. When associated with other developmental defects (e.g., central nervous system, skeletal system, and eye), they are considered part of the epidermal nevus syndrome (see later). They usually occur sporadically.

The lesions are slightly raised, round, oval, or linear circumscribed plaques that vary from pinkish to tan in color and are usually found on the scalp, around the ears, temples, forehead, and central part of the face. At puberty, they become more elevated and thickened. Ulcerated or exophytic lesions suggest malignant degeneration.

Epidermal Nevus Syndrome (Feuerstein–Mims Syndrome)

Epidermal nevus syndrome (Feuerstein–Mims syndrome) comprises an epidermal nevus associated with one or more significant neurologic, ocular, or skeletal deformities. The syndrome is often only fully expressed during childhood.

Epidermal nevi are usually large and quite extensive. Associated abnormalities include angiomatous nevi, hypochromic nevi, café-au-lait macules, congenital melanocytic nevi, dermatomegaly, and alopecia. Uncommonly, keratoacanthomas, squamous cell carcinomas, and basal cell epitheliomas develop in linear epidermal nevi.

Neurologic abnormalities include focal and generalized epilepsy, mental retardation, spastic hemi- and tetraparesis, and hearing loss. The abnormalities arise from vascular malformations, cortical atrophy, hemimegaloencephaly, porencephaly, intracranial hamartomas, and encephaloceles. Skeletal abnormalities include kyphosis and scoliosis, cystic and lytic bone changes, syndactyly, and short extremities.

Other associated abnormalities include bilateral sensorineural deafness, cardiac and genitourinary abnormalities, endocrine disorders, and internal malignancies.

Ocular Features

Ocular abnormalities occur in about one-third of patients. The major ocular abnormality is caused by an epidermal nevus of the eyelid or conjunctiva that may prevent lid closure. Other abnormalities include lid, iris, and retinal colobomas; conjunctival lipodermoids (Fig. 9-7) and choristomas; corneal opacities or dermoids; cataracts; peripapillary atrophy of the optic nerve, unilateral pseudopapilledema, microphthalmia, megalophthalmos; and cortical blindness.

FAT NEVI

Encephalocraniocutaneous Lipomatosis

In encephalocraniocutaneous lipomatosis, multiple unilateral, lipomatous hamartomas are usually present at birth. They appear as soft, skin-colored or yellow, domed-shaped papules, nodules, or plaques, which are confined to the head and neck. Local skin hypoplasia and unilateral alopecia may also be seen.

Associated central nervous system findings include mental retardation; epilepsy; unilateral cerebral hemiatrophy, porencephaly, defective opercularization of the insula; and bony protuberances of the skull.

Ocular Features

Conjunctival choristomas and a cloudy cornea may be found.

HEMANGIOMAS, VASCULAR MALFORMATIONS, AND ANGIOKERATOMAS

Hemangiomas are common, benign neoplasms composed of newly formed mature blood vessels that are present at birth. They are classified as capillary, cavernous, and mixed hemangiomas, and characteristically have a proliferative and an involutional phase.

Vascular malformations represent vascular development defects and, histologically, lack endothelial cell proliferation. They have no tendency to resolve spontaneously and often develop after birth.

Angiokeratomas represent a vascular malformation of the superficial dermal vessels that results in vascular ectasia and some hyperkeratosis.

Hemangiomas

Hemangiomas (angiomatous nevi) are the most common tumors of the newborn. They are sometimes associated with angiomas of other organs, including the eye. Multiple cutaneous hemangiomas occur in about 20% of cases.

Superficial Hemangiomas

Superficial hemangiomas (strawberry hemangiomas or nevi) comprise about 65% of hemangiomas(Fig. 9-8). They are more common in infants of lower gestational age and are more common in girls. About 60% occur on the head and neck. The precursor lesions are often present at birth and appear as a hyperemic macular area (salmon patch) or a macular area of pallor (nevus anemicus). Usually, small strawberry hemangiomas are present at birth; others develop early in life and continue to develop for several years. The lesions usually remain small. They are soft, sharply circumscribed, domed, oval or round, bright-red or purple-red lesions and have many capillaries protruding from the surface. Usually, they begin to spontaneously involute after 1 to 1.5 years, as characterized by the color fading from red to pink to white and the surface becoming wrinkled. About half of the lesions resolve by the age of 5, and 70% to 90% resolve by the age of 7.

Strawberry eyelid hemangiomas are often associated with conjunctival hemangiomas or hemangiomas of the anterior orbit. Retinal capillary hemangiomas appear as globular, red-orange tumors with dilated and tortuous feeder vessels. They are usually found in the von Hippel–Lindau syndrome. Capillary hemangiomas of the optic nerve head associated with central nervous system involvement have also been reported.

Mixed Hemangiomas

Mixed hemangiomas have both superficial and deep elements but may be predominantly deep or superficial. The superficial portion is usually located centrally and has the characteristics of a strawberry angioma. The deep portion is usually evident in the periphery and appears as a round, bluish mass that underlies normal skin.

Cavernous Hemangiomas

Deep hemangiomas (cavernous hemangiomas or deep angiomatous nevi) are located intradermally and subcutaneously. They appear as a round, bluish mass underlying normal skin and on palpation feel like a "bag of worms" with a smooth surface. They are usually small and hardly noticeable at birth, then enlarge rapidly between 1 and 6 months of age (Fig. 9-9). Often they develop after the second decade. Sometimes they involute spontaneously but usually not as completely as strawberry hemangiomas.

Ocular cavernous hemangiomas include the following:

1. Lid hemangiomas similar to other cavernous hemangiomas (Fig. 9-10).
2. Iris cavernous hemangiomas with associated recurrent hyphema.
3. Orbital cavernous hemangiomas usually occurring in middle-aged women, which present as benign, well-encapsulated, slowly progressive neoplasms.

4. Lacrimal fossa hemangiomas presenting as a benign mixed lacrimal gland tumor with progressive proptosis.
5. Retinal cavernous hemangiomas presenting as grapelike clusters of dilated retinal sacs and only minimal alteration of the adjacent arterioles and venules.
6. Optic nerve cavernous hemangiomas. Optic nerve or retinal hemangiomas associated with central nervous system hemangiomas are considered as neuro-oculocutaneous syndromes.

VASCULAR MALFORMATIONS

Vascular malformations present as capillary, mixed, venous, or lymphatic malformations.

Capillary Malformations

Salmon Patch

Salmon patches usually occur on the nape of the neck but may also occur on the forehead, glabella, upper eyelids, upper lip, and, occasionally, other areas. They are irregular, dull, pinkish-red areas that contain fine linear telangiectasia. Most, except the nuchal lesions, fade within 1 year.

Port-Wine Stain (Nevus Flammeus)

Port-wine stains (nevus flammeus) usually involve the face, sometimes the trunk, and, less frequently, other sites. They are usually unilateral and respect the midline. Facial lesions usually correspond to the areas supplied by the sensory branches of the trigeminal nerve. They are pale pink to deep red or purple and progressively darken with time. At first the surface is smooth but later becomes thickened and raised.

Sturge–Weber Syndrome (Encephalofacial Angiomatosis)

The Sturge–Weber syndrome is characterized by a port-wine stain, which almost always involves the area supplied by the ophthalmic and maxillary branches of the trigeminal nerve (Fig. 9-11); vascular malformations of the leptomeninges of the homolateral side; and sometimes vascular malformations of the homolateral eye. The port-wine stain may be only several centimeters in size or it may involve large areas of the scalp, face, neck, trunk (Fig. 9-12), and even the upper and lower extremities. It almost always involves the forehead and upper eyelid (Fig. 9-13). Facial hemihypertrophy often occurs with time. Mucosal lesions of the lips, buccal mucosa, gingiva, and sometimes palate occur in about 25% of patients.

The neurologic findings include a leptomeningeal angioma overlying the occipital and parietal lobe with underlying cerebral atrophy and calcification, epilepsy, mental retardation, macrocephaly, and contralateral hemiplegia.

Ocular Features

The ocular findings include dilated conjunctival vessels or an abnormal plexus of episcleral vessels (69%) (Fig. 9-14), heterochromia irides, coloboma of the iris and optic nerve, glaucoma (71%) (Fig. 9-15), tortuous retinal vessels, retinal aneurysms, retinal detachment, and choroidal angioma (55%). Hemianopia and cortical blindness may occur arising from cerebral atrophy. The choroidal angioma causes retinal elevation and may lead to cystoid macular changes and reduced vision in adults.

The glaucoma often develops before the age of 2.

Klippel–Trenaunay Syndrome (Angioosteohypertrophy Syndrome)

In Klippel–Trenaunay syndrome (angioosteohypertrophy syndrome) one sees a triad of nevus flammeus, venous malformations, and soft-tissue hypertrophy. Parkes–Weber is appended to the diagnosis when there is an associated arteriovenous fistula. The vascular malformation most commonly involves an extremity (Fig. 9-16).

Phakomatosis Pigmentovascularis

The unwieldy term *phakomatosis pigmentovascularis* describes a syndrome manifested by a port-wine stain, oculocutaneous melanosis (nevus of Ota and Ito) (see Chapter 6), café-au-lait spots or nevus spilus, and neurologic involvement manifested by epilepsy and hemiplegia. Iris mammillations in this syndrome are explained by their frequent association with nevus of Ota.

Proteus Syndrome

The Proteus syndrome is characterized by verrucous epidermal and angiomatous nevi, lipoma-like subcutaneous hamartomas, and asymmetric hypertrophy of almost any part of the body. The verrucous nevi of the head and neck are usually sebaceous nevi and in other areas are usually linear verrucous nevi. Other findings include port-wine stains, angiokeratomas, subcutaneous and sometimes dermal angiomatous nevi, cavernous and circumscripta types of lymphangiomas, café-au-lait spots, and areas of hyper- and hypopigmentation. The lipoma-like subcutaneous hamartomas are very common.

The hypertrophy occurs in almost any area of the body and includes facial hypertrophy. Other findings include skeletal abnormalities, myopathy, pelvic lipomatosis, and testicular tumors.

Ocular Features

Ocular abnormalities include epibulbar tumors, macrophthalmia, strabismus, and cataract.

Robert Syndrome (Hypomelia–Hypotrichosis–Facial Hemangioma Syndrome)

Robert syndrome (hypomelia–hypotrichosis–facial hemangioma syndrome) is probably autosomal recessive and is characterized by

1. A pale port-wine stain extending from the forehead onto the nose and philtrum.
2. Cleft lip and often a cleft palate.
3. Silver to blond, sparse hair.
4. Limb reduction syndrome and marked retardation of growth.
5. Ocular findings of hypertelorism, shallow orbits with prominent eyes, and bluish sclera.

Wyburn–Mason Syndrome (Bonnet–Dechaume–Blanc Syndrome)

The Wyburn–Mason syndrome (Bonnet–Dechaume–Blanc syndrome) comprises unilateral retinal arteriovenous (A-V) malformations, ipsilateral aneurysmal A-V malformations usually of the midbrain, and ipsilateral port-wine stains.

Manifestations of central nervous system A-V malformations include headache, seizures, mental retardation, papilledema, optic atrophy, cranial nerve palsies, hemianopia, and hemiparesis.

A-V malformations of nasopharynx may cause epistaxis.

The ocular A-V malformations may involve the following:

1. The lid and orbit, causing ptosis, dilated conjunctival vessels, proptosis, and bruits.
2. The retina, usually in the posterior pole and superior temporal quadrant. The findings are divided into
   a. Grade I, representing anastomosis between a retinal arteriole and venule.
   b. Grade II, representing anastomosis between a branch retinal artery and a branch vein.
   c. Grade III, representing diffuse, marked dilatation and tortuosity of the entire retinal vascular system (Fig. 9-17).
3. The optic nerve, optic chiasm, and optic tract.

Bregeat Syndrome (Ocular Neuroangiomatosis)

The manifestations of Bregeat syndrome include a port-wine stain of the forehead and adjacent scalp; contralateral thalamencephalic angiomatosis, involving the choroidal plexus; angiomatosis, presenting as subconjunctival masses at the limbus; and orbital angiomatosis, causing exophthalmos on the same side as the neurologic lesions.

Von Hippel–Lindau Disease

Von Hippel–Lindau disease is autosomal dominant with variable penetrance and expressivity. It is characterized by bilateral retinal angiomatosis; cerebellar, medullary, or spinal hemangioblastomas; cysts or angiomatous tumors of the viscera; and port-wine stains. Café-au-lait spots may also be found, and patients have a predisposition to develop renal cell carcinoma and pheochromocytomas.

Systemic Findings

The central nervous system hemangioblastomas are sometimes recognized about the fourth decade of life, but often not until after death. Cerebellar hemangioblastomas may cause signs of cerebellar dysfunction or increased intracranial pressure. Medullary hemangioblastomas may compress the brain stem, causing death. The spinal lesions are often asymptomatic or cause symptoms suggestive of syringomyelia.

Visceral abnormalities include renal cell carcinomas; pheochromocytomas; pancreatic carcinoma, hepatic and renal angiomas; cysts and adenomas of the kidney and pancreas; and adenomas of the epididymis.

Ocular Findings

The retinal angiomas develop during early adult life and cause visual impairment and sometimes blindness. They are usually located in the retinal mid-periphery but sometimes are located adjacent to the nerve head (Fig. 9-18). They are 30% to 50% bilateral. Early lesions may appear as a microaneurysm. Mature lesions appear as globular, slightly raised, pink tumors with dilated feeder vessels entering and emerging from the periphery. Lipid is often deposited around the lesion or in the macular area.

Beckwith–Wiedemann Syndrome (Exomphalos–Macroglossia–Gigantism Syndrome)

Beckwith–Wiedemann syndrome (exomphalos–macroglossia–gigantism) is autosomal dominant and has variable expression. It is characterized by overgrowth of the body and viscera. The infant often presents with exomphalos, macroglossia, and large kidneys.

The cutaneous and ocular findings include a port-wine stain of the central forehead and upper eyelids and linear indentations of the earlobes.

MIXED VASCULAR MALFORMATIONS

Mixed vascular malformations comprise disorders in which there are both capillary and venous malformations. They are uncommon and usually are sporadic.

Reticulate Vascular Nevus (Congenital Livedo Reticularis)

In reticulate vascular nevus (congenital livedo reticularis), an unusual condition, small to large areas of skin are pale red to deep purple. Usually, the involved skin has multiple telangiectasias and may be atrophic. Facial hyperemia and port-wine stains often involve the forehead. Congenital glaucoma may be observed. Other abnormalities include macrocephaly, facial hemiatrophy, and shortened and reduced girth of an extremity.

VENOUS MALFORMATIONS

Blue Rubber–Bleb Nevus Syndrome

Blue rubber–bleb nevus syndrome is autosomal dominant, but sporadic cases are common. It is characterized by multiple venous malformations of the skin, gastrointestinal tract, and sometimes other areas.

The cutaneous lesions present as blue or purple, soft, rubbery nodules. Sometimes they are deep and then present with only a bluish discoloration. The lesions look and feel like a rubber nipple and are easily compressed, leaving a flaccid, wrinkled appearance to the overlying skin. They vary in size from pinhead to several centimeters in diameter and may be single or multiple. Lesions occur anywhere on the body surface (Fig. 9-19), the mucosa of the lips, mouth, gastrointestinal tract, and the glans penis. They often become spontaneously painful about the time of puberty, especially at night. Recurrent bleeding may cause severe anemia.

Other venous malformation may occur at other sites, including the brain, meninges, nasopharynx, lungs, heart, liver, spleen, urinary tract, muscles, and joints.

Lesions of the eyelid, conjunctiva, iris, and retina have been observed. Intermittent exophthalmos arising from an orbital lesion has been described.

Riley–Smith Syndrome (Macrocephaly with Pseudopapilledema and Hemangiomas)

Riley–Smith syndrome (macrocephaly with pseudopapilledema and hemangiomas) is autosomal dominant and is characterized by macrocephaly, pseudopapilledema, and multiple, cavernous hemangiomas. The skin lesions usually involve the abdominal wall, hands, feet, and thighs. They are brownish-purple, mobile nodules measuring 0.5 to 2.0 cm in diameter and are located in the dermis and subcutaneously. Sometimes the lesions are tender.

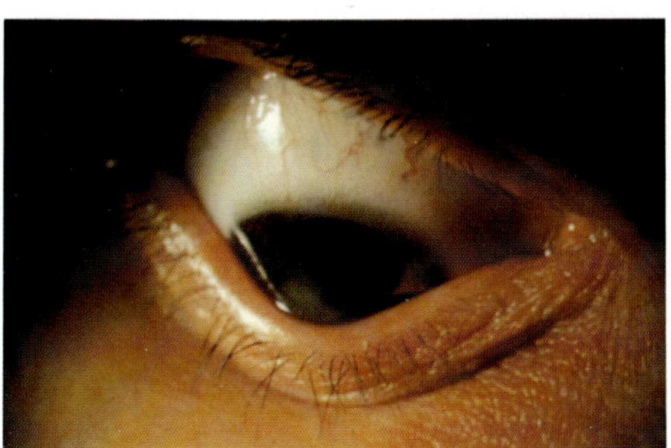

FIGURE 9-1. Keratoconus in Down syndrome. It is manifested in this photograph by the tenting outward of the lower eyelid caused by the cornea (Munson sign). The central opacity has resulted from acute imbibition of aqueous.

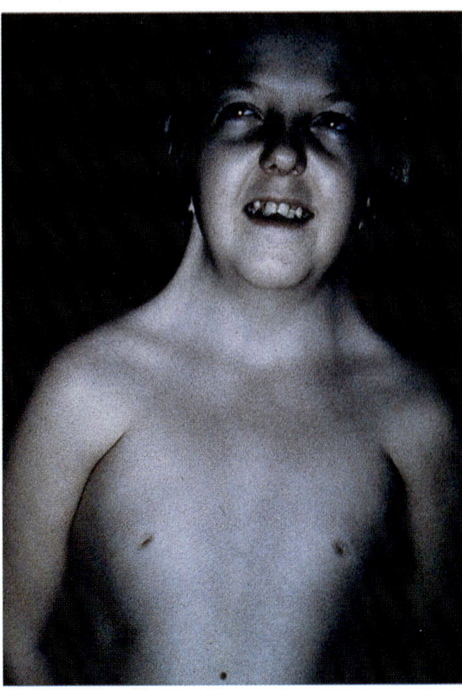

FIGURE 9-2. Turner syndrome. Note striking ebbing of the neck, small mandible, widely spaced nipples and shield chest.

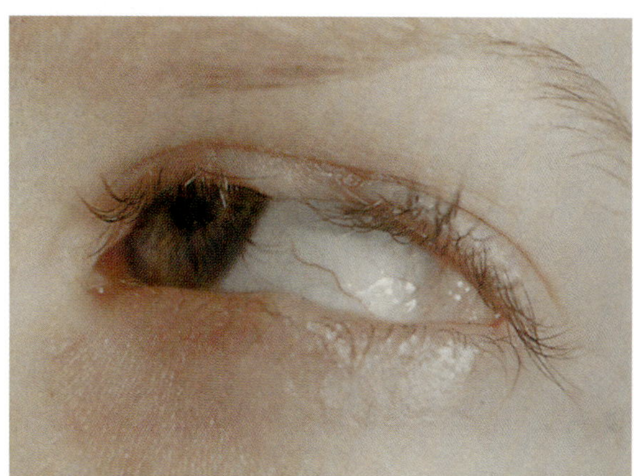
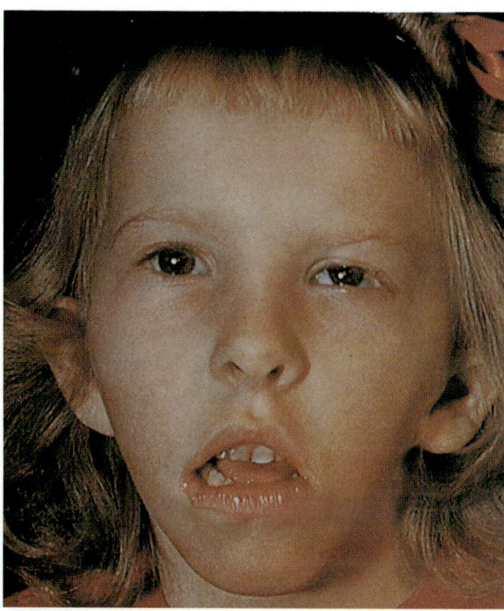

FIGURE 9-3. Orbital distortion with antimongoloid palpebral fissures and ptosis in mandibulo-facial dysostosis.

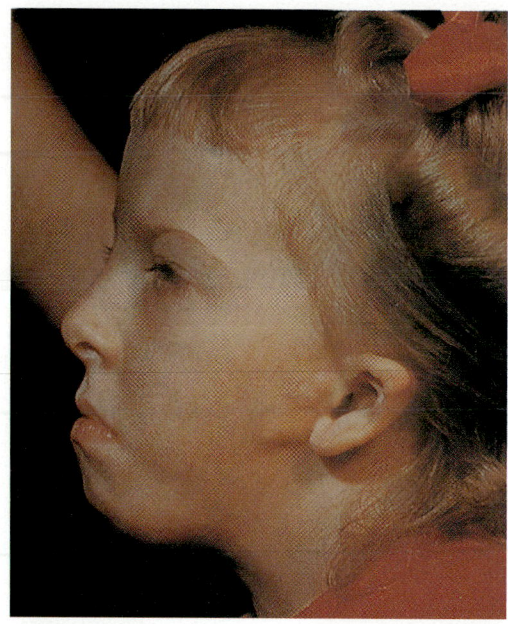

FIGURE 9-4. Malformed ears and hypoplasia of the zygomatic arch in mandibulofacial dysostosis. (Photograph courtesy of Dr. Alson E. Braley.)

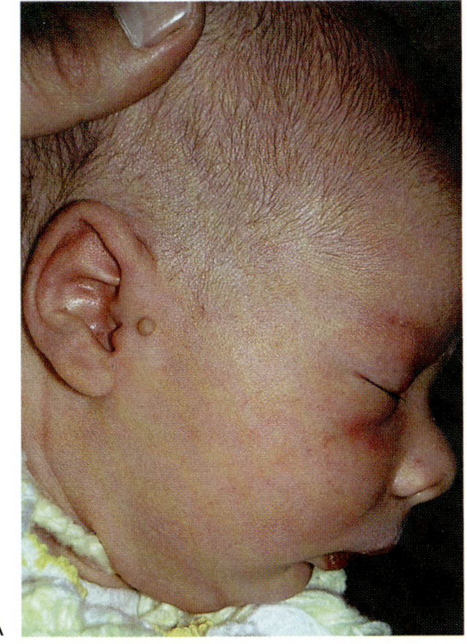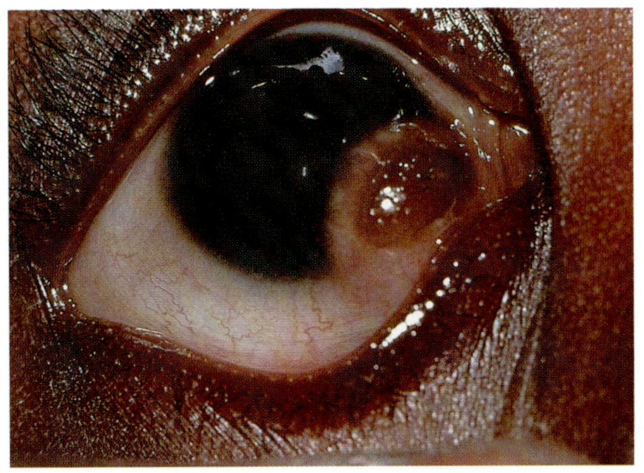

FIGURE 9-5. A: Preauricular skin tag in Goldenhar syndrome. **B:** Epibulbar dermoid. Although usually at the inferior temporal limbus, this dermoid is found in the inferior nasal quadrant. (Photograph courtesy of Dr. Larry Schwab.)

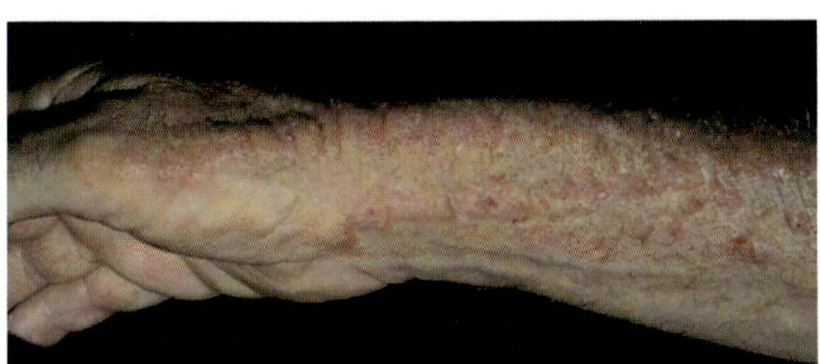

FIGURE 9-6. Verrucous epidermal nevus of the arm.

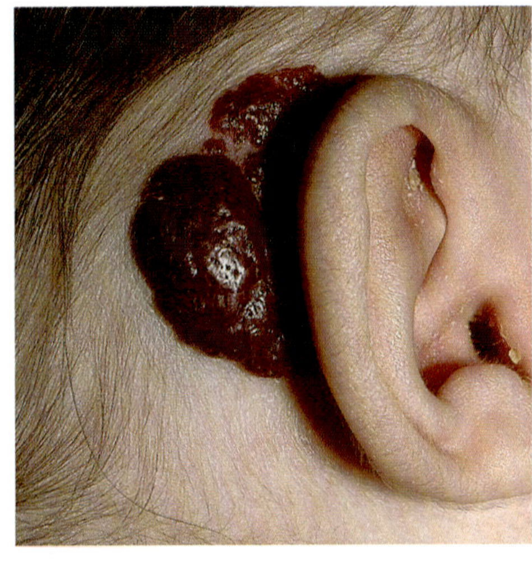

FIGURE 9-7. Strawberry hemangioma in a 10-week-old infant.

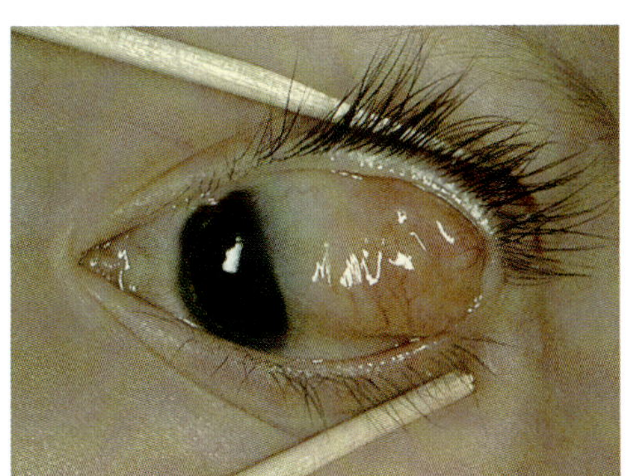

FIGURE 9-8. Conjunctival lipodermoid of the superior–temporal quadrant in a patient with epidermal nervus syndrome.

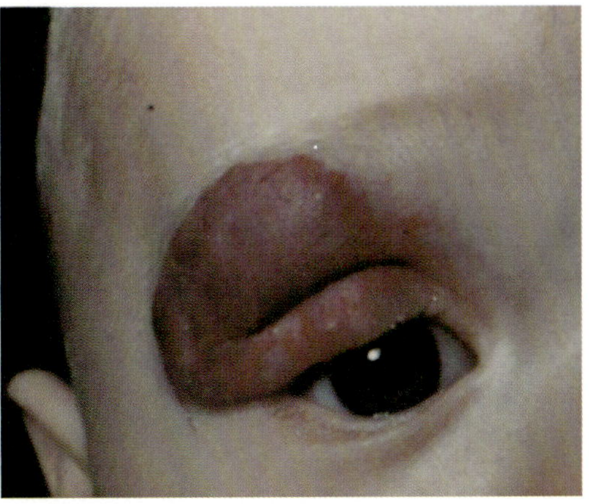

FIGURE 9-9. Cavernous hemangioma of the lid in an infant.

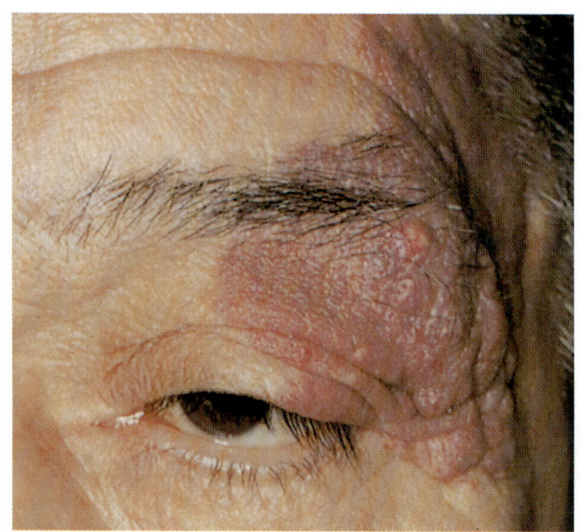

FIGURE 9-10. Cavernous hemangioma of the lid in an adult.

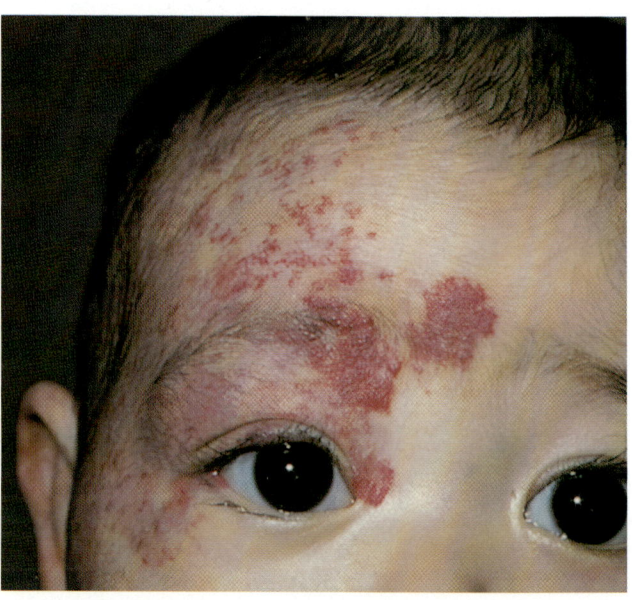

FIGURE 9-11. Sturge–Weber syndrome in an infant.

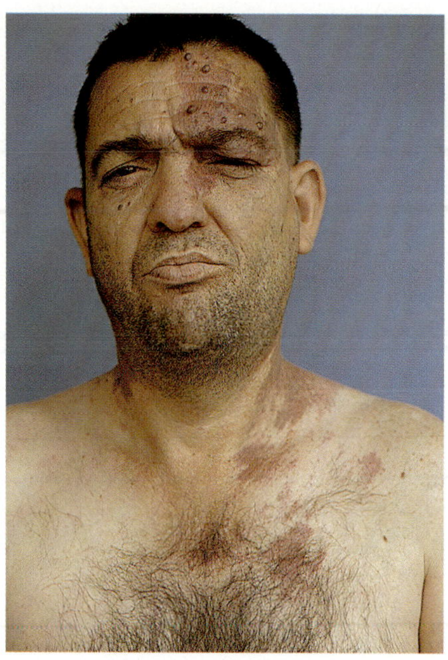

FIGURE 9-12. Sturge–Weber syndrome with lesions extending on the trunk. The patient had epilepsy and mental retardation.

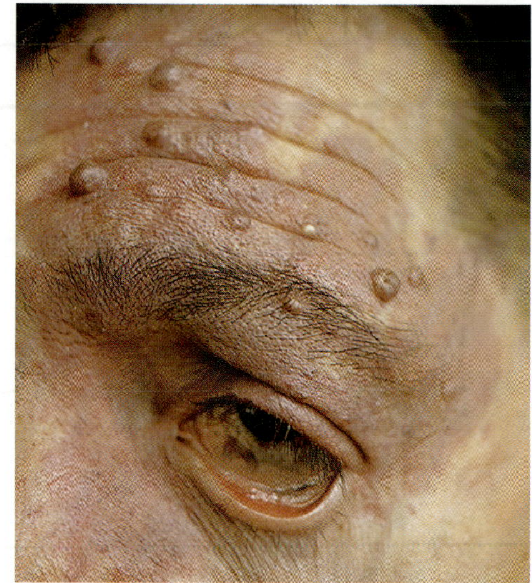

FIGURE 9-13. Close-up of the eye in the same patient as Figure 9-12.

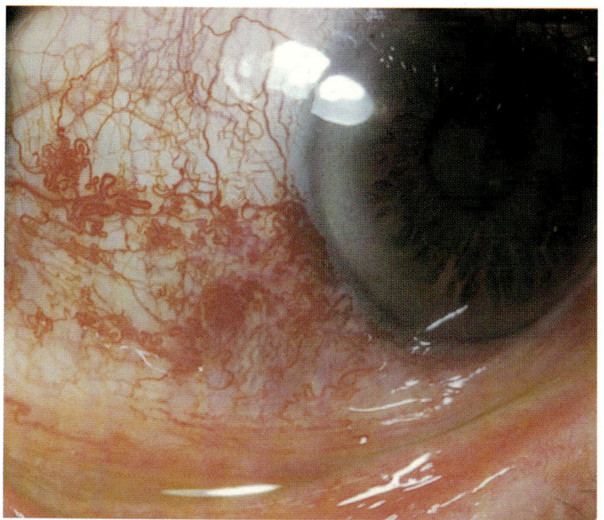

FIGURE 9-14. Hemangioma of the conjunctiva associated with port-wine stain in Sturge–Weber syndrome.

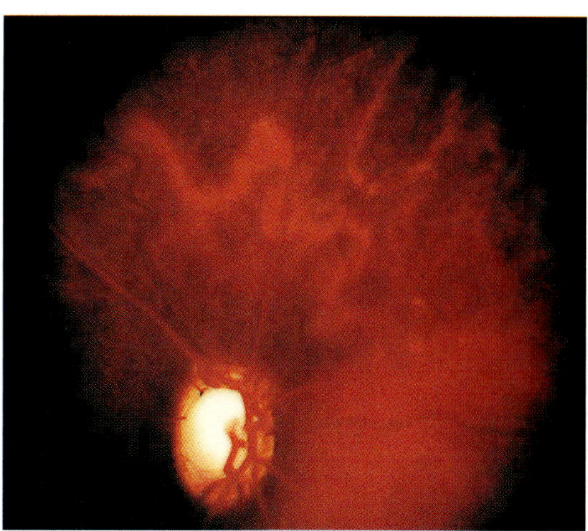

FIGURE 9-15. Glaucomatous cupping in Sturge–Weber syndrome.

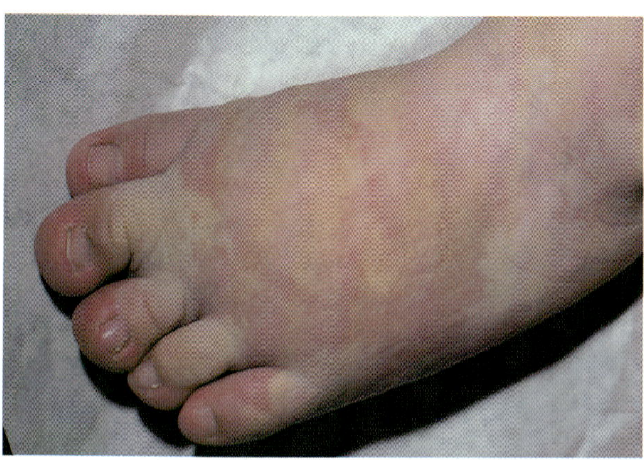

FIGURE 9-16. Klipple–Trenany–Parkes–Weber syndrome showing enlargement of foot and several toes due to arteriovenous shunting.

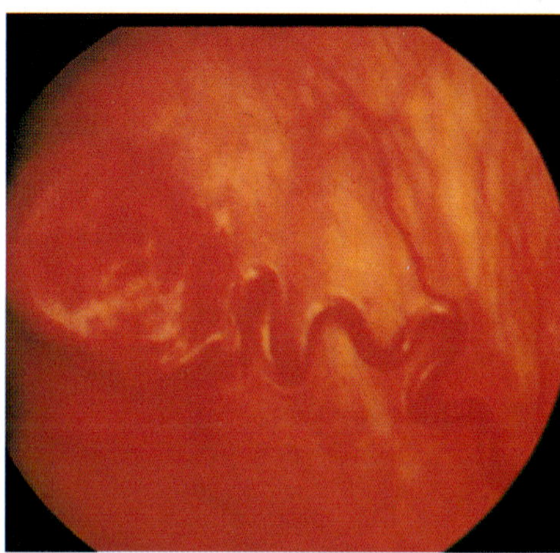

FIGURE 9-17. Grade III retinal changes in Wyburn–Mason syndrome. (Photograph courtesy of Dr. John Belmont.)

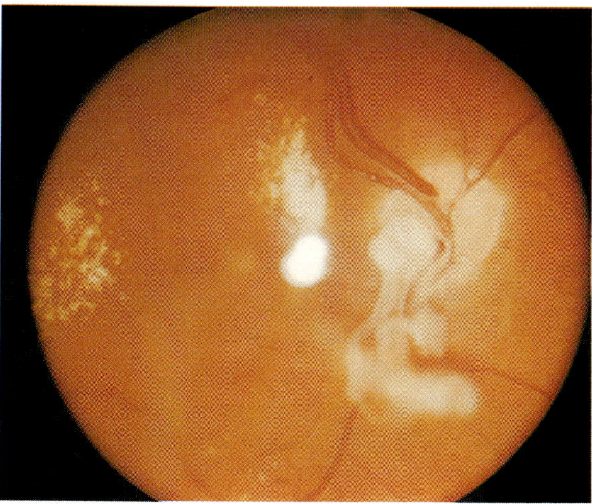

FIGURE 9-18. Feeder vessels and lipid deposition in von Hippel–Lindau disease. (Photograph courtesy of Dr. Alson E. Braley.)

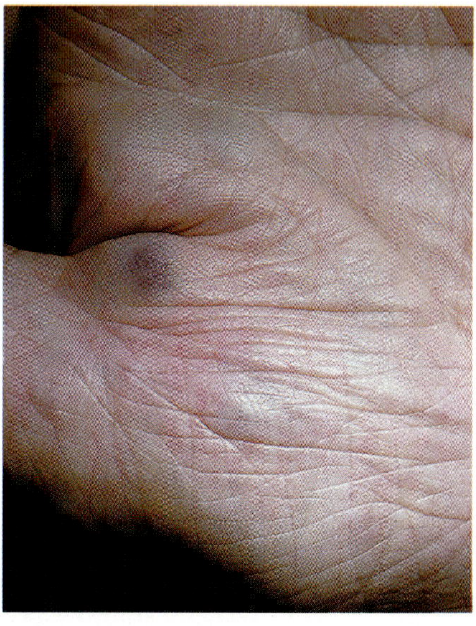

FIGURE 9-19. Blue rubber–bleb nevus of the hand.

THE GENODERMATOSES

The genodermatoses represent hereditary skin disorders that are determined by a single gene.

GENODERMATOSES ASSOCIATED WITH DNA INSTABILITY

Those genodermatoses that share the feature of increased risk of malignancy from chromosomal instability due to irradiation or mutagenic chemicals include Bloom syndrome, Cockayne syndrome, xeroderma pigmentosum, dyskeratosis congenita (Chapter 6), progeria (Chapter 12), ataxia telangiectasia (Chapter 14), and Fanconi anemia.

Bloom Syndrome (Congenital Telangiectatic Erythema and Stunted Growth)

Bloom syndrome (congenital telangiectatic erythema and stunted growth) is autosomal recessive. It is more common in Ashkenazi Jews and is also widely distributed throughout Japan. It is characterized by photosensitivity; telangiectatic facial erythema; pre- and postnatal growth retardation; elongated head; narrow, delicate face; prominent nose; hypoplastic malar and mandibular regions; and an abnormal immune response.

Less common findings include peripheral limb defects, congenital heart disease, pulmonary fibrosis, bronchiectasis, aborted testicular development, and mild mental retardation. Many patients develop malignancies during childhood, and about 25% of adult patients develop lymphoproliferative neoplasms, epithelial neoplasms (especially gastrointestinal), or acute leukemia.

Skin Features

A telangiectatic facial eruption begins during the first two summers as red macules or plaques of the nose and cheeks, and sometimes other exposed areas. Blisters, fissures, and hemorrhages of the exposed skin and the lips may also occur. The skin changes improve with time, leaving mild scarring, depigmentation, and atrophy.

Other skin features include café-au-lait spots, keratosis pilaris, ichthyotic skin, acanthosis nigricans, and hypertrichosis.

Ocular Features

Erythema and telangiectasis of the lower lid and loss of lashes are common. Conjunctival crusting and splitting and chronic conjunctivitis sometimes occur.

Cockayne Syndrome

Cockayne syndrome is autosomal recessive. Its features are usually evident before the age of 3. It is characterized by photosensitivity; dwarfism; decreased or absent subcutaneous fat; extensive CNS demyelinization with ataxia, sensorineural hearing loss, and mental retardation; microcephaly; disproportionately long extremities, large hands and feet; limited joint mobility; retinal atrophy; and intracranial calcification. The patients have small, thin, beaked noses; large, prominent ears; and a small mandible.

Skin Features

Photosensitivity leads to midfacial erythema followed by scarring and pigment alteration, but the risk of skin cancer is not increased. Later, the photosensitivity may disappear. The hair may be sparse and prematurely gray. Delayed dentition and multiple caries are common.

Ocular Features

Ocular findings include photophobia, band-shaped keratopathy, irregular or unresponsive pupils, hypoplastic irides, cataracts, vitreous floaters, nystagmus, and enophthalmos.

Pigmentary retinal degeneration is a cardinal feature and is manifested by fine, granular, pigmented areas scattered throughout the fundus and narrowing of the vessels. There is no perivascular sheathing or bone corpuscle formation. Secondary optic atrophy may occur early in life.

Xeroderma Pigmentosum

Xeroderma pigmentosum (XP) is autosomal recessive. It is characterized by photosensitivity, pigmentary skin changes, telangiectasia, premature skin aging, ultraviolet-induced neoplasia, and abnormal DNA repair. There are eight subtypes: complementation (XP, A through G) and subtype (XP variant). About 20% of patients develop progressive neurologic degeneration leading to mental retardation, sensorineural deafness, speech difficulties, ataxia, spasticity, and hyporeflexia. (The *de Sanctis–Cacchione syndrome* is characterized by XP, severe mental deficiency, microcephaly, dwarfism, hypogonadism, deafness, ataxia, and choreoathetosis.) Death often occurs by the age of 20 and, occasionally, by the age of 10 from metastases of squamous cell carcinomas or malignant melanomas.

Skin Features

XP progresses relentlessly in an orderly fashion through six successive stages. The child appears normal at birth.

Stage 1. The erythematosquamous stage occurs during infancy. Sun exposure causes erythema, inflammation, and bullae of the skin.

Stage 2. The pigmentation stage develops between 6 and 36 months of age. Freckles develop on the face and hands and other exposed areas. At first they are small and may fade; later, they increase in size and number and become permanent.

Stage 3. The telangiectatic stage develops soon after stage 2 and is manifested by telangiectases, small angiomas, and sometimes vesiculobullous lesions in areas between the freckles.

Stage 4. The atrophic stage is characterized by atrophic, hypopigmented areas; superficial ulcers that heal by scarring; moderate to marked deformity, especially of the midfacial region; and thin, dry skin (Fig. 10-1).

Stage 5. The benign keratoses stage.

Stage 6. The malignant stage is characterized by malignancies in the sun-exposed areas. They include basal cell epitheliomas, which occur early in life (median age, 8); squamous cell carcinomas; malignant melanomas; isolated metastatic lesions with undetermined primary sites; angiosarcomas, fibrosarcomas, and oral cancers such as squamous cell carcinoma of the tongue.

Ocular Features

Ocular involvement follows very closely stages 1 through 6 (see the preceding).

Stage 1. Photophobia, blepharitis, conjunctivitis, and sometimes keratitis and iritis.

Stage 2. Freckles and achromic spots on the skin of the lids and conjunctiva.

Stage 3. Telangiectasis of the lid and conjunctiva and corneal neovascularization.

Stage 4. Atrophy of the lid skin, sometimes of the entire lower eyelid; ectropion; madarosis; conjunctival exposure, drying, and scarring; and corneal scarring and opacity.

Stage 5. Benign keratosis, papillomatous growths, and angiomas of the skin of the lid. Lid-margin papillomatous lesions may cause irritation and severe photophobia. Other findings include pterygium, pinguecula, symblepharon, ankyloblepharon, corneal staphylomas, and iris fibromas and papillomas. Lower lid destruction may lead to lagophthalmos.

Stage 6. Superficial ulcerations and carcinomatous degeneration (basal cell epitheliomas; occasionally, squamous cell carcinomas) of the lids. Ectropion occurs from contraction of scars. Malignant melanomas of the iris may be extensive. Conjunctival and corneal neoplasms include intraepithelial epitheliomas, squamous cell carcinomas, sarcomas, malignant melanomas, and malignant fibrous histiocytomas.

ECTODERMAL DYSPLASIA

Ectodermal dysplasia (ED) comprises a group of heterogeneous and complex disorders with various inheritance patterns and abnormalities of one or more ectodermal structures (hair, nails, teeth, and sweat glands.) It is usually classified by the absence or presence of sweating and the inheritance pattern.

Hypohidrotic Ectodermal Dysplasia

Christ–Siemens–Touraine Syndrome

The Christ–Siemens–Touraine syndrome is X-linked recessive. Patients have hypotrichosis, hypodontia, and partial or complete absence of sweat glands. Less common features include mild mental retardation, atrophic rhinitis, asthma, chronic obstructive airway disease, failure of breast development, and depression of cell-mediated immunity.

Patients with the complete syndrome (Fig. 10-2) have prominent frontal ridges; large ears; saddle nose; high cheekbones; thick, everted muscular lips; and a prominent chin. The skin is soft, dry, thin; appears atrophic; and has a tendency to peal. Fine wrinkles, especially around the eyes, are common, and patients often have atopic eczema. Palmar and plantar hyperkeratosis may be evident. Sparseness of all hair is an essential feature of hypohidrotic ectodermal dysplasia. The scalp hair is fine, is dry, and remains short.

Most patients have dental anomalies, including decreased number of teeth; small, pointed, peg-shaped teeth (Fig. 10-3); atrophic gums; and salivary gland hypoplasia with reduced salivation (Fig. 10-3). Five percent of these patients have thin, brittle, or ridged nails.

Ocular Findings

The eyebrows are sparse or absent, but the lashes are usually normal. The meibomian glands are reduced or absent. The conjunctiva is dry, and conjunctivitis is common. Decreased or absent tearing arises from lacrimal gland hypoplasia.

Corneal changes include a circumferential pannus; punctate epithelial keratopathy; intraepithelial cysts; and corneal thinning with stromal opacification. Congenital cataracts also occur.

Ectrodactyly–Ectodermal Dysplasia–Cleft Lip/Palate (EEC) Syndrome

The ectrodactyly–ectodermal dysplasia–cleft lip/palate (EEC) syndrome is autosomal dominant, has variable expression, and, in some families, shows lack of penetrance. It is characterized by ectrodactyly (lobster claw deformity) of the hands (Fig. 10-4); sparse, wiry, and hypopigmented hair; peg-shaped teeth with deficient enamel; and a cleft-lip (Fig. 10-5). Some patients have normal sweating.

Ocular Features

The ocular features include photophobia, absence or decreased numbers of meibomian glands, blepharitis (Fig. 10-5), absence of the lacrimal puncta, lacrimal duct stenosis, corneal scarring, and vascularization.

Rapp–Hodgkin Syndrome

The Rapp–Hodgkin syndrome is autosomal dominant. The general features include hypohidrosis; a high forehead; narrow nose; maxillary hypoplasia; small mouth; cleft lip, palate, or uvula; atretic ear canals; dysplastic eustachian orifices; hypospadias; and hypogenitalism.

The hair is sparse, brittle, and light-colored, with a "steel-wool" texture. Pili torti may also be present. Cicatricial scalp atrophy and a chronic palmar keratoderma have been observed. The nails are narrowed and dystrophic. The teeth are few in number and conical in shape.

Ocular Features

Ocular features include lacrimal punctal aplasia and ptosis.

Ectodermal Dysplasia, Greither Type

Greither type ectodermal dysplasia is autosomal dominant and is characterized by hypohidrosis, almost total alopecia, dystrophic nails, tooth loss, and palmoplantar keratoderma that progressively encroaches on the arms and legs, forming irregular keratotic patches by the time of puberty.

Ocular Features

The eye changes comprise corneal and lenticular opacities.

Ankyloblepharon–Ectodermal Defects–Cleft Lip and Palate (AEC Syndrome)

The ankyloblepharon–ectodermal defects–cleft lip and palate syndrome (AEC syndrome) is autosomal dominant with variable penetrance. It is characterized by fused eyelids (ankyloblepharon); cleft lip and palate; diminished sweating; absent or sparse and coarse hair; absent or dystrophic nails; and widely spaced, pointed teeth. The patients have a broad nasal bridge and sunken maxilla. Less common defects include supernumerary nipples, syndactyly, and heart deformities.

Ocular Features

The ocular abnormalities include ankyloblepharon, microphthalmia, ptosis, lacrimal duct stenosis, and Waardenburg syndrome (Chapter 6).

Ectodermal Dysplasia (Hay–Wells Type)

The ectodermal dysplasia (Hay–Wells type) syndrome is similar to the AEC syndrome. It is characterized by congenital threadlike lid adhesions (ankyloblepharon filiform adnatum); blepharitis; maxillary hypoplasia; cleft lip and palate; slight hypohidrosis; scalp infections; coarse, wiry, sparse hair; dystrophic nails; and hypodontia.

Hidrotic Ectodermal Dysplasia (Clouston Syndrome)

Hidrotic ectodermal dysplasia (Clouston syndrome) is autosomal dominant. It is characterized by normal sweating; nail dystrophy; skin thickening over the free edge of the nails, the finger joints and knuckles, and sometimes the knees and elbows; diffuse palmoplantar hyperkeratosis and fissuring; sparse, fine, pale, dry, brittle hair; and sometimes total alopecia. The outer two-thirds or all of the eyebrow is absent or sparse; the lashes and the vellus, pubic, and axillary hair are fine and sparse or absent.

Ocular Features

Ocular anomalies include conjunctivitis, pterygium, bilateral premature cataracts, and strabismus.

Dwarfism–Alopecia–Pseudoanodontia–Cutis Laxis

Dwarfism–alopecia–pseudoanodontia–cutis laxis is a rare autosomal recessive syndrome characterized by normal sweating, dwarfism, generalized alopecia, failure of both dentitions to erupt, cutis laxa and fragile skin, and hyperconvex nails. Other abnormalities include supraorbital ridges, a depressed nasal bridge, micrognathia, protruding lips, skeletal abnormalities, delayed bone maturation, and choanal atresia.

Ocular Features

The ocular findings include keratoconus and glaucoma.

Oculo-Dento-Digital Dysplasia (Oculo-Dento-Osseous Dysplasia, Gorlin Syndrome)

Oculo-dento-digital dysplasia (Gorlin syndrome) is autosomal dominant and has variable expressivity. The facies is manifested by small, closely set eyes; a thin nose without alar flare; a small mouth; and overlapping upper lip. The tooth enamel is hypoplastic, and the teeth are yellow. The scalp hair is sparse, short, dry, and lusterless. Digital syndactyly associated with camptodactyly of the radially deviated fifth finger is also present.

Ocular Features

Ocular abnormalities include hypertelorism, sparse or absent brows and lashes, microcornea, and iris malformation.

Tricho-Oculo-Dermo-Vertebral Syndrome

Tricho-oculo-dermo-vertebral syndrome is characterized by kyphoscoliosis; short stature; sparse, dry, and brittle hair; dystrophic nails; and plantar keratoderma. Ocular findings include cataracts.

Curly Hair–Ankyloblepharon–Nail Dysplasia Syndrome (CHANDS)

The curly hair–ankyloblepharon–nail dysplasia syndrome (CHANDS) is probably autosomal recessive. The patient has curly hair and hypoplastic nails. The teeth are normal.

Ocular Features

The ocular findings are restricted to ankyloblepharon (fused eyelids).

Dento-Oculo-Cutaneous Syndrome

The dento-oculo-cutaneous syndrome is characterized by skin pigmentation and induration over the interphalangeal joints of the fingers, dystrophic nails with longitudinal ridging and distal splitting, taurodontia, pyramidal or fused molar roots, and a wide, thick filtrum.

Ocular Features

Ocular anomalies include lower lid ectropion.

Ectodermal Dysplasia with Cataracts and Hearing Defects (Marshall Syndrome)

The syndrome of ectodermal dysplasia with cataracts and hearing defects (Marshall syndrome) is characterized by mild tooth defects, deafness, mental and growth retardation, an underdeveloped maxilla, a saddle nose, and bilateral cataracts.

Growth Retardation–Alopecia–Pseudoanodontia–Optic Atrophy (GAPO Syndrome)

The syndrome of growth retardation, alopecia, pseudoanodontia, and optic atrophy (GAPO syndrome) is autosomal recessive and is characterized by hydrocephalus, almost complete alopecia, growth retardation, and a peculiar geriatric facial appearance, with low-set ears; high, arched palate; and unerupted teeth (pseudoanodontia).

Ocular Features

Ocular findings include keratoconus, papilledema associated with the hydrocephalus, secondary optic atrophy, and glaucoma.

Cowden Syndrome (Multiple Hamartoma Syndrome)

Cowden syndrome (multiple hamartoma syndrome) is an uncommon autosomal dominant syndrome with variable expressivity. It is characterized by mucocutaneous papillomatosis, fibromatosis, fibrocystic breast disease with massive breast hyperplasia, and often breast cancer, as well as hamartomas of many organ systems, such as thyroid adenomas or goiters. Craniomegaly may also occur.

Skin Features

Skin-colored lichenoid papules (trichilemmomas or related benign tumors) (Fig. 10-6) develop on the lids, nose, ears, and areas around the eyes and mouth, usually during the second or third decade. The lesions often give a cobblestone appearance.

Acrokeratosis verruciformis-like lesions (warty keratosis of the extremities) or translucent keratoses develop on the palms and soles and on the palmar and plantar aspects of the fingers and toes. Other skin findings include ganglioneuromas, hemangiomas, multiple angiomas, angiolipomas, lipomas, epidermoid cysts, vitiligo, café-au-lait spots, and, rarely, malignant melanomas and squamous cell carcinomas. Verrucous or papillomatous lesions also develop on the oral, oropharyngeal, and laryngeal mucosa.

Ocular Features

Lichenoid papules often occur on the eyelids. Infrequently, retinal gliomas are also found.

Nail–Patella Syndrome [Hereditary Osteoonychodysplasia (Fong Syndrome)]

The nail–patella syndrome [hereditary osteoonychodysplasia (Fong syndrome)] is autosomal dominant and has variable expressivity. The nails, especially the thumbnails, are dystrophic (absent, small, thickened, or depressed). Some patients have palmar–plantar hyperhidrosis. Skeletal defects include aplasia, subluxation or absence of the patella, posterior iliac horns, dislocation of the head of the radius, scoliosis, and thickening of the scapulae. Renal abnormalities include renal dysplasia, glomerulonephritis, and Goodpasture syndrome.

Ocular Features

Hyperpigmentation of the pupillary margin (Lester iris), cataracts, and heterochromia iridis may be seen.

Primary Pachydermoperiostosis (Touraine–Solente–Gole Syndrome)

Primary pachydermoperiostosis is autosomal dominant and has variable expressivity. Some patients are mentally retarded. Thickening and folding or furrowing of the facial, scalp, and forehead skin occurs soon after puberty. The folding produces a form of cutis verticis gyrata on the scalp and may be severe on the forehead and cheeks. It is often associated with hyperplasia and oversecretion of the sebaceous glands of the face and scalp. Hyperhidrosis of the hands and feet may also occur. The facial and pubic hair may be sparse. The bones of the extremities and phalanges are thickened. Clubbing of the fingers (Fig. 10-7) and toes as well as arthralgias and arthritis may be seen. In acquired pachydermoperiostosis, clubbing may be the result of chronic low-grade anoxemia due to cardiac or pulmonary disease. It is important to rule out bronchogenic carcinoma in these patients.

Ocular Features

Ocular features include heavy, thickened lids and ptosis.

Acromegaloid Phenotype with Cutis Verticis Gyrata and Corneal Leukoma (Rosenthal–Kloepfer Syndrome)

Acromegaloid phenotype with cutis verticis gyrata and corneal leukoma (Rosenthal–Kloepfer syndrome) may be part of pachydermoperiostosis. The patients have acromegaloid features (large hands and feet, tall stature, and prominent frontal bones). The sella turcica appears normal.

Hornlike projections that are covered by skin extend from the lateral half of the supraorbital ridges. The scalp and jaw are enlarged and are covered by gyrate folds of skin.

An opacity of the cornea develops during the first decade of life. It begins in the epithelium, later involves Bowman's layer, and eventually affects the entire cornea except for the extreme periphery.

Acrocephalosyndactyly

Acrocephalosyndactyly comprises Apert syndrome, which is autosomal dominant; Vogt cephalodactyly; the Pfeiffer syndrome; and Saethre-Chotzen, all of which are characterized by a tower skull.

Patients with Apert syndrome have a broad, flat face; prominent eyes; shallow orbits; hypertelorism; an antimongoloid slant of the palpebral fissures; and a small nose and maxilla. Less common features are mental retardation, impaired hearing from fixation of the stapes, a high-arched palate, a cleft soft palate or bifid uvula, and short humeri together with ankylosis of the shoulder, elbow, and vertebrae.

Skin Features

Skin features include a transverse frontal skin furrow that overhangs the upper frontal area; syndactyly of both skin and bone of the second to fifth digits (resulting in mitten hands and hooflike feet); severe acne vulgaris developing after puberty (the comedones are extensive and may even involve the arms and forearms); malocclusion; retarded dental eruption with crowding of the teeth; and nail dystrophy.

Ocular Features

The ocular features include prominent eyes, hypertelorism, antimongoloid slant of the palpebral fissures, ptosis, keratoconus, exposure keratitis, strabismus, and secondary optic atrophy. Unusual ocular features include ocular albinism, megalocornea, iris colobomas, congenital cataract, lens subluxation, nystagmus, medullated nerve fibers, and retinal detachment.

Cephalodactyly

Vogt cephalodactyly has syndactyly and a facies suggestive of Crouzon syndrome, Saethre–Chotzen syndrome has cranial asymmetry and minimal syndactyly, and Pfeiffer syndrome is characterized by mild syndactyly, broad thumbs, and broad toes.

Acrocephalopolysyndactyly

The acrocephalopolysyndactyly syndromes are characterized by a tower skull and duplication of the phalanges. In the Carpenter syndrome there is duplication of the thumbs, congenital heart disease, dystopia canthorum, hypertelorism, microcornea, and those ocular features described under Apert syndrome

Cornelia de Lange Syndrome (Brachmann–de Lange Syndrome; Amsterdam Dwarf)

Patients with Cornelia de Lange syndrome (Brachmann–de Lange syndrome; Amsterdam dwarf) have a low birth weight, growth retardation, feeding and respiratory difficulties, and mental retardation. Most die during infancy. The child has a feeble, low-pitched, growling cry. The head, hands, and feet are small; the head is shortened in the anteroposterior dimension (brachycephaly). The facial characteristic are quite distinctive (Fig. 10-8). The face has a grim, expressionless, masklike appearance with hirsutism; the hairline is low on the neck and forehead; the eyebrows are confluent and bushy; the eyelashes are long; the nose is small with anteverted nostrils, a long prominent philtrum, and a depressed bridge; the upper lip is long, and both lips are thin; the angles of the mouth turn down; the chin recedes.

Skeletal anomalies include webbing; short, broad, first and fifth metacarpals; hyperextensibility of the digits; shortening of the extremities (micromelia); and flexion contractures of the elbows and knees.

Skin Features

Skin features include marbling and a bluish tinge around the eyes, nose, and mouth; keratosis pilaris; atypical and hypoplastic dermatoglyphics; prominent hypertrichosis of the forehead, sides of the face, back, shoulders, and extremities; and delayed eruption of widely spaced teeth.

Ocular Features

Ocular features include confluent, bushy eyebrows (Fig. 10-8); long lashes; and myopia.

Cleft Lip/Palate, Mucous Cysts of the Lower Lip, Popliteal Pterygium, Digital and Genital Anomalies (Popliteal Web Syndrome)

Cleft lip/palate, mucous cysts of the lower lip, popliteal pterygium, digital and genital anomalies (popliteal web syndrome) may be autosomal dominant or recessive. This syndrome is characterized by bilateral popliteal pterygium (webs of skin), intercrural pterygium, valgus or varus foot deformities, digital hypoplasia or agenesis, inguinal hernia, absent or a cleft scrotum and cryptorchidism, or aplasia of the labial majora.

The facial features include a cleft lip and/or palate, lower lip pits, and congenital bands of mucous membranes between the jaws.

Ocular Features

The ocular features include filiform adhesions of the eyelids (ankyloblepharon filiform adnatum).

Pachyonychia Congenita

Pachyonychia congenita is a rare autosomal dominant condition. It is characterized by palmar and plantar hyperkeratosis, follicular hyperkeratosis of the elbows and knees, and oral leukokeratosis. The nails are thickened, are hard, and have raised distal margins.

Ocular Features

The ocular features include corneal dyskeratosis and cataracts.

Dubowitz Syndrome

The Dubowitz syndrome is autosomal recessive. It is characterized by microcephaly, mental retardation, a low birth weight, a slow growth pattern, and dwarfism. The patient has sparse hair; high, sloping forehead; ptosis; epicanthic folds; a broad nasal bridge; and micrognathia.

The Broad Thumb–Hallux Syndrome (Rubinstein–Taybi Syndrome)

The broad thumb–Hallux syndrome (Rubinstein–Taybi syndrome) is autosomal recessive and is characterized by physical and mental retardation, broad thumbs and great toes, and dermatoglyphic abnormalities. The head is small, the nose often is beaked, the palate is high and narrow, and the ears are malformed and low-set. Congenital heart defects, cryptorchidism, an enlarged fontanelle, and ureteral reduplication may also be seen.

Skin Features

The skin features include hypertrichosis, especially of the back; a capillary nevus of the forehead, nape of the neck, or lumbar region; seborrhea or atopy; exuberant keloids; and irregular and crowded teeth.

Ocular Features

The ocular features include heavy, greatly arched eyebrows; long lashes; an antimongoloid slant of the palpebral fissures, strabismus, and high refractive errors. Ocular colobomas and glaucoma have been described.

Marinesco–Sjögren Syndrome

The Marinesco–Sjögren syndrome is autosomal recessive and is characterized by cerebellar ataxia, dysarthria, and a rotary and horizontal nystagmus. Skeletal defects are common.

Skin Features

Skin features include brittle, short, sparse, fine, and fair hair; malformed teeth and sometimes absent lateral incisors; and thin, fragile nails.

Ocular Features

The ocular features include the nystagmus and congenital cataracts.

Focal Dermal Hypoplasia (Goltz Syndrome, Goltz–Gorlin Syndrome)

Goltz syndrome is X-linked dominant. It comprises focal skin defects and dental, skeletal, and ocular abnormalities. Mental retardation and seizures sometimes occur.

The patients have a characteristic facies with a small, rounded skull; pointed chin; a triangular facial outline; protruding ears; and sometimes an asymmetrical alae nasi. The stature is slender and short. Sometimes the face, trunk, and extremities are asymmetric. Microcephaly has been observed.

Digit deformities include syndactyly (especially between the third and fourth fingers), polydactyly, absence of one or more digits, claw deformity, and hemimelia. Spinal deformities (including scoliosis, kyphosis, spina bifida, and fusion of the vertebrae) have also been observed.

Skin Features

Skin lesions are present at birth and comprise patchy, asymmetric, linear streaks of atrophy and telangiectasia that follow Blaschko lines. In darker skin, the linear streaks may be hypo- or hyperpigmented. Subcutaneous fat often herniates into atrophic areas, forming soft, reddish-yellow nodules. Verrucous (raspberry-like) papillomas may develop on the lips, perineum, ears, phalanges, buccal mucosa, and esophagus, and, in some patients, there is an initial inflammatory or bullous phase with urticaria and hyperkeratosis.

Scalp and pubic hair is sparse and brittle, and sometimes there are patches of alopecia. The nails may be dystrophic, spoon-shaped, or absent. Hypodontia, microdontia, defective enamel, and retarded tooth eruption occur.

Ocular Features

The ocular features include ptosis; strabismus; blue sclera; coloboma of the iris, choroid, retina, and optic nerve; and keratoconus. Less common ocular abnormalities include microphthalmos, anophthalmos, cloudy corneae, aniridia, subluxation of the lens, retinal pigment epithelial abnormalities, and cloudy vitreous.

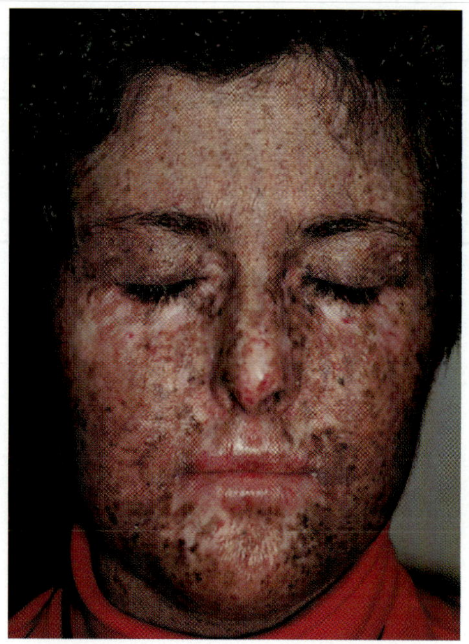
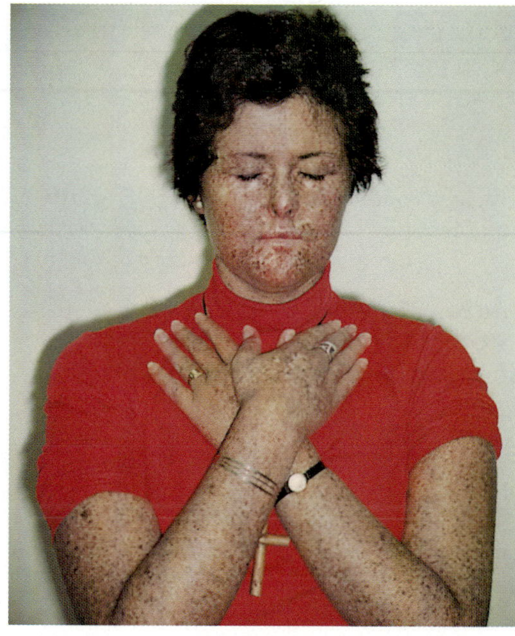

FIGURE 10-1. Stage 4 xeroderma pigmentosum in an 18-year-old woman. Multiple hyperpigmented and depigmented patches are evident as well as erythematous areas on the left upper lid and left tip of the nose suggestive of neoplastic changes.

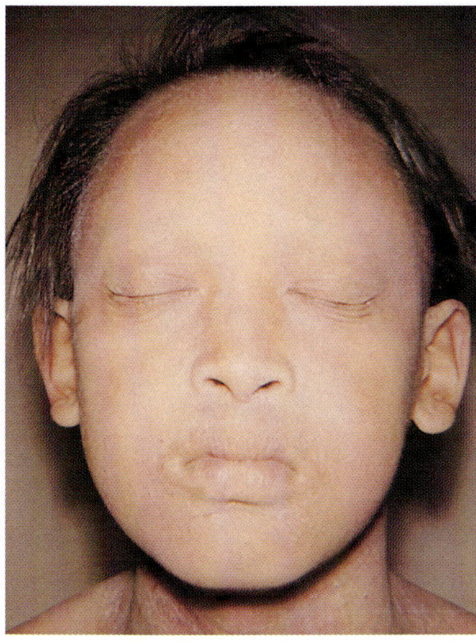

FIGURE 10-2. Sparse eyelashes and scalp hair in hypohidrotic ectodermal dysplasia.

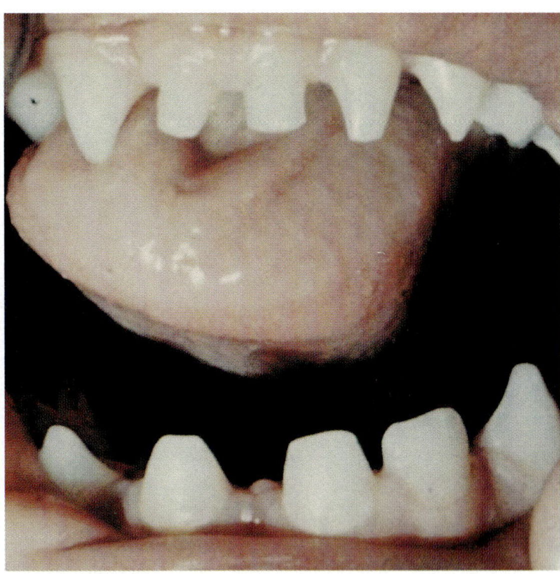

FIGURE 10-3. Wide-spaced peg-shaped teeth in hypohidrotic ectodermal dysplasia.

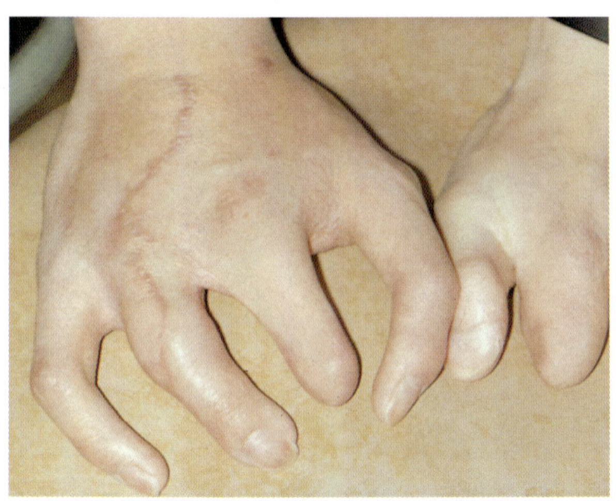

FIGURE 10-4. Lobster-claw deformity of the hands in ectrodactyly ectodermal dysplasia (EEC syndrome). (Photograph courtesy of Suzanne Banuvar.)

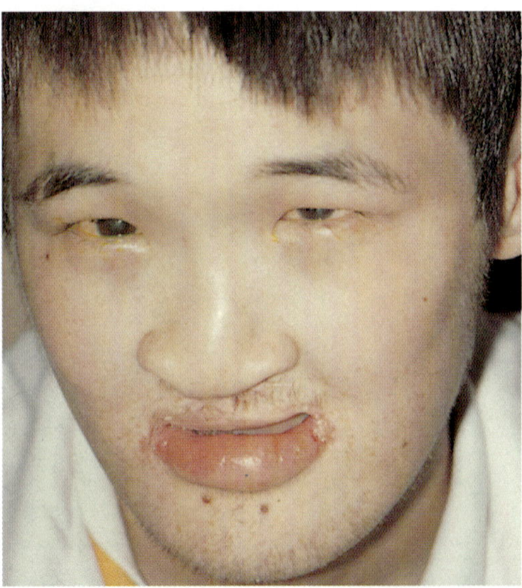

FIGURE 10-5. Cleft lip and blepharitis in patient with ectrodactyly ectodermal dysplasia (EEC syndrome). (Photograph courtesy of Suzanne Banuvar.)

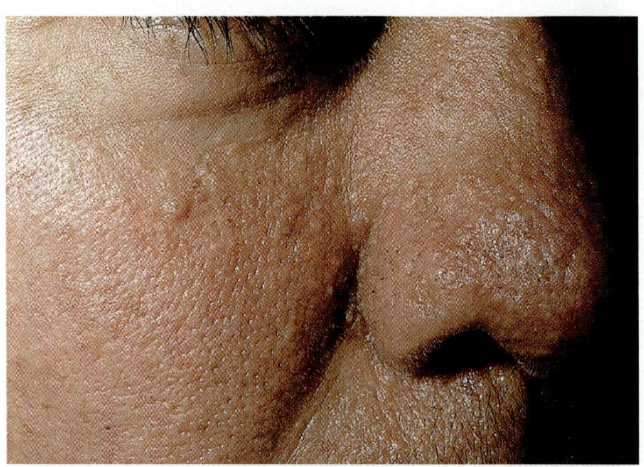

FIGURE 10-6. Trichilemmomas in Cowden syndrome. Note multiple small flesh-colored papules on cheeks and nose, which is the most common location for these benign neoplasms of hair follicles. (Courtesy of John Reeves.)

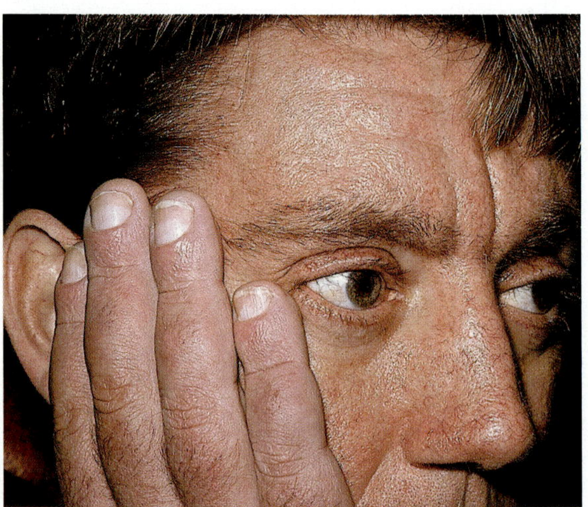

FIGURE 10-7. Pachydermoperiostosis. Note thickened fingers with mild clubbing, furrowed brow, and oily skin.

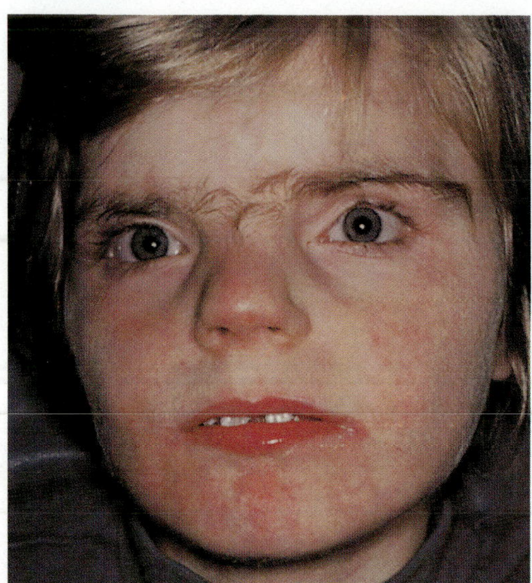

FIGURE 10-8. Facial characteristics of the Cornelia de Lange syndrome.

THE PHAKOMATOSES

The phakomatoses (Greek for "mother spot") comprise syndromes with glial overgrowth and proliferation or malformations involving the brain and retina. Many neurocutaneous syndromes represent phakomatoses such as neurofibromatosis (von Recklinghausen disease), tuberous sclerosis, Von Hippel–Lindau disease, Sturge–Weber syndrome, and Wyburn–Mason (Bonnet–Dechaume–Blanc) syndrome. The latter three are discussed in Chapter 9.

NEUROFIBROMATOSIS

Neurofibromatosis is autosomal dominant and comprises two genetically distinct forms: a peripheral form (type I von Recklinghausen disease) and a central form (type II neurofibromatosis).

Neurofibromatosis Type I (Von Recklinghausen Disease)

Neurofibromatosis type I (Von Recklinghausen disease) is autosomal dominant and has incomplete penetrance. It is characterized by pigmented skin lesions, skin tumors that develop along peripheral nerves, multiple spinal and cranial nerve tumors and associated gliomas, and intracranial meningiomas.

Two or more of the following findings are sufficient for diagnosis:

1. Six or more café-au-lait-spots.
2. Two or more Lisch nodules (Fig. 11-1).
3. Two or more skin or subcutaneous neurofibromas.
4. A plexiform neurofibroma.
5. An optic nerve glioma.
6. Bony defects involving the tibia or sphenoid.
7. Axillary freckling.

Other findings may include the following:

1. Facial weakness and numbness from 5th and 7th cranial nerve involvement and hemilateral facial atrophy from plexiform neuromas that cause overgrowth of the skin and subcutaneous tissue.
2. Neurologic features of macrocephaly, mental retardation, speech impediment, intracranial tumors, epilepsy, and spinal cord and peripheral nerve tumors.
3. Endocrine abnormalities such as acromegaly, Addison disease, hyperparathyroidism, precocious puberty, gynecomastia, pheochromocytoma, and medullary thyroid carcinomas.
4. Skeletal changes (Fig. 11-2) in von Recklinghausen disease include bony overgrowth, fibrous dysplasia, osteomalacia, vertebral anomalies, and pseudoarthrosis of the tibia or radius.
5. Malignant changes (malignant neurofibrosarcoma, Wilms' tumor, fibrosarcoma, rhabdomyosarcoma, leukemias, and retinoblastoma).

Other findings include renal vascular lesions causing hypertension, cystic lung disease, and gastrointestinal neurofibromas with chronic blood loss.

Skin Features

The various skin features include the following:

1. Nodular cutaneous and subcutaneous neurofibromas (Fig. 11-3) develop on the trunk during adolescence in von Recklinghausen disease. They are sessile, dome-shaped, or pedunculated and increase in number throughout life.
2. Café-au-lait spots (Fig. 11-4) appear as sharply defined, light brown patches and occur on the trunk, axilla, and occasionally, face.
3. Smaller freckles of the axilla, Crowe sign (Fig. 11-5), and other intertriginous areas are common and are almost pathognomonic for neurofibromatosis.
4. Subcutaneous plexiform neuromas are usually located along the trigeminal nerve (Fig. 11-6) or in the peripheral nerves (Fig. 11-7). They have indistinct margins, they feel soft like "a bag of worms," and the overlying skin is hyperpigmented or is covered by excessive hair.
5. Other skin features include elephantiasis neurofibromata; papillomatous tumors of the palate, buccal mucosa, tongue, and lips; and macroglossia.

Ocular Features

The ocular features include the following:

1. Lid or eyebrow involvement (Fig. 11-6) includes hyper-pigmentation, neurofibromas, plexiform neuromas of the upper eyelid, ptosis, trichiasis, and thickened skin (fibroma molluscum), especially temporally. When the eyelid is involved there is often an "S" configuration to the eyelid margin because of the weight of the plexiform neuroma.
2. Conjunctival hyperpigmentation; thickening; and isolated neurofibromas on the limbus, tarsus, or bulbar conjunctiva.
3. Corneal nodules (neurofibroma) and thickening of the corneal nerves.
4. Pulsatile exophthalmos or orbital asymmetry from sphenoidal bone defect; exophthalmos and evidence of a space-occupying lesion; enlargement of the optic canal; and enophthalmos from bony defects.
5. Lisch nodules (Fig. 11-1) and choroidal melanocytic lesions represent uveal tract changes in neurofibromatosis. Lisch nodules are round, dome shaped, brownish-colored iris lesions, measuring less than 1 mm.
6. Benign astrocytic growths of the retina similar to tuberous sclerosis and dense macular pigmentation.
7. Optic nerve involvement at the chiasm, optic pathway, or optic nerve; papilledema and optic atrophy.
8. Other ocular features include neuromas of the ciliary body leading to buphthalmos and glaucoma (Fig. 11-8).
9. Café-au-lait spots in fundus can be seen as well-demarcated, nonelevated areas of localized pigmentation or abnormalities in pigment distribution.

Neurofibromatosis Type II

Neurofibromatosis type II is autosomal dominant, has a high degree of penetrance, and is characterized by bilateral acoustic neuromas. Often there are other central nervous system tumors (e.g., meningiomas, Schwannomas, and ependymomas) that involve the cranial nerves, spinal cord, and nerve roots.

Café-au-lait spots and cutaneous neurofibromas are uncommon and few in number.

Ocular Features

The ocular features are limited to posterior subcapsular cataracts, which develop during adolescence or young adulthood.

Tuberous Sclerosis (Bourneville Disease)

Tuberous sclerosis (Bourneville disease) is autosomal dominant and has variable penetrance; new mutations are found in about 50% of patients. It is characterized by hamartomas of the skin, eye, brain, heart, kidney, and other organs. Skin changes and epilepsy usually develop before the age of 5. The epilepsy is usually focal in nature and occurs in about 80% of patients. Severe mental retardation is found in about one-half of patients and may be progressive.

Less common features include rhabdomyomas of the heart; angiomyolipomas of the kidney; renal cysts or renal cell carcinoma; hamartomatous colonic polyps with malignant potential; cystlike lesions and irregular thickening of the bony cortex; dyspnea; spontaneous pneumothorax; and localized giantism.

Skin Features

About 70% of patients have skin involvement, and many of the lesions are almost pathognomonic when accompanied by epilepsy. They include the following:

1. Ash-leaf-shaped white macules (Fig. 11-9) occur in a dermatomal distribution on the trunk or extremities.
2. Facial angiofibromas (adenoma sebaceum) (Fig. 11-10) characteristically develop during early childhood and appear as firm, discrete, red/brown, telangiectatic papules.
3. A shagreen patch or collagenoma appearing as an irregularly thickened, soft, skin-colored plaque in the lumbosacral area, forehead, or eyelids.
4. Subungual and periungual fibromas (Fig. 11-11).
5. Other skin lesions, such as soft, pedunculated fibromas around the neck and axillae, and diffuse cutaneous reticula.
6. Fibromas of the gums, palate, tongue, larynx, or pharynx.

Ocular Features

The ocular features include the following:

1. Poliosis and a shagreen patch of the lid.
2. Pedunculated white or gray conjunctival tumors.
3. Opacities of the cornea and lens.
4. Hypopigmented lesions of the iris and choroid.
5. Single or multiple, unilateral or bilateral astrocytic retinal hamartomas usually occur in the posterior pole, are slow growing, and have a mulberry appearance (Fig. 11-12). They eventually calcify, giving a glistening or cottage cheese appearance, as can be seen at the edge of this lesion.
6. A second form of retinal hamartomas is flat, smooth-appearing, and semitranslucent with poorly defined boundaries (Fig. 11-13). These lesions are more common but usually are missed because their presence is not considered.
7. Keratoconus, strabismus, nystagmus, visual field loss, tilted discs, myelinated nerve fibers, depigmented areas of retinal pigment epithelium, peripapillary veils, optic atrophy, papilledema, and ocular colobomas have been reported.

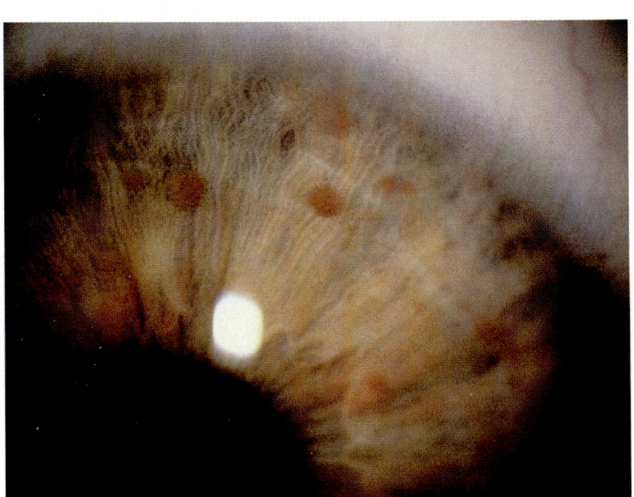

FIGURE 11-1. Lisch nodules evident in the mid portion of the iris stroma in a patient with neurofibromatosis.

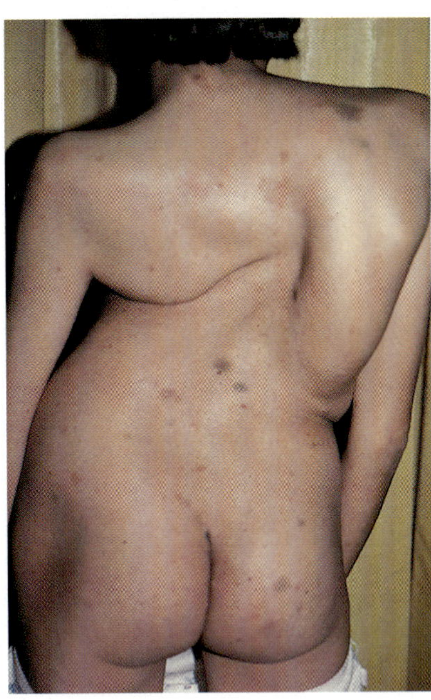

FIGURE 11-2. Von Recklinghausen disease with severe kyphoscoliosis. Multiple café-au-lait spots are evident over the skin.

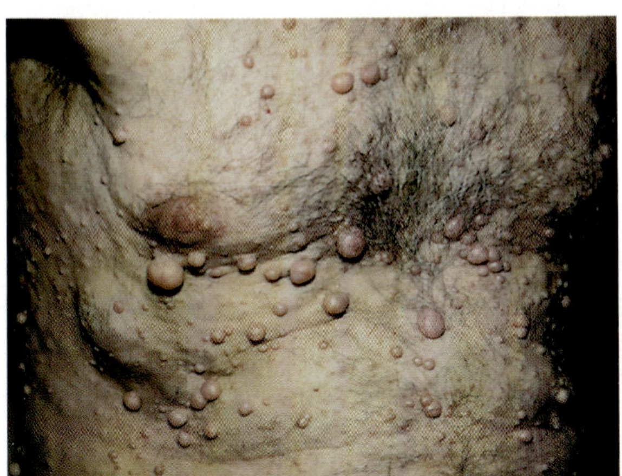

FIGURE 11-3. Von Recklinghausen disease with multiple nodular cutaneous and subcutaneous neurofibromas of the trunk. A plexiform neuroma is located below the right breast.

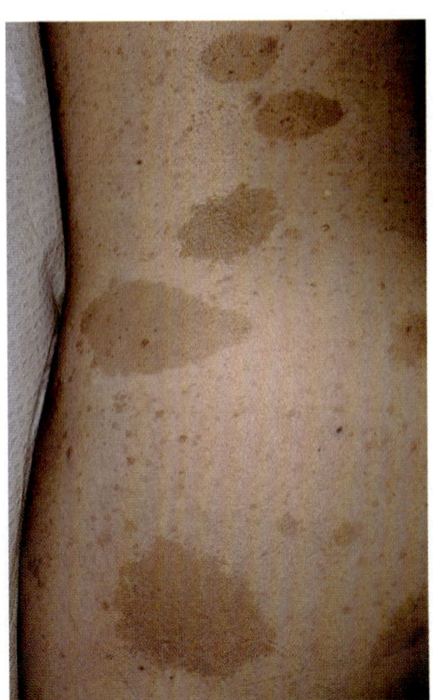

FIGURE 11-4. Café-au-lait spots—uniformly pigmented, pale brown rounded macules noted at birth or by first year of life as a significant cutaneous marker of von Recklinghausen neurofibromatosis.

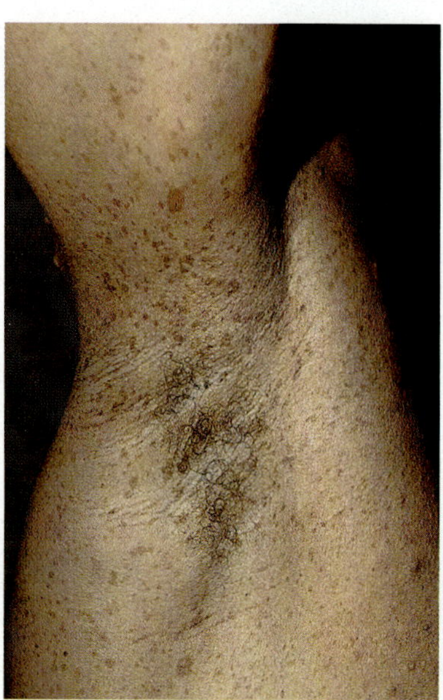

FIGURE 11-5. Axillary freckles (Crowe sign) in neurofibromatosis.

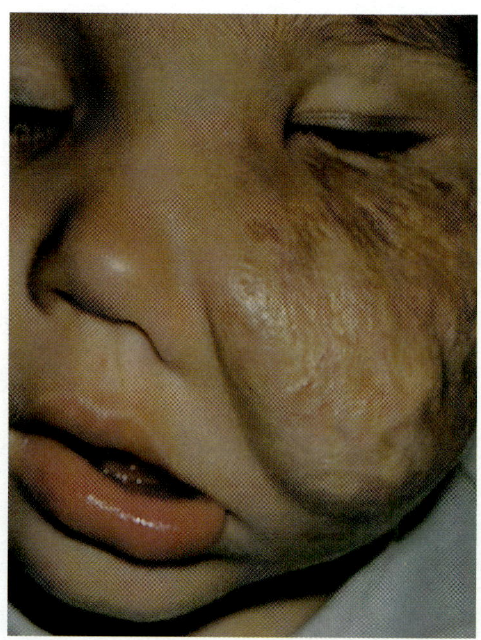

FIGURE 11-6. Large plexiform neuroma of the lower lid and cheek in a young child with neurofibromatosis.

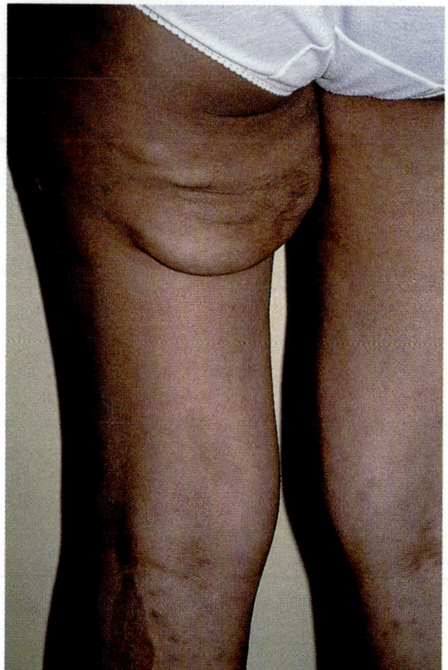

FIGURE 11-7. Plexiform neuroma of thigh in patient with neurofibromatosis.

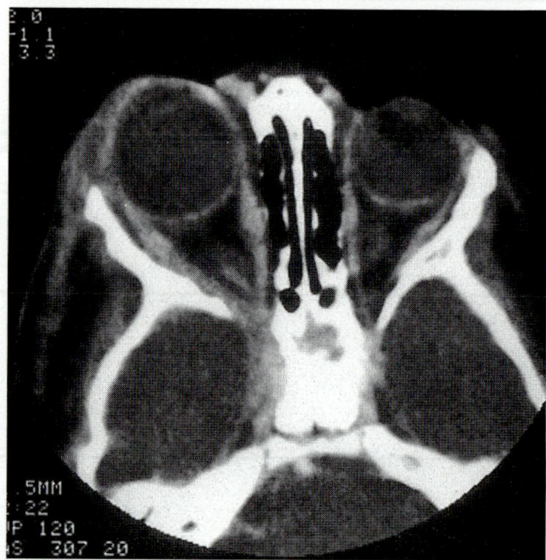

FIGURE 11-8. Computerized axial tomography of patient with ciliary body neuroma and juvenile glaucoma with buphthalmos.

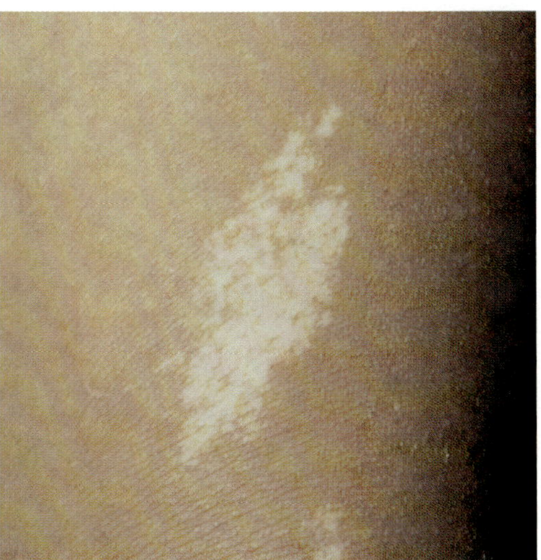

FIGURE 11-9. Ash-leaf-shaped white macules on the trunk in tuberous sclerosis. Three members of the immediate family—the mother, son, and daughter—had tuberous sclerosis.

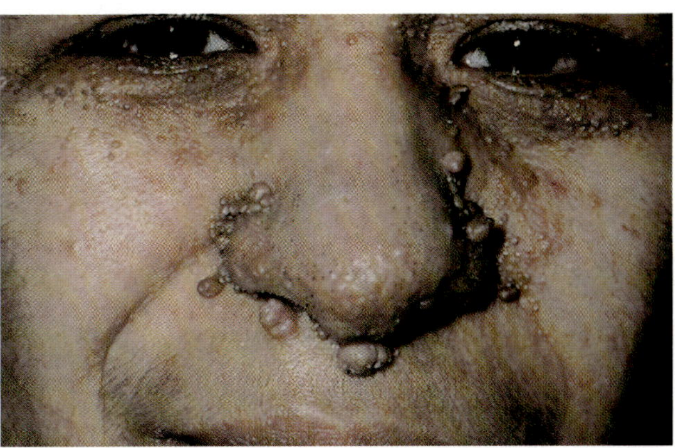

FIGURE 11-10. Multiple facial angiofibromas (adenoma sebaceum) in tuberous sclerosis. Multiple facial angiofibromas can be seen, especially perinasally, but are also present on the lower lid. This young woman had suffered many epileptic seizures and was mentally retarded.

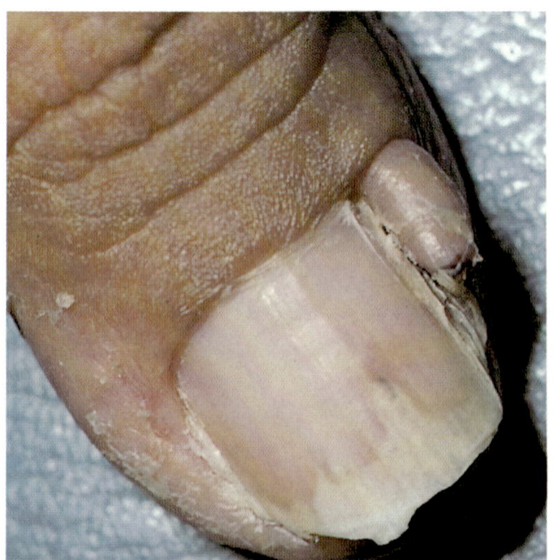

FIGURE 11-11. Subungual and periungual fibromas (Koenen tumors) of the thumb in a patient with tuberous sclerosis. The periungual fibroma is very obvious; the subungual fibroma is located adjacent to it and is partially hidden by the nail.

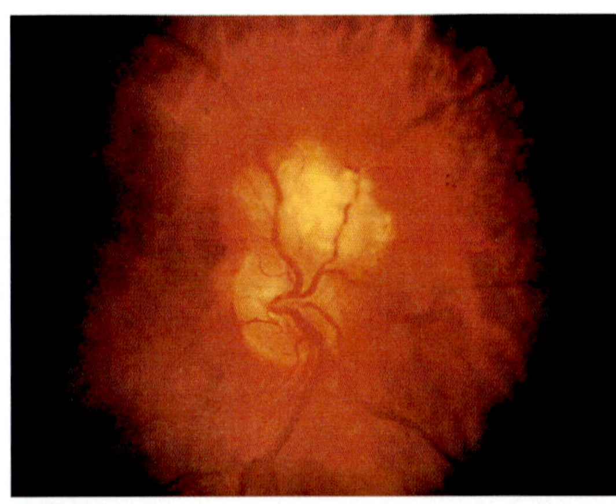

FIGURE 11-12. Astrocytic hamartoma of the retina in tuberous sclerosis.

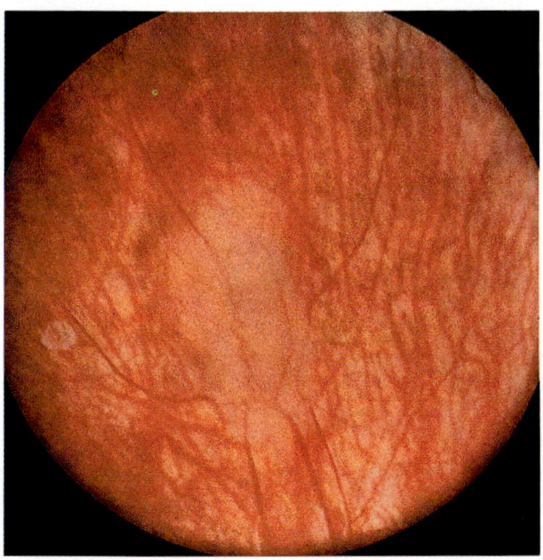

FIGURE 11-13. Flat, semitranslucent astrocytic hamartoma of the retina, which is much more common and more subtle than the "classic" astrocytic hamartoma seen in Fig. 11-12.

GENETIC AND DEGENERATIVE CONNECTIVE TISSUE DISORDERS

Cutaneous connective tissue is composed of elastin, collagen, and ground substance. In this chapter we discuss the collagen and elastic tissue disorders that involve the skin and eye.

ELASTIC TISSUE DISORDERS

Generalized Cutis Laxa (Generalized Elastolysis, Generalized Dermatochalasis)

Generalized cutis laxa (generalized elastolysis, generalized dermatochalasis) is autosomal dominant or recessive, occurs as part of deBarsey syndrome, or is acquired in diseases such as amyloidosis, complement deficiency, systemic lupus erythematous, drug hypersensitivities (e.g., penicillamine), or inflammatory skin disorders.

Cutis laxa is characterized by generalized, loose, pendulous skin, especially of the face, which causes the palpebral fissures to slant downward and the cheeks to sag (Fig. 12-1); prominent skin folds about the abdomen, thighs, and knees; and pulmonary emphysema from loss of pulmonary elastic tissue.

deBarsey syndrome is characterized by a generalized cutis laxa, retarded growth and psychomotor development, pseudoathetoid movements, and corneal clouding.

Blepharochalasis (Fig. 12-2) and dermatochalasis (Fig. 12-3) represent localized areas of cutis laxa but differ significantly in epidemiology. Blepharochalasis is idiopathic or sometimes autosomal dominant. It occurs in young adults and may represent a localized angioedema. It is characterized by intermittent, recurrent episodes of bilateral lid edema lasting 2 to 3 days. The upper lid skin eventually becomes thinned, stretched, wrinkled, and redundant, and may have some increased pigmentation and telangiectasis. Blepharochalasis also occurs in Ascher syndrome, characterized by progressive upper lid enlargement and labial salivary gland and occasionally accessory lacrimal gland inflammation.

Dermatochalasis usually occurs in aging patients and may be associated with keratoconjunctivitis sicca–type symptoms. It is manifested by redundant, excess skin overlying the upper tarsus.

Facial Hemiatrophy (Parry–Romberg Syndrome)

Facial hemiatrophy (Parry–Romberg syndrome) is characterized by progressive facial hemiatrophy, exophthalmos, epilepsy, and sometimes atrophy of the underlying cartilage and bone of one side of the face (Fig. 12-4). It may represent a severe variant of linear scleroderma (en coup de sabre).

Skin Features

The skin features in Parry–Romberg syndrome include hypo- or hyperpigmentation of the forehead, cheek, or jaw. The cutaneous changes are characterized by dry, atrophic, and sometimes adherent skin with progressive atrophy of the underlying subcutaneous tissue, muscle, and bone. These changes eventually lead to a sunken-appearing, hyperpigmented, hemiatrophic face. In some instances, there are also localized canities and alopecia of the frontoparietal region. The changes may be limited to a small area, may occur bilaterally, or may be associated with atrophy of the ipsilateral or contralateral half of the body.

Lipodystrophy (Lipoatrophy)

Lipodystrophy (lipoatrophy) is a rare disorder that is actually a widespread mesodermal atrophy, but we include it here because of its appearance. There is gradual symmetric loss of the subcutaneous fat of the face (Fig. 12-5), and sometimes the upper-half of the body. (Occasionally, it involves only half of the face or body.) Sometimes there is hypertrophy of the subcutaneous fat in the lower part of body. Most patients develop progressive membranous mesangiocapillary glomerulonephritis. Diabetes may also be associated. Retinitis pigmentosa has occasionally been described.

Pseudoxanthoma Elasticum (Grönblad-Strandberg Syndrome)

Pseudoxanthoma elasticum (PXE) (Grönblad-Strandberg syndrome) represents generalized elastorrhexis of the elastic tissue of the dermis, blood vessels, and Bruch membrane of the retina, followed by calcium deposition in the resulting abnormal fibers (Figs. 12-6 to 12-8). It is divided clinically into autosomal dominant types I and II, and autosomal recessive types I, II, and III. PE affects all arteries by the age of 30, causing intermittent claudication, diminished peripheral pulses, and narrowing or occlusion of the peripheral, visceral, and coronary arteries. By age 30, many patients have hypertension and epistaxis.

Skin Features

A linear or reticular pattern of small, yellowish papules develops before the age of 30 and may become confluent on the neck (Fig. 12-6), the area below the clavicles, and the axilla. The skin of elderly patients is usually soft, is loose, and hangs in folds, giving a "plucked chicken" appearance at the neck and axillae (Fig. 12-7). The buccal mucosa may show discrete and confluent small pale yellowish maculo-papules (Fig. 12-8).

Ocular Features

Retinal angioid streaks, named for their resemblance of blood vessels, represent focal breaks in Bruch membrane. Usually appearing in PXE patients during the third and fourth decade, the streaks are deep to the retinal vessels and commonly radiate outward from the optic nerve head (Fig. 12-9). The association of the classic skin lesions of PXE with angioid streaks is called the Gronblad–Stranberg syndrome. Other ocular findings include small retinal and optic nerve head drusen, speckled yellowish mottling of the posterior pole, and subretinal neovascular membranes, which, if near the macula, can lead to severe loss of vision.

Actinic Elastosis

Ultraviolet (UV) radiation causes degenerative elastic tissue skin changes, which are cumulative and usually more severe in fair-skinned patients. These changes are most apparent on the forehead and back of the neck (Fig. 12-10), appearing as wrinkled, thickened yellow skin. Other changes include poliosis, scaling solar keratoses, alopecia, and malignant degeneration. Pinguicula, pterygia, conjunctival intraepithelial neoplasia, and senile scleral plaques may also be related to UV radiation.

Marfan Syndrome

Marfan syndrome, which is relatively common, represents an autosomal dominant connective tissue disorder with variable expressivity. The full syndrome has skeletal, cardiovascular, and ocular components; patients rarely survive beyond the fifth decade of life.

The skeletal features of Marfan syndrome include a dolichocephalic skull; large paranasal sinuses; high, arched palate (Fig. 12-11); pectus excavatum; kyphoscoliosis; long extremities; arachnodactyly (Fig. 12-12); flat feet; and

hyperextensible or unstable joints. The cardiovascular features include aneurysmal dilatation of the ascending aorta, mitral valve prolapse, and aortic and mitral valve incompetence. The subcutaneous fat is sparse; striae are commonly seen (Fig. 12-13); serpiginous perforating elastosis is occasionally found.

Ocular Features

The ocular features of Marfan syndrome include superotemporal subluxated lenses (Fig. 12-14), diffuse and focal iris transillumination defects, glaucoma, myopia, and retinal detachment. Heterochromia iridis and blue sclerae have been uncommonly reported.

COLLAGEN DISORDERS

Ehlers–Danlos Syndrome (EDS) (Cutis Hyperelastica)

Ehlers–Danlos syndrome (EDS) (cutis hyperelastica) is characterized by skin and blood vessel fragility, skin hyperelasticity, and joint hypermobility. The 10 separate genetic and clinical forms have some overlap. Types I, II, and VI have skin and ocular features.

EDS Type I (Gravis) and EDS Type II (Mitis)

EDS type I (Gravis) and EDS type II (Mitis) are autosomal dominant. The findings are similar, except that type II is much milder. Skin changes and joint changes are very characteristic.

Skin Features

The skin in Ehlers–Danlos syndrome types I and II is soft, velvety, hyperextensible, and often redundant, especially in later life, and can be found on the neck, elbows (Fig. 12-15), and around the eyes. A common complaint is easy bruising at sites of pressure (Fig. 12-12). Pseudotumors may develop in these same areas (Fig. 12-16).

Joint hypermobility (Fig. 12-17) is evident, and when present in the lower extremities often makes walking difficult, especially during pregnancy. Congenital hyperextension of the knee joint, subluxation of large joints, and kyphoscoliosis may be seen.

Ocular Features

Widely spaced eyes, epicanthal folds, a wide nasal bridge, and redundant skin folds around the eyes are quite distinctive. The sclera are sometimes blue.

EDS Type VI (Ocular)

EDS type VI (ocular) is autosomal recessive. The skin feels soft and velvety, and patients have scoliosis. Keratoconjunctivitis and intraocular hemorrhages are common. Spontaneous corneal rupture with brittle, thin corneae have been reported.

BONY-TISSUE DISORDERS

Osteogenesis Imperfecta

Osteogenesis imperfecta represents a group of inherited disorders characterized by fragile bones, progressing skeletal deformities, generalized osteoporosis, and short stature, which arise from defective collagen production. It is divided on a clinical and hereditary basis into four types. Types I and III have eye involvement.

Type 1: Mild Form with Blue Sclerae

Type I osteogenesis imperfecta is autosomal dominant. It is characterized by easy bruising, abnormal teeth (dentinogenesis imperfecta), joint laxity, fractures causing minimal or no skeletal deformity, deafness, and cardiac involvement with thin, incompetent aortic valves and mitral valve prolapse. The sclerae are usually blue or gray in color (Fig. 12-18). The sclerae appear blue in childhood but normal in adulthood.

Progressive Deforming Form

The inheritance pattern for the progressive deforming form is unknown. Fractures may occur *in utero* or during delivery. The bones are thin and occasionally cystic, causing progressive scoliosis, bowing of the long bones, and crippling deformity. The sclerae appear blue in childhood but normal in adulthood.

CARTILAGINOUS DISORDERS

Relapsing Polychondritis (Atrophic Polychondritis; Systemic Chondromalacia)

Relapsing polychondritis (atrophic polychondritis; systemic chondromalacia) is characterized by relapsing inflammation and destruction of cartilaginous structures, especially of the ear, nose, and upper respiratory tract. The inflammatory episodes progressively destroy many organs.

The acute inflammatory stage is characterized by pain, tenderness, swelling, and eventual destruction of the involved cartilage with permanent deformity and atrophy. Usually the inflammation is limited to one or two sites, but recurrences often involve new areas. The inflammation may last months, and relapses vary in frequency and severity.

Laryngeal, tracheal, and bronchial inflammation may lead to difficulty in speech, respiratory embarrassment, and asphyxiation. Nonerosive, migratory and asymmetric inflammatory polyarthritis of the small joints, parasternal articulations, and rib cartilage is common and often leads to a deforming arthritis. Immune-complex glomerulonephritis is common. Vasculitis of the central and peripheral nervous system may lead to seizures; involvement of the 2nd, 6th, 7th, and 8th cranial nerves; encephalopathy; ataxia; hemiplegia; mixed motor sensory neuropathy; and mononeuritis monoplex.

Skin Features

Cutaneous or systemic vasculitis and toxic erythema are uncommon. Erythema, swelling, pain, palpable purpura, urticaria, angioedema, erythema multiforme, livedo reticularis, panniculitis, and erythema nodosum have been described.

Involvement of the pinna in relapsing polychondritis is characterized by redness, swelling, and pain centered around the cartilage, while the ear lobe is characteristically spared (Fig. 12-19). It is sometimes bilateral and leads to deformity. Cochlear and vestibular damage may lead to tinnitus, vertigo, and sensorineural deafness.

Nasal cartilage involvement begins as rhinorrhea followed by redness, swelling, pain, nasal obstruction, and eventually collapse of the nasal cartilage, resulting in saddle nose deformity (Fig. 12-20).

Ocular Features

As many as 65% of patients eventually develop ocular findings. These include the following:

1. Bilateral periorbital lid edema.
2. Bilateral conjunctival infiltration and chemosis.
3. Mild keratoconjunctivitis sicca.
4. Corneal edema, peripheral infiltration and vascularization, thinning, ulceration, and perforation. All are usually associated with the scleritis.
5. A nonspecific episcleritis or scleritis. The episcleritis is simple or diffuse, bilateral or unilateral, and recurrent. The scleritis may be anterior and diffuse or necrotizing, causing marked scleral thinning. The scleritis is frequently simultaneously bilateral and difficult to control. Occasionally, proptosis occurs from posterior scleritis.
6. Dacryocystitis secondary to collapse of the nasal bridge.
7. Orbital and peribulbar chemosis with proptosis.
8. A nongranulomatous iridocyclitis or a chorioretinitis, which often accompanies the scleritis.
9. Exudative and sensory retinal detachments, retinal infiltrates, flame-shaped hemorrhages, cotton-wool spots, and microaneurysms.
10. Palsy of the 3rd or 6th cranial nerve, ischemic optic neuritis, papilledema, ischemic optic neuropathy, and field defects.
11. Cataracts and secondary glaucoma.

CONNECTIVE TISSUE DISORDERS

Juvenile Fibromatosis

Juvenile fibromatosis is uncommon but comprises a broad group of benign fibrous tissue proliferations that occur in infants and children under the age of 16. The lesions tend to recur locally following removal.

Infantile Myofibromatosis (Solitary or Multicentric; Congenital Generalized Fibromatosis)

Infantile myofibromatosis (solitary or multicentric; congenital generalized fibromatosis) is the most common of the juvenile fibromatoses. It is characterized by single or multiple lesions that usually occur on the head, lid, and neck. They are often present at birth, and new lesions may develop for several months. The lesions are poorly circumscribed, hard, or rubbery nodules that involve the subcutaneous tissue, including muscle and bone. Bony lesions appear as lytic areas on X-ray. Visceral lesions (heart, lungs, liver, and intestine) may also occur.

Ocular Features

Ocular findings include nodular lesions, a corneal fibroma, and an intraorbital mass.

Juvenile Hyaline Fibromatosis (Systemic Hyalinosis; Pruritic Syndrome)

Juvenile hyaline fibromatosis (systemic hyalinosis; pruritic syndrome) skin lesions are present at birth or develop in early childhood. The skin lesions of the face and neck usually appear as small, pearly papules or nodules. Those on the scalp are more common and usually appear as large subcutaneous tumors that feel soft or hard, fixed or mobile, and that in some instances are ulcerated. Other features include gingival hypertrophy; flexion contractures of the elbows, fingers, hips and knees; osteolytic lesions of the skull, long bones, and phalanges; and poorly developed muscles. A localized lesion has been described in the orbit. Skin lesions may be found on the upper or lower eyelid.

Winchester Syndrome

The Winchester syndrome is a rare mucopolysaccharidosis that develops during infancy. It is characterized by diffusely thickened, hyperpigmented, and hypertrichotic skin; gingival hypertrophy; joint contractures; small joint arthritis; dwarfism; and corneal opacities.

Premature Aging Syndrome

Premature skin aging and eye involvement occur in a number of conditions.

Pangeria (Werner Syndrome; Adult Premature Aging Syndrome)

Pangeria (Werner syndrome; adult premature aging syndrome) is autosomal recessive and is characterized by early aging that begins soon after puberty. Intelligence is usually normal.

The skin of the feet, forearms, hands, face, and neck is tense, shiny, adherent, and dry. It has multiple areas of telangiectasia and mottled hyperpigmentation together with loss of subcutaneous tissue. The skin of the pinnae becomes atrophic and is tightly bound down. Keratoses may develop over pressure points on the feet and ankles and sometimes break down to form indolent ulcers. The hair becomes prematurely gray, and progressive alopecia may also develop. The axillary and pubic hair is sparse.

The loss of subcutaneous tissue and atrophic skin gives a birdlike facies. The legs appear spindly, whereas the trunk appears normal or obese. Patients develop joint contractures and, in some instances, sclerodactyly. Many patients have a short stature. There is a high prevalence of malignancy (10%), especially fibrosarcoma, and occasionally melanomas, leukemia, meningiomas, and astrocytomas. Other findings include early onset of atheromas and X-ray evidence of calcifications of the arteries, ligaments, tendons, and subcutaneous tissue. Death usually occurs between the fourth and the sixth decade of life. Posterior subcapsular cataracts often develop between the third and the fourth decades of life. Keratopathy may occur especially following cataract surgery, and glaucoma may be seen.

Progeria (Hutchinson–Gilford Syndrome)

Progeria (Hutchinson–Gilford syndrome) is autosomal dominant; however, patients fail to mature sexually. They appear normal at birth, but growth is retarded during the first year of life. By the second year; there is profound growth failure. The intelligence is normal.

The skin becomes thin, taut, and shiny in some areas, whereas in other areas it is lax and finely wrinkled. The veins are prominent and there is a history of easy bruising. The subcutaneous fat of the face and extremities is decreased. Eccrine sweating is reduced. There is no evidence of photosensitivity, but exposed areas of skin become hyperpigmented. Thickened sclerotic areas may be found on the lower trunk and thighs.

The scalp hair, the brows, and the lashes are sparse and downy; generalized alopecia begins during the first year of life. The nails are small and thin; sometimes they are dystrophic. The teeth are abnormal and dentition is delayed. The facies is quite distinctive. The cranium is large; the fontanelles are patent; the scalp veins are prominent. There is frontal bossing with prominent eyes, centrofacial cyanosis, micrognathia, a beaked nose, and thin lips.

Joint contractures, dystrophic clavicles, and coxa valga may be present, and fractures are common as a result of progressive bone resorption. Death usually occurs during the second decade of life from cardiovascular abnormalities.

MISCELLANEOUS DISORDERS

Colloid Milium (Colloid Degeneration of the Skin)

The juvenile form of colloid milium (colloid degeneration of the skin) develops before puberty and may be familial. The lesions present as myriads of small, 1- to 2-mm, yel- lowish-brown, sometimes translucent, dermal papules on the face, especially periocularly.

The adult form is often related to sun exposure. The lesions may also occur on the back, sides of the neck, back of the ears, and dorsum of the hands. They develop slowly, are fewer in number than in the juvenile form, and may increase in number over a period of several years before remaining stationary.

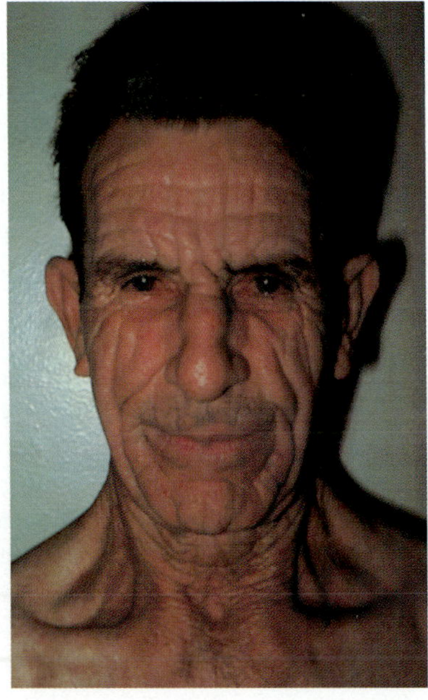

FIGURE 12-1. Cutis laxa in a 60-year-old male.

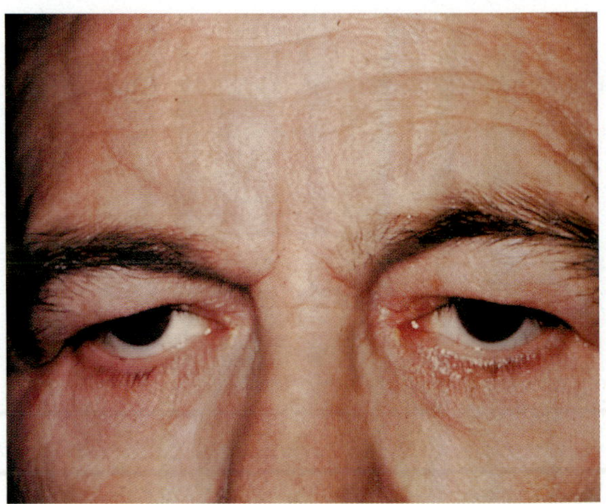

FIGURE 12-2. Blepharochalasis. (Courtesy of Dr. John Belmont.)

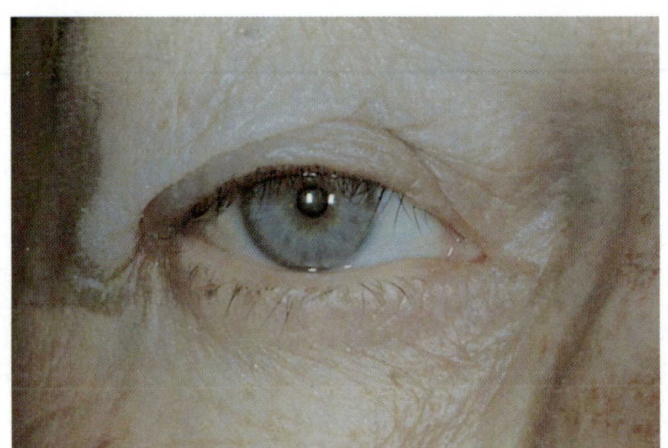

FIGURE 12-3. Dermatochalasis. The redundant skin is readily evident superiorly and on the lateral aspect of the lids.

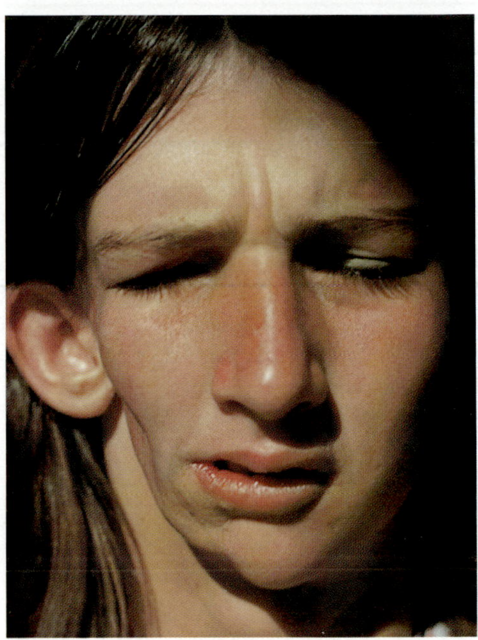

FIGURE 12-4. Hemifacial atrophy due to scleroderma.

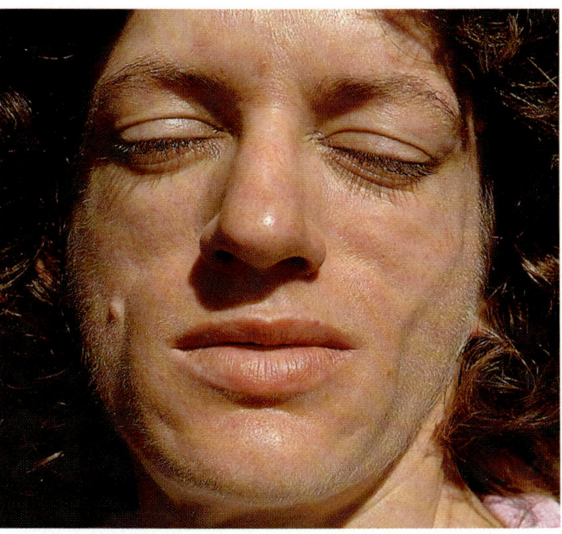

FIGURE 12-5. Progressive lipoatrophy in a patient with insulin-resistant diabetes.

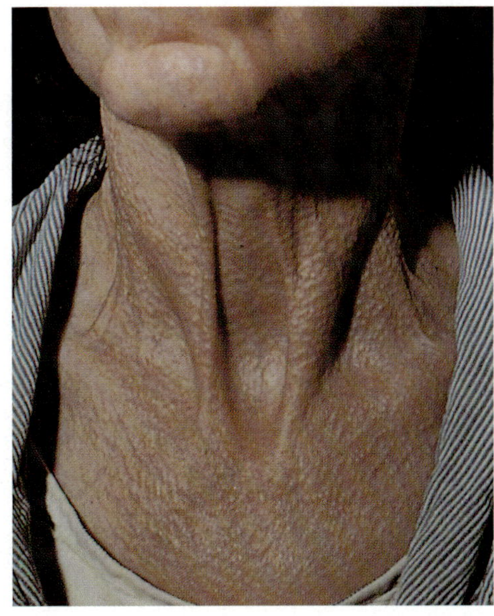

FIGURE 12-6. Reticular pattern of small yellowish papules on the neck of this patient with pseudoxanthoma elasticum.

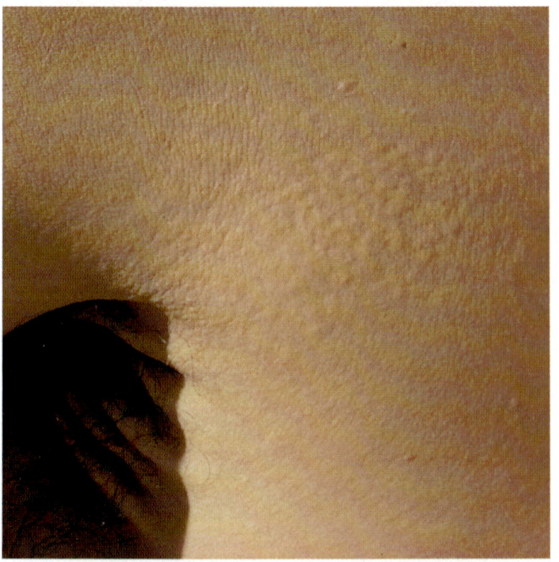

FIGURE 12-7. Pseudoxanthoma elasticum of the axilla showing the "plucked chicken" appearance in this 31-year-old man who already had significant visual impairment.

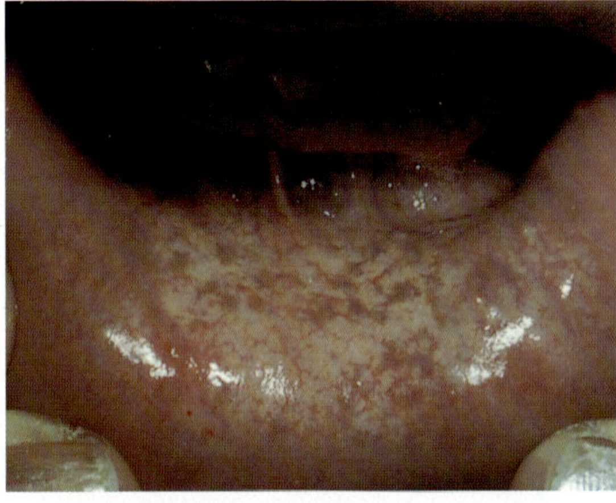

FIGURE 12-8. Buccal mucosal lesions in a 50-year-old woman with pseudoxanthoma elasticum.

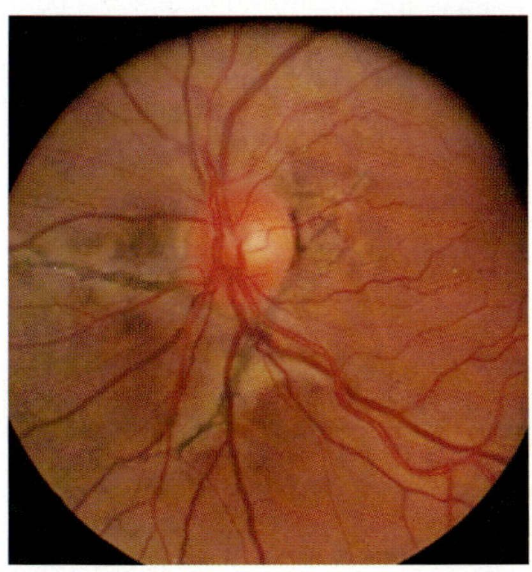

FIGURE 12-9. Angioid streaks in pseudoxanthoma elasticum. Angioid streaks lying deep to the retinal vessels are readily apparent. (Courtesy of Dr. John Belmont.)

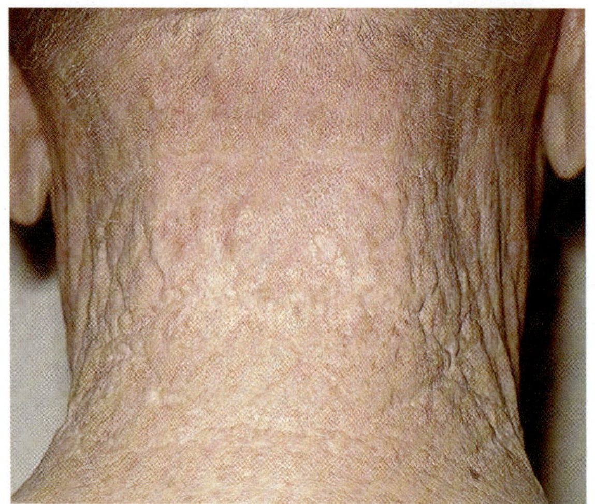

FIGURE 12-10. Actinic elastosis with the nape of neck showing thickened pale yellowish wrinkled skin.

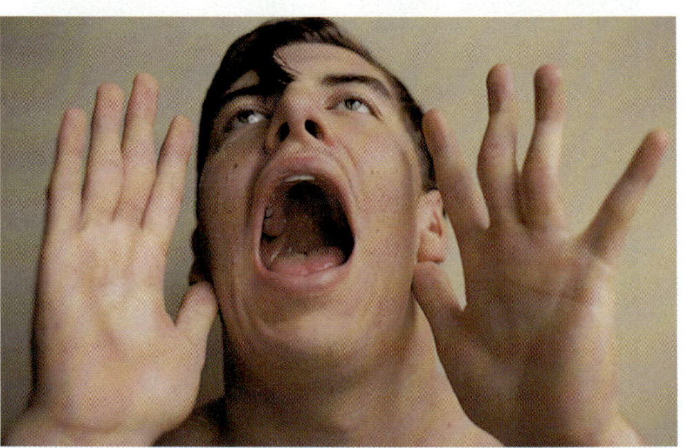

FIGURE 12-11. Marfan syndrome with evidence of a high, arched palate, arachnodactyly, and hyperextensible joints.

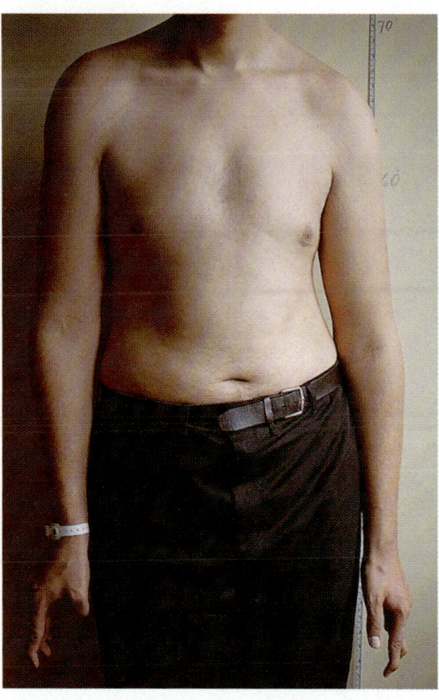

FIGURE 12-12. Marfan syndrome (same patient as in Fig. 12-11) showing pectus excavatum, long arms, and tall stature (almost 7 feet).

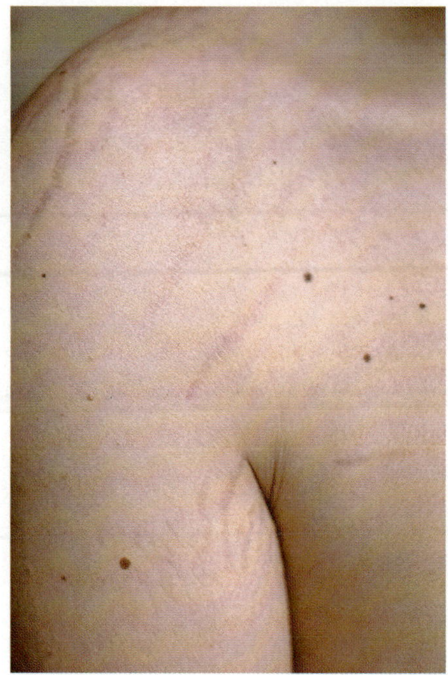

FIGURE 12-13. Marfan syndrome (same patient as in Fig. 12-11) demonstrating striae—a common cutaneous finding in Marfan's.

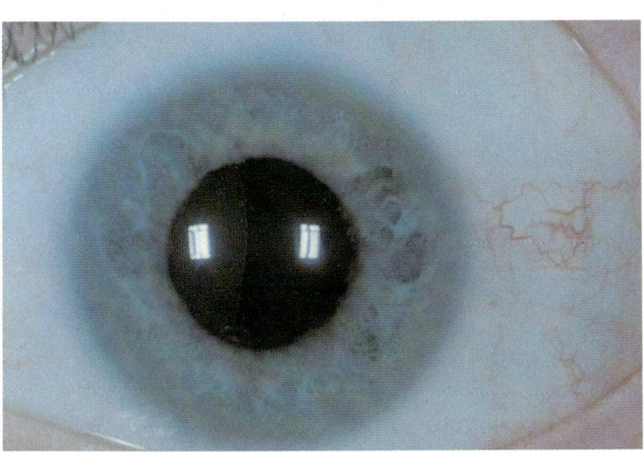

FIGURE 12-14. Supertemporal subluxation of the lens in Marfan syndrome. The edge of the lens is evident in the center of the pupil.

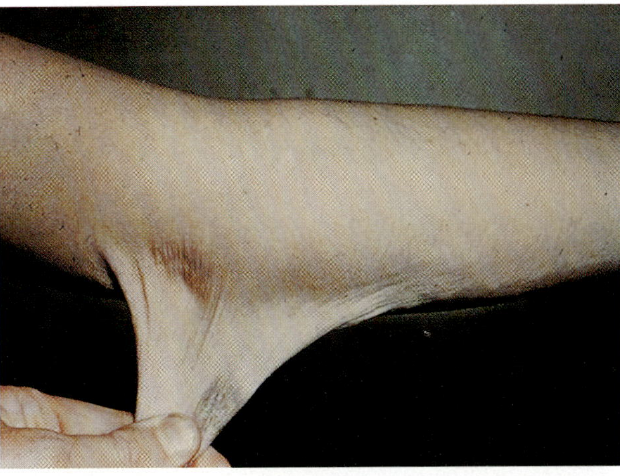

FIGURE 12-15. Ehlers–Danlos syndrome showing hyperelastic skin and easy bruising.

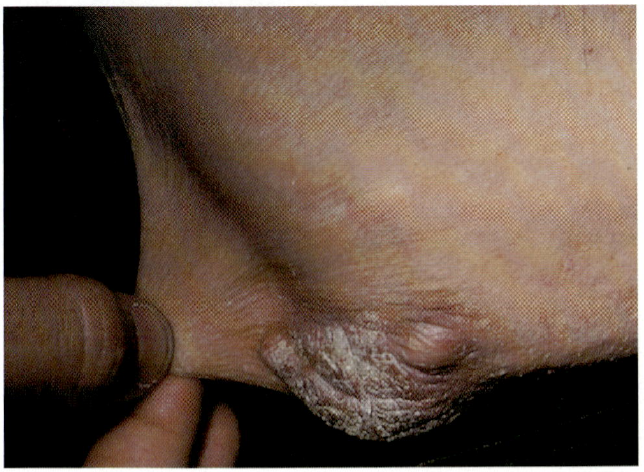

FIGURE 12-16. Hyperelastic skin and pseudotumors of elbow in patient with Ehlers–Danlos syndrome.

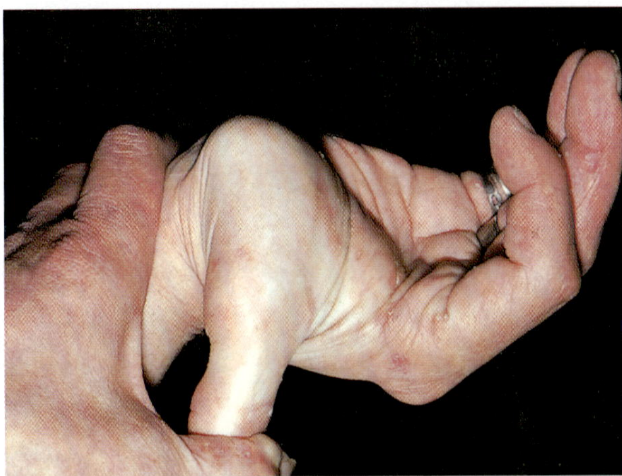

FIGURE 12-17. Ehlers–Danlos syndrome demonstrating extreme hyperextensible joints.

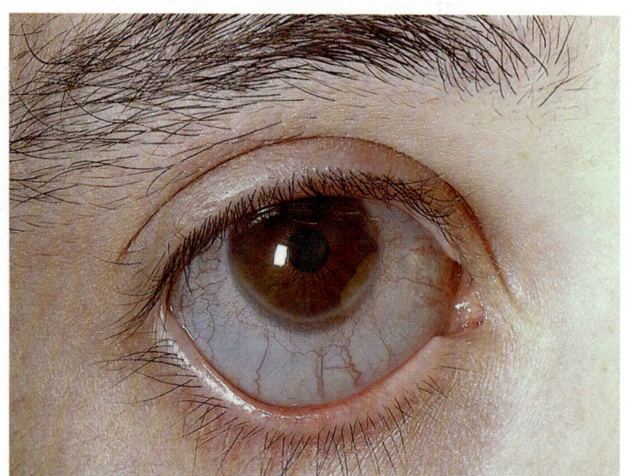

FIGURE 12-18. Blue sclera in an adult with osteogenesis imperfecta.

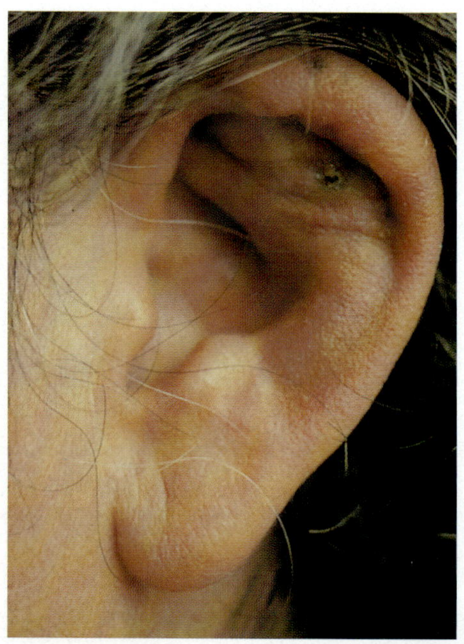

FIGURE 12-19. Relapsing polychondritis. This 48-year-old woman had fever, malaise, polyarthralgia, and recurrent erythema, edema, and pain of the ears for more than 6 months. Note sparing of the ear lobe, a helpful feature differentiating relapsing polychondritis from cellulitis.

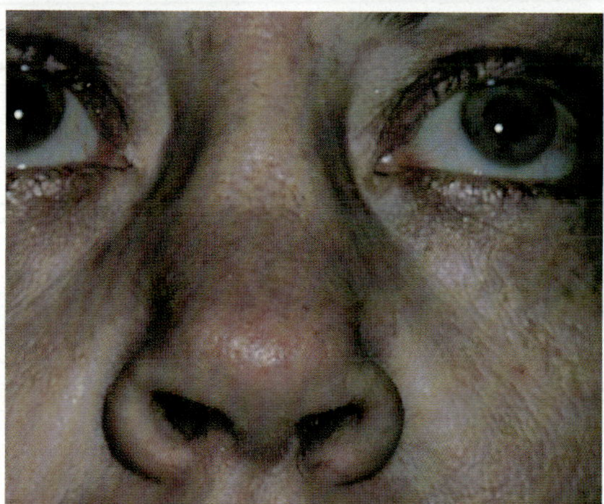

FIGURE 12-20. Saddle nose in relapsing polychondritis.

CONNECTIVE TISSUE DISEASES

Many connective tissue diseases have common features, such as widespread vascular and connective tissue damage. Systemic lupus erythematosus, chronic discoid lupus erythematosus, systemic sclerosis (scleroderma), and scleroderma (morphea) are considered in this chapter. Rheumatoid arthritis is considered in Chapter 22.

LUPUS ERYTHEMATOSUS

Systemic Lupus Erythematosus

Systemic lupus erythematosus (SLE) represents a systemic autoimmune process that involves virtually any organ system. It may be precipitated by ultraviolet (UV) light, bacterial infections, mental or physical stress, or ingestion of various drugs.

Clinical Features

SLE has many protean manifestations, especially arthralgias and arthritis. Initial symptoms include fever, malaise, arthralgia, and sometimes anorexia, and weight loss. Swelling of the hand and wrist joints and dorsa of the hands is common. Muscle pain, weakness, and tenosynovitis also occur.

Cardiopulmonary abnormalities include Libman–Sacks endocarditis, and, in neonatal lupus erythematosus (LE), congenital heart block. Pleurisy, pleural effusion, bronchopneumonia, pneumonitis, and restrictive lung disease are common.

Hepatosplenomegaly is common. Other gastrointestinal manifestations include nausea, vomiting, anorexia, pain, diarrhea, malabsorption, esophageal motility impairment, ileus, peritonitis, abdominal pains, and a nonspecific reactive hepatitis or pancreatitis. Renal findings include a diffuse or membranous glomerulonephritis, nephrotic syndrome, and renal vein thrombosis. The neurologic findings encompass pseudotumor cerebri, seizures, psychosis, severe depression, cranial nerve abnormalities, transverse myelitis, multifocal microinfarcts, cerebral angiitis, multifocal and peripheral neuropathies, and the Guillain–Barre syndrome.

Skin Features

Photosensitivity is common in SLE. There is often erythema and scaling in the form of a "butterfly" rash (Fig. 13-1) and erythematous lesions in other sun-exposed areas. The eruption is maculopapular, bullous, and urticarial; in a few cases, there are hemorrhagic bullae. Facial edema, diffuse pigmentation, or sometimes large areas of scaring with hypopigmentation may occur.

Other skin changes include erythema multiform-like lesions; annular erythema; lesions resembling toxic epidermal necrolysis; persistent nonitching urticarial wheals; lesions resembling chronic discoid erythematosus; a reticulate telangiectatic erythema, especially of the thenar and hypothenar eminences, vasculitic lesions of the fingers (Fig. 13-2), telangiectasia of the nail beds (Fig. 13-3); widespread purpura; *atrophe blanche*; and *livedo reticularis*. Scarring of the skin is common (Fig. 13-4).

Subcutaneous nodules similar to rheumatoid nodules may develop over the dorsa of the phalangeal joints and wrists, elbows, knee, and occiput. Panniculitis leading to subcutaneous atrophy may be seen in lupus profundus (Fig. 13-5). The hair is often dry and brittle, producing irregular, difficult-to-manage hair. Diffuse or cicatricial alopecia (Fig. 13-6) is common.Painless ulcers of the palate, buccal mucosa (Fig. 13-7), or gums as well as nasal septal ulcers may occur during periods of exacerbation.

The skin lesions of neonatal lupus erythematosus are evident at birth or before 3 months of age. They include facial macular erythema, which may be slightly elevated and annular or bullous in character. The lesions are often periocular or involve the chest, back, or extremities. Scaling is common. Delayed healing may occur with alopecia, scarring, and telangiectasia, especially of the scalp and temples.

Ocular Features

Many patients have photophobia, irritation, conjunctival redness, transient blindness, blurred vision, lid involvement (Fig. 13-8), and conjunctival, corneal, scleral (Fig. 13-9), and other changes. Lid changes in SLE include erythema, scaling, telangiectasis, edema, scarring, lash loss, subcutaneous nodules, and ptosis.

Conjunctival findings include papillary conjunctivitis; chronic conjunctivitis associated with keratoconjunctivitis sicca; recurrent attacks of velvetlike edema and congestion of the bulbar conjunctiva; subconjunctival hemorrhages; focal nodules suggestive of phlyctenules; and mild or considerable scarring, arising from the inflammatory conjunctival reaction.

Corneal findings consist of punctate epithelial keratitis with symptoms of recurrent erosions: vascularized, peripheral keratitis associated with conjunctival scarring, peripheral furrows, and deep interstitial keratitis. Scleral involvement in SLE is manifested as episcleritis: a diffuse anterior, nodular, or rarely, necrotizing nodular scleritis. Orbital features include a pseudotumor with proptosis or myositis. Uveal tract involvement is in the form of an iridocyclitis and in some instances grayish-white or yellowish miliary choroidal foci.

Retinal findings include arteritis, vascular occlusions, microaneurysms, and venous engorgement, secondary hypertensive retinal changes, cotton-wool spots (cytoid bodies) usually near the posterior pole, Roth spots, retinal edema, and retinal pigment epithelial disturbance with loss of pigment, gliosis, and detachment.

The neuroophthalmic findings encompass papilledema, optic atrophy, optic nerve ischemia, optic neuritis, decreased accommodation, mydriasis, gaze palsies, intranuclear ophthalmoplegia, third-nerve palsy, nystagmus, homonymous hemianopsia, and visual loss.

Chronic Discoid Lupus Erythematosus

Skin Features

Skin lesions seen in chronic discoid lupus erythematosus are similar in appearance and distribution to those found in systemic lupus erythematosus. Most characteristic is a butterfly pattern over the cheeks and bridging the nose, often extending to other light-exposed sites such as the V of the chest (Fig. 13-10), ears, and dorsac of forearms and hands.

The skin lesions are well defined, dusky red, circumscribed, single or multiple patches at times with dry adherent scales and atrophy (Figs. 13-11 and 13-12). Atrophy with hyper- and hypopigmentation is of significant cosmetic concern, especially in dark-skinned patients (Fig. 13-13). Follicular plugging and dilated follicles are characteristic, especially on the external ears (Fig. 13-14) and in atrophic patches of the scalp (Fig. 13-15). Other skin lesions include the following:

1. A tumid form characterized by large, swollen, brawny, tense, and warm areas on the cheek or arm. The skin surface is reddish and appears mottled because of scarring. Sometimes epidermal atrophy with dilatation of superficial skin vessels causes a reticulated telangiectasia.

2. A rosacea-like skin rash of the midfacial area, forehead, and sometimes chin. The lesions appear as reddish nodules associated with diffuse erythema but no pustules.
3. Annular lesions of the face, mouth, neck, and chest resembling erythema multiforme.
4. Dull erythema, itching, pain, and swelling (chilblainlike lesions) of the toes, fingers, heels, calves, knees, knuckles, elbows, nose, and ears.
5. Lupus erythematosus profundus (panniculitis) of the face, arms, hands, breasts, trunk, buttocks, or legs with or without other skin lesions. The cutaneous infiltrate is deep and persistent, causing nodular, sharply defined lesions. Healing leads to a sunken area and, occasionally, to soft, slightly pink areas of anetoderma (Fig. 13-5).
6. Nail changes include subungual hyperkeratosis red-blue coloring of the nail plate, longitudinal stria, and crumbling.

Mucous membrane lesions may involve the nose, buccal mucosa, palate, vulva, and anal area. They are hyperkeratotic, lichen planus–like plaques (nasal and oral lesions), erythematous patches with a depressed center and superficial ulceration (tongue, buccal mucosa, and palate), leukoplakia (oral lesions), or erythematous lesions (vulva and anus). The lips may be slightly thickened, with superficial ulceration and crusting.

Ocular Features

The skin rash usually involves bilateral inferior lids and lid margins (Fig. 13-16), although unilateral lid involvement is occasionally observed. The lid margins are erythematous, are often telangiectatic, and have fine, adherent scales. Madarosis (lash loss) eventually occurs, and the lid margin becomes irregular in appearance. Scarring may cause lash distortion and restricted lid movement.

A fine papillary conjunctivitis with marked redness and conjunctival scarring sometimes occurs, and a superficial punctate keratitis, stromal keratitis, and neovascularization have been reported.

SCLERODERMA

Scleroderma constitutes a localized or generalized hardening of the skin. It is found in systemic sclerosis, cutaneous forms of sclerosis (localized or generalized morphea), lupus erythematosus, and dermatomyositis.

Systemic Sclerosis (Scleroderma)

Systemic sclerosis (scleroderma) is characterized by fibrous and degenerative changes in skin and internal organs, vascular insufficiency, and vasospasm. It usually affects women in the fourth to sixth decade of life. Raynaud phenomenon often precedes the skin changes (Fig. 13-17). Pain, polyarthralgia, weight loss, and progressive weakness are noted. Infrequently, early symptoms include dysphagia, gastroesophageal reflux, abdominal pain, and constipation or diarrhea. Bony changes consist of mild to severe absorption of the terminal phalanges, erosive arthropathy, intraosseous deposition of calcium, osteopoikilosis, and osteolysis.

Gastrointestinal involvement includes esophageal dysfunction with difficulty swallowing and gastroesophageal reflux, gastrointestinal hypomotility, paralytic ileus, steatorrhea, malabsorption, and diarrhea.

Cardiopulmonary involvement encompasses cystic lung changes, pneumothorax, pneumonia, pulmonary fibrosis, and pulmonary hypertension. Cardiac involvement includes arrhythmias, mitral valve prolapse, and general enlargement of the heart.

Renal disease is the major cause of death and is often associated with malignant hypertension and renal failure. Central nervous system involvement is manifested by cranial nerve involvement and autonomic neuropathy.

Skin Features

The skin at first becomes edematous, followed after several weeks or months by a feeling of tightness, loss of mobility due to contractures, and thickening or induration. It usually involves the fingers, arms, and face but may be generalized. Ultimately, the skin appears glossy and hard; frequently, there are small, matlike telangiectases of the face, lips, upper trunk, and hands (Fig. 13-17). Ulceration of the finger pulp, knuckles, and lower legs, as well as gangrene of the digits may occur.

The facies in scleroderma is distinctive (Fig. 13-18). The forehead appears smooth, the facial wrinkles are "ironed out," the skin is bound down, the nose is small and pinched, radial furrows are evident around the mouth, and opening of the mouth is restricted. Pigmentation often occurs that may be generalized or in an Addisonian pattern without mucous membrane involvement. Sometimes the pigmentation involves primarily the face and extremities. Calcinosis cutis may occur on the phalanges (Fig. 13-19), occasionally around the elbows and knees, along the iliac crest, between the vertebrae, and on the dorsa of the feet.

Ocular Features

Lid skin changes result in lagophthalmos, blepharophimosis, ptosis, and eventually skin atrophy. The lower lids cannot be pulled down because of skin atrophy.

Keratoconjunctivitis sicca (15% of patients), conjunctival edema, foreshortening of the fornix, conjunctival telangiectasis, vascular dilatation, and vascular varicosities may all occur. In the later stages, there is a fine, subepithelial fibrosis beneath the bulbar conjunctiva as well as abnormal conjunctival vessels.

Failure of lid closure may lead to exposure keratitis and shallow indolent ulcers that heal without neovascularization. Periorbital edema is uncommon. Retinal edema, exudates, hemorrhages, central retinal vein occlusion, and cotton-wool patches are usually caused by hypertension but occasionally arise from primary vascular involvement. The cataractous changes appear as fine dots or streaks in the form of a star, situated beneath the anterior and posterior capsule.

Localized Morphea (Localized Scleroderma; Circumscribed Scleroderma)

Skin Features

Localized morphea (localized scleroderma, circumscribed scleroderma) consists of localized sclerosis of the skin. The lesions appear as circumscribed plaques or band lesions (Fig. 13-20), beginning as indurated, purplish or mauve-colored plaques. Guttate lesions are smaller and more numerous but are otherwise similar to plaque lesions. Linear lesions (Fig. 13-21) are similar to plaque lesions except that only the advancing border has a lilac color. Frontoparietal lesions (Fig. 13-22) are often associated with facial hemiatrophy.

Ocular Features

Ocular involvement is uncommon but includes enophthalmos, lash loss, lid edema, heterochromia, atrophy of the medial part of the iris, and myopathy of the extraocular muscles.

Generalized Morphea (Generalized Scleroderma)

Generalized morphea (generalized scleroderma) constitutes sclerosis of widespread skin areas. It begins insidiously and is often relatively mild and slowly progressive, resulting in calcinosis (deposition of calcium salts in subcutaneous nodules, tendons, or muscles); telangiectasia; Raynaud phenomenon; and esophageal dysfunction. There are no systemic abnormalities. It begins between the third and fourth decade of life and is more common in females.

Large plaques occur that are otherwise similar to those in localized morphea. Favored sites include the upper trunk, breasts, abdomen, upper thighs, arms, and hands, and occasionally the scalp, face, neck, and legs. Infrequently, they involve the entire body surface. The skin appears shiny, is indurated, and may be brown in color; the trunk and extremities may have brawny, nonpitting edema.

The face may be expressionless and opening of the mouth restricted. Scalp involvement leads to cicatricial alopecia. Trunk lesions occasionally cause respiratory difficulty and may lead to death.

Lichen Sclerosis [Lichen Sclerosus et Atrophicus (LS and A)]

Lichen sclerosis [lichen sclerosus et atrophicus (LS and A)] is an uncommon disease that usually occurs in females and frequently develops following menopause. It is characterized by small, white skin areas; an atrophic condition of the vulva (Fig. 13-23) and perianal skin in females; and balanitis xerotica obliterans in males.

Skin Features

Nongenital skin lesions occur on the trunk; neck; axilla; flexor surfaces of the wrists, palms, and soles; and around the eyes. They are small, white, shiny, round maculas or papules, which are usually aggregated into plaques. In some instances, they are associated with bullae, purpura, or telangiectases. The orifices of the sebaceous glands and sweat glands contain yellow or brown, horny plugs. The lesions lead to atrophy, characterized by wrinkling and depression of the skin.

Oral lesions are characterized by bluish-white plaques on the inner surface of the cheek or palate. Sometimes they ulcerate or occasionally have a reticulate appearance simulating lichen planus.

The most common sites are vulvar and anal. Itching is frequent and distressing. Lesions have a characteristic hourglass configuration because of sparing of the perineum (Fig. 13-24), although lesions may extend to the inner aspects of the thighs. They appear as ivory-colored, atrophic papules with follicular hyperkeratosis and plugging, often breaking down with a macerated appearance. Intense pruritus irritation, soreness, pain, and dyspareunia may occur along with atrophy and severe shrinkage of the vulva. Many patients develop leukoplakia that is precancerous.

Balanitis xerotic obliterans (Fig. 13-25) begins with an acquired phimosis or recurrent balanitis, which causes itching, soreness, and pain on erection. Later, the prepuce becomes sclerotic and cannot be retracted. The glans and the undersurface of the prepuce are shiny and bluish-white (Fig. 13-26). The skin lesions may involve the lid and periocular area.

Scleredema (Scleredema Adultorum; Scleredema of Buschke)

Scleredema (scleredema adultorum; scleredema of Buschke) is characterized by indurated skin areas that eventually clear. It is usually preceded by infection (e.g., influenza, measles, mumps, tonsillitis, scarlet fever, impetigo, or cellulitis) or trauma. Prodromal symptoms include slight fever, malaise, and muscle and joint pain. It is characterized by nonpitting, poorly circumscribed induration of the forehead; face; occasionally of the tongue and pharynx; later of the shoulders, arms, hands, and upper trunk; and infrequently of the

abdomen and legs. Rarely, it involves the parotid glands and skeletal and cardiac muscles, causing arrhythmias. Myelomas are occasionally seen. Sometimes the involved area is brownish in color. The lesions persist for months or years before receding spontaneously. A second type of scleredema is associated with late-onset insulin-dependent diabetes and is seen more frequently in men than women (Fig. 13-27). Occasionally, scleredema involves the lids.

Dermatomyositis

Dermatomyositis is a systemic vascular disorder characterized by skin and muscle inflammation with acute or insidious onset. It or a dermatomyositis-like picture may be associated with or induced by various medications (e.g., penicillamine and tamoxifen), some viral illnesses, and various collagen diseases, especially Sjögren syndrome. In adult males, an underlying pulmonary carcinoma is sometimes present (Fig. 13-28), and in women, an underlying breast or ovarian cancer; in both males and females, an underlying lymphoma may occur.

The proximal muscle groups of the extremities usually ache and are atonic and weak. Later, they become atrophic and develop contractures (Fig. 13-28). Sometimes the affected muscles are painful and tender. Dysphagia occurs from involvement of the muscles of the tongue, pharynx, and upper third of the esophagus. In the juvenile form, calcification of the subcutaneous tendons may be found. Joint symptoms may also be present. (Muscle involvement without skin involvement is termed *polymyositis.*)

Skin Features

Dermatomyositis is characterized by telangiectasia and skin rash in the butterfly region of the cheeks, on the neck, shoulders, upper chest, and back. Often there is a heliotrope erythema of the face that may involve the upper cheeks, forehead, and temples (Fig. 13-29). Heliotropic telangiectasis of the eyelids is characteristic in dermatomyositis (Figs. 13-30 to 13-32). Scaly areas occur on the backs of the hands, knuckles, elbows, and knees. Flat-topped erythematous papules over the knuckles (Gottron papules) are felt to be diagnostic of dermatomyositis (Fig. 13-31). Diffuse shininess of the nails and subungual erythema caused by dilated capillary loops of the nail folds also occurs. The cuticles are thickened, rough, hyperkeratotic, and irregular. Diffuse pigmentation may be associated with the skin lesions. Rarely, there is scalp alopecia and diffuse erythema. Raynaud phenomenon is common.

Ocular Features

Conjunctival chemosis is common (Figs. 13-32 and 13-33). The disease may cause a nonspecific conjunctivitis; rarely, a pseudomembranous conjunctivitis; and in some instances, bilateral vascular conjunctival lesions distinguished by a small (0.5 cm), circular, avascular zone in which the vessels surrounding the zone terminate in small arteriovenous loops. Occasionally, the vessels have irregular digitations.

Other ocular findings include a nonspecific episcleritis or scleritis, exophthalmos, anterior uveitis, retinopathy with cotton-wool spots, late sequelae of pigmentary maculopathy and optic atrophy, and extraocular muscle paralysis and nystagmus.

SJÖGREN SYNDROME

Primary Sjögren Syndrome

Primary Sjögren syndrome is characterized by dryness of the eyes and mouth without clinical findings of connective tissue disease. Sometimes, at a later date, the patient develops signs of systemic disease such as arthritis, central and peripheral nervous system disease, vasculitis, myositis, pneumonitis, and renal abnormalities. Occasionally, a chronic bilateral anterior and posterior uveitis with pars plana exudates occurs. Usually, primary Sjögren syndrome runs a rather benign course.

Secondary Sjögren Syndrome

About half of Sjögren patients have secondary Sjögren syndrome with dry eyes and mouth, as well as manifestations of connective tissue disease (e.g., rheumatoid arthritis, systemic lupus erythematosus, scleroderma, polymyositis, systemic lupus erythematosus, scleroderma, polymyositis, vasculitis, polyarteritis nodosa, sarcoid, chronic hepatobiliary disease, chronic pulmonary fibrosis, purpura, Hashimoto thyroiditis, hyperglobulinemia, Raynaud phenomenon, Waldenström macroglobulinemia, or lymphoproliferative disorders).

Clinical Manifestations

The patient experiences a loss of taste and smell and a dry mouth. Other symptoms encompass dryness of the lips, tongue, nasopharynx, vagina, and skin; fissuring of the corners of the mouth; and achlorhydria.

The saliva is at first thick and mucoid in character; later, it is reduced in amount. The tongue appears red, smooth, and dry. Dental caries occur and are severe and progressive (Figs. 13-34 and 13-35). The lips are dry and scaly. Cracks occur at the corners of the mouth and are often associated with candidiasis. There is often a history of recurrent episodes of parotid, submaxillary, or sublingual salivary gland swelling.

Involvement of the nasal, pharyngeal, laryngeal, and pulmonary mucous membranes is characterized by decrease in the sense of smell, nasal crusting, dryness, and atrophic rhinitis, hoarseness of aphonia, pulmonary infiltration, atelectasis, and fibrosis. Vaginal and rectal involvement causes pruritus, vaginitis, and dryness of the anal and rectal mucosa.

Skin Features

Dryness of the skin occurs in about 50% of patients (Fig. 13-36), and partial or complete loss of sweating are often seen in Sjögren syndrome. Recurrent episodes of non-thrombocytopenic purpura appearing as round, pink lesions in the dependent areas may also occur. The lesions resolve after several days, leaving brown pigmented stains. The hair is dry, sparse, and brittle; diffuse alopecia of the scalp, axillae, pubis, and limbs may occur.

Ocular Features

Ocular manifestations include reduced aqueous tear production, abnormal accumulation of tear mucus (Fig. 13-37), conjunctival and corneal epithelial filaments (Figs. 13-38 and 13-39). The keratoconjunctivitis sicca causes a foreign-body sensation, irritation, pain, redness, and often blurred vision resulting from the abnormal tear film interface. Interpalpebral epithelial keratitis, corneal erosions, and microbial conjunctival and corneal infections are common. Typically, the devitalized conjunctival and corneal epithelium stain with rose bengal (Figs. 13-40 and 13-41). A papillary response is seen on the tarsal surfaces but is a nonspecific sign.

GRAFT-VERSUS-HOST DISEASE

Graft-versus-host disease (GVH) develops in patients who are unable to reject incompatible lymphoid cells received from an immunocompetent donor. The severity of reaction is graded from 1 to 4, and the prognosis for life is less than 25% for patients who have a grade 2 to 4 reaction. GVH may be acute (developing between 1 week to 3 months after transplant) or chronic (developing after 3 months).

Acute Graft-Versus-Host Disease

Symptoms of acute GVH usually develop within 60 days (often 7 to 12 days) following bone marrow transplantation. This disease is manifested by mild fever, skin rash, watery or bloody diarrhea, and liver involvement.

The skin rash accompanies the fever and varies from a malar flush and erythema of the palms and soles to a generalized erythematous morbilliform or scarlatiniform rash. Sometimes erythematous or violaceous follicular papules are found. Infrequently, toxic epidermal necrolysis or a severe exfoliative erythroderma develops. The mucous membranes are often involved, and, in some patients, the hair follicles are also involved. Diarrhea develops soon after onset of the skin rash; the degree of severity is similar to the severity of the skin rash. It is sometimes prolonged.

Chronic GVH

Chronic GVH often follows acute GVH. It usually develops within 100 days after transplant and involves the skin, liver, mouth, upper respiratory tract, esophagus, lower gastrointestinal tract, skeletal muscles, and eyes. Infrequently, it causes autoimmune hemolytic anemia. Death occurs in about 10% of patients.

Skin Features

Chronic GVH patients often develop a generalized or localized lichenoid eruption mimicking lichen planus and leading to hyper- or hypopigmentation of the skin, nail involvement, and cicatricial alopecia (Fig. 13-42).

The skin reaction may resemble lupus erythematosus or dermatomyositis. During the late phase of chronic GVH (about 1 year later), the patient often develops a severe poikiloderma associated with widespread cutaneous sclero-sis (especially of the face, hands, and feet), contractions, ulcerations, and alopecia. Reticulate, patchy hyperpigmentation or, less commonly, hypopigmentation, vitiligo, erythema, atrophy, cicatricial alopecia, and deep ulceration of the legs and buttocks may also occur. In some instances, the nails are dystrophic.

White plaques on the tongue and white streaks on the buccal mucosa may develop and are similar to those seen in lichen planus. There is usually xerostomia. Gastrointestinal involvement leads to esophageal changes and may lead to malabsorption and wasting. Upper respiratory tract involvement leads to pulmonary fibrosis and obstructive bronchiolitis. A primary biliary cirrhosis with abnormal liver function tests may also occur.

Ocular Features

Ocular findings include lid changes and Sjögren syndrome. The signs and symptoms of keratoconjunctivitis are usually severe and difficult to treat. Conjunctival intraepithelial neoplasia and frank squamous cell carcinoma of the ocular surface have been seen in association, presumably because of decreased immune surveillance.

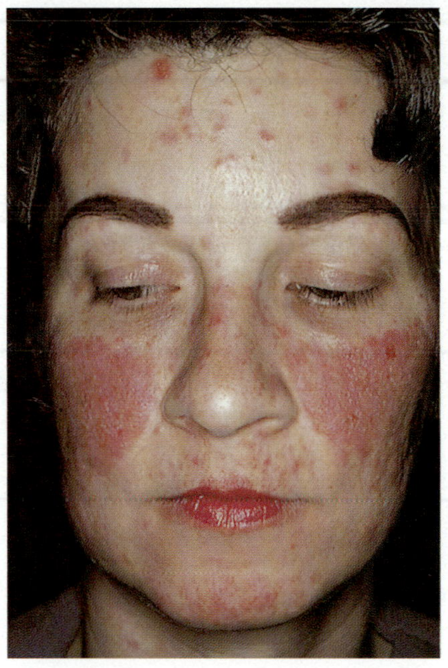

FIGURE 13-1. Butterfly rash in SLE. This 33-year-old woman developed a rash over the face, ears, and arms 10 days after taking Butazolidin for arthralgias. She first noticed marked photosensitivity during the previous spring and summer.

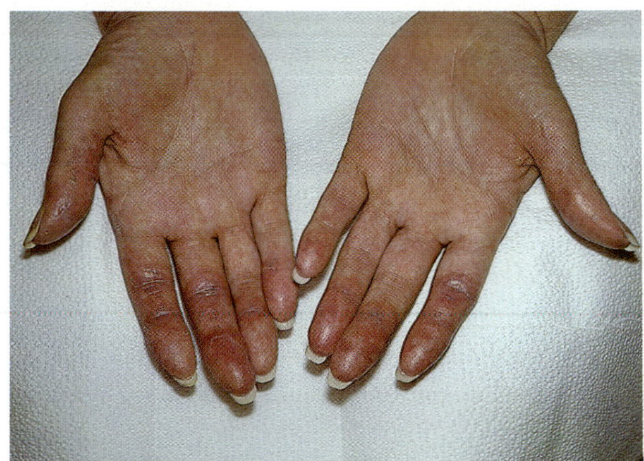

FIGURE 13-2. Vasculitis of palmar aspects of fingertips in the patient shown in Fig. 13-1.

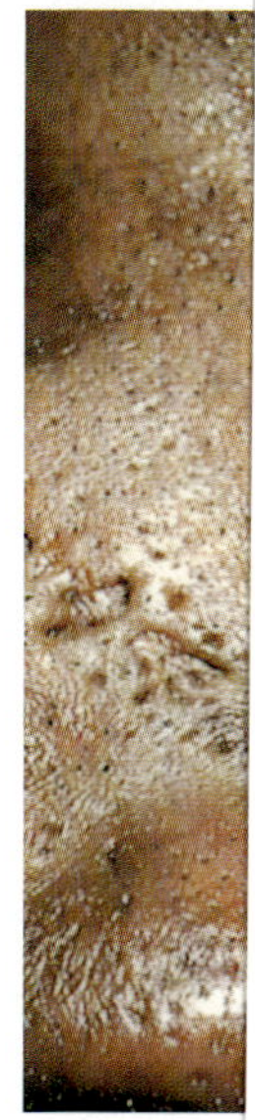

FIGURE 13-1
hyper- and hy
thematosus,
caused him gr

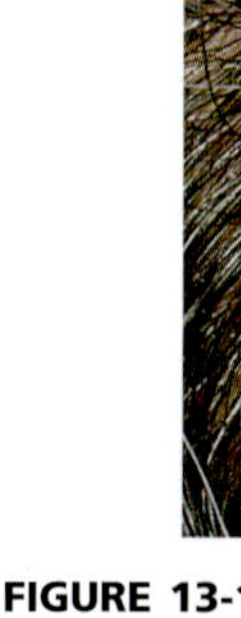

FIGURE 13-1
in discoid lup

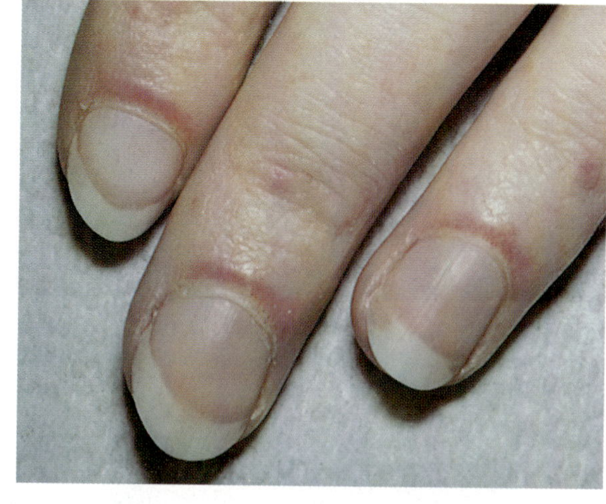

FIGURE 13-3. Telangiectasia of the nail beds in systemic lupus erythematosus.

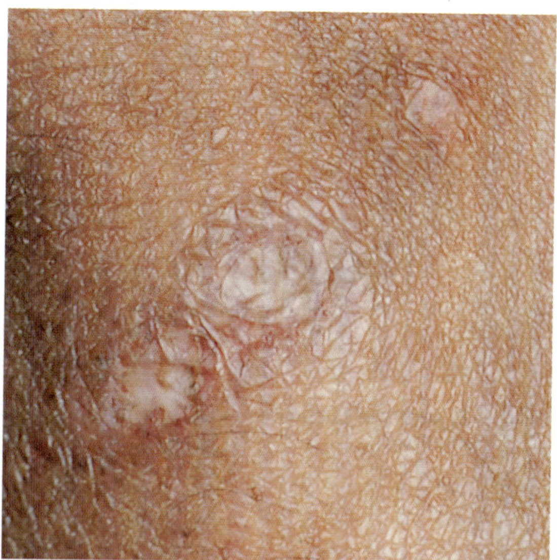

FIGURE 13-4. Scarring of the skin in systemic lupus erythematosus.

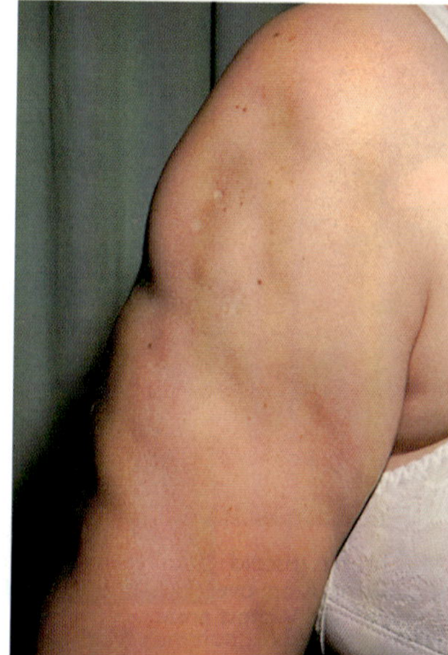

FIGURE 13-5. Panniculitis and subcutaneous atrophy in lupus erythematosus profundus.

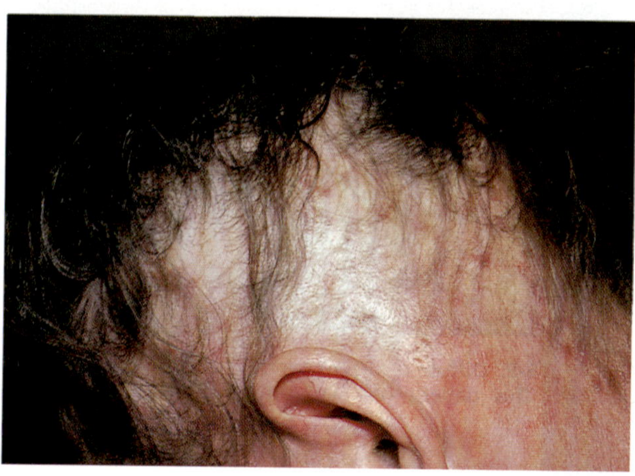

FIGURE 13-6. Extensive cicatricial alopecia in a patient with systemic lupus erythematosus.

   Diseases of the Eye and Skin

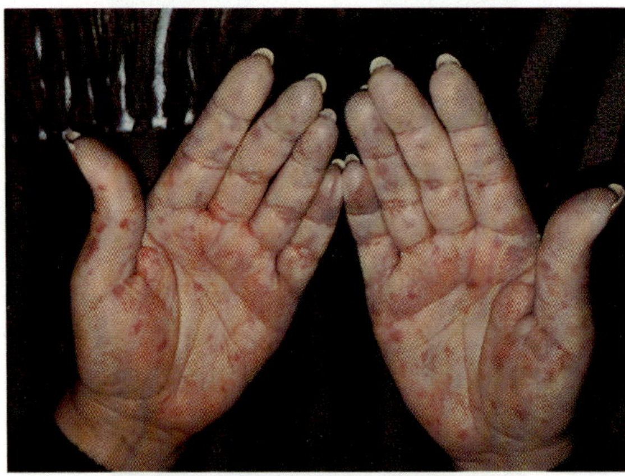

FIGURE 13-17. Telangiectasis and Raynaud phenomenon in scleroderma (CREST syndrome—calcinosis, Raynaud disease, esophageal involvement, sclerodactyly, and telangiectasias).

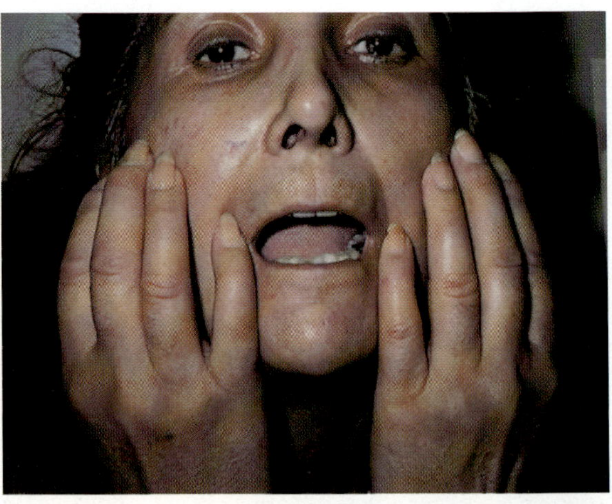

FIGURE 13-18. Acrosclerosis (note the shiny tight skin over the fingers) and decreased ability to open the mouth in systemic scleroderma. The patient also experienced esophageal dysmotility.

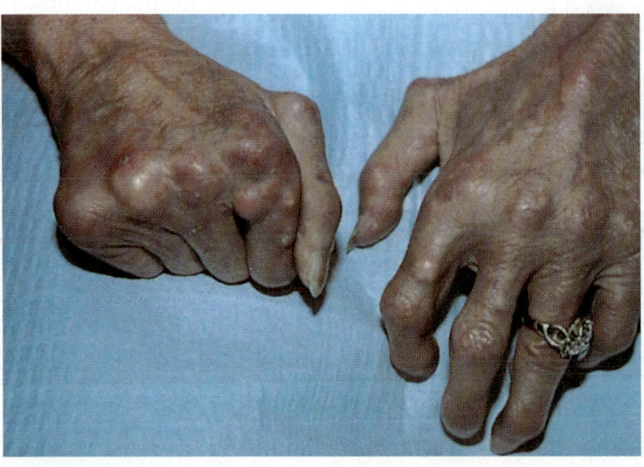

FIGURE 13-19. Calcinosis cutis in scleroderma. The lesions are evident on the dorsum of the middle digit and the index finger of the right hand. Painful extrusion of calcium salts occurred repeatedly in this patient.

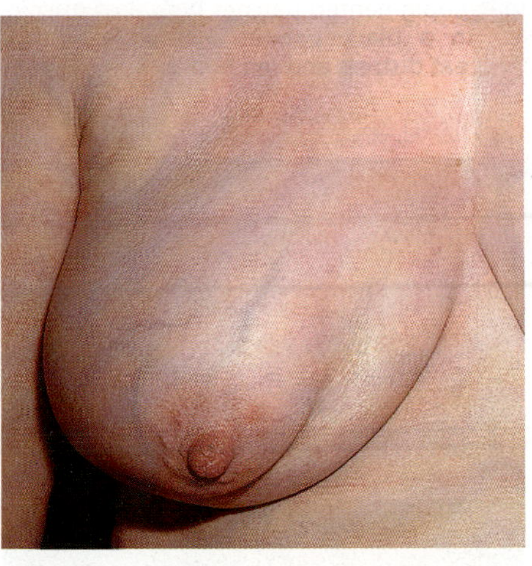

FIGURE 13-20. Scleroderma of the breast. Note annular lesions with pale violaceous margins and central cigarette paper–like appearance. Because of the striking retraction of the skin, the patient feared she had breast cancer.

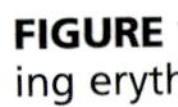

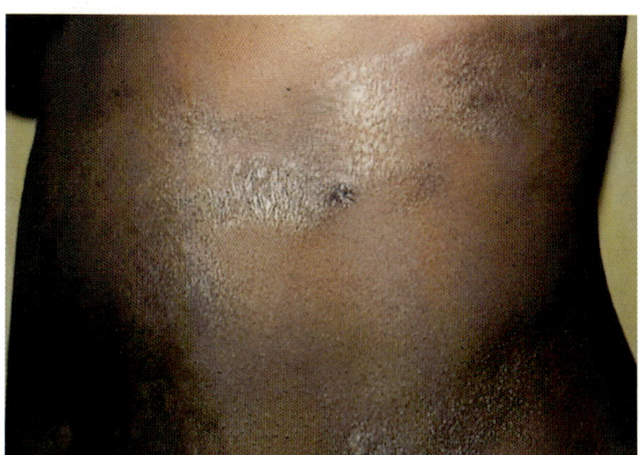

FIGURE 13-21. Linear scleroderma of the trunk.

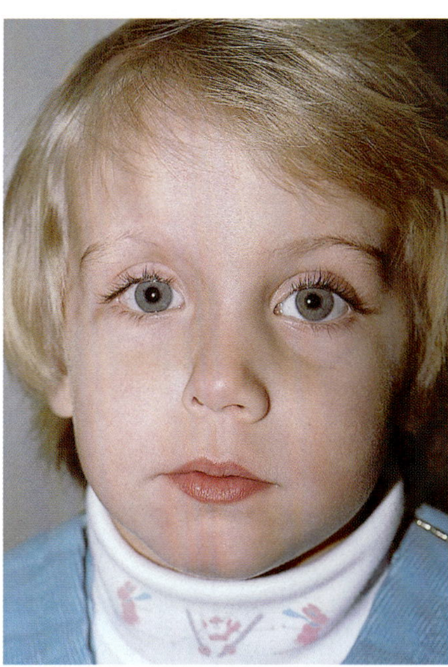

FIGURE 13-22. Frontoparietal scleroderma ("en coupe de sabre") with early hemiatrophy in a 3-year-old girl.

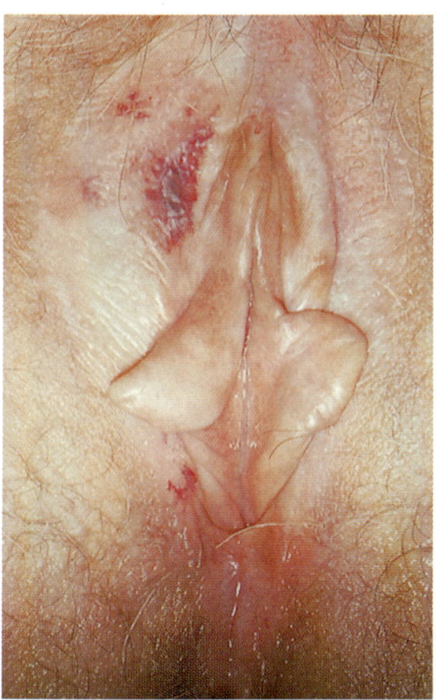

FIGURE 13-23. *Lichen sclerosis et atrophicus* (LS and A) of the vulva. This patient experienced severe itching resulting in hemorrhagic lesions. Because of its sometimes posttraumatic appearance *lichen sclerosis et atrophicus* has been misdiagnosed as sexual abuse in young females.

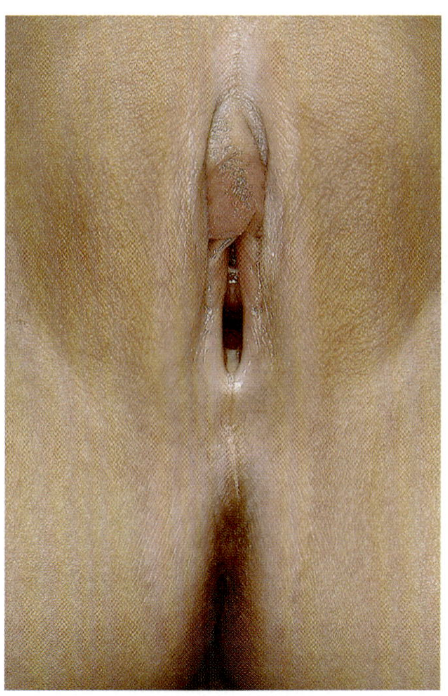

FIGURE 13-24. *Lichen sclerosis et atrophicus* (LS and A) in a 5-year-old girl showing "hourglass" pattern of hypopigmented atrophic lesions.

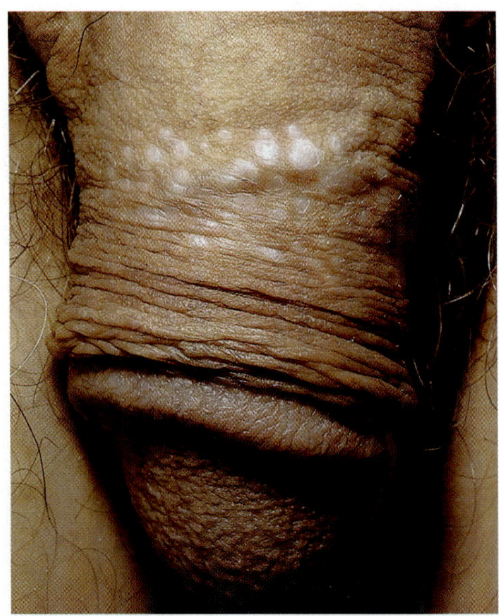

FIGURE 13-25. Lichen sclerosis of penile shaft showing classic ivory-white flat-topped papules.

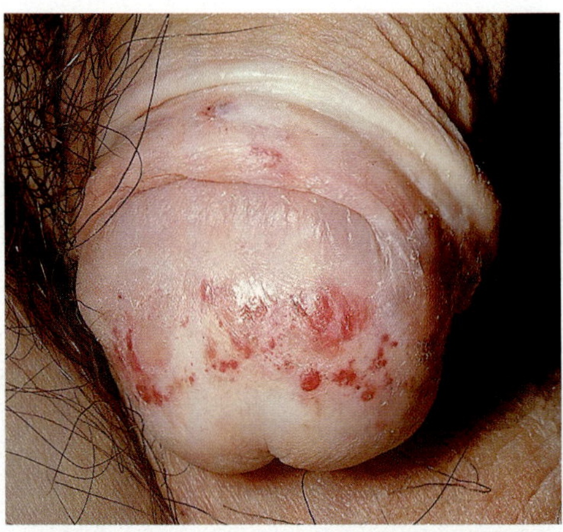

FIGURE 13-26. Lichen sclerosis (balanitis xerotica obliterans) with hemorrhagic lesions of glans penis.

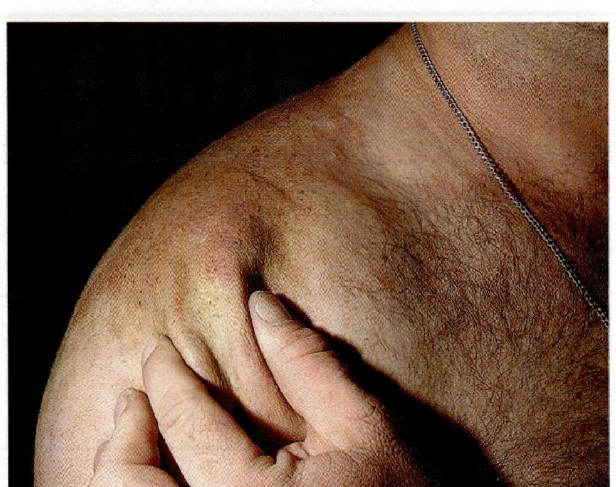

FIGURE 13-27. Scleredema adultorum demonstrating striking woody induration of the skin. He had noticed gradual asymptomatic thickening of his upper back. Further evaluation revealed insulin-resistant diabetes (scleredema diabeticorum).

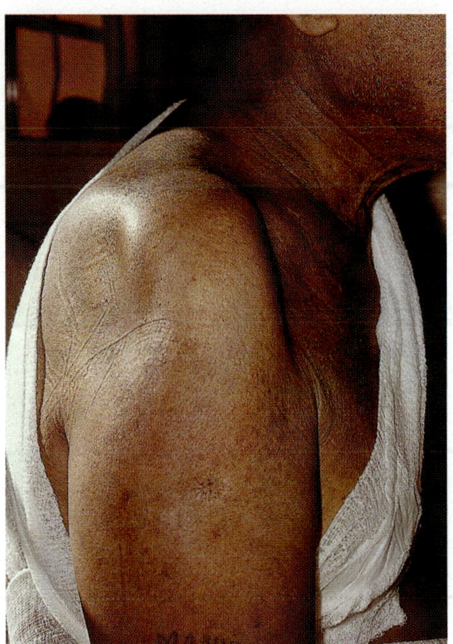

FIGURE 13-28. Marked atrophy of shoulder muscles in patient with dermatomyositis and carcinoma of lung. He died 3 months after this photograph was taken.

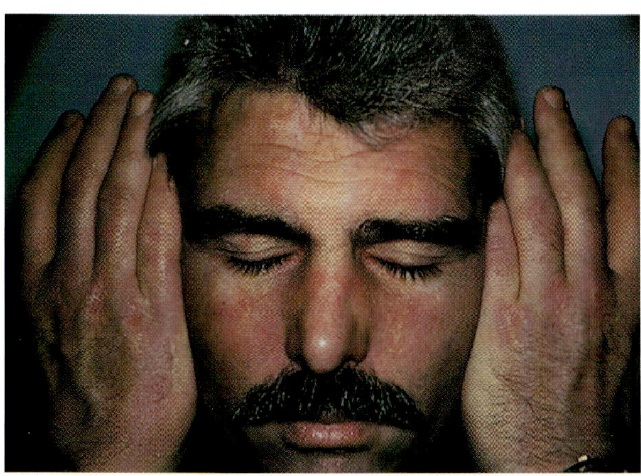

FIGURE 13-29. Dermatomyositis with initial complaint of severe pain and weakness in the hands and arms. Note a pattern of photo dermatitis resembling systemic lupus erythematosus.

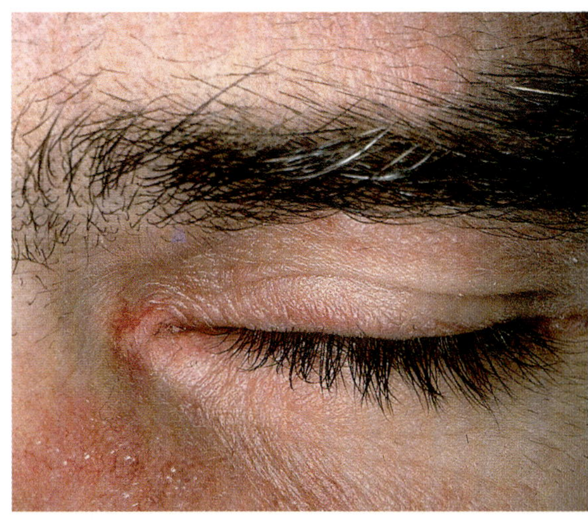

FIGURE 13-30. Heliotropic telangiectasia of eyelids. Close-up of patient pictured in Fig.13-29. This is a classic sign in dermatomyositis.

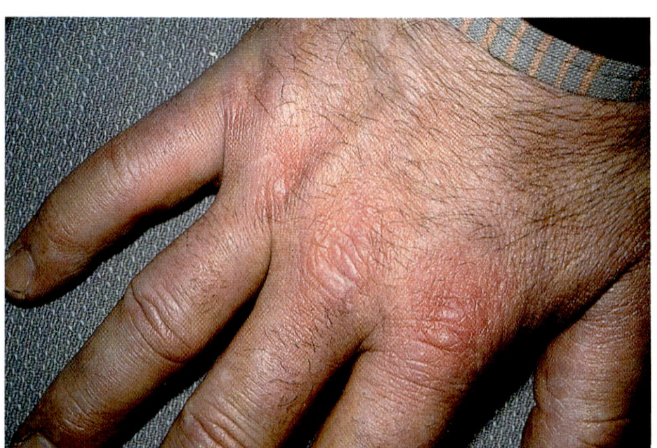

FIGURE 13-31. Gottron papules (flat-topped erythematous papules over the knuckles) highly suggestive of dermatomyositis.

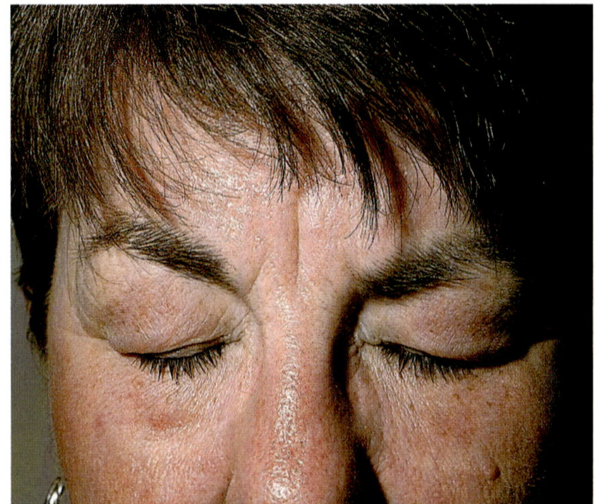

FIGURE 13-32. Lid edema with fine confluent telangiectasia (heliotrope) in patient with dermatomyositis. She had complained of increasing difficulty climbing stairs. Her physician had told her this was because she was aging.

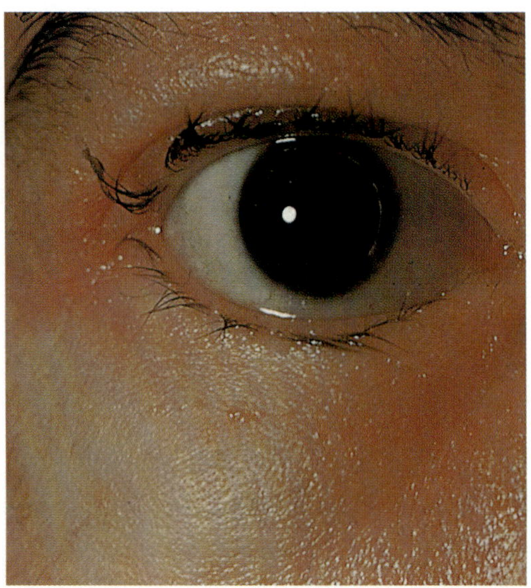

FIGURE 13-33. Upper lid edema and heliotrope erythema of the eyelids is evident in this patient with dermatomyositis. Other lid findings in dermatomyositis include ptosis.

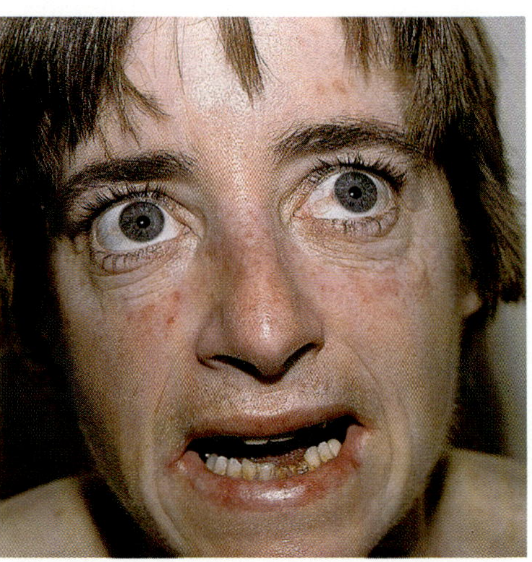

FIGURE 13-34. Sjögren associated with systemic lupus erythematous. Inadequate production of saliva has led to this patient's dental decay. Patient complained of dry mouth, dry eyes, joint pains, and photosensitivity.

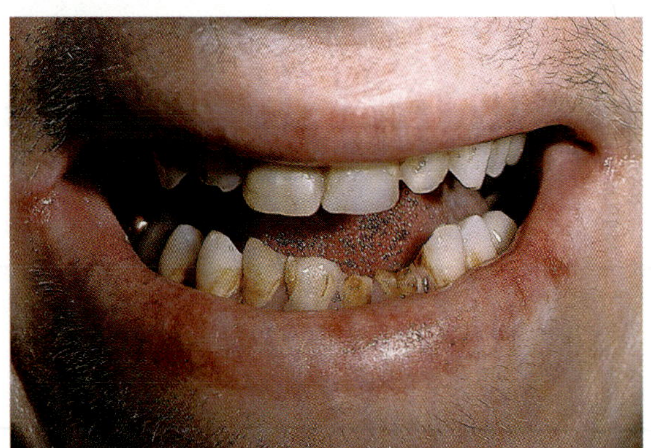

FIGURE 13-35. Close-up of patient in Fig. 13-34 showing severity of tooth decay as well as angular cheilitis.

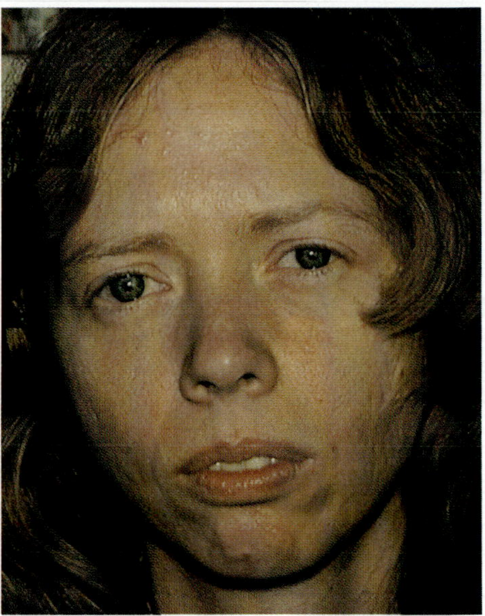

FIGURE 13-36. Facial features in early Sjögren syndrome. Note dry skin and lips.

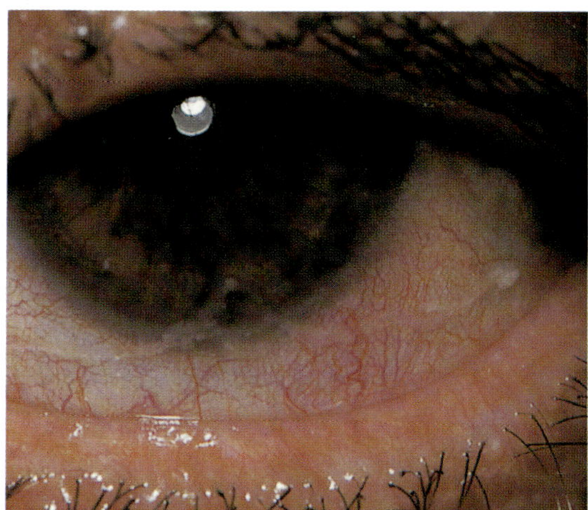

FIGURE 13-37. Abnormal mucus in Sjögren syndrome. A large strand of mucus is evident in the interpalpebral fissure of this patient with Sjögren syndrome. The abnormal mucus often causes blurred vision and foreign body sensation.

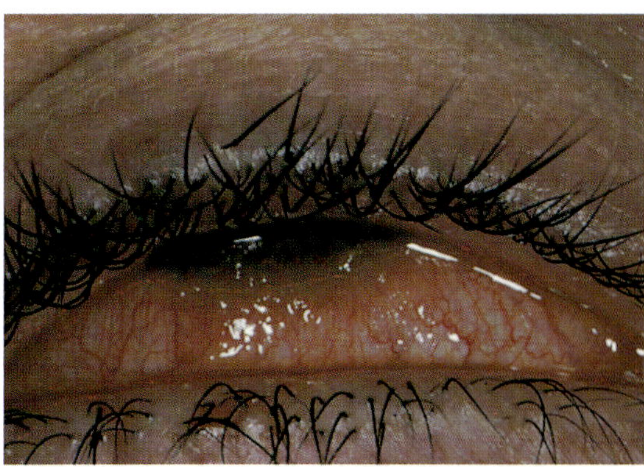

FIGURE 13-38. Conjunctival filaments in Sjögren syndrome. Conjunctival filaments in Sjögren syndrome are uncommon, but when then occur, they are often associated with severe manifestations of dry eye.

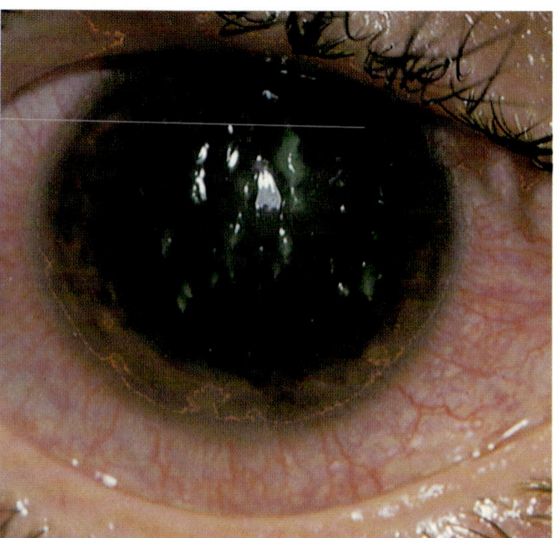

FIGURE 13-39. The corneal filaments are readily seen over the center of the cornea. They have been stained with fluorescein and therefore have a greenish color.

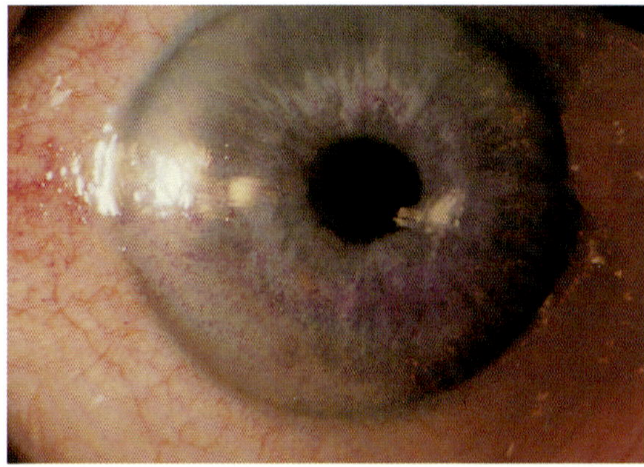

FIGURE 13-40. Staining of the conjunctiva and cornea with rose bengal in Sjögren syndrome. A marked staining of the interpalpebral conjunctiva and cornea is evident in this patient with moderate to marked Sjögren syndrome.

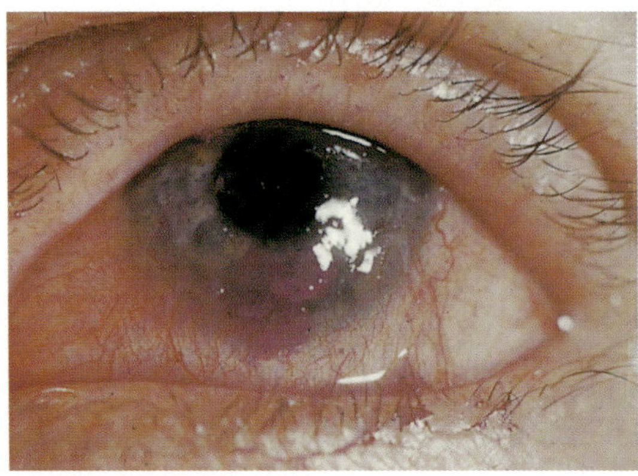

FIGURE 13-41. Rose bengal staining and peripheral corneal scarring in Sjögren syndrome.

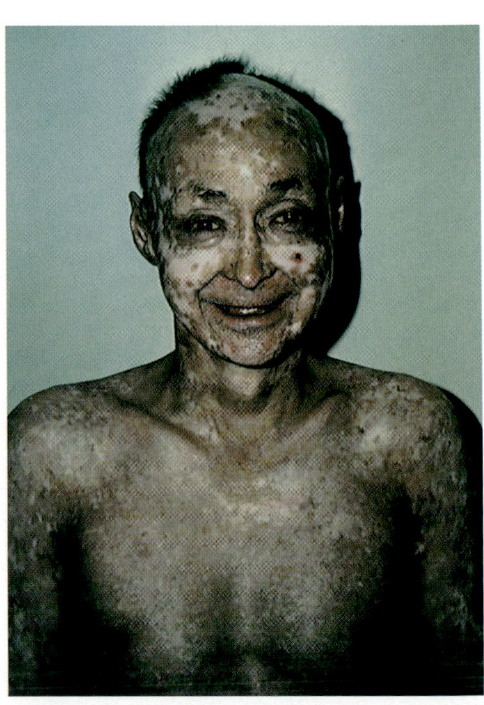

FIGURE 13-42. Chronic GVH disease. Scarring and hypopigmentation are evident in this patient who had received a bone marrow transplant for leukemia.

BLOOD VESSEL DISORDERS

TELANGIECTATIC SYNDROMES

Telangiectases are small vascular lesions produced by the confluence of dilated small venules, arterioles, capillaries, or lymphatics. They appear as dull red, stellate, punctate, or linear blemishes of the skin or mucous membranes.

Secondary Telangiectases

Secondary telangiectases arise secondary to other processes. They are especially common in atrophic skin, such as occurs from prolonged ultraviolet light exposure, irradiation, trauma, use of topical glucocorticoids, and poikiloderma. They develop in various dermatologic diseases, such as xeroderma pigmentosum, lupus erythematosus, dermatomyositis, scleroderma, and mastocytosis.

Spider Telangiectases (Arterial Spider; Spider Nevus; Nevus Araneus)

In spider telangiectases (arterial spider; spider nevus; nevus araneus), the vessels radiate outward from a central arteriole, and the central arteriole usually pulsates when viewed with diascopy. The lesions often develop during pregnancy but usually disappear within 6 weeks following delivery. They are often seen in patients with liver disease (Fig. 14-1). The lesions occur on the face, neck, hands, and the mucous membranes of the lips and nose.

Rothmund–Thomson Syndrome (Poikiloderma Congenitale)

The Rothmund–Thomson syndrome (poikiloderma congenitale) is autosomal recessive and is more common in females. Dwarfism; various skeletal defects; a small, bird-like face; and uncommonly, neurologic changes may be found.

The telangiectasia is prominent on the face, especially the cheeks. In children, photosensitivity may be a prominent manifestation that leads to bullous lesions, which progresses to poikiloderma. The photosensitivity tends to diminish with age. In some patients, hyperkeratotic lesions develop on the elbows, knees, hands, palms (Fig. 14-2), and soles around the time of puberty.

Ocular Features

The eyebrows and lashes are sparse or absent. Degenerative changes may be seen in the cornea. Lamellar cataracts develop by the fourth or seventh year of life in 50% of patients, beginning in the anterior and posterior cortex. In some instances, strabismus also occurs.

Primary Telangiectasia

Primary telangiectasia are those telangiectatic lesions for which there is no known cause. They are seen in the primary telangiectatic syndromes.

Angioma Serpiginosum (Hutchinson Disease)

Angioma serpiginosum is an uncommon disorder that usually begins in childhood and is most common in females. It is characterized by a diffuse erythematous background and minute (up to 1 mm in diameter) red or purple, punctate lesions that are often grouped into lesions several centimeters in diameter and sometimes into larger plaques. The lesions usually develop on the buttocks and lower legs and gradually enlarge over a period of months or years, then cease to enlarge until adulthood, when they may again increase in size. A single case of retinal angiomata together with spinal nerve root angiomata has been observed in this condition.

Hereditary Hemorrhagic Telangiectasis (Osler–Rendu–Weber Disease)

Hereditary hemorrhagic telangiectasis (Osler–Rendu–Weber disease) is autosomal dominant. It is characterized by development of skin and mucous membrane telangiectasis, arteriovenous malformations, and larger aneurysms. It involves both sexes equally. The lesions usually become manifest after puberty. The presenting symptom is often that of recurrent epistaxis, usually beginning at puberty but sometimes sooner. The nasal hemorrhage may lead to hemoptysis, hematemesis, and melena.

Dilated capillaries and telangiectasis develop over the entire body, especially on the upper body (face, ears, lips, forearm, hands, fingers, nail beds, and trunk), usually beginning during the third or fourth decade of life (Fig. 14-3). Individual lesions have a linear or punctate shape. Dilated capillaries and telangiectasis also develop on the mucous membrane, especially the nasal, oral, and gastrointestinal mucosa. Telangiectasis lesions of the tongue are quite characteristic, appearing as a single, dilated vessel that causes the involved fungiform papillae to be greatly enlarged (Figs. 14-3 and 14-4.)

Pulmonary arteriovenous fistulas occur in some families, causing dyspnea, cyanosis, clubbing, and polycythemia. Hepatic arteriovenous aneurysms, hepatomegaly, cirrhosis, aneurysms of the aortic arch and splenic artery, and multiple cerebral angiomas have all been observed.

Ocular Features

The skin of the eyelid may have a violaceous discoloration, and multiple dilated vessels may cover the lid, especially near the lid margin. The palpebral and tarsal conjunctiva (Fig. 14-5) are sometimes involved by scattered, small telangiectasias, varicosities, and star-shaped angiomas. The centers of the angiomas appear bright red, and the lesion has fine vessels that radiate outward in a straight line. Retinal varicosities and hemorrhages and varicose branching of the veins near the optic disc have all been observed.

Ataxia Telangiectasia (Louis-Bar Syndrome)

Beginning in early childhood, ataxia telangiectasia (Louis-Bar syndrome) is an autosomal recessive, progressive neurologic disease characterized by cerebellar ataxia, increasing tremor, deterioration of mental function, immune dysfunction, and risk of cancer.

Clinical Manifestations

A recurrent or chronic sinusitis, bronchitis, and bronchiectasis commonly occur because of the combined immunodeficiency that is present. Characteristically, patients develop progressive cerebellar ataxia by the age of 2 years with ataxia of the trunk and extremities, dysarthria, myoclonic jerks, areflexia, and distal sensory deficits that become severe by the age of 12. Mental deterioration may also occur.

Patients have about a 10% risk of developing a lymphoreticular system neoplasm before the teenage years. The incidence of breast cancer is significantly increased. Severe pulmonary infections and progressive bronchiectasis occur in many patients. Thymic abnormalities and abnormalities of humoral including an IgA deficiency and cell-mediated immunity may also be found.

Skin Features

The skin features include progressive telangiectasia of the malar eminences, ear lobe, and upper neck. Café-au-lait spots (Fig. 14-6), which are mottled, hypo-, and hyperpigmented areas arranged in a dermatomal distribution; photosensitivity; acanthosis nigricans; eczema; premature graying; and granulomatous lesions have also been observed.

Ocular Features

Progressive telangiectasia of the bulbar conjunctiva occurs before any skin changes (Fig. 14-7) and may be the first sign of the disease. Conjugate gaze disturbances and nystagmus are usually observed following development of the ataxia. Ocular motor apraxia is common. Blepharitis is often seen probably because of the associated IgA deficiency.

Generalized Essential Telangiectasia

Generalized essential telangiectasia begins in late childhood or early adulthood. It is more common in females and is characterized by development of extensive sheets of telangiectases on the extremities or trunk that are usually linear. Small angiomas may also be found. There are no other skin changes. The lesions sometimes cause recurrent hemorrhages into the skin, mucous membranes, or eye.

LYMPHATIC VESSEL DISORDERS

Lymphedema

Lymphedema may be primary or secondary and is caused by inadequate lymphatic drainage. It is characterized by epidermal thickening and a firm, nonpitting swelling, with the latter arising from organization of retained edema fluid.

Primary lymphedema usually involves the legs, although other common areas are the arms, face, and genitalia. Pitting, which disappears following elevation of the involved area, can be demonstrated early in the disease process. Later, the swelling does not pit or disappears following elevation, and the skin cannot be picked up in folds. The epidermis is usually thickened (Fig. 14-8).

Secondary lymphedema arises from lymphatic obstruction as a result of damage to the lymph nodes or lymphatic channels by filariasis or surgery. The skin is usually edematous (Fig. 14-8).

Lymphangiectasis

Lymphangiectasis represents dilated lymph capillaries and occasionally occurs in the skin. The dilated vessels are translucent and sometimes ooze lymph spontaneously or following trauma.

Conjunctival lymphangiectasis may develop in the bulbar or tarsal conjunctiva soon after birth or during childhood. They are usually limited to the conjunctiva but are sometimes associated with lid or orbital lymph channel abnormalities. Once fully developed, the lesions have the appearance of irregular cysts in the superficial conjunctiva.

Occasionally, bulbar conjunctival lymphatic channels become intermittently dilated and filled with blood. The surrounding conjunctiva is edematous, and subconjunctival hemorrhages may be seen. In some instances, the abnormality is associated with trauma or mild inflammation; in other instances, the condition occurs spontaneously.

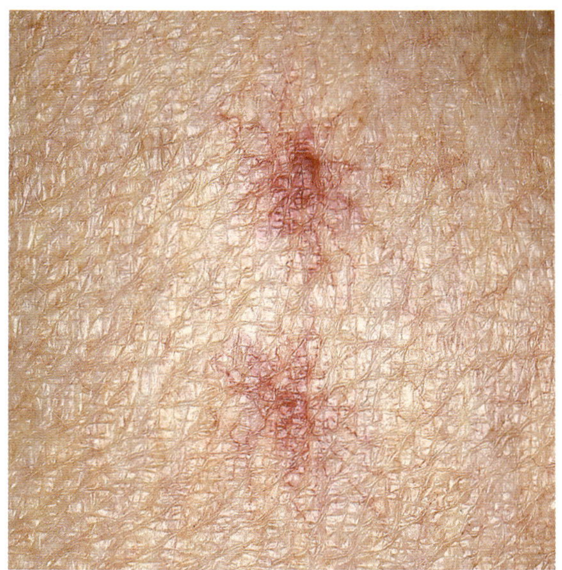

FIGURE 14-1. Spider telangiectasis of the skin arising in cirrhosis.

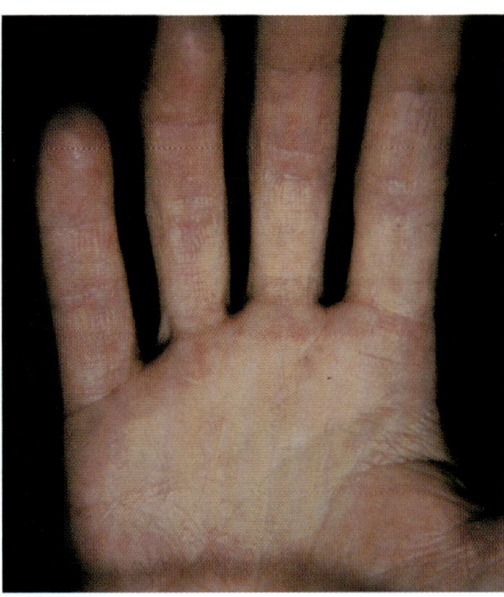

FIGURE 14-2. Hyperkeratotic lesions of the palms in the Rothmund–Thomson syndrome.

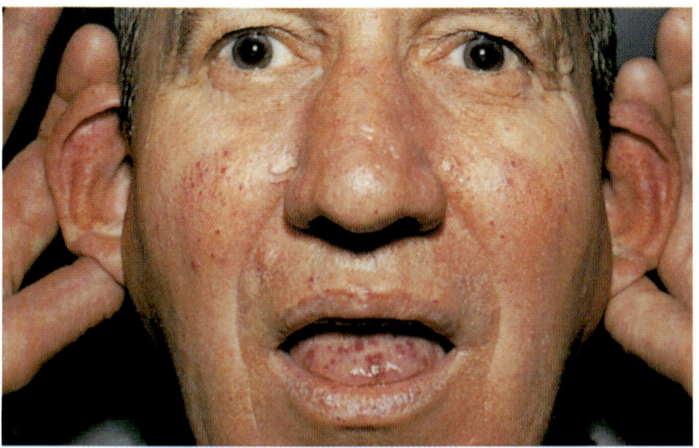

FIGURE 14-3. Telangiectasia of the face, ears, and tongue in hereditary hemorrhagic telangiectasia. This patient had periodic bouts of epistaxis.

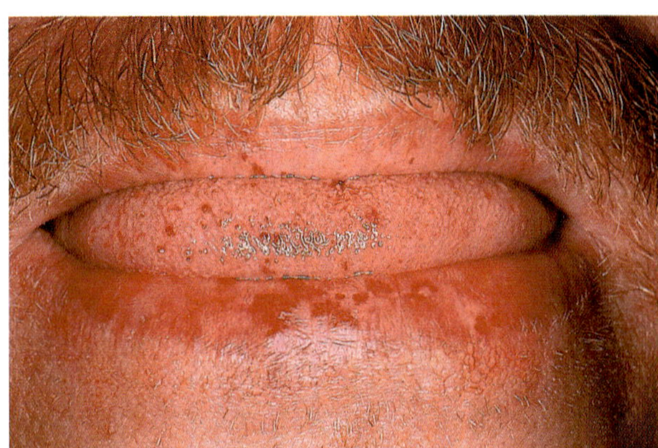

FIGURE 14-4. Telangiectasia of the lips and tongue in a patient with hereditary hemorrhagic telangiectasis. This patient also was found to have a pulmonary arteriovenous fistula.

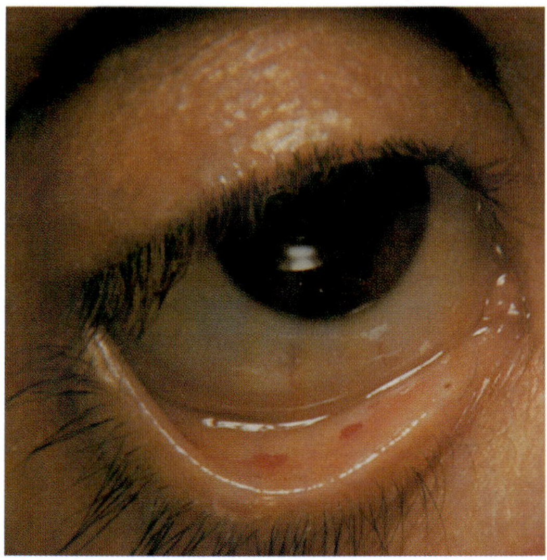

FIGURE 14-5. Telangiectasia of the tarsal conjunctiva of the lower eyelid in hereditary hemorrhagic telangiectasis.

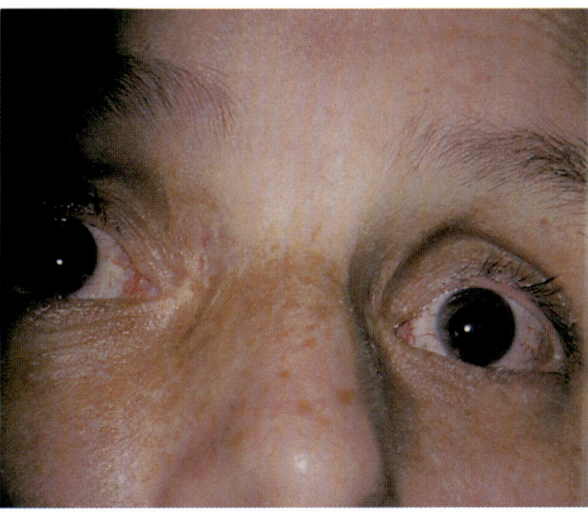

FIGURE 14-6. Skin changes in ataxia telangiectasia. Small café-au-lait spots are evident over the nose and in the area supplied by the maxillary branch of the trigeminal nerve.

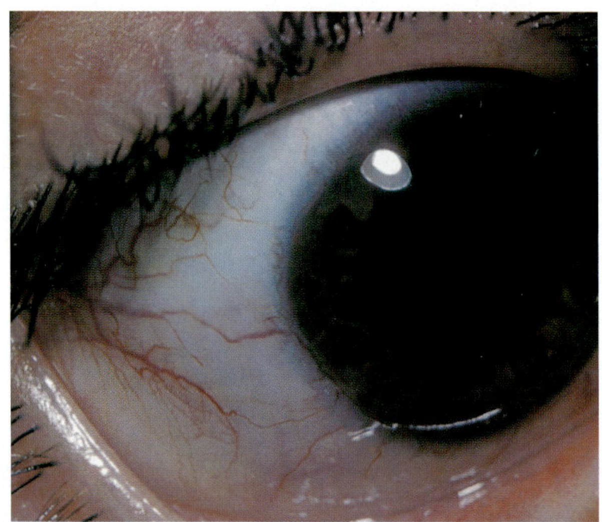

FIGURE 14-7. Early telangiectatic changes of the conjunctiva in ataxia telangiectasia.

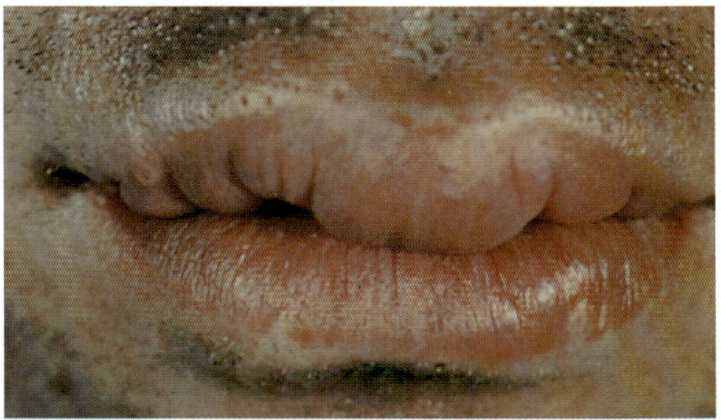

FIGURE 14-8. Chronic lymphedema of the lips. The cause was not discovered in this young patient.

VASCULITIS AND NECROBIOTIC DISORDERS

Vasculitis represents blood vessel inflammation. It may be primary or arise from neighboring tissue inflammation. Cutaneous vasculitis describes inflammation of the small and medium-sized vessels of the dermis, visceral vasculitis (inflammation of the vessels supplying one or more of the viscera), and mixed vasculitis (inflammation of the blood vessels of both skin and viscera). In many diseases, such as polyarteritis nodosa, the vasculitis is confined to the skin or an organ or group of organs and is then considered a limited vasculitis. At other times in the same disease, the vasculitis extends beyond the confines of the skin, organ, or group of organs and is then considered complicated vasculitis.

CUTANEOUS VASCULITIS (LEUKOCYTOCLASTIC ANGIITIS; CUTANEOUS SYSTEMIC ANGIITIS–URTICARIAL VASCULITIS; NECROTIZING VASCULITIS)

Cutaneous vasculitis (leukocytoclastic angiitis; cutaneous systemic angiitis–urticarial vasculitis; necrotizing vasculitis) is caused by infection, an untoward reaction to drugs, lupus erythematosus, or malignancy. The symptoms include headache, malaise, fever, arthralgia, and gastrointestinal symptoms.

Acute cutaneous vasculitis is characterized by the sudden onset of purpura (Fig. 15-1), hemorrhagic vesicles and bullae, and necrotic lesions. It usually affects the legs, thighs, buttocks, and arms; occasionally, it affects other areas. The lesions subside within 2 to 3 weeks, but new crops of lesions often occur for a period of time. Occasionally, atypical erythema multiform-like lesions also occur.

Subacute vasculitis is characterized by purpura, urticaria, papules, maculoerythematous lesions, nodules, and necrotic lesions (Fig. 15-2). The lesions may become confluent, forming plaques, or sometimes developing a vesiculohemorrhagic crust.

Chronic cutaneous vasculitis usually causes minimal constitutional symptoms. The patient develops intermittent eruptions of erythematous macules, papules, modules, and urticarial and purpuric lesions on the legs, arms, and occasionally, other areas. Systemic involvement occurs in many cases and is manifested by vasculitis of the kidney, lung, joints, gastrointestinal system, central nervous system, and retina.

ERYTHEMA MULTIFORME

Erythema Multiforme Minor (Von Hebra)

Erythema multiforme minor (Von Hebra) is often recurrent and is often triggered by herpes simplex infection. There is no distinct prodrome.

Skin Features

The skin eruption begins as a maculopapular rash that progresses to irislike or targetlike lesions (the central area appears purpuric; the peripheral area appears red) (Figs. 15-3 and 15-4). The lesions may be urticarial. Sometimes they are vesiculobullous and present as erythematous plaques with a central bullae surrounded by a marginal ring of vesicles. They are usually symmetric and involve the extensor surfaces of the hands, forearms, elbows, knees, and feet; sometimes the palms; and, less frequently, the face, neck, and trunk. Successive crops develop over several days. Individual lesions fade after 1 to 2 weeks. Recurrent episodes may occur. Mucosal involvement is minimal, if at all.

Erythema Multiforme Major (EM) (Erythema Multiforme Bullosum; Stevens–Johnson Syndrome)

The most frequent causes of erythema multiforme major (EM) (erythema multiforme bullosum; Stevens–Johnson Syndrome) are drug reactions, especially to sulfonamides, other antibiotics, nonsteroidal anti-inflammatory drugs, allopurinol (Fig. 15-5), and anticonvulsants. Other triggers include *Mycoplasma pneumoniae* and radiation therapy.

A prodromal stage with headache, chills, fever, malaise, tachycardia, tachypnea, upper respiratory infection, and prostration usually precedes the skin and mucous membrane eruption by several days. The fever is usually high and often persistent. Marked hemorrhagic crusting lesions are seen on the buccal mucosa, lips, conjunctiva, and occasionally, anogenital area. The untreated disease is frequently fatal because of severe leukopenia.

Skin Features

EM usually involves two or more mucous membranes (Figs. 15-6 and 15-7). It begins as erythematous macules that progress to vesicles, to bullae, and eventually to round or oval ulcers covered by a white membrane and surrounded by a red halo. Oral involvement causes increased salivation, inflammation, crusting, and ulceration of the lips, tongue, buccal mucosa, and palate (Fig. 15-7). Urethral, genital, and anal involvement causes vulvovaginitis, balanitis, and dysuria. Other areas of mucous membrane involvement include, the pharynx, anus, and bronchial tree.

Ocular Features

Photophobia is common. Lid edema may be the earliest manifestation of erythema major. Typical targetlike lesions, flaccid bullae, and epidermal loss may affect the lids; lid margin ulceration, discharge, erythema, and edema are frequently associated with conjunctival involvement. Entropion, trichiasis, scarring of the meibomian orifices, and ankyloblepharon may occur. Lid margin ulceration may cause lacrimal punctual occlusion.

A catarrhal, purulent, or pseudomembranous conjunctivitis is common. The catarrhal conjunctivitis causes tearing, mild photophobia, itching, intense hyperemia, focal areas of infiltration, and in rare instances, vesicle formation. It spontaneously subsides as the skin manifestations disappear. The purulent conjunctivitis is characterized by severe chemosis, hyperemia, occasional subconjunctival hemorrhages, and moderate to severe purulent discharge. Lid margin ulcerations and corneal involvement are common. The pseudomembranous conjunctivitis, with marked discharge, is the most common ocular manifestation of EM (Fig. 15-8). It is usually preceded by severe lid edema and conjunctival chemosis. The pseudomembrane usually involves the tarsal and often the bulbar conjunctiva, which may lead to chronic scarring and symblepharon formation (Fig. 15-9). Conjunctival cicatrization leads to loss of goblet cells, accessory lacrimal glands, and occasionally, scarring of the orifices of the lacrimal gland ductules, resulting in profound keratoconjunctivitis sicca (Fig. 15-10). In severe cases, ankyloblepharon is an unfortunate sequela (Fig. 15-11).

Corneal involvement varies according to the severity of the conjunctivitis. A catarrhal conjunctivitis is usually associated with a few punctate epithelial erosions; the purulent and pseudomembranous conjunctivitis are associated with a scattered or confluent epithelial keratitis that may progress to corneal ulceration, neovascularization, opacification, perforation, and blindness. SJS leads to corneal epithelial stem cell failure and resultant conjunctivization of the cornea. Foreshortening of the fornix, entropion and trichiasis, distichiasis, marked corneal scarring, and severe keratoconjunctivitis often with associated surface keratinization are important sequelae leading to profound visual loss. An anterior uveitis is usually associated with the keratitis. It is manifested by a moderate number of cells and flare.

Purpura

Purpura embodies skin discoloration caused by extravasation of blood into the skin. It includes petechiae (small, purpuric lesions measuring up to 2 mm in diameter) and ecchymoses, which are large extravasations of blood. The purpuric areas may assume various colors as the heme is broken down. It is classified into the following:

1. Idiopathic thrombocytopenic purpura (ITP), which is more common before the age of 21 and is characterized by petechiae or ecchymosis in skin, occasionally in other organs, and infrequently, in joints. Acute ITP usually occurs in children from viral antigen–antibody reactions that induce platelet destruction. Chronic ITP usually occurs in adults and arises from antiplatelet antibodies.
2. Secondary (symptomatic thrombocytopenia) is caused by platelet destruction or prevention of platelet formation by chemicals or drugs that directly or allergenically depress the bone marrow. The platelets may be selectively affected, or all the blood-forming elements may be affected.
3. Vascular or nonthrombocytopenic purpura arises from prolonged coughing, vomiting, straining, Valsalva maneuver, strangulation, gravity, venous stasis, or suction devices used around the mouth. It usually involves the face and neck.
4. Purpura arising from decreased vascular support occurs in scurvy and in atrophic skin as caused by age, ultraviolet exposure, irradiation, and use of topical or systemic glucocorticoids. The purpura appears as irregular spots and is not associated with inflammation or varying color changes.
5. Purpura caused by direct or allergic damage to capillary walls form toxic substances or drugs may be limited or massive.
6. Purpura caused by thrombocytopenia, disseminated intravascular coagulation, or direct or allergic damage to vessel walls from infections.
7. Purpura that arises from vascular damage in systemic disease usually presents with petechiae, ecchymoses,

and/or mucosal bleeding. The causes include renal and liver disease, diabetes mellitus, malnutrition, amyloidosis, fat embolism, hemochromatosis, carcinomatosis, Cushing disease, and ovarian endocrinopathies. The purpura arising in dysproteinemia (Waldenström, sarcoid, lupus erythematosus, myeloma) usually begins as crops of small, irritable, erythematous papules on the legs, which then form punctate purpuric lesions. The lesions usually disappear after a few days but occasionally persist and become confluent.

8. Henoch–Schönlein purpura is a small-vessel vasculitic disorder that involves multiple organs. It occurs most commonly in young children, often triggered by viral infections or streptococcal pharyngitis. It is probably caused by immune complex deposition in the walls of arterioles and venules. The constitutional symptoms include malaise, headache, anorexia, and fever. Abdominal pain and arthralgias, most often of the knees and ankles, precede the cutaneous manifestations by several weeks in about half the patients.

   The skin rash in Henoch–Schönlein purpura begins as a crop of erythematous macules that become purpuric or progress to form papules. The purpura is sometimes urticarial, and the purpuric lesions appear preferentially on the extremities but may also involve the palms and soles (Figs. 15-12 and 15-13). The head is usually spared. Edema of the hands, feet, scalp, and periorbital area is common in younger children.

   Lid edema, hemorrhages into the skin of the lids, subconjunctival hemorrhages, and intraocular hemorrhages may occur, and a keratitis and iritis may be associated with the intraocular hemorrhages (Fig. 15-14). Episcleritis and retinal hemorrhages are uncommon.

9. Infantile acute hemorrhagic edema may represent the infantile analog of Henoch–Schönlein purpura. It occurs in children between the ages of 4 months and 2 years, and is associated with mild fever. Edema and/or ecchymotic symmetric plaques with scalloped margins develop suddenly on the face and extremities, and are especially prominent on the lids, cheeks, ears, hands, and feet. Larger lesions may also occur and have a reticulated pattern. Purpura of the oral mucosa, scrotal edema, urticarial skin lesions, and necrotic ear lesions has been observed. The lesions resolve spontaneously after about 3 weeks, but sometimes crops of lesions recur.

10. Purpura fulminans is characterized by fever and the sudden development of confluent ecchymosis without petechiae. The ecchymosis is well defined and usually occurs on the extremities, especially over points of pressure. The lesions enlarge by coalescence and may lead to hemorrhagic bullae with central necrosis. Internal hemorrhage, shock, and death may eventuate.

Pyoderma Gangrenosum (Phagedena Geometric; Dermatitis Gangrenosa; Phagedenic Pyoderma)

Pyoderma gangrenosum (PG) (phagedena geometric; dermatitis gangrenosa; phagedenic pyoderma) occurs in association with many other conditions, most frequently with inflammatory bowel disease (both Crohn and ulcerative colitis) and seronegative arthritis. Associations have also been reported with leukemias, myeloproliferative diseases, monoclonal gammopathies, dysproteinemias, chronic active hepatitis, hepatitis C, HIV infection, and systemic lupus erythematosus.

Clinical Manifestations

PG may be associated with a high fever and constitutional symptoms of toxicity. The skin lesions usually occur on the legs, often at sites of trauma (pathergy). The ulcerative form of pyoderma gangrenosum is characterized by painful, deep dermal lesions, which begin as tender pustules with an erythematous margin (Fig. 15-15). After several days painful ulcerations ensue. These may gradually enlarge resulting in indolent painful lesions with a characteristic rolled violaceous undermined margin and a granulomatous base (Fig. 15-16). There is no lymphadenopathy.

   Vesiculo-bullous types of pyoderma gangrenosum are less destructive and more superficial than the ulcerative form. A vegetative variant is the least aggressive, not painful, with cribriform lesions usually on the trunk. Occasionally, the lesions develop on the lips, lid, conjunctiva, and oral mucosa.

Acute Febrile Neutrophilic Dermatosis (Sweet Syndrome)

Acute febrile neutrophilic dermatosis (Sweet syndrome) more frequently occurs in middle-aged women and is often preceded by an upper respiratory tract infection or inflammatory bowel disease. Hematoproliferative disorders or solid tumors may be associated. It consists of a sudden eruption of one or more painful, dull-red or plum-colored nodules or plaques on the extremities, neck, or face associated with a high, persistent fever and malaise. Erythema nodosum on the legs may also be found. The nodules or plaques enlarge and persist for several weeks but characteristically do not ulcerate, although they sometimes develop pseudovesicles or pustules on their surface. Infrequently, Sweet syndrome presents as a nonscarring granulomatous facial eruption that may be recurrent. Some cases are associated with arthralgia, and many are associated with a conjunctivitis or episcleritis. In some instances, oral ulcerations also occur.

Granuloma Faciale (Facial Granuloma with Eosinophilia)

Granuloma faciale (facial granuloma with eosinophilia) represents a focal vasculitis. Single or multiple granuloma faciale lesions occur on the face, especially the forehead, nose, and cheeks (Fig. 15-17). Sometimes they occur in other areas, including the back. They are usually asymptomatic but occasionally are tender or cause itching or burning. They are soft, red brown, or violaceous, sharply circumscribed nodules or plaques. The follicular orifices are prominent, and scaling and telangiectasis may be found. Differential diagnosis includes sarcoidosis, infectious granulomata (especially leprosy and cutaneous tuberculosis), lymphoma cutis, and lupus erythematosus.

Polyarteritis Nodosa (Periarteritis Nodosa)

Polyarteritis nodosa (periarteritis nodosa) is an uncommon autoimmune disease characterized by widespread focal or segmental vasculitis of the small and medium-sized muscular arteries and, rarely, phlebitis. The lesions are typically in various stages of development—acute, healing, and healed. Areas that surround bifurcations and branches of vessels are preferentially involved. The renal and visceral arteries are characteristically involved, but the pulmonary circulation is usually spared; however, virtually any organ may be affected.

Clinical Manifestations

The clinical manifestations are variable and protean in nature, often beginning abruptly with chills, fever, and tachycardia. Occasionally, they begin insidiously with low-grade fever, arthralgia, myalgia, anorexia, abdominal pain, weight loss, and nonspecific fatigue and weakness. Kidney involvement often occurs from thrombosis, cortical infarction, or glomerulosclerosis. Testicular involvement may also occur.

Arthralgias, pain, weakness, and muscle tenderness arise from involvement of vessels supplying the muscles or joints. Heart failure is a common cardiac finding. Other findings include pericarditis, intrapericardial hemorrhage, myocarditis, arrhythmia, myocardial infarction, and coronary vasculitis and thrombosis. About 25% of patients have pulmonary manifestations of asthma, bronchitis, and pneumonia.

The most common manifestations of gastrointestinal involvement are abdominal pain, nausea, vomiting, and sometimes diarrhea and intestinal bleeding. Cholecystitis, intestinal obstruction, appendicitis, pancreatitis, hepatitis, gangrene, perforation, intraabdominal hemorrhage, perihepatitis, perisplenitis, and occasionally peritonitis may also occur.

Central nervous system abnormalities may develop late in the course of the disease from cerebral infarction or subarachnoid hemorrhage. The manifestations include headache, dizziness, cerebellar ataxia, vomiting, delirium, and other mental changes, convulsions, difficulty with speech, hemiplegia, homonymous hemianopsia, cortical blindness, bulbar disturbances, and bilateral pyramidal tract disturbances. Encephalopathy and myelopathy may be seen, and the visual and oculomotor pathways are also frequently involved.

Skin Features

About 25% of patients develop skin abnormalities that follow the course of superficial arteries. Skin findings include palpable purpura (Fig. 15-18), petechiae, urticaria, ulceration, painful cutaneous or subcutaneous nodules, and mucous membrane lesions. The nodules usually occur around the knee, the anterior aspect of the lower leg, and the dorsum of the foot or hand. They arise from focal arterial wall necrosis at areas of bifurcation.

Tissue infarction arising from peripheral embolization results in splinter hemorrhages, Osler nodes (tender purple swellings), absorption, and gangrene, especially in the fingers and toes. Skin infarcts appear as purpuric plaques or hemorrhagic bullae.

Ocular Features

Conjunctival hyperemia, chemosis, subconjunctival hemorrhages, and indurated violaceous conjunctival nodules occasionally develop; late in the disease process, a keratoconjunctivitis sicca may also occur. Nodular or diffuse, unilateral or bilateral, scleritis may be one of the earliest manifestations of polyarteritis nodosa and arises from involvement of the scleral vessels (Fig. 15-19). Polyarteritis nodosa may be associated with Cogan syndrome, and by that relationship may be related to peripheral interstitial keratitis and partial or total deafness.

Vasculitis of the limbal vessels may lead to marginal corneal ulceration and necrotizing sclerokeratitis (Figs. 15-20 and 15-21). The peripheral margin of the ulcer often shows signs of healing, whereas the central margin remains active, leading to progressive infiltration and vascularization. Eventually, the cornea perforates or becomes completely scarred. Dacryoadenitis manifested to lacrimal gland swelling has been observed and verified at autopsy. Sjögren syndrome may also occur.

Arteritis of the vessels of the orbit or extraocular muscles may simulate an orbital cellulitis or orbital pseudotumor with signs of proptosis, lid edema, and chemosis. Uveal tract involvement in the form of recurrent iridocyclitis and choroiditis may occur. The iridocyclitis is bilateral, is recalcitrant, and may be mild or severe. A complicated cataract and glaucoma are common sequelae of the iridocyclitis. Choroidal lesions may not be seen because of the presence of a hypertensive retinopathy, retinal involvement from the disease itself, or serious retinal detachment. They appear as yellow or whitish foci of edema and inflammation with fairly well-defined borders that gradually clear, leaving white-pigmented scars.

Hypertensive retinal changes include retinal edema, flame-shaped hemorrhages, exudates, retinal artery spasm, occlusion of the retinal arteries, arteriolar sclerosis, and papilledema. Direct retinal artery involvement may cause cotton-wool spots (cytoid bodies), aneurysms, fusiform dilatation of the arterioles, round and linear hemorrhages, retinal detachment, and massive intraocular hemorrhages. Papilledema, papillitis, optic atrophy, loss of convergence, extraocular muscle palsies, Horner syndrome, and nystagmus may also occur.

Erythema Nodosum

Erythema nodosum represents a symptom complex characterized by erythematous, exquisitely tender nodules that are usually located on the extensor surfaces of the legs. Erythema nodosum occurs with various bacterial, viral, chlamydial, and fungal infections; sarcoidosis; and some drug sensitivities. It arises from immune-complex deposition around venules. (Erythema nodosum leprosum in leprosy is clinically and histologically distinct from erythema nodosum.) A sore throat, fever, malaise, fatigue, loss of weight, and cough often precede the nodules by 1 or 2 weeks. Arthralgias may also occur.

Skin Features

The subcutaneous nodules occur on the extensor surface of the tibia (Figs. 15-22 and 15-23) and less frequently on the knees, ankles, thighs, forearm, arms, trunk, and face. They may number more than a dozen, are located in the deep dermis and adipose tissue, and are hard and extremely tender. At first they are pink. Then they become red before fading with varying hues of color over a 6-week period. The lesions do not suppurate.

Ocular Features

Tiny cherry-red conjunctival nodules with a triangular shape located over the insertion of all four rectus muscles and hyperemia of the surrounding conjunctiva may precede the subcutaneous nodules. Erythema nodosum in children, particularly when associated with arthritis of the larger joints, should raise the consideration of familial granulomatosis, or Blau syndrome, which includes panuveitis with multiple choroidal granulomata, associated vitreitis, and mild iridocyclitis.

VASCULITIS WITH GRANULOMATOSIS

This section includes those vasculitides associated with granulomas and lung disease, namely, Wegener granulomatosis, allergic granulomatosis, and giant cell arteritis.

Wegener Granulomatosis

Wegener granulomatosis is a multisystem disease characterized by a necrotizing granulomatous vasculitis. The generalized form is manifested by glomerulonephritis and necrotizing granulomatous vasculitis of the small and medium-sized arteries and veins of the lungs, and mucosa of the paranasal sinuses, nose, and nasopharynx, and other organs, including the eyes. The limited form usually involves a single organ, especially the skin, while sparing the pulmonary and renal system.

Clinical Manifestations

Wegener granulomatosis is often triggered by a flulike illness in a patient with a concomitant upper and lower respiratory tract disease. It causes fever, malaise, weakness, and weight loss. In some instances, symptoms arising form one organ system (e.g., dyspnea, chest pain, cough, and hemoptysis) dominate the picture. Without treatment, the granulomatous inflammation progresses into a generalized vasculitis with an associated glomerulonephritis resulting in rapid decline in renal function and death.

Wegener granulomatosis involves the nose and paranasal sinuses about 90% of the time. Nasal stuffiness, epistaxis, and purulent rhinorrhea occur; eventually, there is destruction of the soft tissue, cartilage, and bone of the soft palate. In some instances, there is destruction of the midfacial region.

Shortness of breath, persistent cough, pleuritic pain, and hemoptysis with chest x-ray evidence of multiple bilateral infiltrates occur in 50% to 95% of cases, but usually late in the course of the disease. Renal involvement occurs in up to 85% of patients, but usually late in the disease process. Arthritis occurs in about one-third of patients.

Neurologic involvement arises in three different ways:

1. Continuous invasion of the nervous system may cause exophthalmos (Fig. 15-24), and signs of involvement of the optic nerve or chiasm, pituitary, base of the brain and meninges, cranial nerves (producing ophthalmoplegia, facial neuritis, and 8th nerve deafness), and skull.
2. Central nervous system vasculitis, with signs of mononeuritis multiplex (fleeting muscular pains and tenderness), polyneuritis, intracerebral and subarachnoid hemorrhage, arterial and venous thrombosis, and myopathies.
3. Remote granulomatous cranial nerve involvement from multiple intracerebral granulomas and granulomas of the skull.

Skin Features

About 45% of patients develop skin manifestations. The early skin lesions are usually vesicular or papulonecrotic and are distributed symmetrically on the extremities and especially over the elbows, knees, and buttocks. Occasionally, an erythematous, urticarial maculopapular eruption occurs. Pyoderma gangrenosum lesions of the neck, scaphoid region, buttocks, or thighs occasionally occur, and subcutaneous nodules may be seen. A generalized erythematous, purpuric, or vesicular eruption may occur in the late stages of Wegener granulomatosis. Oral ulcers are almost a constant feature at some stage of the disease. Gingivitis, septal and palatal perforation, and necrosis of the alveolar ridge may be seen. A prominent feature of the disease is the absence of cervical lymphadenopathy.

Ocular Features

Ocular involvement occurs in about 50% of patients and in some instances arises as a limited form of the disease. Lid edema is common, and occasionally the lids are involved and destroyed by contiguous spread of the necrotizing process itself, or a necrotizing lid lesion may begin in the lid as a subcutaneous nodule and may be mistaken for a chalazion. A conjunctivitis with nodule formation sometimes occurs in Wegener granulomatosis. Conjunctival chemosis occurs with orbital involvement.

Corneal involvement is occasionally the first manifestation of Wegener granulomatosis. A granuloma develops at the limbus, then progresses to form a marginal furrow that may or may not be associated with a necrotizing scleritis (Fig. 15-25). The marginal furrow usually spreads superficially and circumferentially to form a ring ulcer; the surrounding stroma is moderately infiltrated and vascularized. Eventually, the lesion progresses centrally, suggesting a sclerosing keratitis. (This form of keratitis, in many respects, resembles that seen in polyarteritis nodosa.) Infrequently, the furrow progresses into the deep cornea, suggesting a Mooren ulcer. Other corneal changes include superficial corneal edema and punctate blotchy epithelial lesions.

The sclera and episclera may be involved in the form of nonspecific episcleritis or anterior or posterior scleritis, granulomatous necrotizing scleritis, or sclerokeratitis. The scleritis is usually difficult to manage without immunosuppression and may be nodular, sectoral, or diffuse. It may be unilateral (more commonly) or bilateral.

The orbit is usually involved by contiguous spread of inflammation from the paranasal sinuses and nose or, occasionally, from the lid. Sometimes the lesion begins in the orbit and presents as a pseudotumor and may be bilateral. Orbital involvement is characterized by edema, conjunctival chemosis, pain, limited movement, and relentless progression, with necrotizing granuloma formation and ulcerations.

The lacrimal system may be involved by the granulomatous processes that sometimes destroy the midline structures of the face. A bilateral dacryoadenitis simulating an acute infection or a chronic dacryoadenitis may occur. Increased tearing, nasolacrimal duct obstruction, and a dacryocystitis may develop from nasal mucous membrane involvement.

Iritis is often associated with corneal involvement, and a posterior uveitis usually occurs with the necrotizing scleritis. Retinal edema, vasculitis, congestion of the retinal veins, and retinal granulomas may be found. Papilledema, hemorrhages involving the nerve head, primary optic atrophy, and ischemic optic neuritis (from involvement of the posterior ciliary arteries) may develop from granulomatous lesions of the central nervous system or nasopharynx.

Ocular involvement may be the only sign of disease. In many instances, the ocular involvement is soon followed by necrotizing granulomas in the upper and/or lower part of the respiratory tract, focal inflammatory lesions of the arteries and veins, and focal glomerulonephritis.

Lethal Midline Granuloma

Lethal midline granuloma is often confused with Wegener granulomatosis. This rare disease begins with symptoms of watery or serosanguinous nasal discharge of variable duration followed by nasal obstruction and, eventually, induration, inflammation, and swelling of the external tip of the nose, upper lip, cheek, and, sometimes lower eyelid. Ulceration usually occurs in the midline structures of the face. Symptoms of fever, malaise, and eventual exhaustion occur; death often supervenes within 18 months.

Skin Features

Papulonecrotic lesions may develop in the midline areas of the face, which then progress to destruction of the underlying tissue (Fig. 15-26). A small ulcer may develop on the inferior concha or nasal septum followed by ulceration of the hard palate and abscess formation. Destruction of the involved area results in sloughing that usually involves the nose, upper lip, cheeks, orbit, and eye. Sometimes the hard and soft palate are also destroyed (Fig. 15-27).

Ocular Features

Corneal involvement is occasionally the first manifestation of lethal midline granuloma (Fig. 15-28). A granuloma develops at the limbus, then progresses to form a marginal furrow. The marginal furrow usually spreads superficially and circumferentially to form a ring ulcer, and the surrounding stroma is moderately infiltrated and vascularized. Symptoms of fever, malaise, and eventual exhaustion occur; death often supervenes within 18 months.

Allergic Granulomatosis (Churg–Strauss Angiitis)

Allergic granulomatosis (Churg–Strauss angiitis) is an uncommon condition characterized by asthma, recurrent cutaneous vasculitis, and eosinophilia. Prodromal, infiltrative, and vasculitis phases occur. The prodromal phase may persist for years and is manifested by symptoms of allergic disease with rhinitis, nasal polyps, bronchitis with shortness of breath, and fever. Arthralgia may also occur. The infiltrative phase is manifested by a peripheral blood eosinophilia and eosinophilic infiltration of the skin, lungs, and gastrointestinal tract. The vasculitis phase is characterized by weight loss, malaise, lassitude, fever, and skin lesions. Other manifestations of this phase include cardiac and renal failure, central nervous system involvement with convulsions and coma, and peripheral neuropathy with foot drop from peripheral involvement.

Skin Features

Eosinophilic infiltration of the skin occurs during the infiltrative phase; erythema multiforme–like lesions form during the vasculitis phase. The lesions occur in crops over several months and involve the trunk and extremities.

Ocular Features

The conjunctiva becomes involved during the infiltrative phase of the disease. It presents as bilateral, slowly progressive waxy nodules of the bulbar and palpebral conjunctiva (Fig. 15-29). The disease may cause a unilateral marginal corneal ulceration and a severe unilateral episcleritis. Panuveitis, scattered retinal infarctions, and branch retinal artery occlusion are sometimes seen. Other findings consist of a superior oblique muscle palsy and ischemic optic neuropathy.

Giant Cell Arteritis (Temporal Arteritis; Polymyalgia Rheumatica)

Giant cell, or cranial, arteritis (temporal arteritis; polymyalgia rheumatica) causes multiple symptoms and may lead to blindness within a period of weeks. It represents an inflammation of any large or medium-sized artery and especially affects the cranial arteries. The presenting complaints include those associated with the following:

1. Classical temporal arteritis, with red, tender nodules over the temporal arteries.
2. Headache and tender scalp.
3. Stroke with meningeal signs.
4. Amaurosis fugax.
5. Blindness.
6. Visual hallucinations.
7. Mental aberrations.
8. Facial neuralgia.
9. Ear pain with vertigo and deafness.
10. Polymyalgia rheumatica with jaw pain claudication as an early feature.
11. Coronary artery disease.
12. Polyarteritis.
13. The aortic arch syndrome.
14. Vomiting, asthenia, and cachexia.
15. Low-grade fever of unknown origin.

Giant cell arteritis begins with headaches, low-grade fever, lassitude, depression, anorexia, malaise, weight loss, and aching pain in the extremities. Often the constitutional symptoms precede the clinical findings by as much as 5 months.

Several weeks after onset of general symptoms, unilateral or bilateral frontal, temporal, or occipital head pains and scalp tenderness may occur. The pain is usually severe and boring in character. The temporal, occipital, and facial arterial systems may be involved. The pain and tenderness occur in the regions of involvement. The pain and tenderness last several weeks or longer and may be so severe as to make touching the head or combing the hair impossible. The involved arteries are thickened and often palpable as tender cords. Pulsation is diminished or absent in the involved vessels. Ischemic ulcers sometimes occur.

Occasionally, polymyalgia rheumatica—characterized by gradual onset of jaw claudication and pain in the muscles of the neck, shoulders, upper arms, thighs, and buttocks—is the major manifestation of giant cell arteritis. Jaw claudication (manifested by difficulty in opening the mouth and pain on eating) may be pathognomonic of giant cell arteritis.

Carotid artery involvement may occur and is manifested by central nervous system findings of bulbar palsy and dysphagia. The coronary, celiac, and mesentery arteries are sometimes involved and cause symptoms referable to their distribution.

Skin Features

Purpura often occurs during the prodromal phase. The skin overlying the involved scalp arteries may be red, inflamed, and tender. Occasionally, bullae, ulcers, or massive necrosis occurs in those areas. Other features include purpura, ulceration, or gangrene of the legs. The hair is often thin or absent in areas of involvement. About 10% of patients develop pain and a glossitis of the anterior two-thirds of the tongue manifested by redness, desquamation, blistering, or gangrene.

Ocular Features

Visual loss occurs in about 10% to 60% of patients. At first, the loss is transient but soon becomes total and permanent. A mild ptosis may accompany other cranial nerve abnormalities. Chemosis and conjunctival inflammation accompany anterior segment ischemia. In the exceptional case, anterior segment ischemia occurs and is associated with severe transient corneal edema. Marginal corneal ulceration may also occur; episcleral and scleral nodules occasionally occur.

Rubeosis iridis is occasionally found and may lead to glaucoma. An iritis is generally associated with anterior segment ischemia. Central retinal artery occlusion, narrowing of the retinal arteries, striate hemorrhages and cotton-wool spots, retinal edema, and ischemic retinopathy may be observed.

Anterior ischemic optic neuritis occurs in about one-third of patients and is the most common cause of blindness. It is often bilateral. Initially, the optic nerve appears pale and swollen; later, the swelling disappears, leaving a pale nerve head. Small hemorrhages may be evident in the adjacent retina.

Diplopia probably results from ocular muscle ischemia or 3rd or 6th cranial nerve palsy. Ophthalmoplegia may also occur. Altitudinal hemianopsia, homonymous hemianopsia, sector-shaped defects, and large central scotomata are occasionally found.

NECROBIOTIC DISORDERS

The necrobiotic disorders are characterized by a partial, focal necrosis of the dermal connective tissue resulting in a histiocytic and granulomatous response. We consider granuloma annular and necrobiosis lipoidica next.

Granuloma Annulare

Granuloma annulare represents a granulomatous reaction of unknown cause that is associated with altered collagen metabolism. The generalized form of granuloma annulare, which is seen more often in middle-aged women, may be associated with diabetes in up to 20% of patients. Sun exposure may trigger generalized granuloma annulare.

The localized form of granuloma annulare is the most common, especially in children. Areas of minor trauma such as the dorsal aspects of hands or feet are the most frequent sites. Granuloma annulare is characterized by development of a ring of small, smooth, firm, skin-colored or slightly pink, flattened papules. Single or multiple lesions develop on the dorsal surface of the feet, hands (Fig. 15-30), fingers, and, less commonly, extensor surfaces of the extremities. Infrequently, they occur in other areas, including the scalp and near the eye (Figs. 15-31 and 15-32). They usually spontaneously disappear within 2 years, but recurrence is common.

A linear form of granuloma annulare occasionally occurs that affects the trunk or the finger. A subcutaneous form is uncommon and is usually found in children, where it affects the scalp, palms, buttocks, and legs. The perforating form of granuloma annulare is rare; it is characterized by papules on the hand that develop a yellowish center that drains a clear, viscous fluid, causing crusting before healing with a hypo- or hyperpigmented scar.

Necrobiosis Lipoidica (Necrobiosis Lipoidica Diabeticorum)

Necrobiosis lipoidica (necrobiosis lipoidica diabeticorum) occurs more frequently in women than in men. About 75% of the patients are diabetics, and many of the others are pre-diabetics.

The earliest lesions begin as papules or firm, dull, yellowish-red plaques (Fig. 15-33). They slowly enlarge and coalesce to form an oval or irregular, sharply demarcated plaques of yellowish skin. The skin in the center of the lesion is usually atrophic and has a glazed appearance with prominent telangiectatic vessels (Fig. 15-34). Sometimes the lesion ulcerates and is painful. The affected skin is anesthetic, and hypohidrosis may be demonstrated.

Eighty-five percent of lesions are seen on the shins; less commonly, they occur on the thighs, backs of the legs, ankles, feet, and heels. Infrequently, they occur on the hands, arms, trunk, scalp, and face (Fig. 15-35). Scalp lesions may cause alopecia. Sometimes there are multiple lesions that are scattered over several areas of the skin. Atypical forms may occur on the scalp and upper face. These lesions usually do not scar but may be depigmented centrally and tend to follow the outline of the scalp margin.

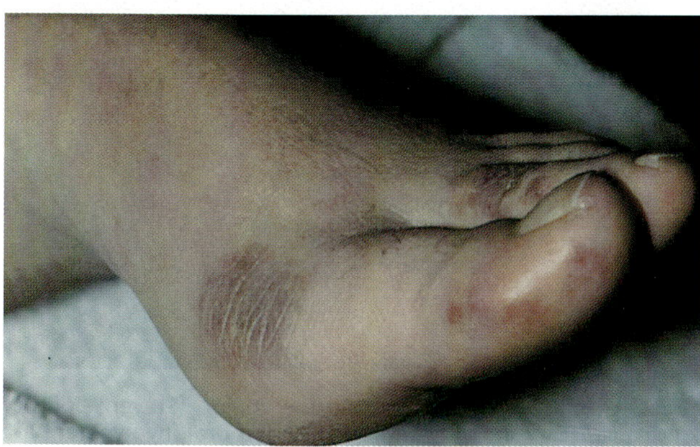

FIGURE 15-1. Cutaneous vasculitis of the foot, causing purpura. Pain was a prominent symptom in this patient.

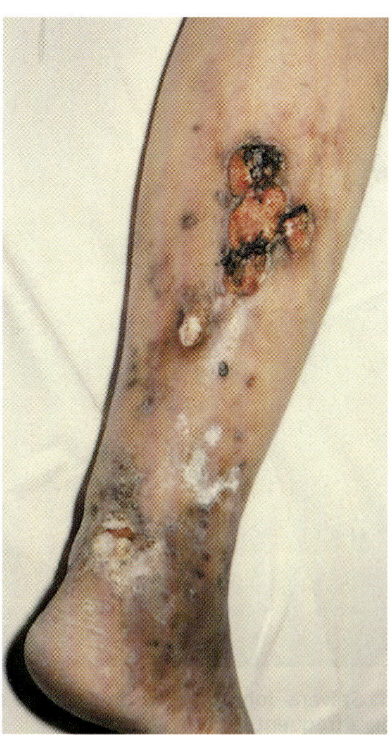

FIGURE 15-2. Subacute vasculitis and necrotic lesions on the leg.

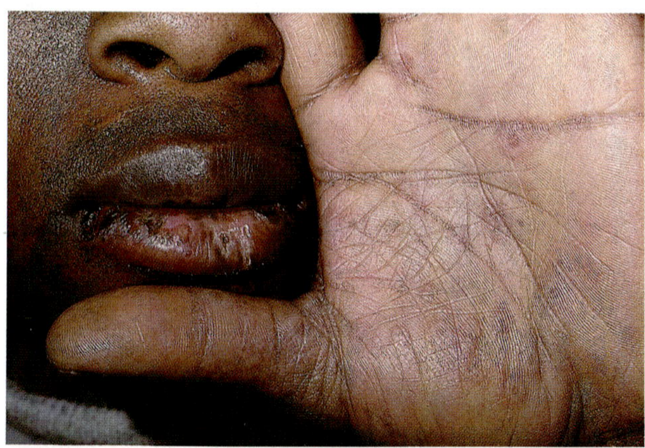

FIGURE 15-3. Erythema multiforme minor. Note characteristic "iris" or "target" lesions of palm and resolving herpes of lips. This patient has had recurrent episodes of erythema multiforme minor, usually appearing 7 to 10 days after onset of herpes simplex labialis. Prophylactic treatment with acyclovir suppressing his herpes problem also stopped his recurrent EM.

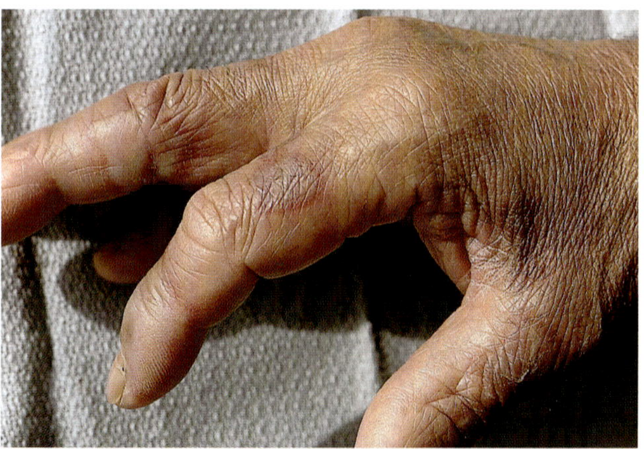

FIGURE 15-4. Early lesions of erythema multiforme minor showing characteristic dusky to pale violaceous bullae with erythematous margins. The most frequent sites of lesions are the dorsum of hands and fingers, as seen in this patient.

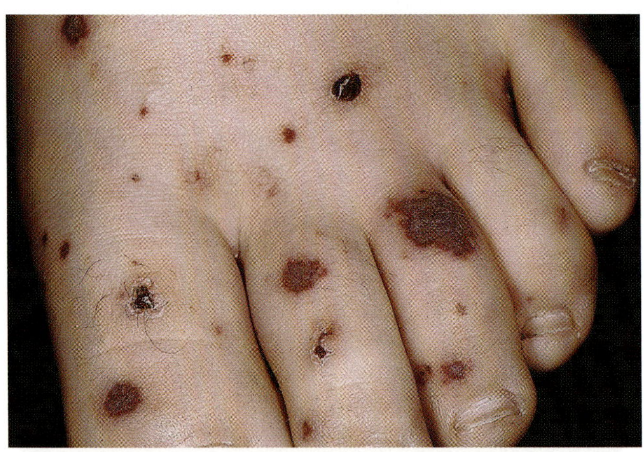

FIGURE 15-13. Henoch–Schönlein purpura of dorsum of foot and toes showing petechiae and early necrotic purpura.

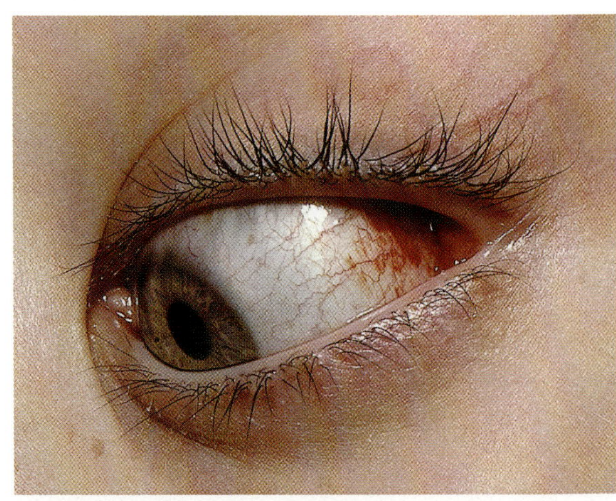

FIGURE 15-14. Henoch–Schönlein purpura showing subconjunctival hemorrhage (same patient as shown in Fig. 15-13).

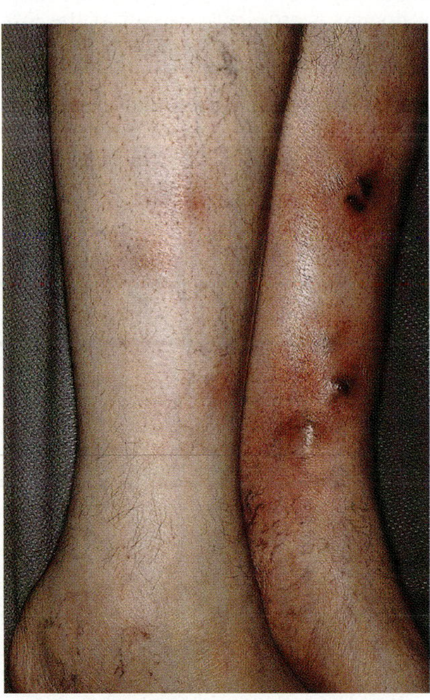

FIGURE 15-15. Early lesions of ulcerative pyoderma gangrenosum. The patient presented with a 1-week history of painful, dusky, faintly palpable subcutaneous nodules that were thought initially to be erythema nodosum. Small vesiculopustules soon appeared as seen here.

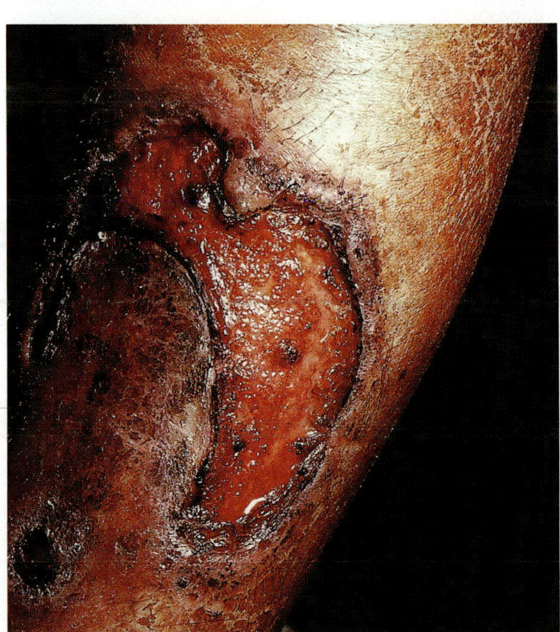

FIGURE 15-16. Pyoderma gangrenosum demonstrating a large ulcer on the calf with typical rolled undermined dusky margins. Factitious ulcers may closely mimic such a lesion.

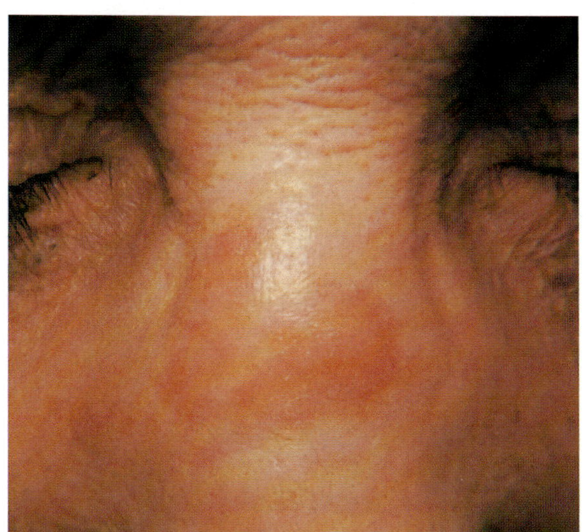

FIGURE 15-17. Granuloma faciale of the nose.

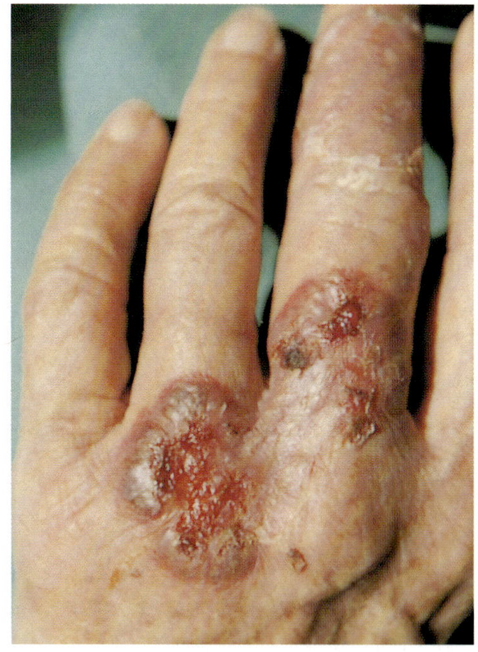

FIGURE 15-18. Palpable purpura of the hands as may be seen on polyarteritis nodosa. This patient was found to have 3+ cryofibrinogen.

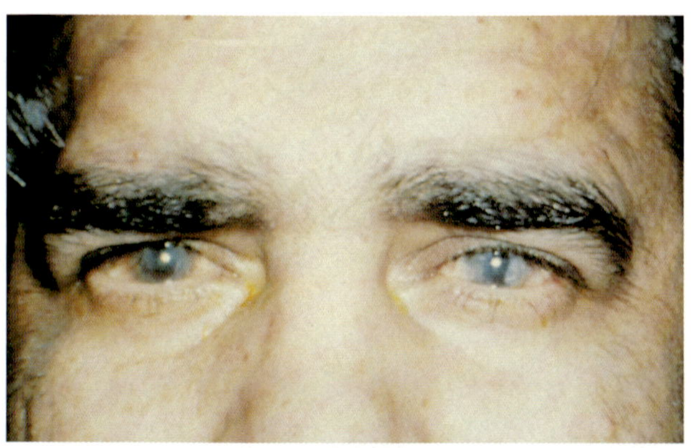

FIGURE 15-19. Scleritis and peripheral corneal involvement in polyarteritis nodosa. A persistent low-grade scleritis is evident in the left eye of this 47-year-old Pakistani male who has had polyarteritis nodosa for more than 8 years.

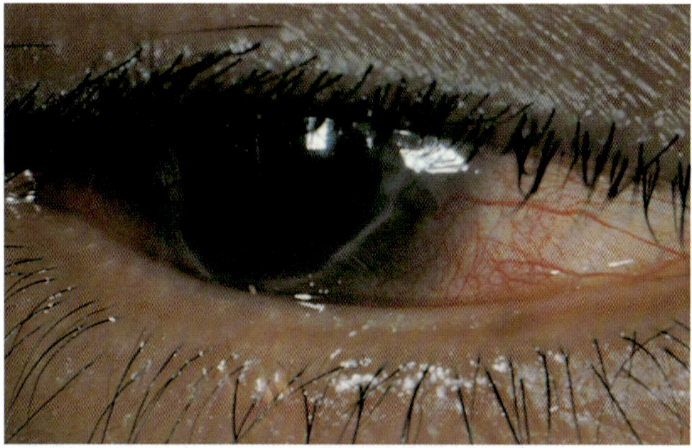

FIGURE 15-20. Perilimbal scleritis with marginal corneal ulceration.

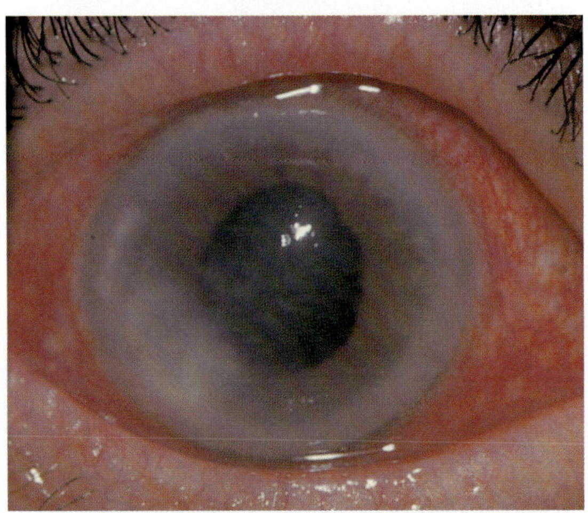

FIGURE 15-21. Peripheral corneal infiltration with central corneal edema in polyarteritis nodosa.

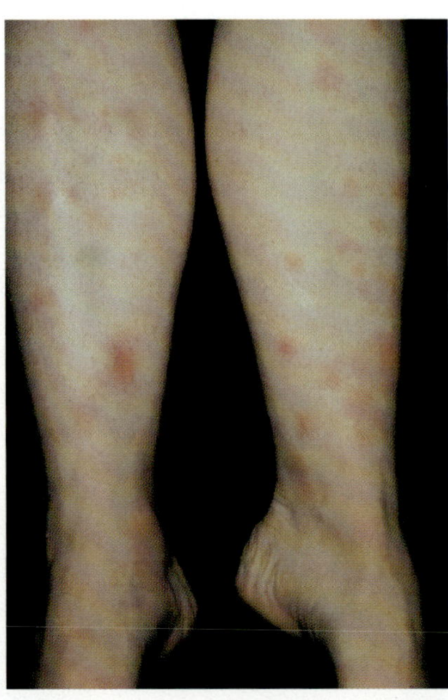

FIGURE 15-22. Erythema nodosum on the shins due to birth control pills. Sensitivity reactions to drugs are a common cause of erythema nodosum.

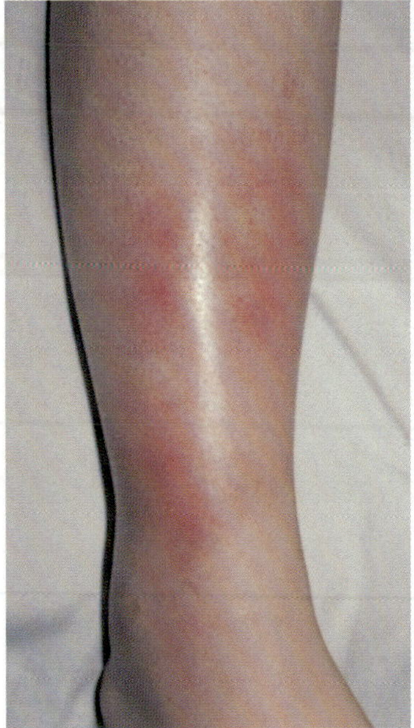

FIGURE 15-23. Erythema nodosum in patient with sarcoidosis. Note the dusky contusiform appearance often seen in erythema nodosum. These lesions were quite tender.

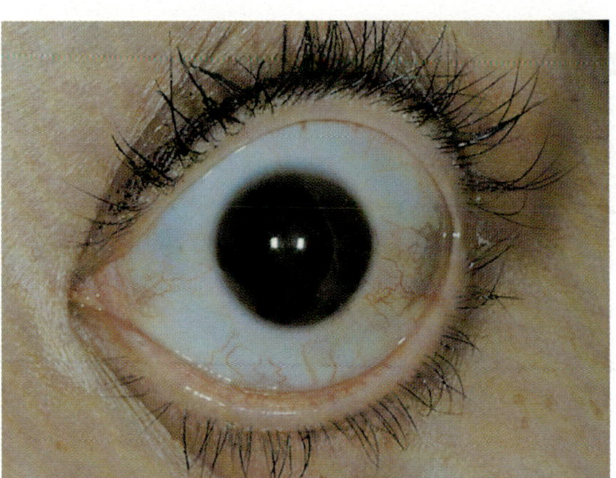

FIGURE 15-24. Exophthalmos in Wegener granulomatosis. This 27-year-old woman has had Wegener granulomatosis for 3 years. She was well controlled until stopping her medication. She then began to develop exophthalmos and some neurologic signs. CT scan revealed infiltration in the region of the lacrimal gland.

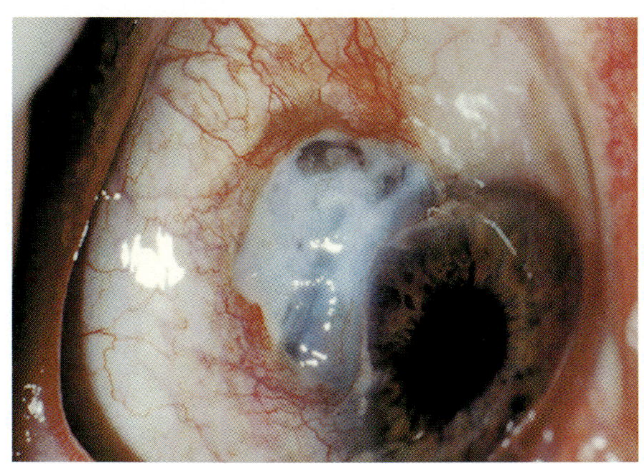

FIGURE 15-25. Necrotizing scleritis with marginal corneal involvement in Wegener granulomatosis. Severe scleritis is evident in this patient; a marginal furrow is readily apparent at the superior edge of the scleritis.

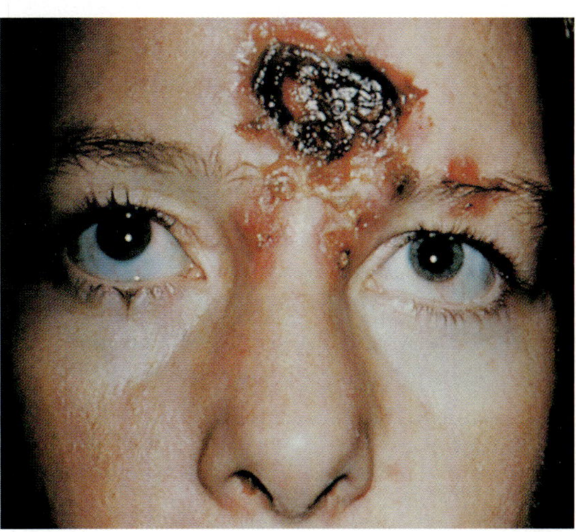

FIGURE 15-26. Papulonecrotic lesions in the midline area of the face, brow, upper eyelid, and nares, in lethal midline granuloma. Peripheral corneal lesions are also evident (see Fig. 15-28).

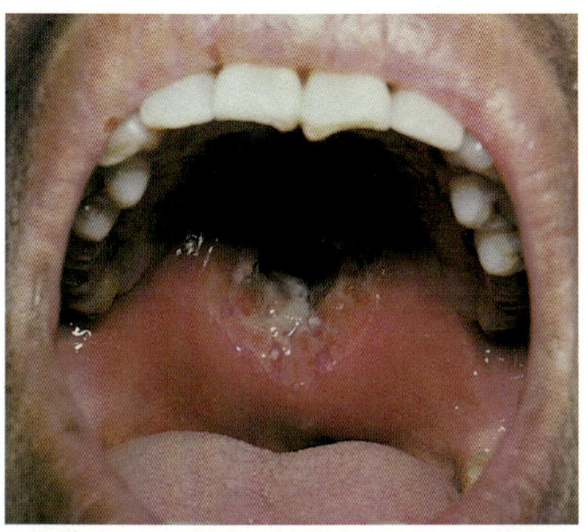

FIGURE 15-27. Lethal midline granuloma with destruction of the soft palate and uvula. The patient had been referred to rule out tertiary syphilis.

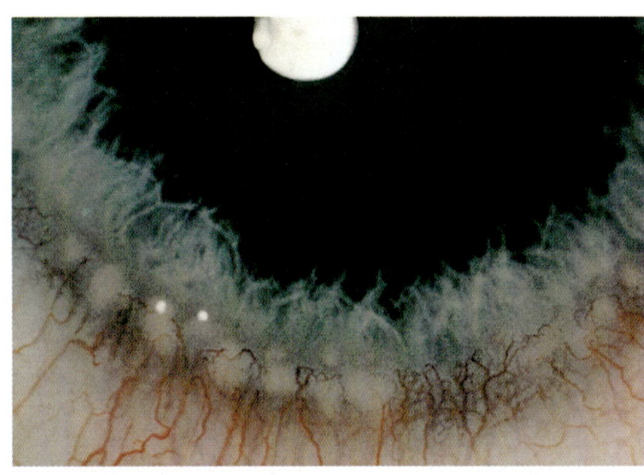

FIGURE 15-28. High-magnification photo of inferior corneal lesions in lethal midline granuloma.

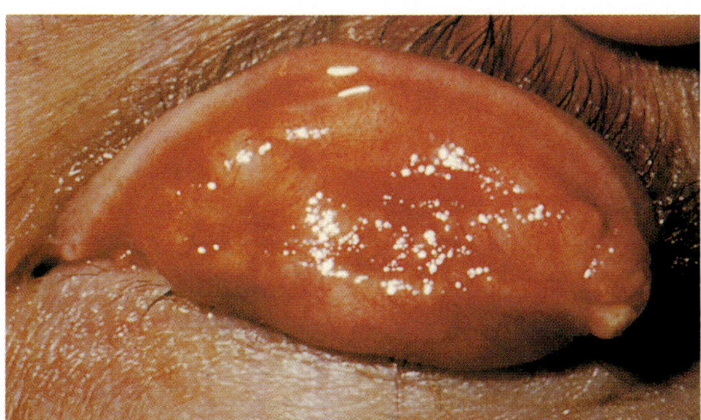

FIGURE 15-29. Superior palpebral conjunctiva in Churg–Strauss syndrome. Granulomatous lesions with marked injection are evident in the upper tarsus. (Courtesy of Dr. Devron Char.)

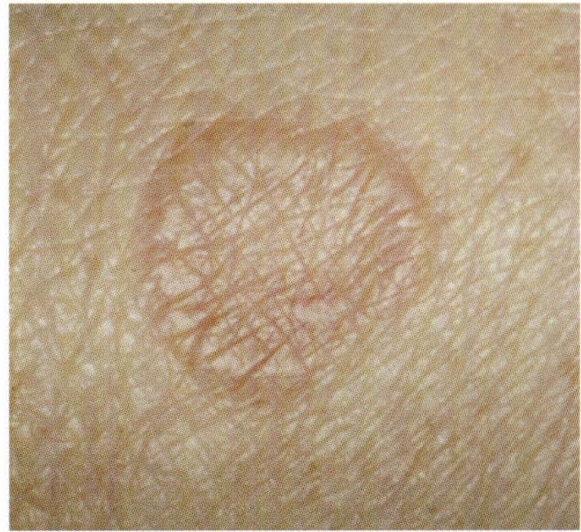

FIGURE 15-30. Granuloma annulare on the dorsum of the hand. Note typical flattened papules producing an annular lesion.

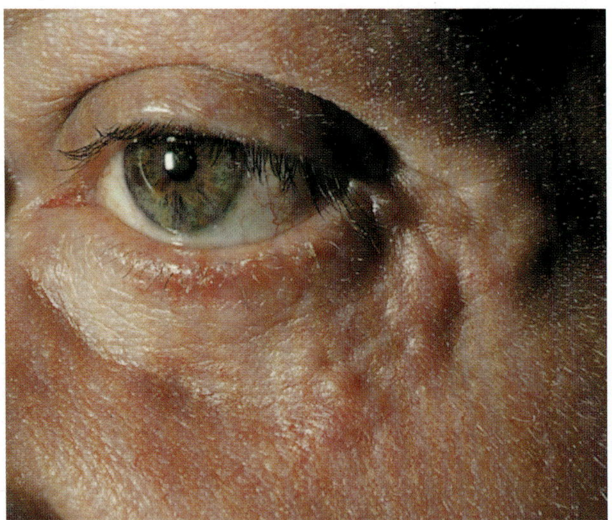

FIGURE 15-31. Granuloma annulare at the lateral margin and below the left eyelid. The patient had been exposed to arc welding, which may have triggered his lesions.

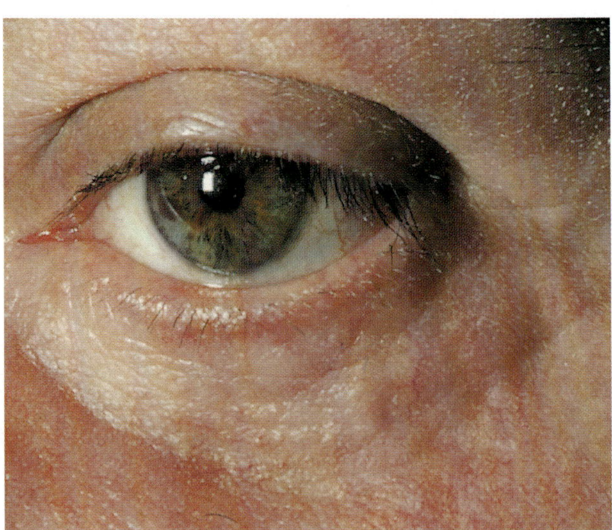

FIGURE 15-32. Spontaneous regression after 3 to 4 years of the lesions in Fig. 15-24.

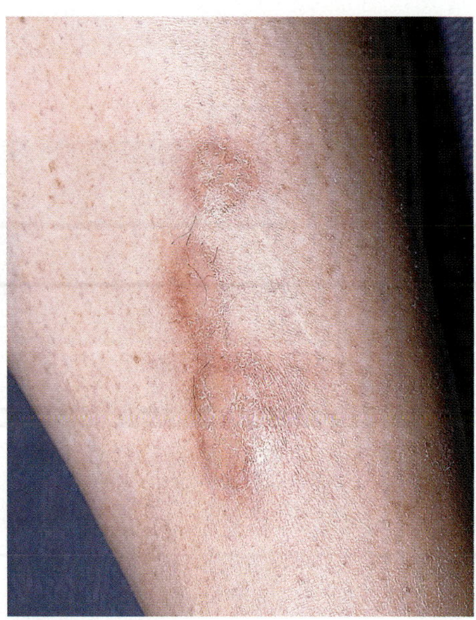

FIGURE 15-33. Early lesions of necrobiosis lipoidica on the shin of a young woman. Note typical dull erythematous yellowish plaques. This patient did not have diabetes.

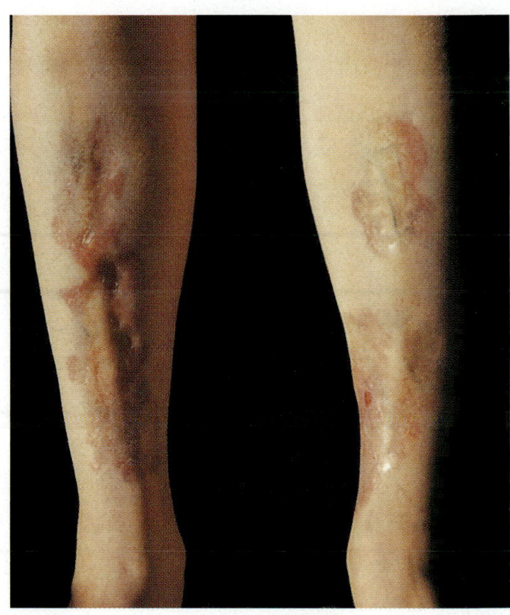

FIGURE 15-34. Necrobiosis lipoidica in a patient who has had diabetes for many years. Note the typical sharply demarcated atrophic patches with glazed appearance and prominent vessels. Early ulcerations have occurred on the right shin.

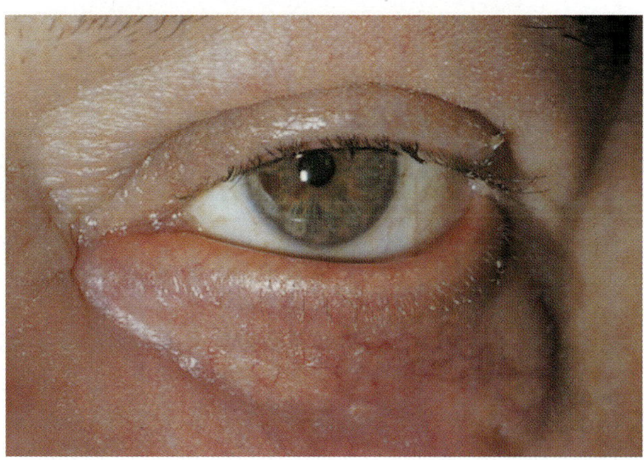

FIGURE 15-35. Necrobiosis lipoidica in a diabetic. There is lower lid laxity with poor apposition of the lid margin to the ocular globe. A slight ectropion is caused by the lid lesion.

16

GRANULOMATOUS DISORDERS

SARCOIDOSIS

Sarcoidosis, a multisystem inflammatory disease of unknown cause, is characterized by noncaseating granulomatous lesions throughout the body. It is usually chronic and self-limited, although death and blindness may occur. Sarcoidosis of the skin and the eye are more common in females and probably in those of African-American descent.

Clinical Manifestations

The constellation of fever, erythema nodosum, iritis, and polyarthritis suggests the presence of acute sarcoidosis, although patients often have various vague symptoms, such as malaise, weakness, fatigue, anorexia, weight loss, night sweats, nonproductive cough, exertional dyspnea, and central nervous system symptoms. Occasionally, there are no symptoms, and the diagnosis is suggested on routine chest x-ray. The disease is usually low-grade and prolonged, with remissions and exacerbations. It may also be self-limited.

Sarcoid affects almost any organ system but most commonly the skin, lungs, eyes, superficial and deep lymph nodes, salivary and lacrimal glands, liver, spleen, small bones of the hands and feet, heart, nervous system, and kidneys. Pulmonary involvement occurs in about 90% of patients. Chest x-ray findings include a normal-appearing chest, bilateral hilar adenopathy, pulmonary infiltration, and pulmonary fibrosis. The lymph nodes are enlarged and are usually discrete and nontender. Salivary gland enlargement is uncommon.

Acute polyarthralgia is commonly associated with erythema nodosum. Chronic polyarthritis occurs in about 15% of patients and involves the hand, wrist (Fig. 16-1), knee, and ankle. Cystic lesions of the small bones of the hands and feet may be seen on x-ray.

Central nervous system involvement is commonly associated with posterior segment eye disease and includes psychiatric changes, meningoencephalitis, multiple sclerosis–like changes, mononeuritis multiplex, and peripheral neuropathy. Facial nerve involvement leads to Bell palsy.

Hepatosplenomegaly occurs in about 20% to 40% of patients. Granulomata of the kidneys are usually asymptomatic.

Skin Features

Skin lesions usually develop on the face, ears, eyelids, and extremities. They may present as

1. Erythema nodosum.
2. Maculopapular eruptions, which may progress to yellow-ochre granulomatous papules and plaques (often in an annular pattern) of the face, ears, nose, eyelids, and extensor surfaces of extremities (Figs. 16-2 to 16-6). Healing occurs with scarring.
3. Nodular sarcoid.
4. Angiolupoid form of sarcoidosis. This form is usually single and occurs at the medial canthal area, below the eyebrow, or on the adjacent cheek. It is often dome-shaped and orange-red or reddish-brown in color. It is more common in women.
5. Subcutaneous sarcoid lesions. These usually occur on the extremities and present as tender or painless persistent nodules (Fig. 16-7).
6. Sarcoid plaques. Plaques usually develop on the extremities, shoulders, and buttocks. They are often diffuse and irregular in shape.
7. Lupus pernio. This form is usually symmetric and has a dusky, erythematous hue. The lesions feel indurated. Rarely, they ulcerate. They frequently involve the cheeks, nose, ears, lower eyelids, fingers, and hands (Figs. 16-6 to 16-9).

   Nodular sarcoid of the face, trunk, and proximal part of the extremities is single and begins as a red or yellow-red nodule that becomes violaceous or purplish-brown in color. The lesion heals with a brownish or yellowish telangiectatic scar with a central depression.
8. Lesions in scar tissue. These occasionally develop in a scar and present as a purplish-red lesion that eventually fades to a brownish color (Fig. 16-10).
9. Cicatricial alopecia.

10. Sarcoid may involve the mucous membranes, especially the buccal mucosa. The lesions are nodular, ulcerative, or plaquelike and are surrounded by a hyperpigmented area.

Ocular Features

Sarcoid involves the eye in up to 50% of patients. In some instances, it is the earliest feature. Lid changes consist of sharply defined, red or brown, asymmetric nodular and papular lesions. Occasionally, the lesions spread diffusely to produce a thickened, plaquelike appearance. Lupus pernio may also involve the lid and is symmetrically dispersed over the cheeks and lower lids. Seventh cranial nerve paralysis produces lagophthalmos. Ptosis is caused by 3rd cranial nerve involvement.

Conjunctival involvement in sarcoid may be in the form of granulomata or appear as conjunctival thickening with injection. The granulomata are often single and are located in the inferior cul-de-sac or on the tarsal conjunctiva of the lower lid (Fig. 16-11). Sarcoid nodules are often mistaken for follicles.

The cornea is only rarely involved if there are no conjunctival changes. Limbic nodules or interstitial keratitis (IK) occasionally develops in association with the uveitis. The IK is almost always inferior and found in the deep stroma. It begins with deposition of keratitic precipitates and corneal thickening along the inferior periphery of the cornea, often barely visible at the slit lamp. The IK will gradually progress superiorly but only rarely interferes directly with vision. Hypercalcemia may lead to band keratopathy. Fifth cranial nerve paralysis may cause corneal anesthesia.

Scleral plaques, a nondescript nodular scleritis, or episcleritis occasionally occurs in sarcoidosis. Lacrimal system involvement in sarcoid includes a unilateral or bilateral dacryoadenitis in which the gland is nontender and feels hard to palpation (Fig. 16-12). Keratoconjunctivitis sicca and occasionally Sjögren syndrome may occur. Nasolacrimal duct obstruction and nonspecific dacryoadenitis may also be seen.

Orbital involvement may suggest a rapidly developing pseudotumor. In some instances, there is a palpable nodule deep to the upper eyelid or within the lower eyelid. Ptosis may also be present. Orbital sarcoid infrequently extends along the chiasm to the cerebrum, destroys the orbital walls, and invades the paranasal sinuses.

Uveal tract involvement occurs in more than 75% of patients with ocular sarcoid and includes the following:

1. Severe acute bilateral iridocyclitis.
2. Iris granulomata (Fig. 16-13).
3. Chronic granulomatous iridocyclitis (Figs. 16-14 and 16-15).
4. Posterior uveal tract involvement in about one-fourth of all patients. The central nervous system and posterior uveal tract involvement are often associated. Vitreous opacities may be seen inferiorly and appear as small globoid bodies, snowballs, or a string of pearls.
5. Retinal findings that include yellow exudates resembling candle-wax drippings that course along the vessels, large chorioretinal granulomata, retinal periphlebitis, edema, preretinal and intraretinal hemorrhage, and retinal pigment epithelial atrophy (Fig. 16-16).
6. Neuroophthalmic findings that include large granulomata of the optic nerve, papillitis, papilledema, neuroretinitis, optic atrophy, and 3rd , 4th, and 6th cranial nerve paralysis (Fig. 16-17).

Specific sarcoid findings associated with eye changes are found in the following conditions:

1. Lofgren syndrome (acute iridocyclitis associated with erythema nodosum and bilateral hilar lymphadenopathy).
2. Heerfordt syndrome (uveitis, parotid gland enlargement, and facial nerve palsy).
3. Keratoconjunctivitis sicca associated with lacrimal gland and parotid gland enlargement (Mikulicz syndrome).
4. Chronic iridocyclitis, lupus pernio, bone cysts, and pulmonary fibrosis.

FAMILIAL GRANULOMATOSIS

Blau syndrome (familial juvenile systemic granulomatosis) is a rare autosomal dominant form of sarcoid or sarcoid-like condition that presents in the first decade of life, usually with erythema nodosum and arthritis of the large joints, such as the knees. It affects the posterior segment much more frequently than other forms of sarcoid, invariably showing multiple choroidal granulomata resembling the pattern seen in birdshot choroidopathy (Fig. 16-18). There is an associated vitreitis and often papillitis. If untreated, this will progress to choroidal and retinal damage, leaving hyperpigmented lesions scattered throughout the retina (Fig. 16-19).

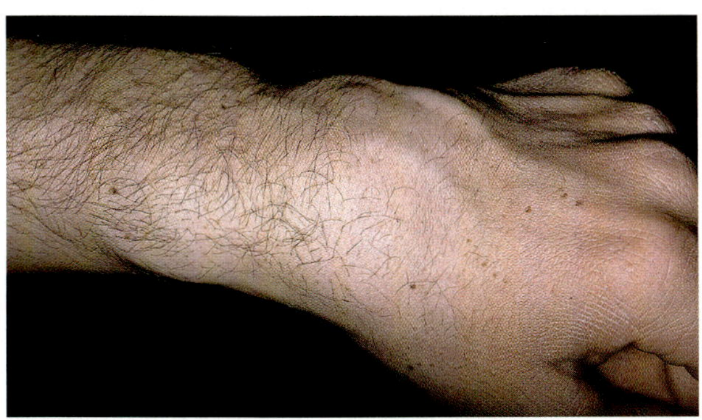

FIGURE 16-1. Chronic arthropathy of wrist and hand in patient with subcutaneous sarcoid pictured in Fig. 16-16.

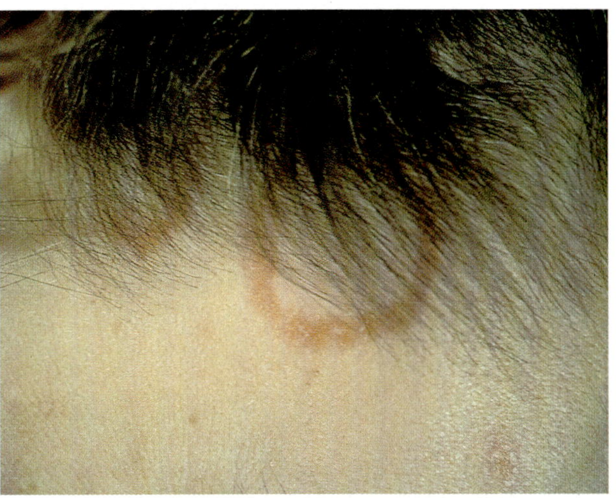

FIGURE 16-2. Annular sarcoid on nape of neck. The dull erythemato-brownish color suggests sarcoidosis. Biopsy is always indicated to rule out other causes of granulomatous disease.

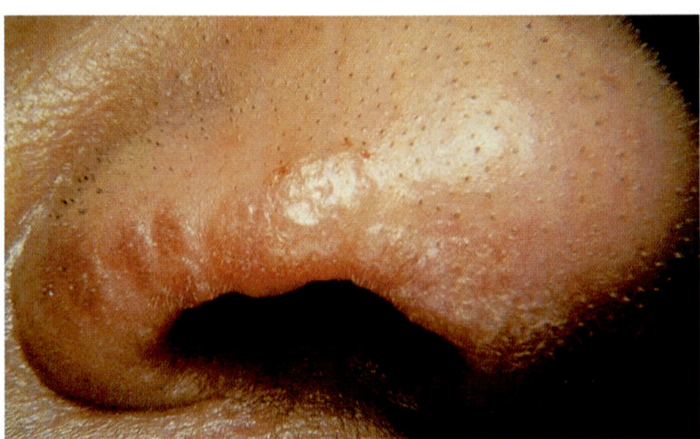

FIGURE 16-3. Firm erythematous papules of cutaneous sarcoidosis on nose. Sun-exposed sites are often favored in sarcoidosis.

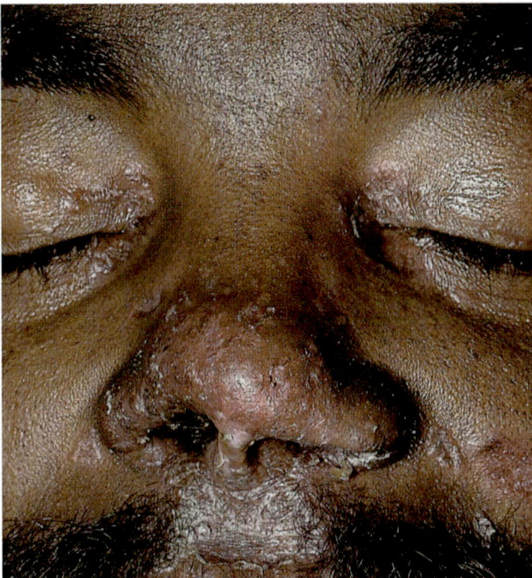

FIGURE 16-4. Small sarcoidal granulomata of medial upper eyelids in patient with extensive cutaneous as well as systemic sarcoidosis. (Courtesy of Richard Odom, M.D.)

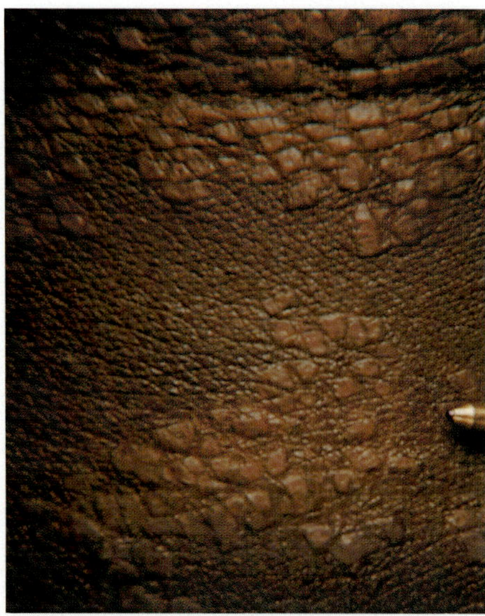

FIGURE 16-5. Lichenoid lesions of the extensor surface of the arm in sarcoid.

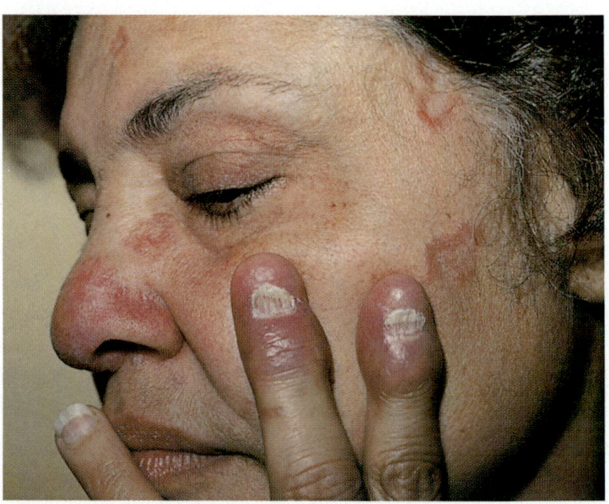

FIGURE. 16-6. Annular lesion of the face together with mild lupus pernio of the nose, and severe involvement of the fingers and nails with sarcoidosis. X-rays of the affected fingers showed classic lytic lesions.

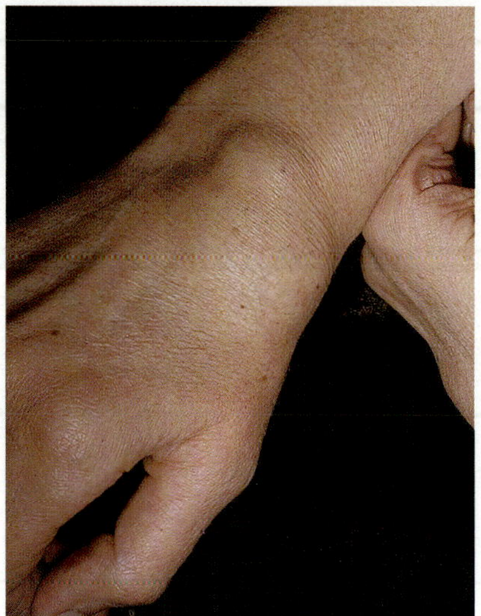

FIGURE 16-7. Subcutaneous sarcoid nodules of wrist. This patient also had chronic arthropathy of wrist and hand as shown in Fig. 16-1.

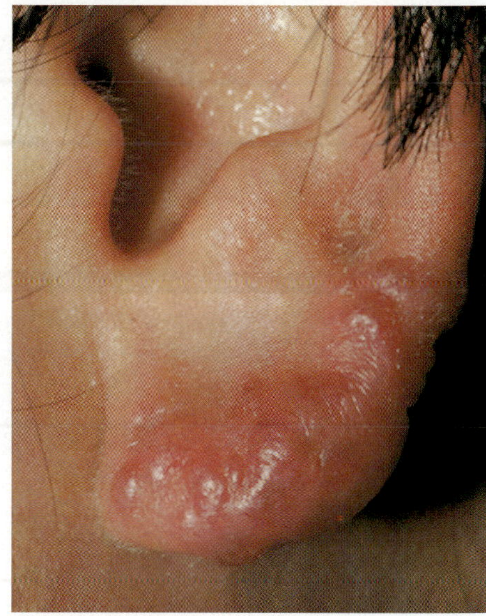

FIGURE 16-8. Lupus pernio (sarcoidosis) of the pinna. Lupus vulgaris (tuberculosis) and lepromatous leprosy must be ruled out in a patient like this one.

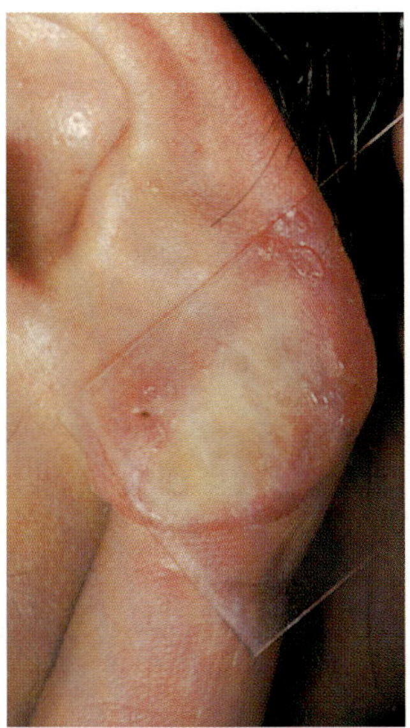

FIGURE 16-9. Diascopy of the lesions in Fig. 16-8 showing "apple jelly nodules." A helpful bedside test for cutaneous sarcoidosis.

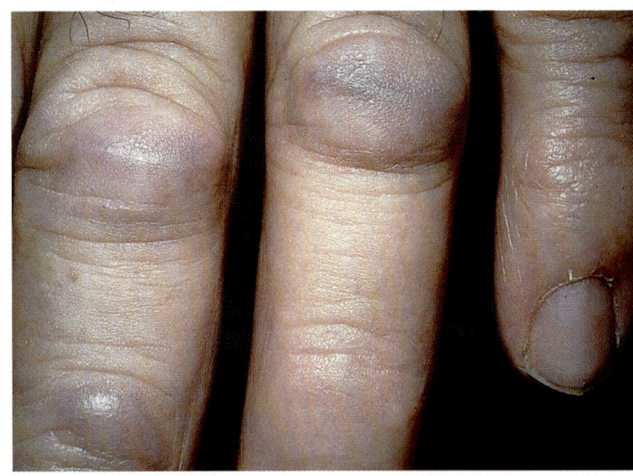

FIGURE 16-10. Sarcoid nodules over knuckles—sites of previous injury some 20 years earlier.

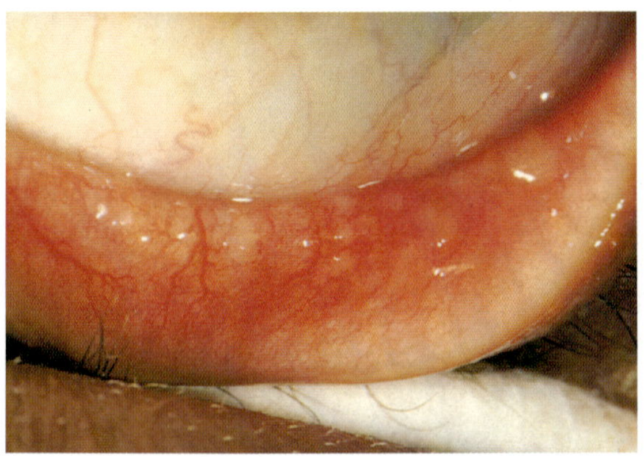

FIGURE 16-11. Multiple sarcoid nodules of the conjunctiva.

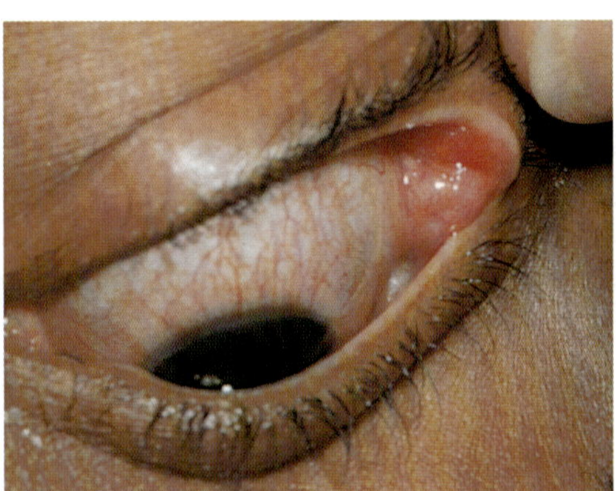

FIGURE 16-12. Recurrent dacryoadenitis in sarcoid. This patient has had recurrent lacrimal gland enlargement over the past 2 years. The conjunctival redness is caused by keratoconjunctivitis sicca. There is a small amount of mucus in the tear film.

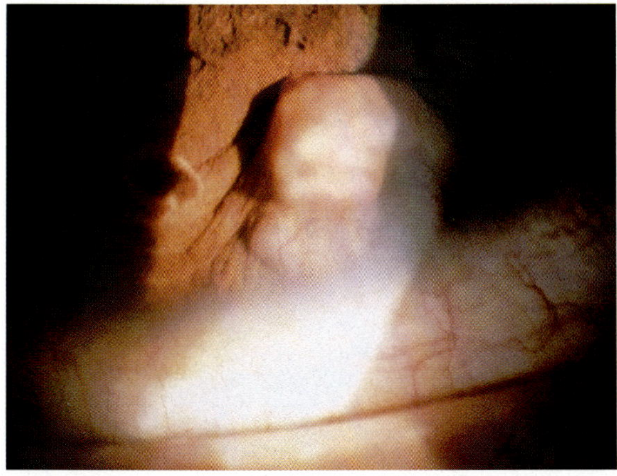

FIGURE 16-13. Iris granuloma in a patient with biopsy-proven sarcoidosis.

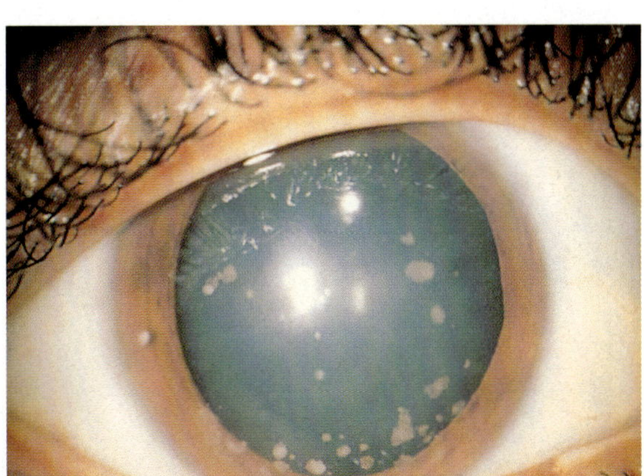

FIGURE 16-14. Large mutton-fat keratic precipitates, many of which are pigmented in the patient with chronic sarcoidal granulomatous iridocyclitis.

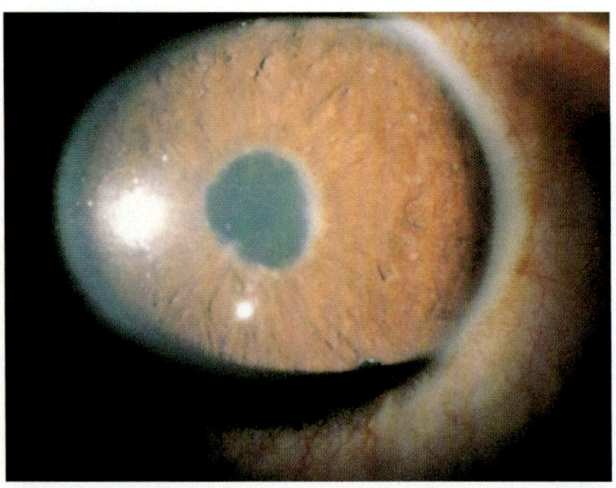

FIGURE 16-15. Posterior synechiae and iris bombé in sarcoid iridocyclitis.

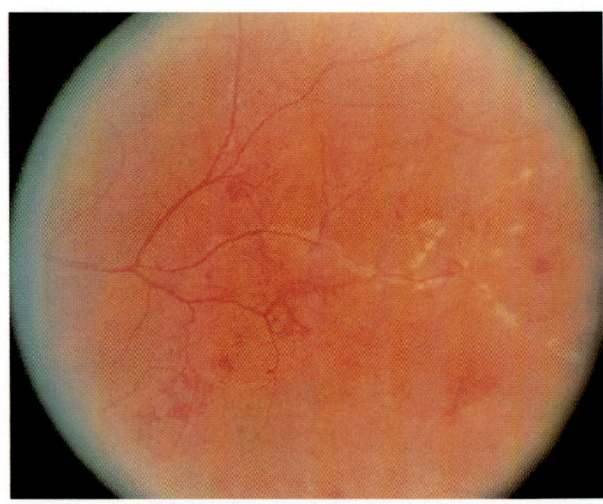

FIGURE 16-16. Retinal changes in sarcoidosis. Candle-wax drippings and intraretinal hemorrhages are evident in this patient. (Courtesy of Dr. John Belmont.)

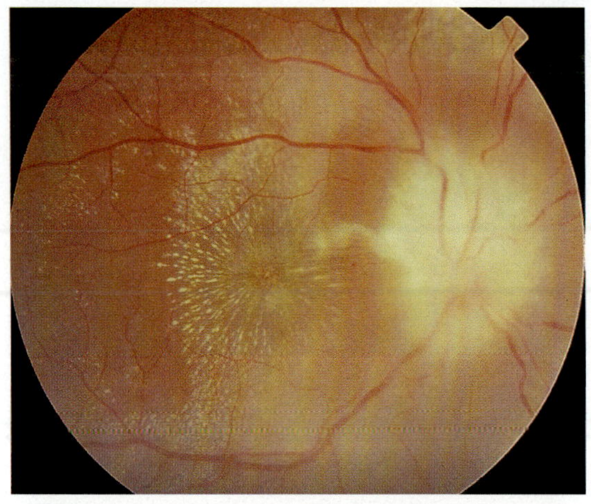

FIGURE 16-17. Optic nerve granuloma in sarcoidosis.

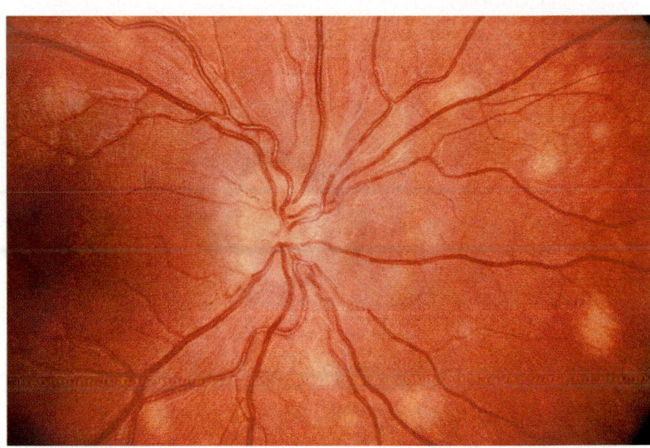

FIGURE 16-18. Choroidal granulomata in a 6-year-old male with familial granulomatosis.

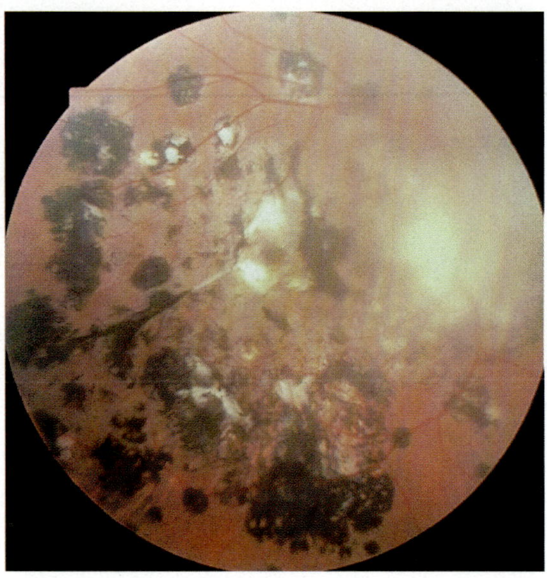

FIGURE 16-19. Fundus of mother of patient illustrated in Fig. 16-17. Note hyperpigmented spots from previous choroidal granulomata.

17

METABOLIC DISEASES

The metabolic diseases represent a diverse group of inherited and acquired diseases that often have dramatic and profound ocular and skin changes. Some of these findings may be pathognomonic and diagnostic, may contribute to the diagnosis, or may help provide a short differential diagnostic list. These diseases may be inborn errors of metabolism, enzymatic deficiencies, or impaired excretion of metabolites. The recognition and early diagnosis of some of these metabolic diseases may change the course of the patient's life, as can be seen with these patients with tyrosinemia.

TYROSINEMIA

Tyrosinemia Type II (Richner–Hanhart Syndrome; Oculocutaneous Tyrosinemia)

Tyrosinemia type II (Richner–Hanhart syndrome; oculocutaneous tyrosinemia) is an autosomal recessive syndrome that is caused by deficiency of tyrosine aminotransferase. This condition leads to increased tyrosine serum levels with aminoaciduria and reducing substances in the urine. The children are often mentally retarded if the condition is not recognized early in infancy and treated with dietary therapy.

During the first year of life, erythematous lesions develop on the palms and soles, followed by painful, circumscribed erosions of the palms, soles, and tips of the digits. The areas later become hyperkeratotic and present as dry lamellar patches or gross keratoderma (Fig. 17-1). Sometimes the lesions are bullous in character and have a linear configuration. Hyperkeratosis of the tongue may also occur.

Ocular Features

Ocular features include long lashes, conjunctival plaques, corneal scarring, nystagmus, strabismus, cataract, and glaucoma. The corneal epithelium often shows ridges that radiate outward from the central cornea, simulating a dendritic ulcer. Peripheral corneal neovascularization may also occur, as well as conjunctival plaques, corneal scarring (Fig. 17-2), long lashes nystagmus, strabismus, cataract, and glaucoma.

MUCINOSIS

Lichen Myxedematosus (Papular Mucinosis; Scleromyxedema)

Lichen myxedematosus (papular mucinosis; scleromyxedema) is a rare idiopathic dermatosis characterized by acid mucopolysaccharides in the skin, which causes discrete or large confluent papules or plaques. It usually develops during the third to fifth decade of life. The thickened skin may cause impairment of joint motility. A progressive generalized skin rash begins on the extremities, then spreads to the trunk and face. It begins as lichenoid papules that coalesce to form hyperpigmented plaques, progressive and extensive skin thickening, and a leonine face (Fig.17-3).

Cardiovascular abnormalities, extreme muscle weakness, and lassitude may be seen.

Ocular Features

Ocular findings include thickening of the lid skin and corneal changes that are characterized by discrete, irregular, gray-white, subepithelial corneal opacities in a whorl pattern over the entire superficial cornea. The overlying epithelium is intact, and deep stroma and Descemet membrane are normal. Other corneal changes include linear refractile crystals in the anterior to mid-stroma; fluffy, somewhat round deposits in the mid-stroma; and diffuse, larger aggregates in the posterior stroma.

THE MUCOPOLYSACCHARIDOSES

The mucopolysaccharidoses are a group of metabolic, inborn errors characterized by mucopolysaccharide accumulation (primarily dermatan sulfate, heparan sulfate, and keratan sulfate) in tissues throughout the body. They are classified according to their clinical manifestations and by the deficient enzymes causing the particular syndrome, namely:

1. Mucopolysaccharidosis I: (a) mucopolysaccharidosis I-H (Hurler's syndrome), (b) mucopolysaccharidosis I-H/S (Hurler/Scheie syndrome), (c) mucopolysaccharidosis I-S (Scheie syndrome)

2. Mucopolysaccharidosis II (Hunter syndrome)
3. Mucopolysaccharidosis III (Sanfilippo syndrome)
4. Mucopolysaccharidosis IV (Morquio-Brailsford syndrome)
5. Mucopolysaccharidosis VI (Maroteaux-Lamy Syndrome)
6. Mucopolysaccharidosis VII

All the mucopolysaccharidoses are autosomal recessive except for Hunter syndrome, which is X-linked recessive. Skin findings occur only in mucopolysaccharidosis I, II, and IV.

Mucopolysaccharidosis I

Patients with mucopolysaccharidosis I are deficient in lysosomal enzyme alpha-*L*-iduronidase, which results in accumulation of dermatan sulfate and heparan sulfate.

Mucopolysaccharidosis I-H (Hurler Syndrome)

Mucopolysaccharidosis I-H (Hurler syndrome) becomes manifest during the first or second year of life. It is also known as gargoylism because of the large head and grotesque facial appearance. Patients are often shorter than normal. Death frequently supervenes before the age of 20.

The tongue is enlarged and protrudes from the mouth. Loss of abdominal muscle tone and hepatosplenomegaly causes the abdomen to protrude. Skeletal abnormalities develop early in life. The supraorbital ridges are heavy; the neck is very short; the back has dorsolumbar kyphosis and is broad and hunched; the limbs and hands are short, the extremities are deformed, and the fingers are stubby and broad. The joints have limited motion. Mental retardation usually develops by the first year of life, and sexual development is retarded and minimal in degree.

Skin Features

Symmetric ivory-white nodules or ridges occur between the angles of the scapula and the posterior axillary lines and occasionally on the arms, pectoral regions, and outer thighs. Hypertrichosis of the face and trunk may be quite conspicuous.

Ocular Features

The eyebrows are thick and bushy. The lids are large, coarse, thickened, and edematous.

The cornea is often grossly cloudy at birth. The opacity is most marked in the subepithelial area and extends posteriorly toward Descemet membrane. In some patients, the cloudiness is most marked in the posterior stroma, whereas gray or yellow foci are evident in the middle layers. Gradually, the cornea becomes completely opaque. The epithelium stains diffusely. There are no vessels. Megalocornea may occur.

Other ocular findings include buphthalmos, hypertelorism, small orbits, enlarged optic foramen, congenital anterior polar cataract, retinitis pigmentosa, retinal detachment, macular edema with loss of the foveal reflex, papilledema and optic atrophy caused by the hydrocephalus, disc hyperemia, nystagmus, anisocoria, convergent squint, decreased visual acuity, and a high degree of refractive error.

Mucopolysaccharidosis I-H/S (Hurler–Scheie Syndrome; MPS I-H/S)

The mental deficiency and dwarfism in mucopolysaccharidosis I-H/S (Hurler–Scheie syndrome; MPS I-H/S) is intermediate between Hurler and Scheie syndrome. A small jaw is unique to this form of mucopolysaccharidosis. Cardiac enlargement and umbilical and inguinal hernias are major manifestations of the syndrome. Multiple skeletal changes may be seen. Severe acne develops early in life.

Ocular Features

The ocular features include the following:

1. Decreased vision caused by the corneal opacity; visual field constriction and night blindness caused by retinal changes.
2. Coarse, bushy eyebrows; coarse lashes; thick, edematous lids; ptosis; and tylosis.
3. Diffuse cloudy cornea; occasionally, punctate corneal opacities, megalocornea, corneal bullae, and corneal thickening.
4. Scleral thickening from acid mucopolysaccharide deposition.
5. Hypertelorism, small orbits, enlarged optic foramen.
6. Iris thickening, distortion, and folding from acid mucopolysaccharide deposits.
7. Other findings include congenital anterior polar cataract, pigmentary retinopathy, tapetoretinal degeneration, retinal detachment, macular edema, optic atrophy or cupping, disc edema, disc hyperemia, buphthalmos, proptosis, anisocoria, convergent squint, and secondary glaucoma.

Mucopolysaccharidosis I-S (Scheie Syndrome)

Mucopolysaccharidosis I-S (Scheie syndrome) is a relatively mild disease. There is no mental retardation or dwarfism, although there is mild facial coarseness. Joint contractures causing clawlike fingers are a major manifestation, and there is often a carpel-tunnel syndrome. Juxtaarticular cystic lesions have been observed. Aortic regurgitation and late cardiac decompensation may be seen. A protuberant abdomen is associated with umbilical and inguinal hernias.

Ocular Features

The eyebrows and lashes are coarse. The brows are bushy. Lid edema and tylosis may be observed. Severe, progressive corneal clouding develops relatively early and is typically more severe in the periphery. Punctate opacities, corneal edema, and increased thickness are common.

Other findings include scleral thickening; iris distortion, folding, and thickening; tapetoretinal degeneration, which is a major manifestation of the syndrome; macular edema with resultant decreased visual acuity; glaucoma; papilledema from increased cerebrospinal fluid pressure; optic atrophy; proptosis; and anisocoria.

Mucopolysaccharidosis II (Hunter Syndrome)

Mucopolysaccharidosis II (Hunter syndrome) is caused by deficiency of iduronate-2-sulfatase that results in cellular accumulation of dermatan sulfate and heparan sulfate. Patients with the mild form of the disease have a longer survival time and no mental retardation, gargoylism, dwarfism, hepatosplenomegaly, or corneal clouding. In the severe form, the mental retardation and neurologic changes are similar to those found in Hurler syndrome. Both forms have early deafness.

The skin changes are similar to those of Hurler syndrome (see earlier).

Ocular Features

The brows are bushy and coarse, and the lashes are coarse. Lid edema, ptosis, and lid thickening occur. Corneal clouding develops relatively late, usually during the fourth decade. Other findings include scleral thickening, proptosis, retinal degeneration, papilledema, optic atrophy, and optic cupping and hyperemia.

Mucopolysaccharidosis IV (Morquio–Brailsford Syndrome)

Patients with mucopolysaccharidosis IV (Morquio–Brailsford syndrome) are deficient in *N*-acetyl-hexosamine-6-sulfatase, which results in keratin sulfate accumulation in the tissues and excretion in the urine.

Progressive clinical manifestations begin by the age of 2, with severe growth retardation and coarse facial features. Some patients exhibit gibbus of the thoracolumbar spine, an awkward gait, knock-knees, sternal deformity, and hearing loss.

Skin and Ocular Features

Skin features include multiple telangiectases and tooth enamel defects that become evident soon after the teeth erupt. Ocular features include bushy, coarse, splayed lashes; corneal clouding evident only at the slit-lamp until after the age of 8; and occasionally, optic atrophy.

THE MUCOLIPIDOSES

The mucolipidoses have clinical and cytologic characteristics of both the mucopolysaccharidoses and the sphingolipidoses as well as many clinical features of Hurler syndrome.

XANTHOMATA AND THE LIPOPROTEIN DISORDERS

Xanthomata are common in primary and secondary lipoprotein disorders and in normolipemic xanthomatous diseases. They are uncommon in individuals without other evidence of disease.

Primary Lipoprotein Disorders

The primary lipoprotein disorders are classified into types I, IIA, IIB, III, IV, and V on the basis of serum levels of cholesterol, low-density lipoprotein (LDL), triglycerides, and the ultracentrifugation pattern of plasma lipoproteins. They are not distinct disease entities, but the classification helps to explain the disease processes and the type of therapy indicated for each disorder.

1. Type I hyperlipidemia (hyperchylomicronemia). (New terminology = familial lipoprotein lipase deficiency.) Type I hyperlipidemia is autosomal recessive, represents a fat-induced hyperlipemia, and is characterized by excess chylomicrons, a triglyceride level of 1,000 to more than 10,000, cholesterol of about 10% of the triglyceride level, and variable LDLs.
2. Type IIA hyperlipidemia. (New terminology = familial hypercholesterolemia or common polygenic hypercholesterolemia.) Type IIA hyperlipidemia is autosomal dominant, usually becoming manifest around the fourth decade of life, when the patient develops coronary artery disease. It is characterized by excess low-density lipoproteins, raised LDL cholesterol, raised cholesterol levels of 300 to more than 600, and normal plasma triglycerides. In type IIA hyperlipidemia, xanthomatous deposits develop in the skin and tendons. Eventually, widespread atheromatous changes occur in the vascular system, especially in the coronary vessels.

   Ocular findings include xanthomata of the lid, an irritative conjunctivitis, xanthomatous conjunctival nodules, arcus lipoides, a hypercholesterolemic lipid keratopathy, and infiltrative scleral plaques.
3. Type IIB hyperlipidemia (mixed hyperbeta- and hyperprebetalipoproteinemia). (New terminology = familial combined hyperlipidemia.) Type IIB hyperlipidemia is autosomal dominant and is characterized by excess low-density and very-low-density lipoproteins, elevated plasma cholesterol to levels of 250 to 600, elevated

triglycerides to about 200 to 600, and elevated low-density cholesterol.

4. Type III hyperlipidemia (hyper-"remnant"-lipoproteinemia or dysbetalipoproteinemia). (New terminology = familial dysbetalipoproteinemia or familial type III hyperlipoproteinemia.) Type III hyperlipidemia is autosomal recessive. Patients may also have hypothyroidism, central obesity, or diabetes mellitus. This type is characterized by excess chylomicron remnants and intermediate-density lipoproteins, variable plasma cholesterol levels from normal to more than 1,000, variable triglyceride levels from 175 to 1,500, low or normal LDLs, and in some instances, hyperglycemia and hyperuricemia.

5. Type IV hyperlipidemia (carbohydrate induced). (New terminology = familial combined hyperlipidemia; familial hypertriglyceridemia or sporadic hypertriglyceridemia.) Type IV hyperlipidemia is autosomal dominant. It is characterized by elevated prebetalipoprotein, which is markedly exaggerated by ingestion of large amounts of carbohydrates, nonketotic glucose intolerance, hyperinsulinemia, obesity, and mild decrease in lipoprotein lipase activity. Laboratory findings include excess very-low-density lipoproteins, plasma triglycerides from 200 to 5,000, cholesterol levels of 300 to 800, and normal LDL cholesterol. A hyperuricemia and carbohydrate intolerance may also be seen.

6. Type V hyperlipidemia (mixed). [New terminology = familial type V hyperlipoproteinemia, familial hypertriglyceridemia, or familial lipoprotein lipase (apo CII) deficiency.] Type V hyperlipidemia is accentuated by excess-alcohol, high-fat, or high-carbohydrate intake. It is characterized by excess chylomicrons and very-low-density lipoproteins, elevated plasma cholesterol levels from 300 to 1,000, triglycerides from 500 to more than 10,000, and normal LDL cholesterol. Mild glucose intolerance is usually evident.

Secondary Hyperlipemias

Various disease entities may induce or exacerbate hyperlipemia, as follows:

1. *Uncontrolled diabetes mellitus*—hyperlipoproteinemia.
2. *Hypothyroidism*—hyperbetalipoproteinemia, dysbetalipoproteinemia, or hyperbetalipoproteinemia, and mixed lipemia.
3. *Nephrotic syndrome*—hyperbetalipoproteinemia or hyperbetalipoproteinemia and mixed lipemia.
4. *Hypopituitarism*—hyperbetalipoproteinemia and mixed lipemia.
5. *Lipodystrophy*—hyperbetalipoproteinemia and mixed lipemia.
6. *Renal failure with azotemia*—hyperbetalipoproteinemia and mixed lipemia.
7. *Hypergammaglobulin disorders*—hyperbetalipoproteinemia and mixed lipemia.

The antihypertensive agents (thiazide and betaadrenergic blockers) may be associated with elevation of the serum lipids.

Secondary hypercholesterolemia is uncommon but may cause corneal involvement.

Normolipemic Xanthomatous Diseases

Xanthomata found in the normolipemic states are similar to other xanthomata.

1. Histiocytoma cutis causes single, well-circumscribed yellow-to-brown nodules or papules. They usually develop during early adulthood.
2. Xanthoma disseminatum occurs in adults and is associated with discrete, multiple, papular, red-yellow or mahogany-brown lesions on the flexor surfaces of the extremities. The lesions do not spontaneously involute. Mucous membrane, conjunctival, corneal, bone, and lung infiltrates may occur, and involvement of the pituitary produces diabetes insipidus.
3. Lipemia retinalis and eruptive xanthoma are seen in hypertriglyceridemia and are proportional to the triglyceride level.
4. Xanthelasma (Figs. 17-4 and 17-5), corneal arcus senilis (Fig. 17-6), and palpebral tuberous xanthoma are related to elevated beta lipoprotein and associated hypercholesterolemia.

Skin Features

Xanthoma of the skin and tendons develop in any of the xanthomatous diseases.

1. Eruptive xanthomata (Figs. 17-7 and 17-8). Eruptive xanthomata occur in types I, III, IV, and V hyperlipidemias and sometimes in secondary hyperlipidemia associated with diabetes mellitus. They appear as multiple small, firm, yellowish-orange papules usually asymptomatic but occasionally pruritic, most commonly over the buttocks, abdomen, and extensor surfaces of the extremities.
2. Tendon xanthomata develop in types IIA, IIB, and III hyperlipidemia, and in secondary hyperlipidemia associated with prolonged cholestasis. They present as asymptomatic nodules that feel hard to palpation and are attached to tendons, ligaments, fascia, and periosteum, especially the extensor tendons of the hands and feet and the Achilles tendon.
3. Planar xanthomata occur in type III and IV hyperlipidemia and in secondary hyperlipidemias associated with chronic biliary obstruction or prolonged cholestasis, as occurs in primary biliary cirrhosis and, rarely, in mono-

clonal gammopathy. They appear as smooth, neoplastic skin plaques. The lesions of the palms are virtually diagnostic. Sometimes they are extensive, involving large areas of the scalp, face, neck, and the skin folds of the extremities. In such instances, they are often associated with myelomas, macroglobulinemia, or lymphomas.

4. Tuberous xanthomata occur in patients with hypercholesterolemia and increased levels of LDL (type II and type III) hyperlipoproteinemia. They also occur in secondary hyperlipidemia arising from hypothyroidism, chronic biliary disease, and, uncommonly, monoclonal gammopathy. The lesions are comparatively acute in onset and usually become widespread, involving the joints and extensor aspects of the extremities. They present as small yellow or orange papules or lobulated tumors, feel firm to palpation, and are often surrounded by erythema (Fig. 17-9).

5. Multiple skin xanthomata occur in xanthoma disseminatum, a rare histiocytic proliferative disorder seen in 5- to 20-year-olds with diabetes mellitus. They are symmetric, have a reddish-yellow color, and resolve completely after several years.

6. Disseminated lipogranulomatosis of Farber represents a slowly progressive disturbance of lipid metabolism. Subcutaneous lesions are common and occur on the flexor surfaces, including the antecubital fossae, sides of the neck, and groin.

7. Xanthoma diabeticorum is associated with diabetes mellitus or biliary cirrhosis with hyperlipidemia. Crops of eruptive xanthoma develop on the skin and usually resolve spontaneously.

8. Mucous membrane xanthomata of the pharynx, larynx, and bronchi may occur in xanthoma disseminatum.

Ocular Features

Xanthomata develop in the skin of the eyelid, the conjunctiva, cornea, sclera, and orbit but are uncommon except in the skin of the eyelid. They cause minimal symptoms except for occasional reduced vision and irritation from corneal involvement. Generally, bilateral lesions are associated with systemic disease.

Lid

Lid xanthomata include the following:

1. Xanthelasma palpebrarum (planar xanthomata) are small intracutaneous, yellow, soft skin lesions, which slowly increase in size and may coalesce to form large, raised, plaquelike lesions. They are usually bilateral and occur on the upper eyelid and at the inner canthus. They cause no symptoms (Figs. 17-4 and 17-5).

   Xanthelasma occurs as an isolated finding without evidence of systemic abnormality but may also occur in types IIA, IIB, and III lipoprotein disorders, hypercholesterolemic xanthomatosis, mixed hyperlipidemia type IV, biliary obstruction, and apolipoprotein E phenotypes, and in association with Schneider crystalline corneal dystrophy. They are more common in older women.

2. Tuberous xanthomata are similar to those in the skin. They are usually located in the inner canthal region or on the lid margin and may be multiple. Sometimes they are tender and cause itching.

3. Eruptive xanthomata are similar to those in the skin.

4. Lid xanthomata may occur in xanthoma disseminatum.

Conjunctiva

Conjunctival xanthomata are similar to xanthomata of the skin and other mucosal areas.

Essential hypercholesterolemic xanthomatosis may be associated with an irritative, persistent conjunctivitis, and occasionally, xanthomatous conjunctival nodules. Disseminated lipogranulomatosis of Farber occasionally produces subconjunctival xanthomata.

Cornea Arcus Senilis

Cornea arcus senilis is common in types IIA and IIB hyperlipidemias (occasionally in type III disease) and in aging patients with normal plasma cholesterol (Fig. 17-6). Young patients with levels of serum cholesterol greater than 350 mg/dL often develop arcus senilis.

Primary lipidosis of the cornea (corneal xanthoma) appears as a solid, yellowish opacity that later becomes gray. It begins in the deep stroma near the limbus, then progressively encroaches on the central cornea; occasionally, it begins in the central cornea. The peripheral corneal rim remains clear. There is deep and superficial vascularization. Eventually, the corneal epithelium and endothelium are involved. Corneal xanthoma occurs in type I (essential hyperlipemic xanthomatosis) (type I hyperlipidemia) and type II disease.

In essential hyperlipemic xanthomatosis, a solid, yellowish opacity develops in the central cornea and involves its entire thickness. Large areas of the cornea, including the peripheral cornea, remain clear, allowing moderate vision. Essential hypercholesterolemic xanthomatosis may produce a hypercholesterolemic lipid keratopathy with opacification of the central or peripheral cornea.

Progressive, diffuse corneal involvement of all layers occurs in secondary hypercholesterolemia and is associated with vascularization. Corneal xanthoma are also seen in xanthoma disseminatum.

Sclera and Orbit

Essential hypercholesterolemic xanthomatosis and xanthoma disseminatum occasionally produce yellow scleral plaques. Localized xanthomata of the orbital roof are extremely uncommon but usually cause proptosis, downward displacement of the globe, and x-ray evidence of rarefaction of the bone.

Uvea and Retina

Iris xanthomata occur in type I disease; choroidal xanthomata, in type I and II disease.

Lipemia retinalis and hyperlipemic retinopathy occur in type I hyperlipidemia when the serum triglycerides exceed a level of 2,500 mg/dL. They may also be seen in types III, IV, and V disease. In lipemia retinalis, the blood vessels appear hazy, milky, flat, and ribbonlike. The vascular light reflex is lost. The fundus and the optic nerve head otherwise appear normal.

Patients with primary hypercholesterolemia may develop glistening crystals in the fundus or small yellowish-white spots associated with the terminal arterioles in the central fundus.

Retinal xanthomata occur in type I (hyperlipemic xanthomatosis) and II disease. A retinal detachment may be caused by xanthoma diabeticorum xanthomatous masses in the posterior eye.

Occasionally, the retina is affected in disseminated lipogranulomatosis of Farber.

LIPID STORAGE DISEASES

The lipid storage diseases also cause xanthomata.

Cerebrotendinous Xanthomatosis (Cholestanolosis)

Cerebrotendinous xanthomatosis (cholestanolosis) is autosomal recessive and probably occurs from defective synthesis of bile. It results in tendon xanthomata, especially of the Achilles tendon, and sometimes xanthelasma and tuberous xanthomata. The patients develop progressive mental deterioration and spasticity. Patients may also have juvenile cataracts. Death occurs from premature arteriosclerosis. The plasma cholesterol levels are low or normal. Plasma cholestanol levels are elevated.

β-Sitosterolemia and Xanthomatosis

β-Sitosterolemia and xanthomatosis is an autosomal recessive disease that becomes manifest in early childhood. It is associated with tendinous xanthomata of the Achilles tendon and extensor tendons of the hand. Sometimes, tuberous xanthomata and xanthelasma occur. Splenomegaly, hemolysis, and premature arteriosclerosis may be found. The patients have elevated plasma cholesterol and the presence of plant sterols.

Tangier Disease (Familial High-Density Lipoprotein Deficiency)

Tangier disease is a rare autosomal recessive disease in which high-density lipoprotein (HDL) is markedly reduced and probably abnormal. The patients have orange-yellow tonsils and adenoids, and many have hepatosplenomegaly and peripheral neuropathy. Corneal infiltrates are sometime seen. The plasma cholesterol is markedly decreased and the triglycerides are elevated.

Lipoid Proteinosis (Urbach–Wiethe Disease; Hyalinosis Cutis Et Mucosae, Lipoglycoproteinosis)

Lipoid proteinosis (Urbach–Wiethe disease; hyalinosis cutis et mucosae; lipoglycoproteinosis) is a chronic dysproteinemia. It is autosomal recessive and is characterized by disturbances in serum proteins and carbohydrate metabolism. Mucopolysaccharides are deposited in the skin and mucous membranes of the mouth and larynx. Intracranial calcification and epilepsy sometimes occur. Diabetes mellitus is occasionally present.

Skin Features

Lipidlike material is deposited extracellularly in the skin and later in the mucous membranes . The deposits occur anywhere, but they are more common on the face (Fig. 17-10), scalp, neck, and axilla. The skin becomes thickened and assumes a pale yellow-brown, pockmarked appearance. Scalp involvement leads to alopecia. At first, the eruption is papular but then becomes confluent. The extensor surfaces, especially the elbows and knees, become hyperkeratotic. The skin may be darkened. Atrophic scars occur late in the disease.

Small yellowish-transparent papules develop in the mucous membranes of the mouth, lips, tongue, epiglottis, and larynx; occasionally, they also develop in the labia and vagina. Hoarseness is an early manifestation of laryngeal deposits. The lip and tongue lesions appear yellow and hard. The tongue becomes markedly thickened, reducing its range of motion. Swallowing may be difficult, especially late in the course of the disease. Parotitis sometimes recurs.

Ocular Features

The patient may complain of a granular or foreign-body sensation. Pathognomonic nodules develop in the region of the lashes. They are discrete, yellow-white, beadlike papillae that often have a yellow, waxy appearance. The lesions cause trichiasis. Small, yellow subconjunctival nodules infrequently develop in the conjunctiva. Other findings consist of a hyalin-like material deposited in Descemet membrane and macular degeneration with reddish-yellow drusenlike deposits.

Farber Disease (Disseminated Lipogranulomatosis)

Farber disease (disseminated lipogranulomatosis) is an autosomal recessive lipid storage disease and leads to death in infancy. There is severe motor and mental retardation. The lymph nodes, lungs, and heart may be involved. Infiltrated, erythematous papules, nodules, and plaques develop near the tendons and joints of the hands and feet, on the ears, the occipital region, and trunk. Laryngeal involvement leads to dysphonia, laryngeal stridor, a hoarse cry, and noisy respirations. Cherry-red spots of the macula may be evident.

Gaucher Disease (Cerebroside Lipidosis)

Gaucher disease (cerebroside lipidosis) is characterized by accumulation of cerebrosides (kerasin) in cells of the reticuloendothelial system. It is autosomal recessive and is more common in patients of Jewish ancestry from Eastern Europe.

Clinical Manifestations

Gaucher disease has three clinical forms: adult, infantile, and juvenile. The infantile form begins acutely about the fourth or fifth month of life and is rapidly lethal. The child becomes apathetic and shows no ability to fixate objects but is not blind. Later, decerebrate rigidity, laryngeal spasms, and death occur. The juvenile form is chronic and relatively benign, lasting for several decades. There is severe splenomegaly with a protuberant abdomen. Spontaneous bone fractures may occur. The adult form usually begins insidiously. Patients may have erosion of the cortex of the long bones, and pain periodically arises from the bone changes. Gross splenomegaly and protuberant abdomen occur. Some patients survive until the seventh or eighth decade.

Skin Features

Skin pigmentation is common in adults but unusual in children. It may be diffuse or in the form of brown patches resembling chloasma on the face, neck, hands, and lower legs, appearing symmetrically with an irregular upper and a sharp lower margin.

Ocular Features

An addisonian type of hyperpigmentation of the lid occurs in the adult form of Gaucher disease. A triangular brown-colored thickening of the nasal and temporal bulbar conjunctiva resembling a pinguecula develops during the second or third decade in the juvenile form. Later, it becomes ocher in color.

Retinal changes include hemorrhages related to the profound microcystic anemia, retinal edema, ring-shaped perimacular degeneration, and, occasionally, a cherry-red spot of the macula. A squint may be seen in the infantile form, and in the juvenile form, there may be impaired abduction and jerky, uncoordinated movements.

Amyloidosis

Amyloidosis may be generalized or localized. It is characterized by impaired organ function caused by deposition of amyloid. The fibrils of amyloid are composed of immunoglobulin light chains or light-chain fragments (designated *AL*) and nonimmunoglobulin protein (designated *AA*).

Amyloid occurs in several forms, namely:

1. Systemic primary amyloidosis, in which amyloid AL is deposited in the tongue, heart, gastrointestinal tract, skeletal and smooth muscles, nerves, ligaments, and skin.
2. Systemic amyloidosis arising in multiple myeloma and related plasma cell dyscrasia, in which amyloid AL is deposited in the liver, spleen, kidneys, and adrenals.
3. Primary localized cutaneous amyloidosis in immunoglobulin light-chain disease with deposition of amyloid AL.
4. Heredofamilial forms of systemic secondary amyloidosis with deposit of amyloid AA.

   Systemic secondary amyloidosis, with deposits of amyloid AA, occurs in several heredofamilial diseases. In familial Mediterranean fever, which is autosomal recessive, amyloid is deposited in the liver, spleen, kidneys, adrenals, and vitreous. In Muckle–Wells syndrome, which is autosomal dominant, amyloid is deposited in the peripheral nerves and kidneys, and is associated with deafness. In amyloid polyneuropathy, which is autosomal dominant and found in Portuguese patients, amyloid is deposited in the peripheral nerves and viscera.

   Familial Mediterranean fever begins in early life. It occurs principally in Sephardic Jews, Armenians, and Arabs of the Mediterranean area. Periodic self-limiting episodes of fever, abdominal pain, chest pain, and joint pain occur. The skin lesions resemble erysipelas, urticaria, Henoch–Schonlein purpura, other forms of purpura, and vasculitic nodules on the legs (Fig. 17-11). The attacks lessen in severity as the patient gets older. Death occurs from renal failure. In the Muckle–Wells syndrome, patients develop urticaria in early childhood, then, later, nerve deafness, pain in the extremities, and nephropathy.
5. Secondary amyloidosis arising from infection (e.g., tuberculosis, leprosy); inflammation (e.g., rheumatoid arthritis, systemic lupus erythematosus); hemodialysis; and intravenous drug abuse is characterized by deposits of amyloid AA at any site. The AA form of amyloid not uncommonly involves the eye.

Clinical Manifestations

Systemic primary amyloidosis usually presents in the seventh decade of life and causes weight loss, fatigue, weakness, dyspnea, dysphonia, paresthesias, and ankle edema. The skin findings are similar to those found in myeloma-associated amyloidosis (see later).

Myeloma-associated amyloidosis causes macroglossia, the carpal tunnel syndrome, hepatomegaly, edema, cardiac arrhythmias, congestive heart failure, peripheral neuropathy, and skin lesions. Many of the skin findings are related to intracutaneous hemorrhage (petechiae, purpura, and spontaneous or trauma-induced ecchymoses). Less frequently, smooth, shiny, waxy-appearing papules or plaques occur, or there are large areas of diffuse infiltration simulating scleroderma or myxedema. The scalp may be thrown into longitudinal folds, and a diffuse or patchy alopecia may be evident. Amyloid infiltration into the nail matrix causes longitudinal striations, crumbling, or brittle nails.

Primary localized cutaneous amyloidosis is characterized by papular (lichen amyloidosis) (Figs. 17-12 and 17-13) or macular (macular amyloid) lesions (Fig. 17-14). The papular form usually occurs on the shins and occasionally on the extensor surface of the thighs, forearms, and upper arms; it presents as discrete, scaly papules that may coalesce into thick plaques. They are often pigmented, and in some instances, areas of hypopigmentation are also seen. The macular lesions usually occur on the back or chest, occasionally on the extensor surfaces of the extremities, and infrequently, around the eyes. The pigmentation in this form of amyloid has a distinctive ripple pattern.

Ocular Features

Lid

The eyelids are involved more frequently than any other part of the eye in amyloidosis (Figs. 17-15 and 17-16). Amyloid deposition in the lids occurs in familial amyloidosis, primary systemic amyloidosis, and secondary systemic and secondary localized amyloidosis. In primary localized amyloidosis, periocular pigmentation also occurs.

Edema, ecchymosis, petechial hemorrhages, ptosis, dermatochalasis, and lid thickening are all seen. Yellow-white nodules (often resembling wax or xanthomata) may occur. Localized ecchymosis or lid or periorbital purpura may follow mild trauma or the Valsalva maneuver.

Conjunctiva

Conjunctival amyloid presents as yellow, structureless, friable masses in the superior tarsal conjunctiva, fornix, and area near the caruncle, and occasionally, on the bulbar and limbal conjunctiva (Fig. 17-17). Subconjunctival hemorrhages and ecchymosis of the eyelids are common. Nodular conjunctival lesions suggest systemic disease such as a systemic lymphoma. Amyloid deposition in the conjunctiva also occurs secondary to trachoma, syphilis, vernal conjunctivitis, pterygium, chronic recurrent uveitis, rheumatoid arthritis, and the Churg–Strauss syndrome. Conjunctival plasmocytomas also causes amyloid deposition.

Amyloid involves the cornea in several ways, namely:

1. Lattice or flat and, occasionally, protuberant subepithelial corneal deposits in association with familial systemic amyloidosis.
2. Secondary localized deposits arising from corneal trauma and inflammation.
3. Lattice dystrophy, polymorphic amyloid degeneration, and gelatinous droplike dystrophy.
4. Decreased corneal sensation from corneal nerve involvement.

Widespread amyloid deposition in the sclera occurs by spread from the conjunctival and subconjunctival tissues.

Primary familial amyloidosis may involve the uveal tract with deposition of amyloid in the sphincter and dilator muscles of the iris, causing anisocoria and pupil irregularity as well as deposition of amyloid in the choroid, occasionally causing occlusion of patches of choriocapillaris.

Infrequently, primary familial amyloidosis causes retinal perivasculitis, retinal vascular occlusion, and retinal hemorrhages and exudates.

Deposition of amyloid in the vitreous causes floaters and slow deterioration of vision. The vitreous opacities are linear, veil-like, glass-wool-like, yellowish spheres with a distinctive white dot, or multiple circumscribed grayish-white opacities. The latter are attached to the posterior surface of the lens by an opaque "foot-plate." Vitreous deposition of amyloid occurs in primary familial amyloidosis and in familial amyloid polyneuropathy.

Amyloid infiltration in the orbit (Fig. 17-18) occurs by spread of conjunctival amyloid, localized primary amyloid deposition, or amyloid infiltration into the extraocular muscles in familial primary systemic amyloidosis. It causes gradual, painless, progressive proptosis and loss of motility. It is bilateral in familial primary systemic amyloidosis and unilateral in localized amyloid infiltration. Amyloid deposition in the lacrimal gland may be isolated or occur in Sjögren syndrome or familial systemic primary amyloidosis. It causes keratoconjunctivitis sicca, ptosis, proptosis, and other signs of an enlarging lacrimal gland or orbital mass. Occasionally, it is bilateral. Secondary glaucoma occasionally occurs from deposition of amyloid in the trabecular meshwork in primary familial amyloidosis.

Angiokeratoma Corporis Diffusum (Anderson–Fabry Disease)

Angiokeratoma corporis diffusum (Anderson–Fabry disease) is sex-linked recessive and represents a hereditary lipid storage disease in which ceramide trihexoside accumulates in the skin and viscera. It involves the skin, myocardium, smooth muscles of the blood vessels, and epithelium of the kidney and cornea. Most female carriers have corneal changes but no skin changes.

Febrile crises, episodic pain, burning of the hands and feet, skin eruptions, and marked proteinuria occur at onset and during exacerbations. The pain is described as lightninglike, occurring in the fingers and toes and occasionally in the abdomen and flanks. Mild hypertension, cardiomegaly, conduction disturbances, and murmurs are often present, especially late in the disease.

Glycolipid is deposited in the central nervous system when the disease is fully established. Lipid infiltration of the glomerular vessels causes albuminuria, hematuria, and specific lipophages in the urine. Cardiomyopathy and renal insufficiency often bring death by the fifth decade.

Skin Features

Affected males, in early life, develop a dark-red or black punctate telangiectatic and papular eruption (Figs. 17-19 to 17-21). Multiple angiokeratomas (the color of red wine) involve the trunk and areas about the genitalia, fingers, lips, and tongue. The skin is often dry, lax, and hypohidrotic. Edema of the hands and feet are common. Generalized lymphadenopathy may be found.

Ocular Features

Lid and periorbital edema may be part of the generalized edema. Nonspecific bulbar and palpebral conjunctival vascular changes consist of many small focal varicosities and dilatations of the smaller venules. Sometimes the vessels are ampulliform or saccular in type.

Cornea

Bilateral corneal epithelial involvement often occurs early in the disease in both males and females (Fig. 17-22). It begins as a diffuse yellow epithelial haziness with mild perilimbal vascular dilatation. The haziness gradually becomes concentrated into dense rays that radiate from the center of the cornea into dense bronze streaks arranged in a vortex or star shape pattern. It is best seen by transillumination.

Retinal vascular changes consist of segmental sausagelike dilatations of the retinal veins near the posterior pole. Retinal hemorrhages, perimacular edema, and hypertensive retinopathy may also be seen. Other ocular findings include a granular anterior or a spokelike posterior subcapsular cataract, edema of the optic nerve resulting from hypertension, and internuclear ophthalmoplegia.

Niemann–Pick Disease

Niemann–Pick disease is a rare autosomal recessive lipidosis that usually leads to death by the second year of life. There are six types. Types B and E have no neurologic manifestations. Within 2 to 3 months, the infant begins to lose weight and develops gross hepatosplenomegaly, generalized lymphadenopathy, and loss of muscle tone. The child has a mongoloid appearance. Deafness is common. A diffuse brown pigmentation occurs on the child's face along with suppurative lesions and indurated discolored patches on the cheeks. The skin is indurated and appears waxy. Purpuric lesions, cafe-au-lait spots, and dark, bluish mongolian spots may be seen on other skin areas and on the oral mucosa. Transient xanthomata develop over the enlarged cervical nodes. Periorbital fullness may be seen. Corneal opacification, brownish discoloration of the lens capsule, and a cherry-red spot of the macula, a macular halo, granular changes in the macula, and vertical ophthalmoplegia have been demonstrated.

Gout

Gout comprises a number of disease entities that arise from abnormal purine metabolism, abnormal uric acid excretion, or a combination of both. It is characterized by elevated levels of serum uric acid, deposition of monosodium urates in the cartilage of the pinna, urate deposits in the skin (tophi), recurrent attacks of acute arthritis, and renal stones. In many instances, it progresses to cause a chronic tophaceous arthritis.

Primary gout is autosomal dominant. Secondary gout is caused by purine metabolism disorders (seen in Hodgkin disease, leukemia, hemolytic diseases, chronic renal disease, lead intoxication, glucose 6-phosphate deficiency, sarcoidosis, psoriasis, and hyperparathyroidism); ingestion of drugs (e.g., pyrazinamide, chlorothiazide, and hydrochlorothiazide); obesity, starvation, and dietary indiscretion.

Gout commonly causes attacks of acute gouty arthritis in males after the fourth to sixth decade of life. It is usually recurrent and self-limited and causes acute pain, swelling, and other inflammatory signs. At first, it usually involves only a single joint, such as the great toe; later, several joints, such as the joints of the feet and ankles, are involved.

Skin Features

Gouty tophi (uric acid deposits) may occur in the pinna (especially the helix and antihelix), on the fingers, subcutaneous regions, joints, and bursae (Figs. 17-23 to 17-25).

Ocular Features

Tophi are rarely deposited near the margin of the eyelid. Gouty conjunctivitis causes burning, itching, and a foreign-body sensation. Occasionally, the patient complains of a "hot eye," especially in the morning, and may have difficulty in opening his eyes because of a feeling of stiffness. Exacerbations of symptoms usually occur during cold, wet weather; on exposure to dust or smoke; and following dietary indiscretion. There is marked hyperemia; dilated, tortuous vessels; and spontaneous ecchymoses. Meibomian froth is frequently present. Sodium urate conjunctival deposits appear as concretions (hard, chalklike deposits) in the bulbar conjunctiva. They cause chronic irritation and a chronic conjunctivitis.

A punctate keratitis, marginal ulceration, and a painful band keratopathy have all been observed. The band keratopathy is similar in appearance to the classical band keratopathy caused by calcium deposition.

Episcleritis and Scleritis

Gout may cause a localized simple episcleritis or scleritis (episcleritis periodica fugax) (Fig. 17-26). It usually develops suddenly, persists 3 to 4 days, then subsides spontaneously. Occasionally, sodium urate crystals are deposited in the sclera or episclera and cause a chronic episcleritis or scleritis.

Gouty iritis is uncommon and is usually associated with episcleral and scleral inflammation. The onset is sudden and associated with severe pain, an intense, deep-red or bluish-red injection, a cloudy cornea, keratic precipitates, and often secondary glaucoma.

THE PORPHYRIAS

Porphyria represents a group of enzymatic disorders of the porphyrin–heme metabolic pathway, which results in an abnormal amount of heme precursors (porphyrins) in the tissues, urine, feces, blood, and bone marrow. All the porphyrias are autosomal dominant except for erythropoietic porphyria, which is autosomal recessive, and porphyria cutanea tarda, which is autosomal dominant. They are classified according to the location of the excessive porphyrin production (i.e., liver or bone marrow).

Hepatic Porphyria

Hepatic porphyria includes acute intermittent porphyria, variegate porphyria, hereditary coproporphyria, porphyria cutanea tarda, and hepatoerythropoietic porphyria.

Acute intermittent porphyria has no skin manifestations.

Variegate Porphyria

Variegate porphyria can be triggered by barbiturates and sulfonamides. The clinical manifestations of variegate porphyria are similar to those of acute intermittent porphyria with abdominal pain, with or without constipation, and neurologic manifestations of seizures, mental depression, confusion, hallucinations, personality changes, and polyneuritis with foot and wrist drop. The manifestations usually begin during the second to third decade of life.

Skin Features

The skin is affected in areas exposed to light or minor trauma such as the face, neck, and dorsal aspects of the hands. Superficial erosions, dermal abrasions, and blister formation occur that heal with slightly depressed tissue-paper-thin scars and milia. On the face and cheeks the scars are thicker and associated with hyper- and hypopigmentation. Hypertrichosis may also be seen.

Ocular Features

Variegate porphyria occasionally causes blindness from corneal or scleral involvement. Photosensitivity, hyperpigmentation of the lids, and hypertrichosis of the forehead are frequent findings.

Conjunctival involvement is manifested by diffuse hyperemia, vesicles, and bulla followed by conjunctival cicatrization. Nodular limbal elevations resembling limbal papillae of vernal keratoconjunctivitis may also occur. Encroachment of scleral inflammation into the cornea may lead to an adherent leukoma and corneal scarring. Infrequently, the scleritis leads to necrosis, scleromalacia perforans, perforation, and uveal prolapse. Other findings include retinal edema, retinal hemorrhages, retinal pigment proliferation, and paralysis of the 3rd, 4th, 5th, and 6th cranial nerves.

Hereditary Coproporphyria

Symptomatic cases of hereditary coproporphyria are more common in women, being precipitated by pregnancy and oral contraceptives. The manifestations of hereditary coproporphyria are milder but otherwise similar to variegate porphyria.

Porphyria Cutanea Tarda

Porphyria cutanea tarda is the most common of the porphyrias. Clinical disease may be triggered by estrogens, naprosyn, barbiturates, phenytoin, and tolbutamide. A toxic form without hereditary factors is caused by chronic ingestion of alcohol, estrogens, iron, or hexachlorobenzene (a fungicidal agent used for wheat).

Skin Features
The findings of porphyria cutanea tarda are limited to the skin (Figs. 17-27 and 17-28). Patients exhibit photosensitivity that leads to vesicles, bullae, and crusting on the exposed areas, such as the back of the hands (Fig. 17-27A), forearms, and face. The lesions lead to scarring, milia, and often hyper- and hypopigmentation. The skin is easily damaged by trauma (Fig. 17-27B). Hirsutism of the forehead, temples, cheeks, and sometimes the arms and trunk occur (Fig. 17-28).

Hepatoerythropoietic Porphyria

Hepatoerythropoietic porphyria is extremely rare. Excess porphyrins are produced in both the liver and bone marrow.

Skin Features

The disease becomes manifest early in life by development of extreme photosensitivity that leads to blistering, scarring, mutilation, hyperpigmentation, hypertrichosis, and sclerodermatous changes. The urine appears dark immediately after birth. Other abnormalities include hemolytic anemia and splenomegaly.

Erythropoietic Porphyria

Congenital Erythropoietic Porphyria (Guenther Disease; Congenital Porphyria; Hematoporphyria Congenita; Erythropoietic Uroporphyria)

Congenital erythropoietic porphyria (Guenther disease; congenital porphyria; hematoporphyria congenita; erythropoietic uroporphyria) usually begins in early infancy but may not become manifest until adolescence. It is often associated with growth retardation and hepatosplenomegaly.

Skin Features

Erythroderma in congenital erythropoietic porphyria is common and is readily detected with a Wood's light. Discrete or confluent skin vesicles (hydroa vacciniforme or hydroa aestivale), followed by crusting, develop on exposed areas (face and hands) (Figs. 17-29 and 17-30) usually about the third or fourth year of life. Lesions occur during the summer, then disappear to return each summer until about puberty. Secondary infection leads to severe scarring and mutilation, especially of the ears, nose, and fingers (Fig. 17-30).

Generalized pigmentation and sometimes hypopigmentation and hypertrichosis may occur. The hypertrichosis appears as lanugo hair on the extremities and coarse hair on the face. Scarring and alopecia of the scalp and more severely involved areas may also occur. The fingernails are often deformed, resembling those of scleroderma patients. Finger deformity may also occur.

The teeth may have a brownish or rose discoloration, which under the Wood's light fluoresces reddish-pink (Fig. 17-30).

Ocular Features

Photophobia is common. Discrete or confluent vesicles develop on the skin of the lids and may lead to severe scarring, ectropion, and deformity. Hyperemia and conjunctivitis are common. The conjunctiva assumes a yellowish appearance, and conjunctival cysts may be noted in the yellowish-colored masses located in the interpalpebral area. Recurrent conjunctival bullae produce cicatrization and progressive shrinkage of the cul-de-sac. Papillae resembling those seen in limbal vernal keratoconjunctivitis may occur at the limbus.

Cornea

The corneal findings include a linear form of epithelial keratitis, corneal vesicles that lead to vascularization, a diffuse keratitis with deep vascularization, and exposure keratitis, arising from conjunctival scarring or eyelid deformity (Fig. 17-31). Both episcleritis and scleritis may occur. The scleritis may lead to scleromalacia perforans and spontaneous perforation. Fundus changes include cotton-wool spots, retinal edema and hemorrhages, choroidal lesions, and pallor of the optic nerve.

Erythropoietic Protoporphyria (Hydroa Aestivale; Erythrohepatic Protoporphyria; Protoporphyria)

When fully developed, erythropoietic protoporphyria (hydroa aestivale; erythrohepatic protoporphyria; protoporphyria) is a milder disease than the other porphyrias. The clinical manifestations are limited to the skin and eyes.

Skin Features

Skin changes usually occur in prepubertal boys but occasionally develop as late as the third or fourth decade. Intense pruritus and pain develop in the exposed areas of skin within only a few hours following sun exposure or sometimes artificial light. Later, edema, erythema, vesicles, and an eczematoid reaction occur. In some instances, linear, crusted, and pitted areas develop over the nose, cheeks, and dorsal aspects of the hands. Spontaneous healing leaves small scars. In hydroa aestivale or the more severe hydroa vacciniforme, pink teeth and bones can be seen.

Ocular Features

The disease leads to photophobia, tearing, and blurred vision. Other ocular features include the following:

1. Scarring, ectropion, and immobilization of the lids.
2. A severe chemosis and papillary hypertrophy at the limbus similar in many respects to vernal keratoconjunctivitis.
3. Hypesthesia, fine-to-medium superficial epithelial keratitis, scarring, and adherent leukoma.
4. Scleral ulceration, necrosis, and occasionally, staphyloma.
5. Orbital cellulitis.
6. Axial, stellate lens opacity of the anterior cortex that may be unilateral.
7. Field changes and optic atrophy.

Alkaptonuria

Alkaptonuria is autosomal recessive and arises from deficiency in homogentisic acid oxidase that results in accumulation of homogentisic acid in various body tissues. Alkaptonuria causes pigmentation of the connective tissue and cartilage, which leads to bluish discoloration of the tendons and later limitation in movement along with periodic inflammatory signs and pain in the larger joints (knees, shoulders, and hips) and vertebral column. A generalized arteriosclerosis, mitral and aortic valve disease, and myocardial infarction often occur. Myocardial disease is one of the major causes of death. Occasionally, deafness is caused by involvement of the ossicles and eardrums by ochronotic changes.

Skin Features

Skin manifestations begin about the fourth decade of life. The skin appears dusky, especially over the forehead, cheeks, axillae, and genital areas. The oral and laryngeal mucosa may also appear to be dusky. The nails may be brownish.

Pigmentation of the pinna is one of the earliest findings, generally beginning about age 20 to 30. The pinna becomes slate blue or gray and feels thickened, rough, and irregular (Fig. 17-32). The cerumen may be brown or jet black. The urine becomes dark on standing, a process that may be hastened by the addition of a few drops of potassium hydroxide or other alkali (Fig. 17-32).

Ocular Features

The skin of the eyelids may be pigmented, and the tarsus may appear blue on transillumination. Black scleral pigmentation usually develops at the insertion of the lateral and medial rectus muscles during the third decade of life (Osler sign) (Fig. 17-33). Amber-colored oil globules may also be seen in Bowman layer.

Homocystinuria

Homocystinuria comprises a group of rare, inborn errors of amino acid metabolism. Most cases are autosomal recessive. Secondary forms may occur in vegetarians with vitamin B12 deficiency or following treatment with isonicotinic acid. The infant is usually normal at birth but over the next few years develops features attributable to the disease.

The patients are often mentally retarded or have chronic personality disorders and chronic obsessive compulsive disorders. A myopathy is common, and osteoporosis of the spine may occur, leading to scoliosis. Other changes include hepatomegaly, genu valgum, growth changes similar to Marfan syndrome, and venous and arterial thrombosis caused by increased platelet stickiness.

The malar area becomes flushed. Livedo reticularis may be seen on the legs, and tissue-paper scars develop on the hands. The hair is sparse, brittle, and fine in texture. Lens subluxation is common (Fig. 17-34). Inferior, nasal, bilateral subluxation of the lens occurs in most patients with homocystinuria.

Hartnup Disease

Hartnup disease is a rare metabolic disorder that arises from failure of the transport of tryptophan across the epithelium of the intestine and kidneys and that results in hyperaminoaciduria, a deficiency of nicotinamide, and resultant pellagra-like findings. It usually becomes manifest between the ages of 3 and 9. Attacks usually arise after sun exposure and are often exacerbated in the spring and summer.

Neurologic involvement includes cerebellar ataxia, tremor of the hands and tongue, minor cognitive defects, and psychiatric disturbances of depression, delusions, and hallucinations. Other findings include fever, diarrhea, atrophic glossitis, and edema.

Skin Features

The skin rash is usually the first manifestation and is characterized by erythema, exudation, and scaling of the exposed areas of the skin (forehead, cheeks, arms, and dorsum of the hands). The lesions have distinct margins.

Ocular Features

A similar skin rash occurs on the eyelids and periorbital region. Nystagmus and diplopia may be associated with the cerebellar ataxia.

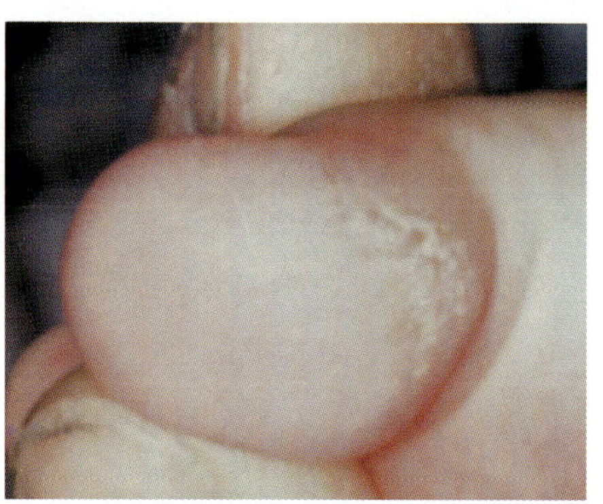

FIGURE 17-1. Hyperkeratotic plaques on the great toe in tyrosinemia.

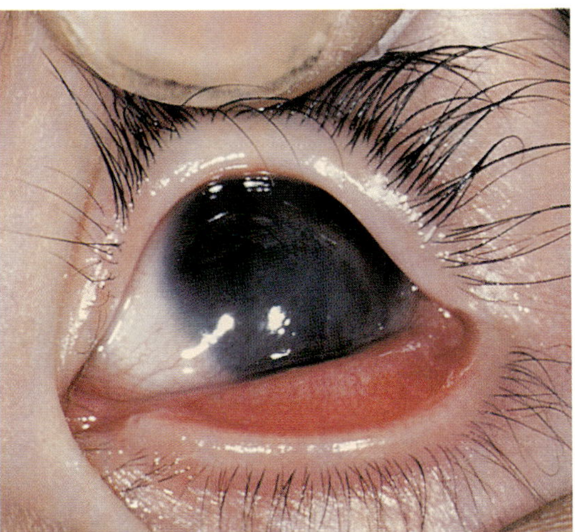 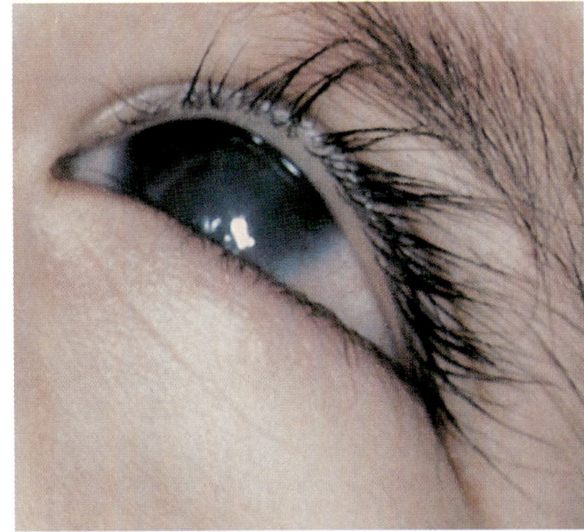

FIGURE 17-2. Corneal scarring and long lashes in patient with tyrosinemia.

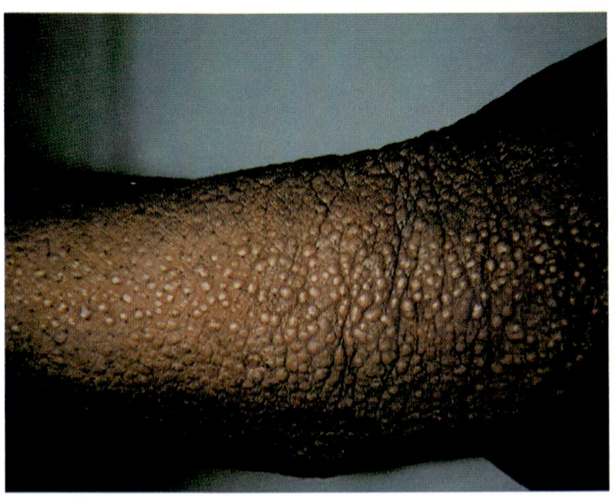

FIGURE 17-3. Papular mucinosis involving the finger.

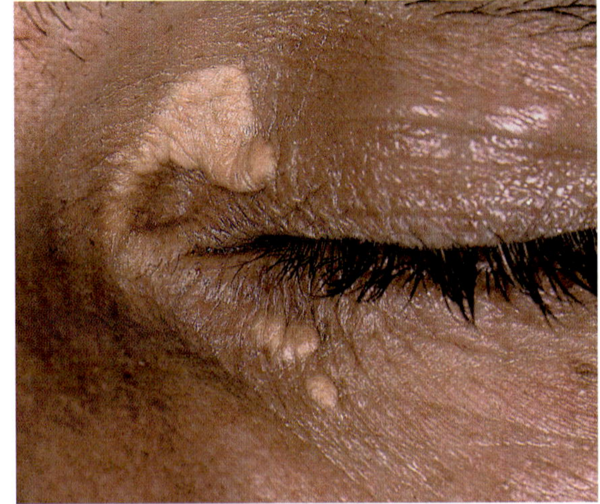

FIGURE 17-4. Xanthelasma of the eyelid.

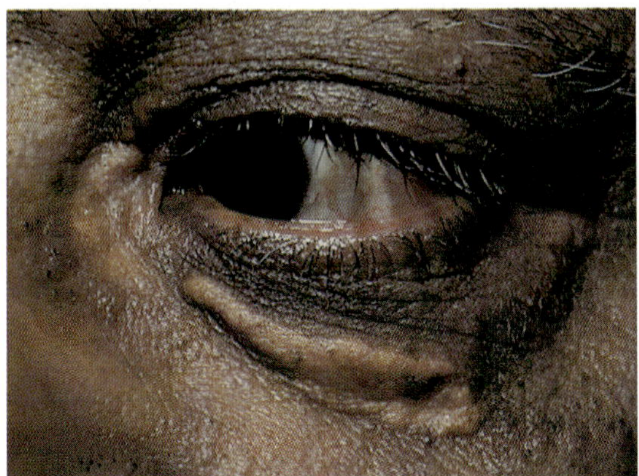

FIGURE 17-5. Xanthelasma of the lid in a patient with a triglyceride level of 300 and a cholesterol of 350.

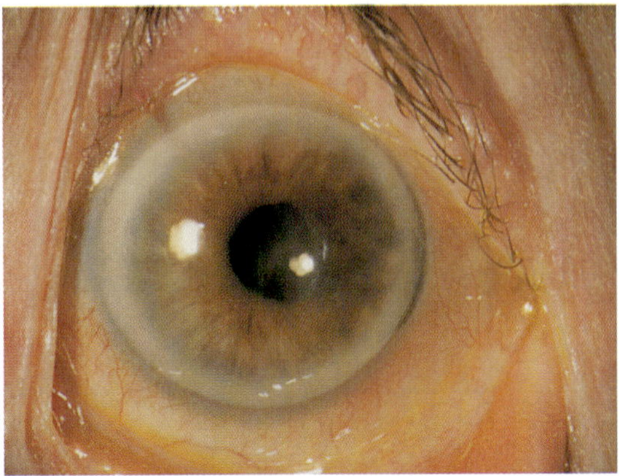

FIGURE 17-6. Arcus senilis.

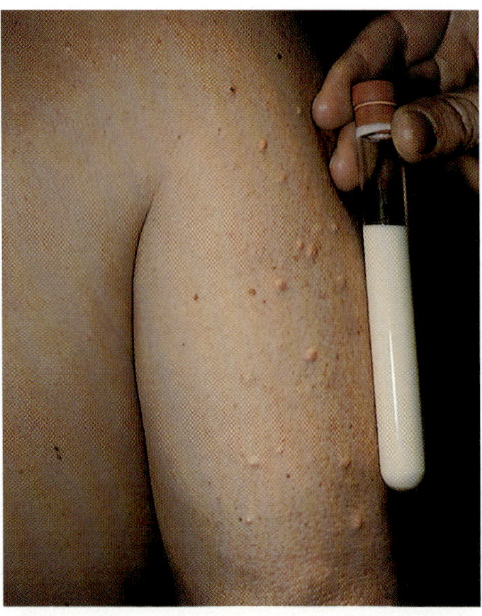

FIGURE 17-7. *Eruptive xanthoma of the extensor surface of the arm. Note the typical orange-yellow color of these papules. The vial contains the patient's serum and shows the amount of lipid present.*

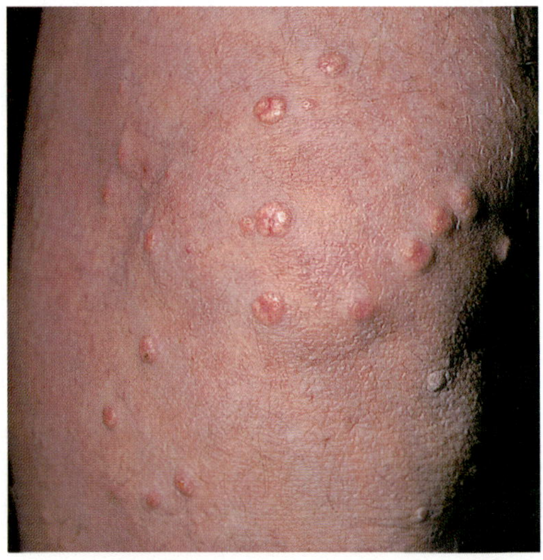

FIGURE 17-8. Eruptive xanthoma on the knee of a diabetic patient. The triglycerides at the time were 4,800; the cholesterol was 550.

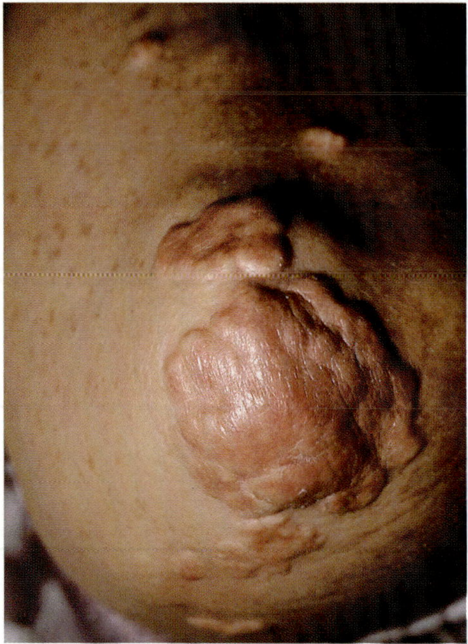

FIGURE 17-9. Tuberous xanthoma of the elbow.

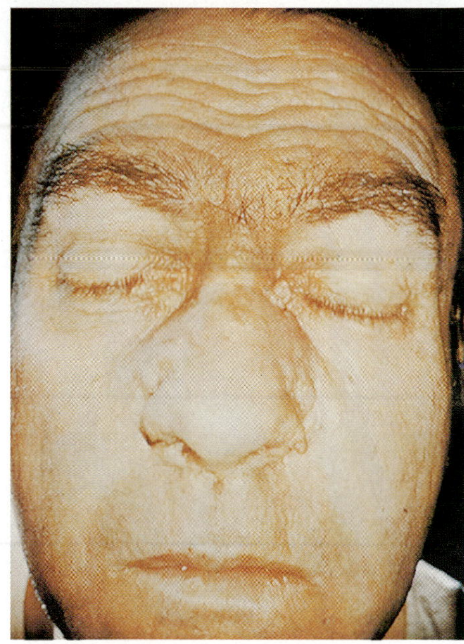

FIGURE 17-10. Lipoid proteinosis with involvement of the lids, nose, and face. (Courtesy of Dr. Lewis Shapiro.)

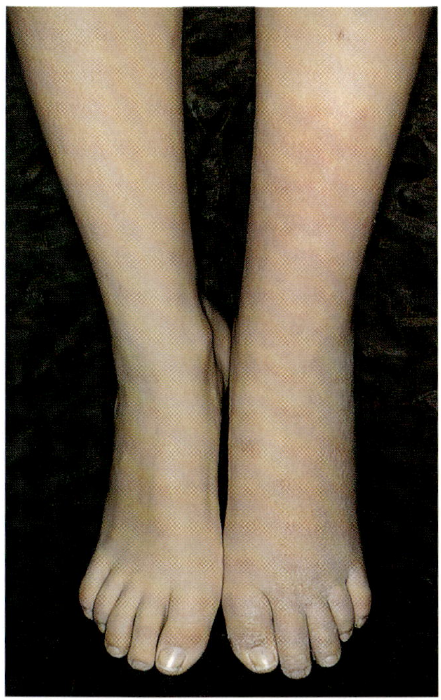

FIGURE 17-11. Familial Mediterranean fever. This 9-year-old boy developed abdominal pain, fever, and painful, swollen ankles and presented with an erysipelas-like area of the calf and foot. His father had undergone several unnecessary abdominal surgeries because the diagnosis of familial Mediterranean fever had not been considered.

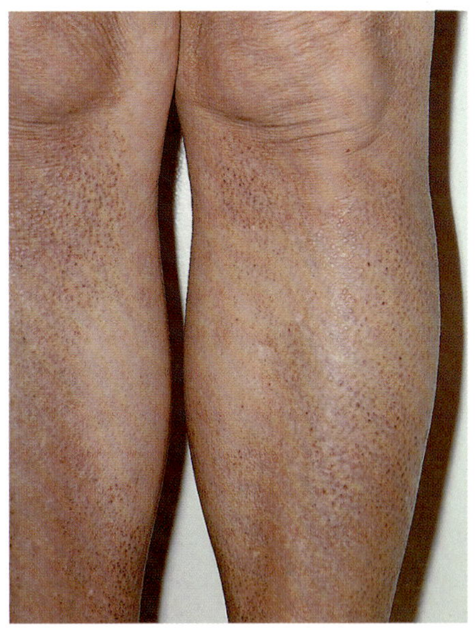

FIGURE 17-12. Lichen amyloidosis secondary to chronic rubbing of shins.

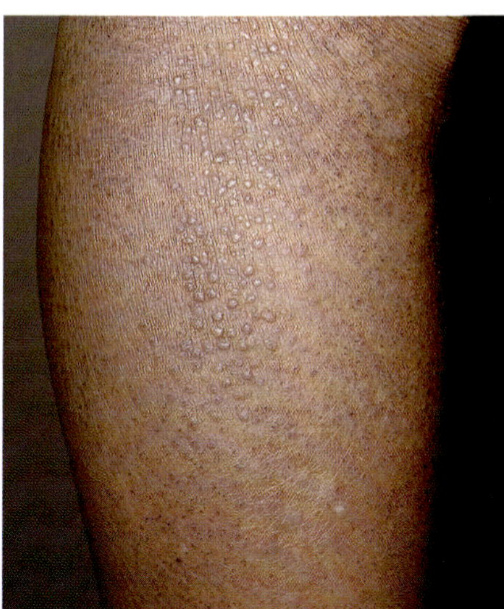

FIGURE 17-13. Close-up of lesions in Fig. 17-12 showing multiple small, flat-topped lichenoid papules.

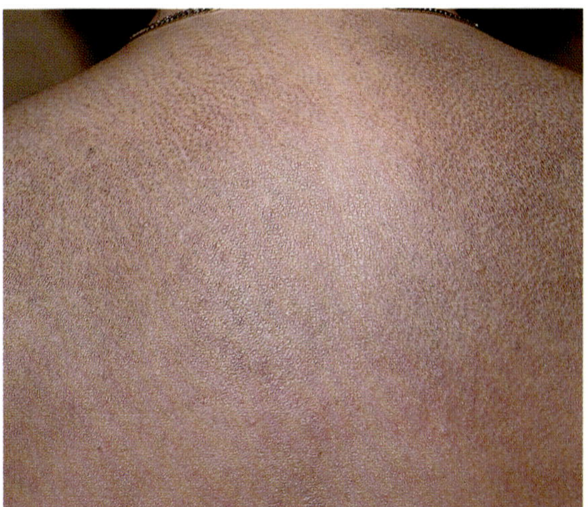

FIGURE 17-14. Macular amyloidosis. Interscapular site is a common location of these small, grouped, brownish maculopapules. Itching in this area may be secondary to notalgia paresthetica.

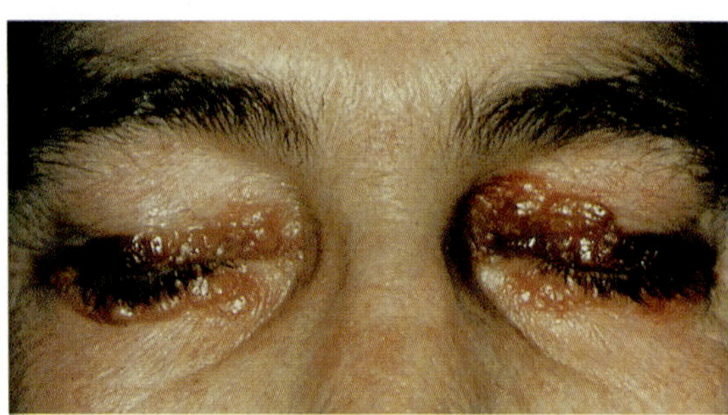

FIGURE 17-15. Primary systemic amyloidosis with characteristic waxy brown erythematous papules and plaques in linear pattern. Note also mild "pinch pupura." (Courtesy of Dr. Robert T. Brodell.)

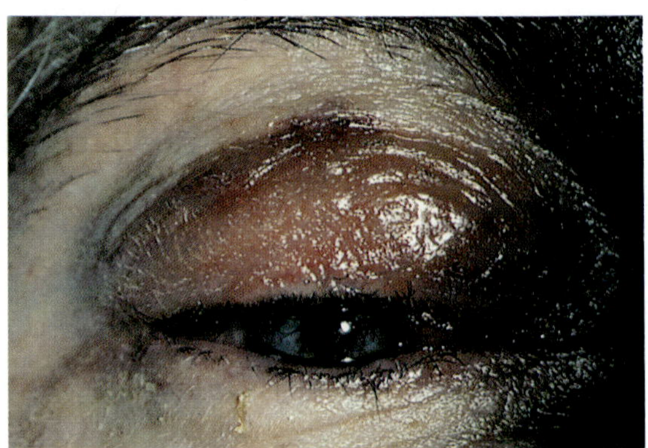

FIGURE 17-16. Amyloidosis of the lids. This patient had primary localized amyloidosis and always wore a wisp of hair over the eye to cover the continued ecchymosis that occurred whenever she rubbed the eye. A large collection of amyloid is seen at the medial angle of the palpebral fissure.

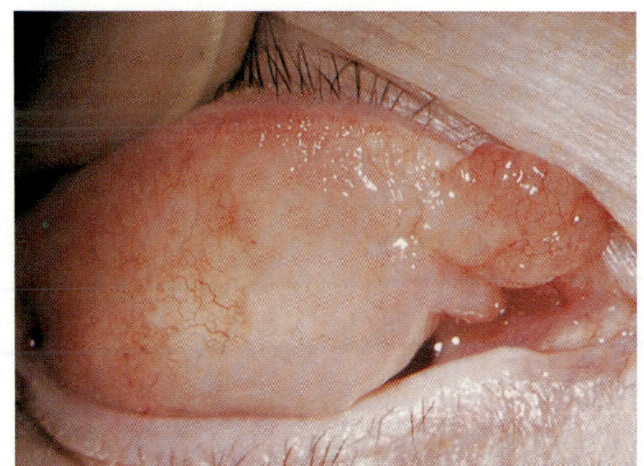

A

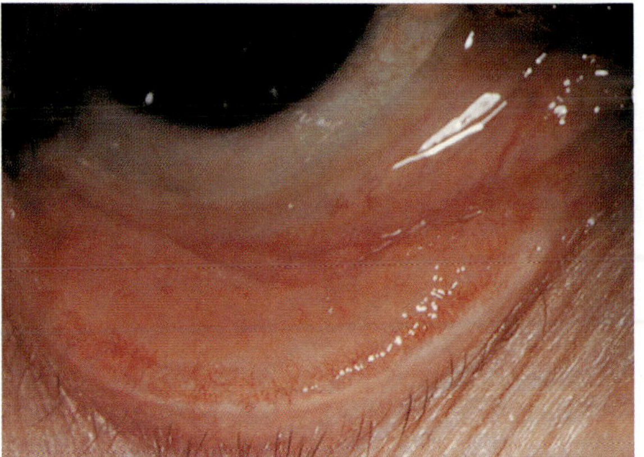

B

FIGURE 17-17. A,B: Conjunctival amyloid deposition. The amyloid mass in this patient replaced most of the tarsus and presented as a small mass at the medial angle of the palpebral fissure.

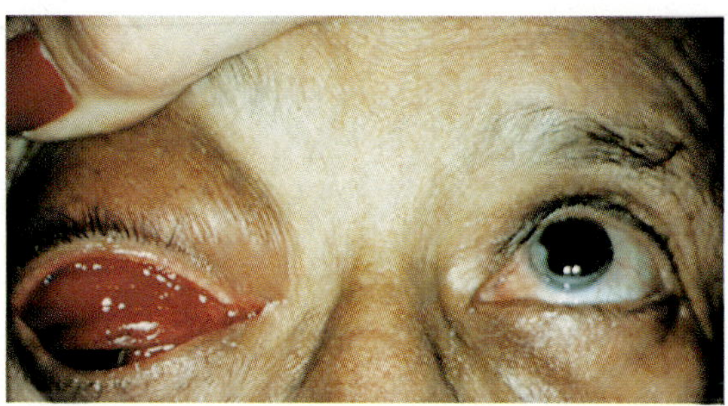

FIGURE 17-18. Amyloid infiltration into the orbit. (Courtesy of Dr. Lee Schwartz.)

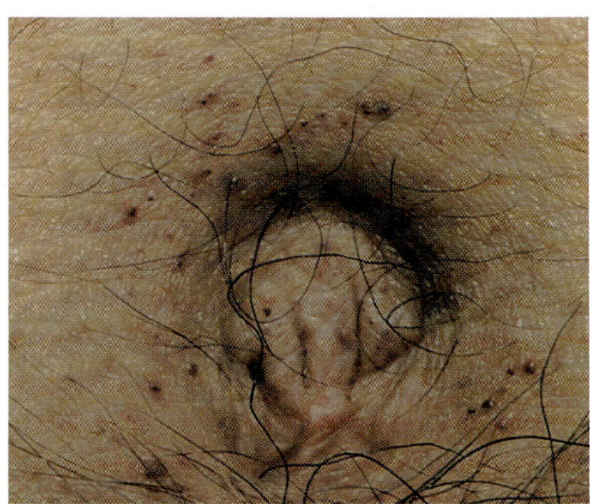

FIGURE 17-19. Multiple angiokeratomas near the umbilicus in Fabry disease.

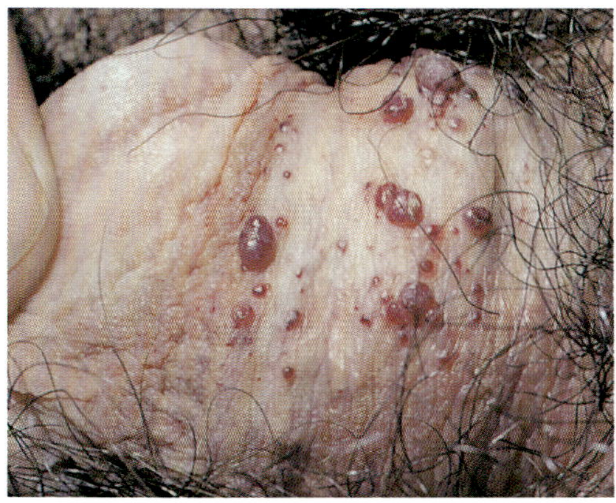

FIGURE 17-20. Multiple angiokeratomas on the penis in Fabry disease.

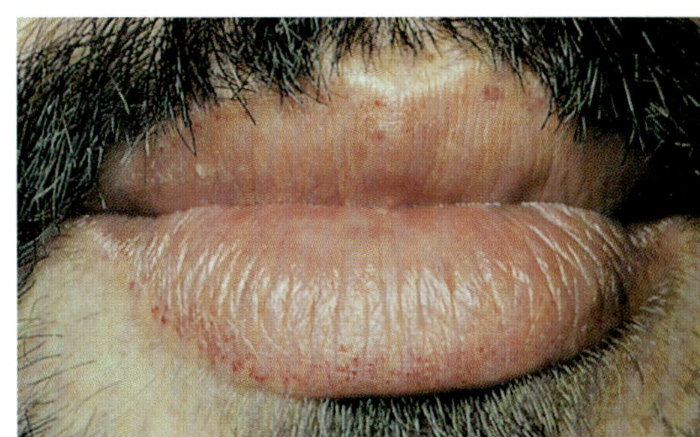

FIGURE 17-21. Subtle angiokeratomas on the lips in Fabry disease.

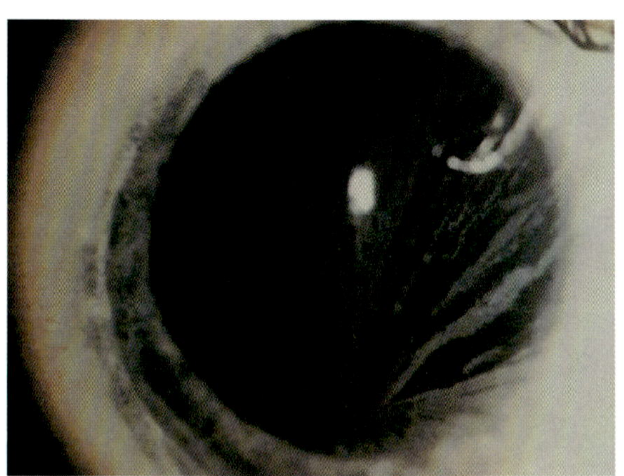

FIGURE 17-22. Corneal involvement in Fabry disease.

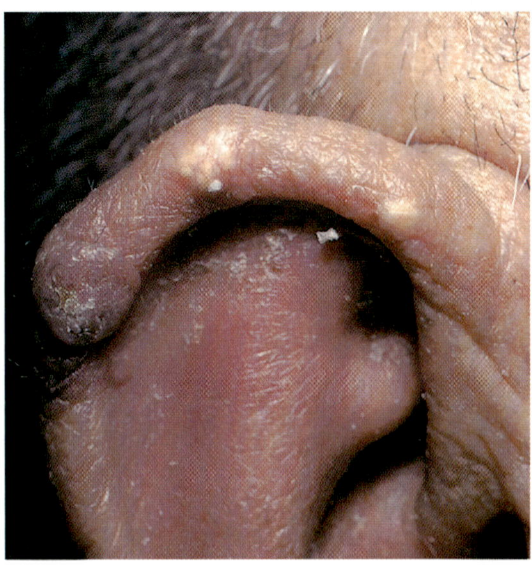

FIGURE 17-23. Tophaceous gout of the helix of the ear.

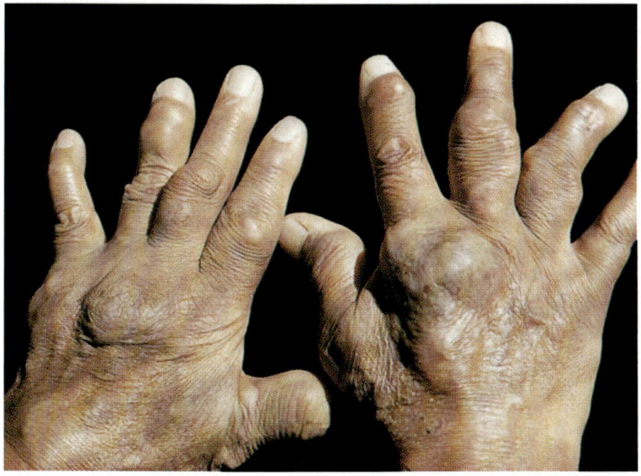

FIGURE 17-24. Gouty arthropathy. The patient experienced pruritusos as well as pain of the hands and fingers.

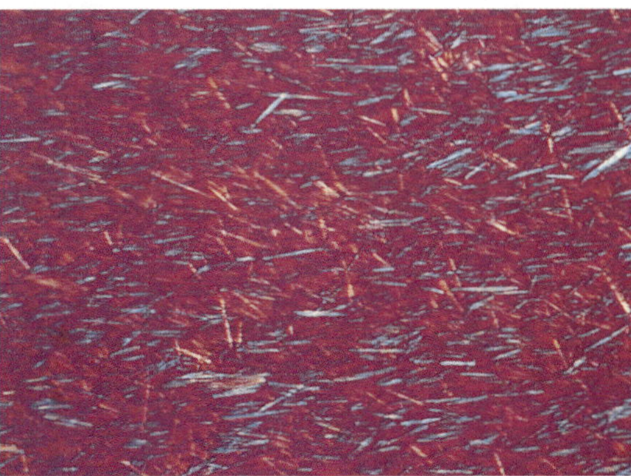

FIGURE 17-25. Uric acid crystals as seen under polarized light. The crystals were recovered from a gouty tophus.

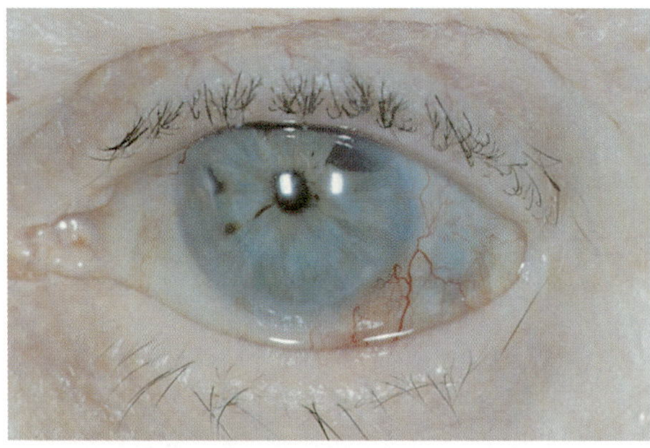

FIGURE 17-26. Recurrent scleritis with corneal infiltrates in gout. Scleral thinning and mild injection are evident laterally.

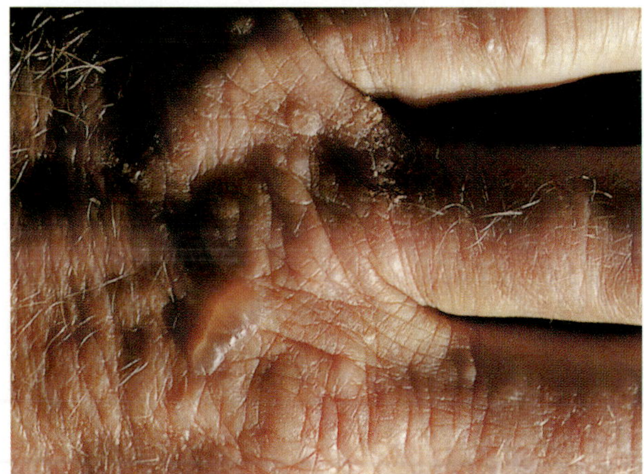

A

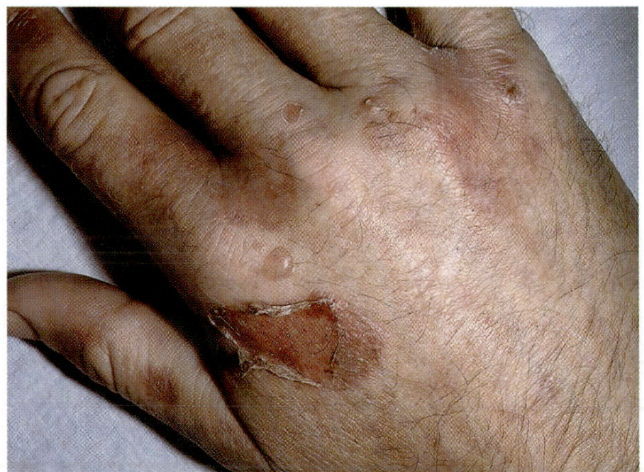

B

FIGURE 17-27. A: Bullae and milia on dorsum of hand in porphyria cutanea tarda. **B:** Small bullae and sloughing of skin after minor abrasion demonstrating the fragility of this tissue in porphyria cutanea tarda.

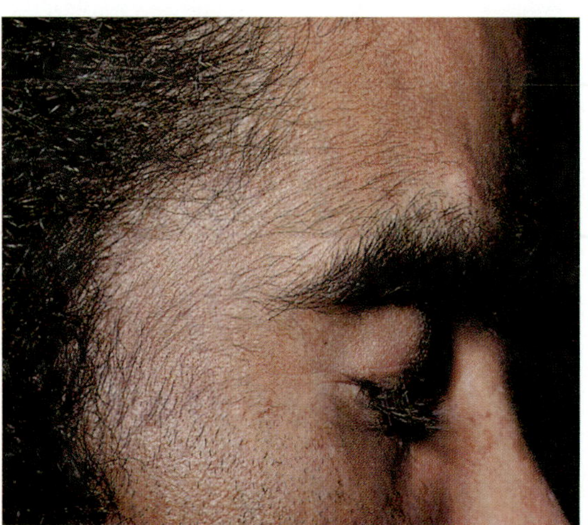

FIGURE 17-28. Hirsutism of the temple and cheek in porphyria cutanea tarda.

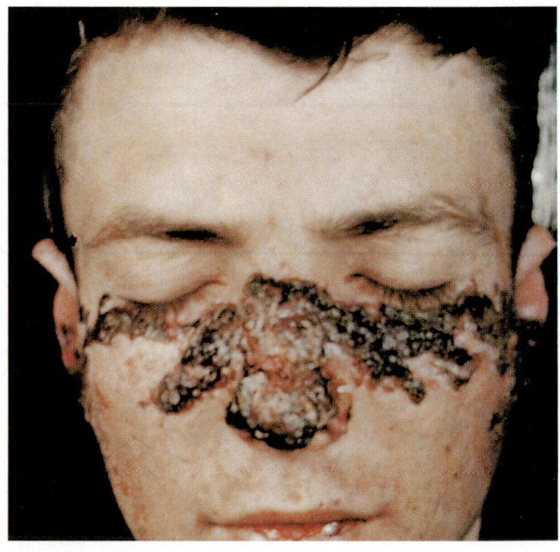

FIGURE 17-29. Hydroa vacciniforme in erythropoietic porphyria. (Courtesy of Dr. Philips Thygeson.)

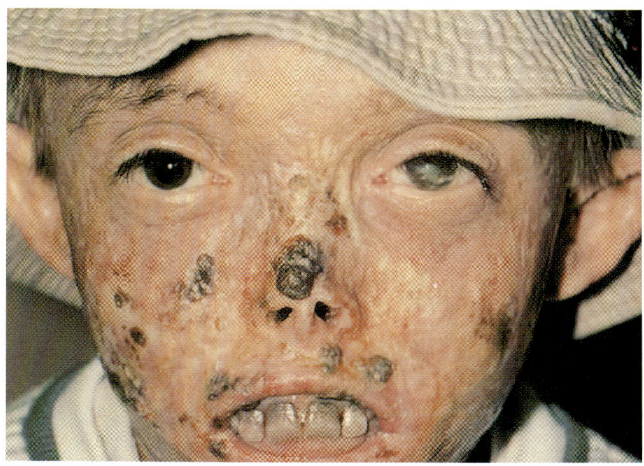

FIGURE 17-30. Congenital erythropoietic porphyria. (Courtesy of Suzanne Banuvar.)

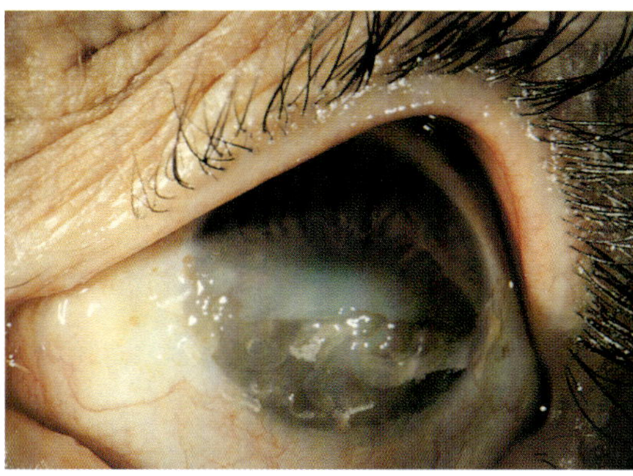

FIGURE 17-31. Cornea in a patient with congenital erythropoietic porphyria. (Courtesy of Suzanne Banuvar.)

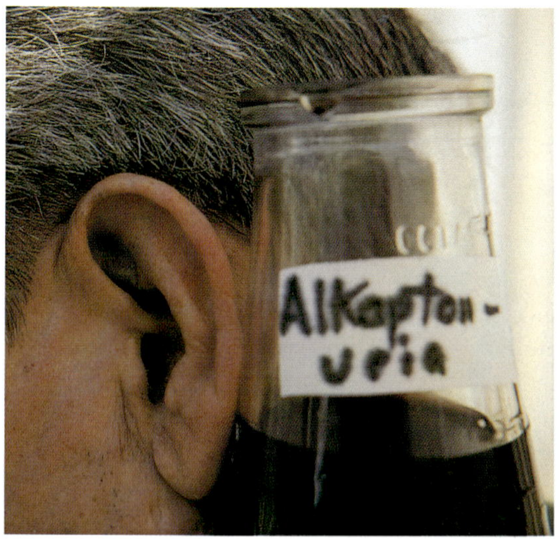

FIGURE 17-32. Darkening of the pinna of the ear in ochronosis. The bottle the patient is holding contains the patient's urine. Addition of a few drops of potassium hydroxide hastened the darkening of the urine. When the patient was an infant his mother complained of dark urine—soaked diapers which became even darker on washing with soap (alkali).

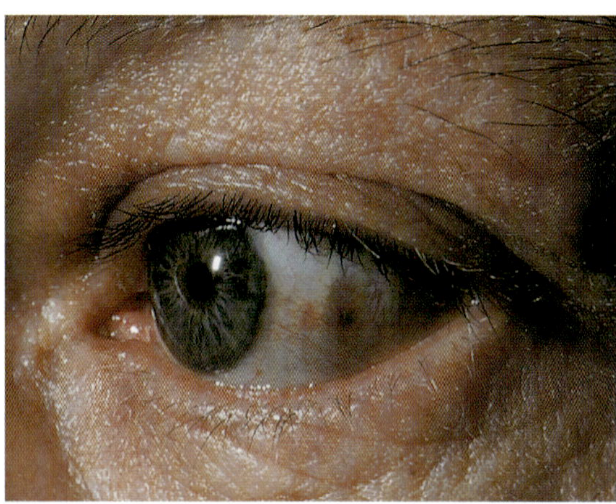

FIGURE 17-33. Scleral pigmentation at the insertion of the lateral rectus muscle (Osler sign) is an early finding in ochronosis.

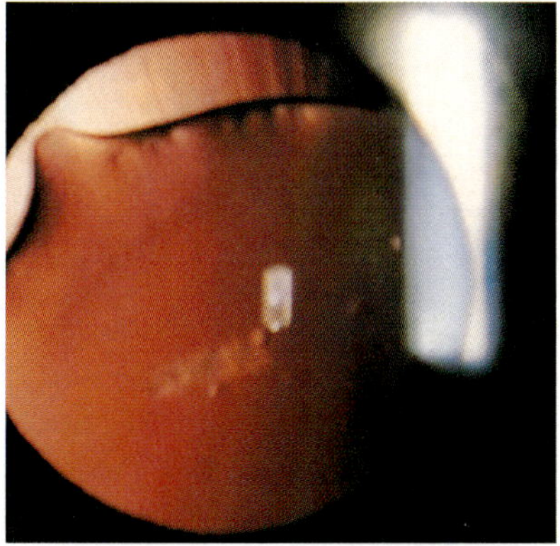

FIGURE 17-34. Lens subluxation in homocystinuria. The edge of the lens is evident at the border of the pupil superiorly. (Courtesy of Dr. John Belmont.)

ENDOCRINE DISORDERS

PITUITARY GLAND DISORDERS

In general, pituitary tumors cause visual symptoms by compression and systemic manifestations by hypersecretion of hormones.

The ocular features of compression encompass the following:

1. Bitemporal hemianopsia.
2. Ipsilateral loss of color vision and central scotoma with an afferent pupillary defect.
3. Optic atrophy late in the disease process.
4. Afferent pupillary defect (Marcus–Gunn pupil), characterized by an ipsilateral afferent pupillary defect from optic nerve compression.
5. Wernicke pupil, characterized by a bilateral hemiafferent pupillary defect from optic chiasm or tract compression.
6. Diplopia arising from 3rd, 4th, or 6th cranial nerve compression.
7. Papilledema arising from compression of the third ventricle and hypothalamus.

Acromegaly

Acromegaly is caused by growth hormone oversecretion from a somatotropic (eosinophilic) adenoma. (Occasionally, the adenoma secretes both growth hormone and prolactin.) Acromegaly is characterized by facial coarseness, tooth misalignment, hand and foot enlargement, and glucose intolerance. Secretion of both growth hormone and prolactin causes arrested puberty in both sexes. In adult women it causes headaches, secondary amenorrhea, galactorrhea, and infertility, and in males, headache, infertility, sexual dysfunction, and gynecomastia.

Some patients develop an addisonian-type pigmentation or, occasionally, acanthosis. The scalp hair is usually coarse, and the nails are flat and wide.

Basophilic Adenomas or Prolonged ACTH Administration

Basophilic, or ACTH-producing, adenomas secrete ACTH leading to bilateral adrenal hyperplasia and Cushing syndrome. Prolonged administration of ACTH may result in the same changes. Cushing syndrome is characterized by truncal obesity, hypertension, muscle weakness, and glucose intolerance. The skin changes include a thin skin, purple-colored striae, and sometimes an addisonian pattern of hyperpigmentation.

Hypopituitarism

Hypopituitarism may be caused by a nonsecretory adenoma. Often it causes no systemic manifestations; at other times it causes hypothyroidism or adrenal insufficiency. Skin features include photosensitivity, generalized hypopigmentation, and fine wrinkling. The face is often expressionless. Terminal hair is often lost, and the nail plates show longitudinal ridging and brownish discoloration.

ADRENAL DISORDERS

Addison Disease (Hypocorticism; Hypoadrenalism)

Addison disease (hypocorticism; hypoadrenalism) is caused by primary adrenal gland insufficiency or hypopituitarism. Primary insufficiency is caused by infections (tuberculosis, histoplasmosis, viral), metastatic malignant diseases, and autoimmune diseases. Acute hypocorticism also occurs in patients who abruptly discontinue glucocorticoids after receiving them for prolonged periods of time. Addison disease causes vague symptoms of malaise, fatigue, wasting, hypotension, dizziness, anorexia, abdominal pain, and, in women, amenorrhea.

Skin Features

Characteristically, Addison disease causes diffuse hyperpigmentation that is accentuated in the flexures, around the nipples, in areas of friction and pressure (Fig. 18-1), and around scars, creases of the palms and soles, the genital region, and areas exposed to light (Figs. 18-2 and 18-3). Hyperpigmented patches also occur in the mouth, vagina, and conjunctiva. Darkening of nevi may be an early cutaneous finding of Addison's (Fig. 18-3). Occasionally, there are also vitiligo-like areas. Hyperpigmentation may occur under the nails. The hair usually becomes darker. In women the pubic and axillary hair becomes sparse, and acne, if present, tends to improve.

Nelson Syndrome

Nelson syndrome may occur following bilateral adrenalectomy. The skin and mucous membranes show striking hyperpigmentation. Multiple lentigines may develop. The hair is dark.

Cushing Syndrome (Hypercorticism)

Endogenous Cushing syndrome (hypercorticism) is caused by adrenal hyperplasia secondary to overproduction of adrenocorticotropic hormone by pituitary chromophobic or, occasionally, basophilic microadenomas. Exogenous Cushing syndrome arises from systemic glucocorticoid administration. Patients have a moon facies caused by fatty facial deposits; a buffalo hump (Fig. 18-4) from fat deposits over the clavicles and back of the neck; an obese trunk (Fig. 18-5); and slender, wasted extremities.

The skin features include the following:

1. Increased fragility, striae (Fig. 18-5), and poor healing.
2. Addisonian pattern of hyperpigmentation.
3. Hirsutism (Fig. 18-4) and acne.
4. Male-pattern alopecia in women.

Pheochromocytoma

Pheochromocytomas are usually found in multiple endocrine neoplasia. They cause hypertension, headaches, profuse sweating, palpitation, apprehension, abnormal catecholamines, and an addisonian pattern of pigmentation.

Ocular Features

Ocular features include thickening of the corneal nerves.

THYROID DISEASES

Hyperthyroidism (Thyrotoxicosis)

Hyperthyroidism (thyrotoxicosis) represents a hypermetabolic state caused by excessive production or ingestion of the thyroid hormones thyroxine (T4) and triiodothyronine (T3), or, infrequently, by increased production of thyroid-stimulating hormone (TSH) or thyrotropin-releasing hormone (TRH). Graves disease (endocrine ophthalmopathy) often occurs in patients with thyrotoxicosis.

In Graves disease, there is often cellular infiltration of the lacrimal gland, orbit, and extraocular muscle. The thyroid gland and sometimes the parotid gland are diffusely enlarged. Unlike thyrotoxicosis, Graves disease occurs about equally in both sexes and usually during the middle years of life.

Clinical Findings

The clinical manifestations of thyrotoxicosis and Graves disease include the following:

1. Weight loss and increased appetite.
2. Heat tolerance and sweating.
3. Fine muscle tremor, weakness, and fatigue.
4. Irritability, nervousness, difficulty sleeping, and gastrointestinal disturbances, especially diarrhea.

The thyroid is usually diffusely enlarged or sometimes feels nodular. Cardiac abnormalities include tachycardia, congestive failure, paroxysmal atrial fibrillation, a pulmonary systolic murmur, and mitral valve prolapse. Splenomegaly and generalized lymphadenopathy may also occur.

Skin Features

Bilateral pretibial myxedema is a hard, nonpitting, symmetric swelling over the anterior surface of the tibia that may later spread to the back of the legs and feet. It occurs in about 10% of patients (Fig. 18-6). It is waxy, yellow, pink or skin-colored. The hair follicles are prominent, and in some cases, there is localized hypertrichosis. Occasionally, the myxedema also involves the arms, shoulders, neck, and pinnae.

Other skin findings include epidermal thickening; addisonian-type hyperpigmentation of the skin; vitiligo (Fig. 18-7); soft, velvety, moist skin; facial flushing; palmar erythema; increased sweating, especially of the palms and soles; and increased skin temperature. Skin appendage findings include rapid nail growth, distal onycholysis, and diffuse thinning of scalp hair.

Ocular Manifestations

Photophobia is a common complaint.
Lid abnormalities include the following:

1. Dalrymple sign (upper eyelid retraction, which is usually bilateral).
2. Von Graefe sign (lid lag in which the upper lid appears to trail behind the eye as the patient looks downward).
3. Boston sign (a jerky movement of the upper eyelid when the patient is instructed to look down).
4. Stellwag sign (incomplete and infrequent blinking). Occasionally, it is unilateral.
5. Lagophthalmos (inability to completely close the lids).
6. Enroth sign (lid edema, which is especially severe near the supraorbital margin).

7. Gifford sign (difficulty in everting the upper eyelid).
8. Jellinek sign (prominent hyperpigmentation of the lids).
9. Other lid changes include loss of lashes and eyebrows, hypertrichosis, angioedema, and chloasma-like pigmentation.

Corneal changes include an epithelial keratitis and epithelial ulceration caused by exposure.

Lacrimal gland enlargement, prolapse of the gland, and excess lacrimation and epiphora may occur.

Exophthalmos develops in more than 70% of patients with Graves disease and is seen in patients who are hyper-, hypo-, or euthyroid (Figs. 18-8 to 18-10). It usually begins gradually and often fluctuates in degree. About 20% of cases of exophthalmos are unilateral, and exophthalmos in one eye often precedes and exceeds that of the other eye.

Conjunctival abnormalities consist of injection and dilatation of the vessels overlying the insertion of the lateral and medial rectus muscles, chemosis (Fig. 18-11), and dryness. The latter is caused by lagophthalmos and prolonged exposure.

Fundus changes comprise chorioretinal folds, edema of the optic nerve and surrounding retina, retinal nerve fiber dropout, tortuous and dilated retinal vessels, ischemic optic neuritis, and optic atrophy. Muscle palsies of any or all of the extraocular muscles, including convergence weakness (Mobius' sign), may be encountered. Limitation of the elevators is usually an early sign.

Classification

The following guide is useful for classifying patients with ophthalmopathy:

Class 0. No signs or symptoms.
Class I. Lid signs only (e.g., lid lag or retraction).
Class II. Soft-tissue involvement.
Class III. Proptosis greater than or equal to 23 mm.
Class IV. Extraocular muscle involvement.

Hypothyroidism (Myxedema)

Hypothyroidism is characterized by a reduced metabolic rate caused by decreased serum free thyroid hormone or peripheral blockage of the hormone's effect. Its causes include autoimmune disease (primary hypothyroidism), iodine deficiency, antithyroid agents, congenital absence of the thyroid (cretinism), pituitary failure (Sheehan syndrome), pituitary tumor or disturbed hormone synthesis (goitrous hypothyroidism), and lack of TSH or TRH production. It is often associated with Graves disease (exophthalmos and dermopathy).

Hypothyroidism begins insidiously. The patient becomes lethargic, gains weight, and complains of loss of appetite, constipation, and intolerance to cold; women often have menorrhagia. Findings include motor weakness and macroglossia.

Features of cretinism include lethargy and somnolence, feeding problems, temperature instability, prolonged physiologic jaundice, macroglossia, umbilical hernia, a hoarse cry, and poor muscle tone. Untreated patients become physically and mentally retarded. The facial features are coarse and associated with a broad, flat nose; the abdomen is protuberant.

Patients who develop juvenile hypothyroidism have abnormal physical and mental development.

Skin Features

The skin of the hands, face, and eyelids become puffy from dermal accumulation of mucopolysaccharides (hyaluronic acid and chondroitin sulfate B) that bind water. Other skin changes include ivory-yellow xanthomas, which develop secondary to hyperlipidemia; dry, pale, cold, scaly, and wrinkled skin; absence of sweating; purpura and ecchymoses; punctate telangiectases of the arms and fingertips; and delayed wound healing. Skin appendage changes include coarse, sparse, and brittle scalp hair; loss of pubic, axillary, and facial hair; loss of the lateral eyebrows; and brittle and striated nails. In cretins, the skin is cold and dry with livedo often present. The scalp hair is coarse and sparse, and the pubic and axillary hair fails to develop.

Patients with juvenile hypothyroidism may have hypertrichosis of the upper back and shoulders.

Ocular Features

Periorbital puffiness is common. A third to a half of the temporal portion of the eyebrows (Hertoghe sign) (Fig. 18-12) and sometimes of the eyelashes is lost. Exophthalmos may be the earliest recognized sign of the disease. Other ocular findings include strabismus, ptosis, corneal edema, keratoconus, cataract, nyctalopia, papilledema, and optic atrophy. In cretinism, the ophthalmic findings include synophrys, hypertelorism, and epicanthus.

Multiple Endocrine Neoplasia Syndrome

Multiple endocrine neoplasia (MEN) syndrome, or adenomatosis, is autosomal dominant and is characterized by medullary thyroid carcinomas and an amine- or peptide-producing tumor. MEN type I and type II are the two major subgroups. MEN type I has aggregations of parathyroid, pancreatic, and pituitary gland tumors. MEN type II (type IIA) has an aggregation of parathyroid, pancreatic, and pituitary tumors. Type IIB (type III) has features of type IIA plus mucosal neuromas. Only type IIB (type III) has ocular features.

MEN type IIB is characterized by multiple mucosal neuromas in organs of neural crest origin. They are present at birth or develop during infancy, causing lid, lip, and tongue enlargement. Individual lesions appear as flesh-colored papules or nodules of the conjunctiva, lips, tongue, and other mucosal surface, including the gastrointestinal tract. The patients have a characteristic appearance: a "starry-eyed gaze"; blubbery, protuberant lips; marfanoid habitus; muscle weakness; and musculoskeletal anomalies with increased joint laxity. Many patients also have prognathism.

Medullary thyroid carcinomas, which are usually bilateral and multifocal in origin and preceded by secretion of calcitonin, often develop late in the second decade of life. About half of the patients have large, multicentric, bilateral adrenal medulla neoplasia, which often are pheochromocytomas.

Skin Features

Skin abnormalities include café-au-lait spots, cutaneous nerve hypertrophy, and progressive striated pigmentary changes of hyperplastic dermal nerves on the trunk.

Ocular Features

Neuromas of the palpebral conjunctiva cause lid thickening, especially near the lid margin.

Conjunctival neuromas are most easily seen at the corneal scleral limbus and appear as enlarged bundles of nerves that extend to the equator. Keratoconjunctivitis sicca may also occur. Corneal findings include prominent, grayish-white corneal nerves evident at the slit-lamp. The nerves form an irregular filigree pattern over the entire cornea and are usually thickest at the areas of branching.

DIABETES MELLITUS

Diabetes mellitus (DM) is characterized by both fasting and postprandial elevated blood glucose and multisystem complications of the skin, kidney, nervous system, and eye. There are three types.

Type I (insulin-dependent or juvenile-onset) begins abruptly and is characterized by severe loss of beta cells, decreased or absent insulin production, dependence on insulin, a predisposition to ketoacidosis, and failure to produce C-peptide.

Type 2 (non–insulin-dependent or adult-onset) is distinguished by a disorder of regulation of insulin secretion and/or its action in peripheral tissue, lack of ketoacidosis except under stress, tendency to obesity, improvement following weight loss, and ability to produce C-peptide.

Type 3 (secondary) represents a complication of pancreatic, genetic, or hormonal disease, or occurs following ingestion of particular drugs or chemicals.

Clinical Manifestations

The many clinical manifestations include myocardial infarction, thrombosis, and nephrosclerosis caused by atherosclerosis.

Skin Features

Skin lesions in diabetes mellitus are often caused by microangiopathy of skin vessels and include the following:

1. Erysipelas-like erythema of the legs or feet of elderly patients, sometimes associated with underlying bone destruction.
2. Wet gangrene of the foot (Fig. 18-13) and occasionally fingers (Fig. 18-14).
3. Rubeosis (a rosy reddening of the face, occasionally of the hands and feet).
4. Diabetic dermopathy (diabetic shin spots) of the shin (Fig. 18-15), forearm, thigh, and bony prominences. It consists of oval, dull-red papules that gradually scale and eventually leave an atrophic brownish scar.
5. Ulceration of the sole of the foot (malum perforans) (Fig. 18-16).
6. Large-vessel disease in diabetes mellitus often leads to intermittent claudication, a pallid, cool skin of the distal extremities, and ischemic gangrenous lesions.
7. Diabetic neuropathy, especially in elderly patients, leads to numbness, tingling, aching, burning, absence of sweating, edema, erythema, atrophy, and indolent perforating ulcers of the sole of the foot [malum perforans (Fig. 18-16)] and other pressure sites. The ulcer is a circular, punched-out-appearing ulcer in the middle of a callous.
8. Skin infections in diabetics are more common than in normal patients, especially from *Staphylococcus aureus* (furuncles, carbuncles, and styes), Gram-negative rods (secondary infection of diabetic ulcers), and *Candida albicans* infections [mouth (Fig. 18-17); intertriginous area; genital region; and nail folds].
9. Other skin maladies include necrobiosis lipoidica (Chapter 15); disseminated granuloma annular (Chapter 15); bullae (Fig. 18-18), waxy, tight skin, and joint limitation of the hands, and vitiligo (Chapter 6); eruptive xanthomas (Chapter 17); skin tags and lichen planus (Chapter 7).
10. Diabetic thick skin (cheiroarthropathy) occurs in about 40% of insulin-dependent diabetics. It is characterized by thick, tight, waxy skin with limited joint mobility.

Ocular Features

A superficial punctate keratopathy, recurrent corneal erosion, persistent epithelial defects, or trophic ulcers may develop following intraocular surgery and arise from delayed healing. Diabetic epitheliopathy can occur spontaneously as a neurotrophic keratopathy. Corneal sensation may be decreased or completely absent, occasionally resulting in a recalcitrant neurotrophic ulcer with a horizontally oval defect somewhat beneath the midline of the cornea. These defects may be resistant to therapy, including tarsorrhaphy.

Orbital cellulitis is more prevalent, especially during periods of ketoacidosis in which the patient is particularly prone to develop mucormycosis. Cataracts are more prevalent in diabetics under the age of 55, and anterior and posterior snowflake opacities located near the lens capsule are probably related to periods of severe hyperglycemia.

There are five basic pathologic retinal processes in diabetes mellitus:

1. Retinal capillary microaneurysm (earliest retinal sign).
2. Excessive retinal vascular permeability resulting in retinal hemorrhages, hard lipid exudates, and in advanced cases, retinal edema (Fig. 18-19).
3. Vascular occlusion characterized by large patches of capillary closure with overlying cotton-wool spots and sur-

rounded by microaneurysms and tiny tortuous vessels. It leads to extensive dark-red-blot hemorrhages and segmental retinal venous dilatations (bending).
4. Proliferation of new blood vessels on the surface of the retina and/or optic disc, which may lead to vitreous hemorrhage and retinal distortion or detachment.
5. Fibrous tissue proliferation on the surface of the retina and optic nerve head arising from, and associated with, proliferation of the new blood vessels as mentioned earlier.

Chronic open-angle glaucoma and neovascular glaucoma are more common in diabetics.

PREGNANCY, MENSTRUATION, AND ORAL CONTRACEPTIVES

Melasma (chloasma), a blotchy pigmentation of the cheeks, forehead, upper lip, and chin, commonly develops in pregnancy, especially in brunettes. In some instances, the neck, nipples, and anogenital skin also become pigmented. A familial form of melasma also occurs and is sometimes more conspicuous just prior to menstruation. Oral contraceptive use has also been associated with melasma.

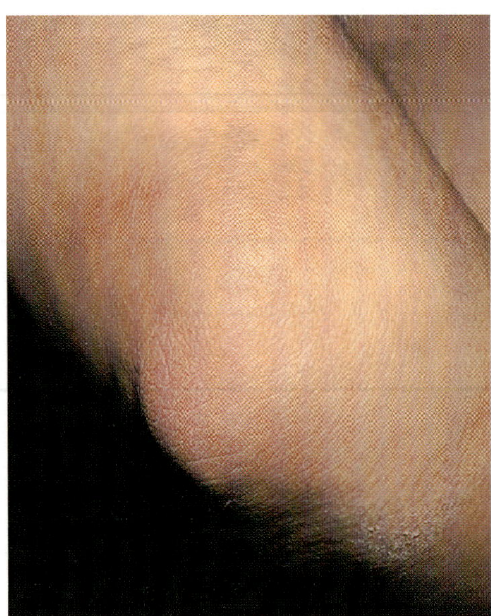

FIGURE 18-1. Hyperpigmentation of the elbow in Addison disease. Sites of recurrent trauma or pressure are often affected.

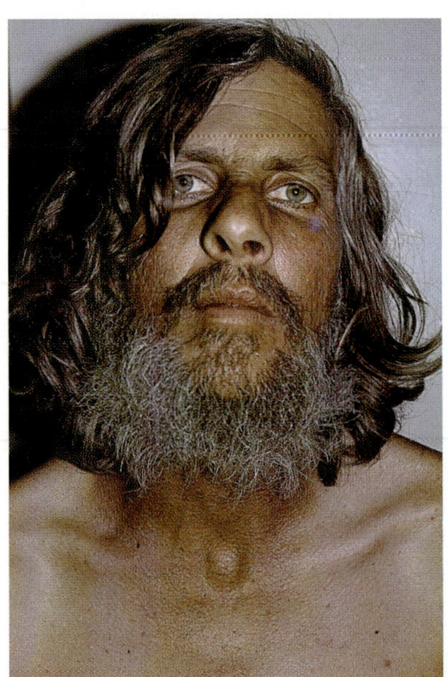

FIGURE 18-2. Addison disease showing darkening of sun-exposed sites (face and V-neck). The patient noticed that he tanned rapidly and felt "woozy."

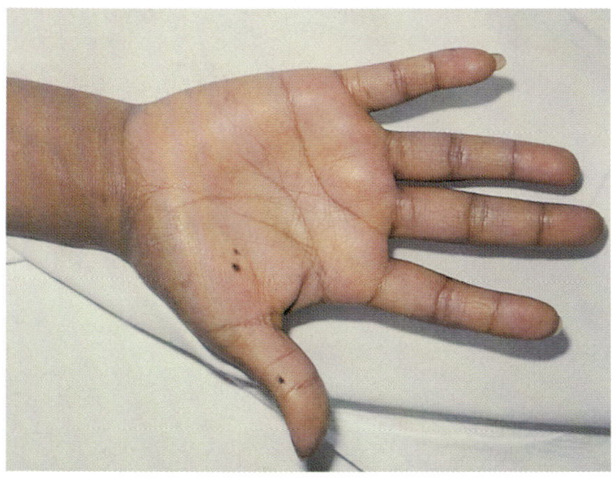

FIGURE 18-3. Increased pigment of the palmar creases in Addison disease. This patient came to this dermatologist because of darkening of the nevi of his palms. (Courtesy of John Reeves, M.D.)

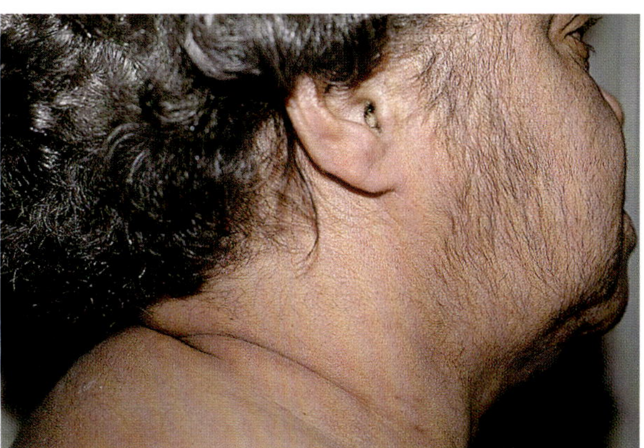

FIGURE 18-4. Cushing syndrome (iatrogenic) resulting from prolonged admnistration of corticosteriods for asthma. Note "buffalo-hump" obesity and hirsutism.

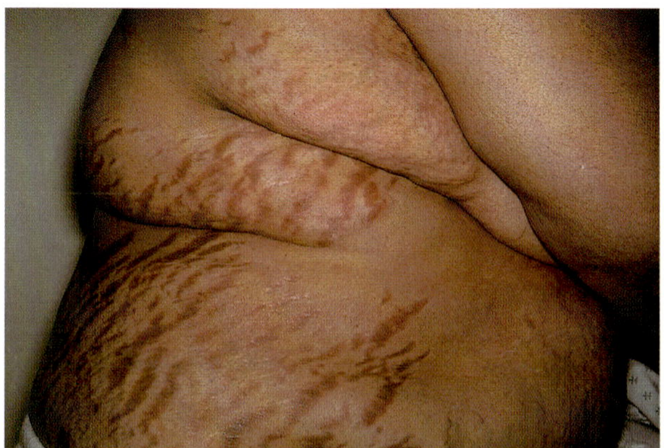

FIGURE 18-5. Cushing syndrome. Same patient as pictured in Fig. 18-4, showing truncal obesity and severe striae.

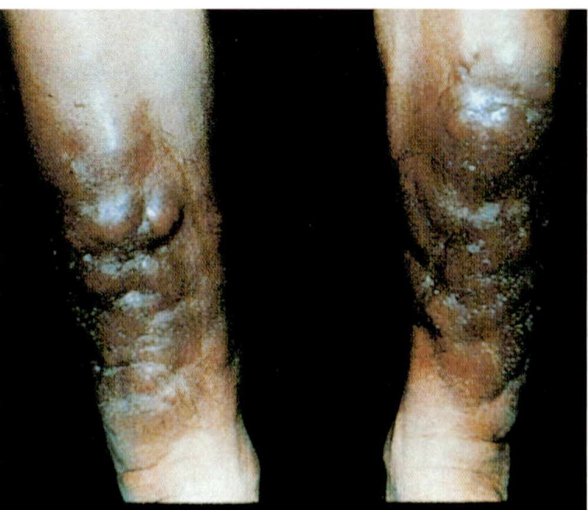

FIGURE 18-6. Severe pretibial myxedema. (Photo courtesy of Dr. Lewis Shapiro.)

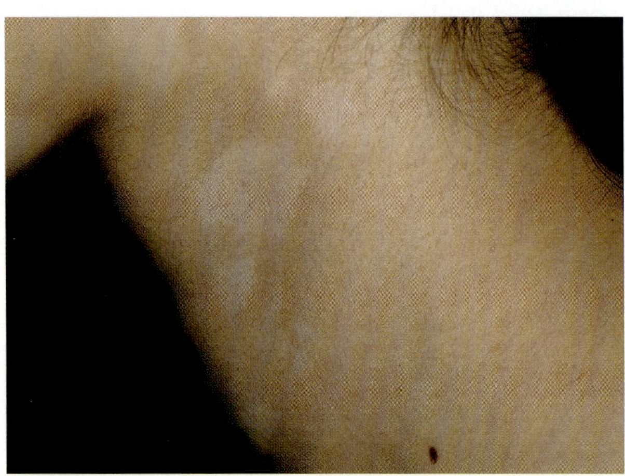

FIGURE 18-7. Vitiligo of the neck in a patient with Hashimoto thyroiditis. Note diffusely enlarged thyroid.

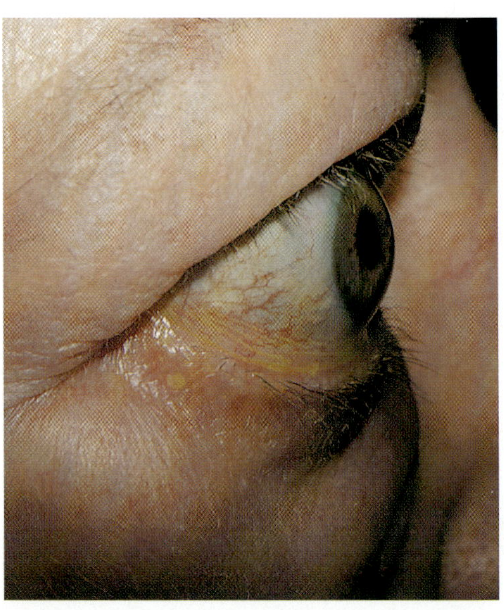

FIGURE 18-8. Exophthalmos. Axial forward displacement of the globe is noted in this patient with thyroid orbitopathy.

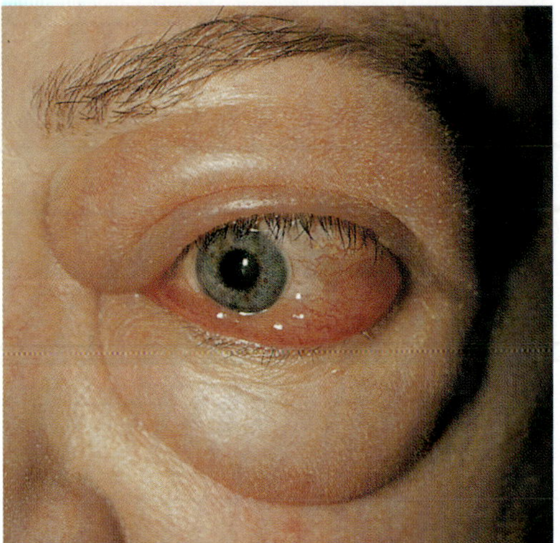

FIGURE 18-9. Exophthalmos. In this patient (the same patient shown in Fig. 18-5), exophthalmus is accompanied by a nonerythematous periorbital edema, and conjunctival chemosis.

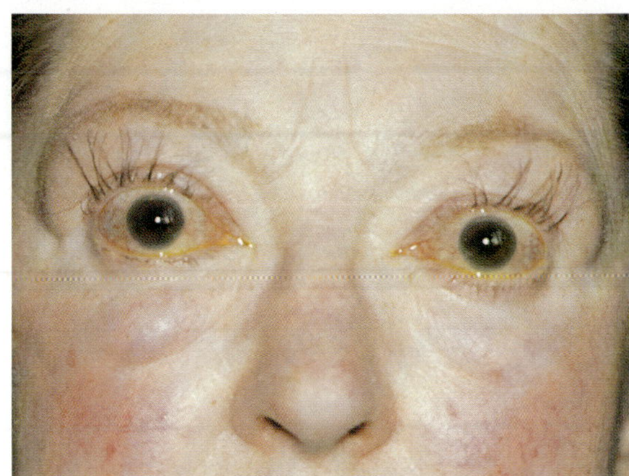

FIGURE 18-10. Bilateral lid retraction. Typical "stare" associated with hyperthyroidism.

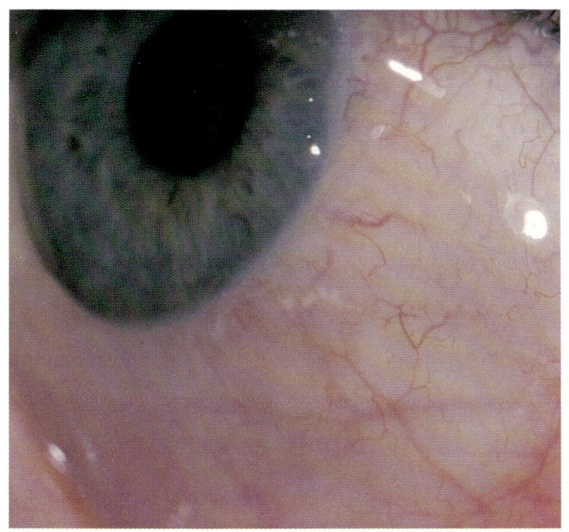

FIGURE 18-11. Bulbar conjunctival chemosis in Graves disease.

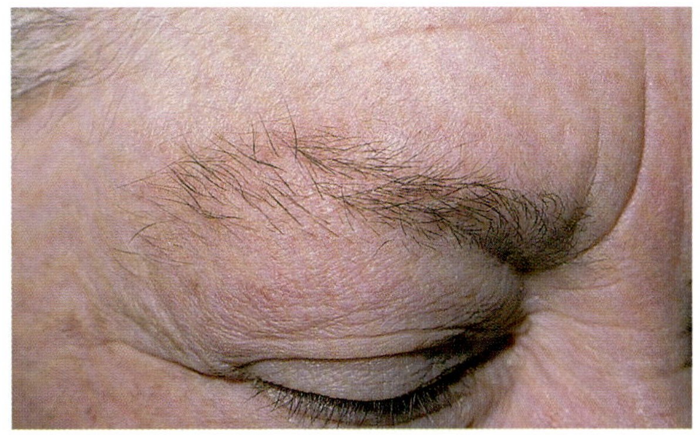

FIGURE 18-12. Hertoghe sign (sparse lateral eyebrows) in hypothyroid patient.

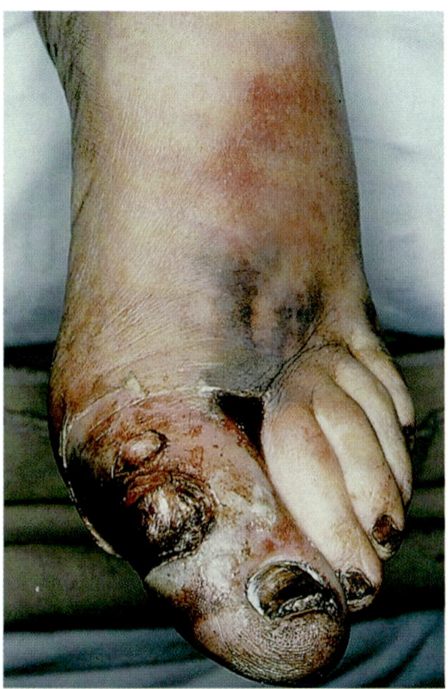

FIGURE 18-13. Gangrene of foot in a patient with diabetes and peripheral neuropathy.

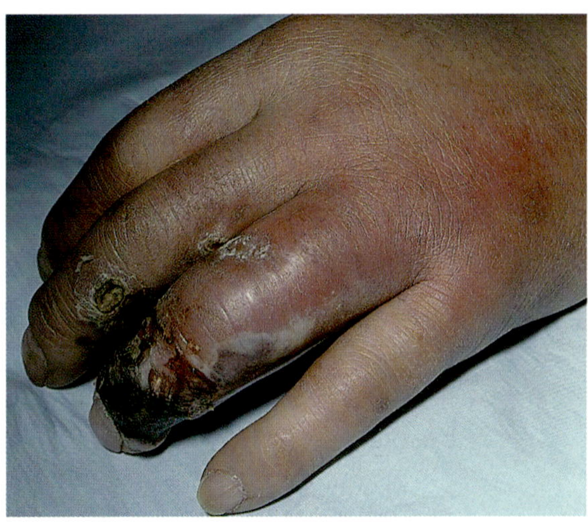

FIGURE 18-14. Gangrene of a finger in a patient with uncontrolled diabetes. Amputation was necessary.

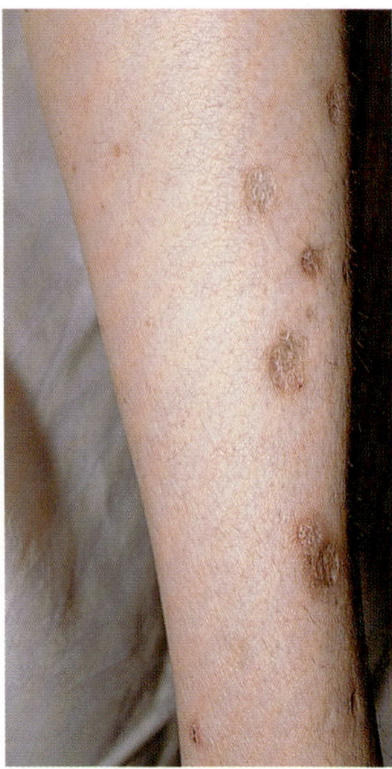

FIGURE 18-15. Diabetic dermopathy in a patient with type I diabetes.

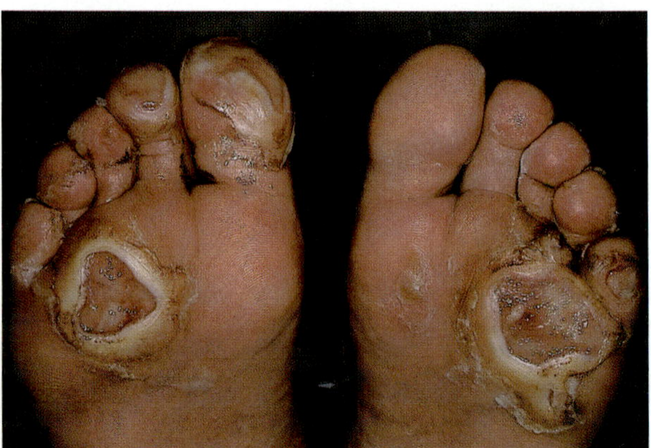

FIGURE 18-16. Malum perforans in a patient with peripheral neuropathy due to diabetes.

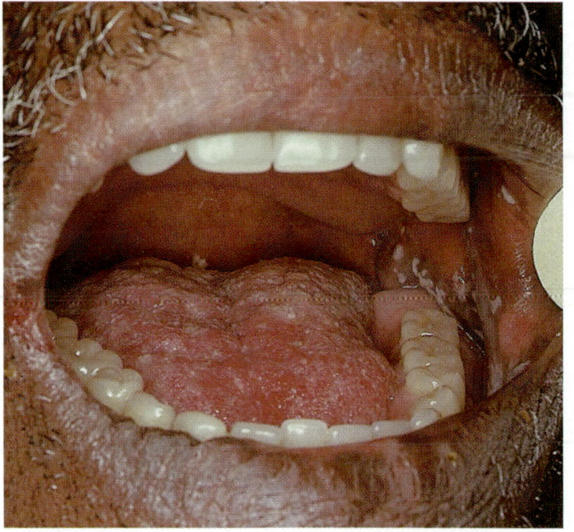

FIGURE 18-17. Yeast stomatitis and glossitis in a patient with uncontrolled diabetes. Note "curd-like" material on inner cheek, white dappling of tongue, and angular cheilitis.

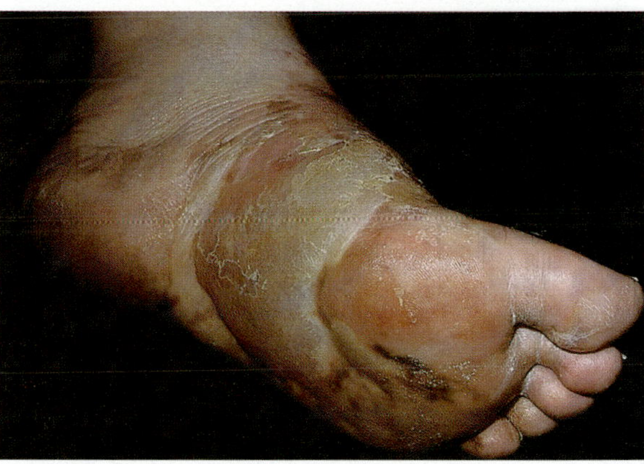

FIGURE 18-18. Painless diabetic bullae are seen arising seemingly spontaneously usually in acral locations as in this patient. Trauma and peripheral neuropathy may be contributing factors.

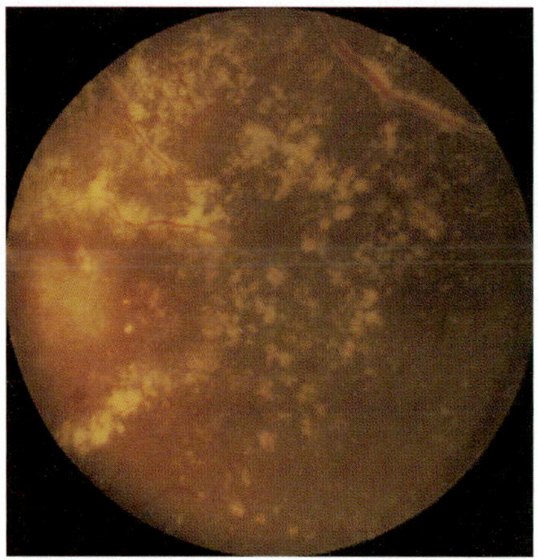

FIGURE 18-19. Hard, yellow retinal exudates in diabetes mellitus.

EPIDERMAL SKIN TUMORS

BENIGN EPIDERMAL TUMORS

Benign tumors have some degree of autonomous control, but these cells differentiate normally. They are localized and have no tendency to metastasize. The lesions are seen frequently and often develop in areas exposed to ultraviolet light. (A hamartoma is composed of more than one cell type and thus differs from a benign tumor.)

Seborrheic Keratosis

Seborrheic keratosis is benign and is composed of epidermal keratinocytes. It is often pigmented and is more common in white patients over the age of 40. Multiple lesions are often autosomal dominant but sometimes follow an inflammatory dermatoses. The sudden appearance of numerous seborrheic keratoses in an adult may indicate internal malignancy (sign of Leser–Trelat).

Seborrheic keratosis is the most frequent benign tumor of the face and lid (Fig. 19-1) and is common in the median area of the trunk. Initially, they are slightly hyperpigmented and appear slightly granular. Later they become elevated, heavily pigmented, and dome-shaped, and the follicular orifices appear occluded. Sometimes they present as dirty yellow-to-black, verrucous plaques with a loosely adherent, greasy keratin surface that often shows small fissures (Fig. 19-2). The lid lesions are often pedunculated and are not keratotic; otherwise they resemble other seborrheic keratoses.

Keratoacanthoma

Keratoacanthoma (KA) may be divided into solitary, multiple, and eruptive types. Of these the most frequently encountered is the solitary one, which begins as a small, firm, dome-shaped, skin-colored papule rapidly evolving as a sun-exposed site usually in middle-aged to elderly males. A central keratin-filled plug is characteristic (Figs. 19-3 and 19-4). Lesions may attain alarming proportions quite rapidly (Fig. 19-5), making early conservative excision or curettage the treatment of choice. Spontaneous resolution occurs after 3 to 6 months in most KAs, leaving variable scars.

Multiple KAs are occasionally seen in association with sebaceous tumors and multiple low-grade malignancies in the Muir–Torre syndrome. A familial type of generalized keratoacanthoma known as the Ferguson–Smith type of self-healing squamous cell epitheliomas may be confused with prurigo nodularis because of severe pruritus.

Eruptive KAs characterized by a generalized, small, dome-shaped skin-colored papule occasionally involving the oral mucous membranes is more often seen in the immune-compromised patients. Pruritus may be severe. Bilateral ectropion and narrowing of the oral aperture are sometimes found.

Ocular Features

Patients give a clear history of progressive unilateral, red, irritated eyes, without exudative discharge, and with no change in visual acuity. A raised, firm, globular, conjunctival lesions can grow rapidly over 2 to 3 months (Fig. 19-6). Treatment is excisional biopsy with 3 to 4 mm of "clinically normal" borders, as the histopathology commonly will show incomplete excision. Positive surgical margins place the patient at risk for recurrence of the lesion.

CYSTIC LESIONS OF THE SKIN AND EYELID

Skin and eyelid cysts include epidermoid and trichilemmal keratinous cysts, dermoid cysts, milia, and eccrine and apocrine hidrocystomas. Eccrine hidrocystomas arise from sweat gland ductules. Apocrine hidrocystomas arise from the glandular portion of a sweat gland.

Epidermoid (Epidermal Inclusion) Cysts

Epidermoid cysts are common in young and middle-aged adults. They arise from squamous metaplasia in a damaged sebaceous cyst developing as a result of inflammation (such as in severe acne vulgaris); from trauma in which epidermis is implanted into the dermis; and as a developmental defect in Gardner syndrome or the nevoid basal cell carcinoma syndrome. They are more common on the mid-face, neck, shoulders, and chest, and lie deep within and elevate the epidermis (Fig. 19-7). The lesions often periodically become inflamed (Fig. 19-8). They vary in size from a few millimeters to 5 cm. Multiple cysts are common, especially when associated with acne vulgaris.

Trichilemmal Cysts

Trichilemmal cysts are autosomal dominant, usually occur on the scalp (Fig. 19-9), and are more frequent in middle-aged women. The cysts arise from remnants of hair root segments during catagen. They appear as smooth, firm, rounded nodules; feel mobile; and may be lobular. They are often multiple.

Dermoid Cysts

Dermoid cysts arise from sequestration of skin during development. They may be found in the upper eyelid, where they often extend into the orbit and are common in the midline of the neck above the mylohyoid muscle.

Milia

A milium represents a small, subepidermal keratin cyst that arises in an undeveloped sebaceous gland, in a hair follicle, or in the proximal part of a damaged sweat gland. They are caused by keratinization within a collar of a vellus hair follicle or from dilatation of a damaged sweat gland. Sometimes milia arise as an eruptive phenomenon, especially in young women. They are 1 to 2 mm, white or yellowish lesions (Fig. 19-10) that are located in or just below the epidermis; they often occur on the face and lids, and seldom recur once expressed.

Miliaria

Miliaria crystallina (sudamina) arise from minimal nonspecific epidermal injury and profuse sweating. They usually occur on the trunk and are small, clear, thin-walled vesicles that occur in crops. The lesions often occur in infancy but are rarely congenital. They may be recurrent during a persistent febrile illness.

Miliaria rubra arise from prolonged exposure to sweat, as in a hot, humid climate or from polyethylene skin occlusion. They are erythematous papules that usually develop in areas of friction from clothing or in flexures. In infants, they occur on the face, neck, groin, and axillae. They often cause an intense prickly sensation ("Prickly heat") (Figs. 19-11 and 19-12).

Miliaria profunda arises from more severe damage to the sweat gland ductules, including irradiation, dermabrasion,

damage associated with acute subepidermal bullae (e.g., second-degree burns), and repeated attacks of miliaria rubra. They cause no symptoms and usually present as firm 1- to 3-mm papules on the trunk and extremities.

PREMALIGNANT SKIN CONDITIONS

Premalignant skin conditions such as actinic (solar) keratosis, cutaneous horn, Bowen disease, radiation dermatosis, and xeroderma pigmentosum (Chapter 10) may involve the lid. Histologically, precancerous skin lesions have an underlying chronic inflammatory cellular infiltrate and an intact basement membrane. When the basement membrane is breached or disappears, squamous cell carcinoma occurs.

Solar (Actinic) Keratosis

Solar (actinic) keratoses are the most common precancerous lesions of the skin. They occur in chronically sun-exposed sites of adults, especially in fair-skinned individuals. Actinic keratoses often involve the face (Fig. 19-13) (especially the cheeks, temples, and forehead), dorsum of the hands (Fig. 19-14), forearms, scalp, lids (Fig. 19-15), side of the neck, pinnae, vermilion border of the lower lip, "V" of the chest, upper back, and sometimes the legs. Untreated lesions may progress to squamous cell carcinomas, but there is little tendency to metastasize, except for lesions of the lips, nose, ears, temple, and dorsum of the hands. Patients may complain of persistent roughness and at times sensitive areas, which are more easily felt than seen. Over time, lesions become more keratotic or verrucous with adherent scale. Color may vary from erythematous to brown. The margins tend to be poorly defined as opposed to the more discrete edges seen in seborrheic keratoses. Multiple lesions are common. Induration and inflammation at its base suggest that transition to squamous cell carcinoma has occured (Figs. 19-13 and 19-14).

Cutaneous Horn

A cutaneous horn represents dysplastic skin changes similar to solar keratosis, and solar skin changes often accompany the lesion. They usually occur on the face (Fig. 19-16), scalp, external ears, eyelids (Fig. 19-17), and hands. Cutaneous horn presents as a horny, skin-colored, or yellowish-brown protrusion of the epidermis with circumferential ridges. Histology may reveal an underlying epithelioma at the base, especially in elderly patients.

Bowen Disease

Bowen disease is squamous cell carcinoma *in situ* and may become invasive. Most lesions occur on the skin of sun-exposed areas in elderly fair-skinned people. Early lesions present as sharply demarcated erythematous patches or plaques with scaling or crusting (Fig. 19-18). Older lesions become more infiltrated (Fig. 19-19). Differential diagnoses include psoriasis, dermatophytoses, actinic keratoses, squamous cell carcinoma, and superficial basal cell carcinoma.

Mucosal sites such as vulvovaginal, nasal, laryngeal, and conjunctival surfaces may be involved. Ulceration, loss of lashes, and nodularity of the lid margin suggest invasion. When Bowen disease affects the penis, it is referred to as erythroplasia of Queyrat (Fig. 19-20). Chronic arsenism may lead to Bowen disease on non–sun-exposed sites and increase the chance of internal malignancies, especially of the gastrointestinal tract and lungs.

Postirradiation Dermatitis

Acute radiodermatitis is seen 1 or 2 days after therapeutic or accidental exposure to radiation. It is followed by a second phase of erythema, which may be accompanied by vesiculation, edema, and erosion, depending on the quality, amount, and duration of exposure (Fig. 19-21). Chronic radiodermatitis is characterized by atrophy, hypopigmentation, and telangiectasia, and may lead to carcinoma of the skin (Fig. 19-22).

Ocular Features

Lid irradiation causes lash loss (Fig. 19-23), chalazia, and chronic conjunctival inflammation with telangiectases, keratinization, and plaques of squamous metaplasia. Keratoconjunctivitis sicca is a common sequela, and scleritis and even scleral necrosis are uncommon complications of radiation.

MALIGNANT EPIDERMAL TUMORS

A malignant skin tumor is capable of metastasizing to lymph nodes and other organs and may cause death. The growth is under autonomous control, and abnormal differentiation occurs.

Basal Cell Carcinoma

Basal cell carcinoma is the commonest malignant tumor of the skin, with more than 1 million patients treated yearly in the United States alone. The tumor is found most frequently in middle-aged or elderly fair-skinned individuals. Genetic predisposition, excessive sun exposure, and chemical carcinogens such as arsenic are risk factors. X-ray treatment for acne, which was popular from the end of World War I through the late 1950s, resulted in many cases of basal cell carcinoma some 20 to 30 years later (Fig. 19-22).

Most basal cell carcinomas (85%) are found on the head and neck. The nose, cheeks, forehead, ears, and periocular areas, especially the medial canthae and lower lids, are com-

mon sites. In general, basal cell carcinomas grow slowly, invade locally, and metastasize only rarely, as in severely neglected cases.

Skin Features

There are a number of clinical presentations of basal cell carcinomas. The most common form (about 50%) is the nodular type. This begins as a small, flesh-colored, or slightly erythematous firm, waxy, or semitranslucent papule, which as it enlarges, assumes a rolled, pearly margin often with telangiectatic vessels (Figs. 19-24 and 19-25). The center may be crusted and eventually ulcerate and bleed (Figs. 19-26 and 19-27). The lesions are usually painless.

A useful clinical procedure to help determine if a suspected lesion may be a basal cell carcinoma is to stretch the area between two fingers, which often will demonstrate the characteristic waxy appearance of this tumor (Figs. 19-28 and 19-29).

Pigmented basal cell carcinomas comprise only 6% of these tumors. They are more often present in darker-skinned patients and may be confused with pigmented nevi, pigmented seborrheic keratoses, and malignant melanomas (Figs. 19-30 and 19-31).

Sclerosing or morphea-like basal cell carcinomas, though comprising only 2% of all basal cell carcinomas, are particularly aggressive. They may be confused with scars or morphea (localized scleroderma) (Figs. 19-32 and 19-33).

Superficial basal cell carcinoma, also known as multicentric, most often present as erythematous plaques on the trunk. Healing with pale white scars may be seen in some areas, whereas progression is visible in others. Close inspection reveals a raised, thready border (Fig. 19-34). Lesions may be confused with psoriasis, Bowen disease of the skin, and extramammary Paget disease.

Untreated or neglected basal cell carcinomas may invade deeply into subcutaneous tissue, nerves, cartilage, and bone. Rarely, they may metastasize and cause death (Figs. 19-35 and 19-36).

Nevoid Basal Cell Carcinoma Syndrome (Basal Cell Nevus Syndrome; Gorlin Syndrome)

Nevoid basal cell carcinoma syndrome (basal cell nevus syndrome; Gorlin syndrome) is autosomal dominant with variable expressivity. It usually occurs in white males and is characterized by multiple skin tumors, which are indistinguishable from basal cell carcinoma.

Other findings include the following:

1. Palmoplantar pits and cysts of the mandible (odontogenic keratocysts).
2. Neurologic manifestations of ectopic intracranial calcification, agenesis of the corpus callosum, mental retardation, and rarely medulloblastomas.

3. Bony abnormalities of multiple dental cysts and defective dentition, spina bifida, kyphoscoliosis, bifid ribs, and abnormal sella turcica.
4. Internal malignancies, such as medulloblastomas, astrocytomas, meningiomas, craniopharyngiomas, fibrosarcomas, and ameloblastomas.

Skin Features

Skin lesions develop during childhood and include tumors, multiple epidermoid cysts, milia, and palmoplantar pits.

The tumors occur haphazardly but may have a zosteriform or quadrant distribution. The most common sites are the lids, cheeks, nose, forehead, neck, trunk, and axillae. (The upper lids are usually involved when tumors occur on the face.) The scalp and extremities are usually spared. Lid, neck, and axillary tumors are often pedunculated; in other areas, they present as smooth, rounded, elevated papules. They vary in size from 1 to 15 mm in diameter; are grayish-white, pearly, or flesh-colored; and have fine telangiectatic vessels. Some are umbilicated. The tumors gradually increase in size. Many behave like benign tumors, whereas others (especially those on the lids and nose) ulcerate and become invasive, leading to severe destructive changes that include orbital invasion and death.

Palmoplantar pits are characteristic and become evident about the second decade of life. They are circular, vary in size from pinpoint to several millimeters in diameter, and are about 1 mm deep. The base is red; the edges are perpendicular. The surrounding skin has diffuse or punctate hyperkeratosis.

Ocular Features

The ocular manifestations include the skin tumors, hypertelorism, strabismus, and congenital, and juvenile cataracts.

Squamous Cell Carcinoma of the Skin

More than 100,000 cases of squamous cell carcinoma (SCC) of the skin are diagnosed annually in the United States, making it the second most common form of skin cancer. Lesions are most commonly seen in the middle to elderly fair-skinned individuals at sites of chronic sun exposure, such as the dorsae of the hands, scalp, face, ears, and lower lip. Patients who were treated with x-ray or radium 20 to 40 years ago are at higher risk for SCC (Fig. 19-22), as are persons who are immunosuppressed.

Early SCC may be difficult to differentiate from hyperkeratotic actinic keratosis but generally are more infiltrated and erythematous (Figs. 19-37 to 19-39). When SCCs arise from preexisting actinic keratoses in most skin sites, the risk of metastasis is low, about 5%. When, however, they arise from the lip (Fig. 19-40), pinnae, penis, scrotum or anus, they carry a much higher risk, as do those arising from chronic ulcers or old burn sites (Fig. 19-41).

Rapid growth may cause confusion with keratoacanthoma (Fig. 19-42). SCC may occasionally be misdiagnosed and treated as warts (Fig. 19-43). SCC may involve the eyelids (Fig. 19-44).

Merkel Cell Tumors (Trabecular Carcinoma)

Merkel cell tumor (trabecular carcinoma) is an uncommon, potentially life-threatening neoplasm, which may be of neuroendocrine origin, as evidenced by neurosecretory granules seen within the neoplastic cells on electron microscopy.

It occurs most often on sun-exposed sites in elderly patients and is more common in women. The tumor is most often found on the head and neck (Fig. 19-45) but is also seen on the extremities. The lesion presents as a violaceous or reddish-blue nodule, which may resemble an angiomatous lesion. Local recurrence as well as metastasis is common, with a 5-year survival of only 30% to 60%, giving this rare tumor a prognosis worse than that of malignant melanoma.

TUMORS OF THE SKIN APPENDAGES

This section discusses tumors that arise from the pilosebaceous unit and the eccrine sweat glands. Most are benign but can recur; they rarely metastasize.

Inverted Follicular Keratosis

Inverted follicular keratosis is a benign tumor. It is a hyperkeratotic papule arising from abnormal growth of hair follicle epithelium. It presents as a scaling papule, a nodular or wartlike mass or a cutaneous horn of the lid margin, head, or neck. Sometimes it is inflamed and causes pruritus. Most dermatologists consider this common lesion to be an irritated seborrheic keratosis. Recurrences are common.

Tricholemmoma (Trichilemmoma)

A tricholemmoma (trichilemmoma) is an organized benign tumor that develops by proliferation of the lower part of the outer sheath of the hair follicle. It presents as a small, asymptomatic, solitary papule on the face, most often on the nose or cheeks and sometimes on the brow or lid. Usually, the lid margin is not involved. Clinically, it may be confused with a wart of basal cell carcinoma.

COWDEN SYNDROME (MULTIPLE HAMARTOMA SYNDROME)

Multiple trichilemmomas of the head and neck are an important cutaneous marker of Cowden disease, an uncommon autosomal dominantly inherited condition with multiple benign and malignant tumors. Among the benign features are oral and acral papules, lipomas, gastrointestinal polyps, and fibrocystic disease of the breast. Carcinoma of the breast may occur in approximately one-third of women, with carcinoma of the thyroid and colon also being more common.

It is important for the physician to detect this syndrome so that patients can be evaluated for possible cancers, especially of the breast and thyroid. A retinal angioma has been reported in this disease.

Trichofolliculoma

Trichofolliculoma is derived from a pilosebaceous unit. It contains abortive hair roots located in the large sinus and presents as a small, slightly elevated, dome-shaped solitary nodule with a central pore from which a fine white hair (or hairs) protrudes. Sebum-like material may intermittently drain from the opening (Fig. 19-46). Trichofolliculomas usually develop on the head, face, and neck, especially during middle age, but have been seen in childhood.

Trichoepithelioma

A trichoepithelioma is a deeply seated hamartoma of the pilosebaceous unit inherited as an irregular autosomal dominant trait. It presents as a small, firm, elevated, skin-colored nodule that usually involves the face, including the forehead and lids.

Multiple trichoepitheliomas (epithelioma adenoides cysticum) are autosomal dominant with incomplete penetrance (Fig. 19-47). They develop during adolescence and resemble the single lesion or may be more translucent. Larger lesions are flesh colored or pale yellow. They involve the forehead, lids, cheeks, nasolabial folds, and other parts of the face in a symmetric fashion. Occasionally, they involve the scalp, neck, upper trunk, and arms.

Pilomatricoma (Pilomatrixoma)

Pilomatricoma (pilomatrixoma) is a hamartoma that develops from the hair matrix, usually in children. It presents as a freely movable, single, solid, or cystic subcutaneous lesion. The overlying skin appears normal. It is found on the face and upper extremities, and preferentially involves the eyebrow and upper lid. Malignant pilomatricoma is rare.

SEBACEOUS GLAND TUMORS

Sebaceous gland tumors occur on the face, chest, and upper back. We consider benign sebaceous cysts, chalazia, sebaceous adenomas and epitheliomas, and sebaceous carcinoma under this heading.

Sebaceous Cysts

Sebaceous (pilar) cysts are clinically similar to epidermoid cysts but usually develop in the scalp and brow region. (In the lids they are called meibomian gland cysts.) They are firm, slowly progressive, rounded lesions that involve the dermis (Fig. 19-48).

Meibomian gland cysts occur in the lid from retention of meibomian gland material. They usually occur spontaneously but may arise secondary to inflammation or tumor. Sometimes they are associated with a chalazion.

Chalazion

A chalazion represents a localized lipogranulomatosis inflammation of a meibomian gland or gland of Zeis (Figs. 19-49 and 19-50). It is more common in the upper lid and is characterized by a painless, localized swelling. Usually there are no acute inflammatory signs. The overlying skin is freely movable and sometimes becomes stretched as the chalazion increases in size. The conjunctiva is usually injected, thickened, and elevated near the lesion. A chalazion usually gradually increases in size, causing the overlying conjunctiva to become thinned, revealing a grayish mass. Eventually, the chalazion may drain, exuding a turbid fluid and leaving an area of spongy granulation tissue or a polypoid mass. Sometimes the chalazion subsides spontaneously.

Infrequently, a chalazion develops in a gland of Zeis (a marginal chalazion) and presents at the lid margin. There are usually mild signs of inflammation. Occasionally, a sebaceous gland carcinoma may be misdiagnosed as a recurrent chalazion (Fig. 19-51).

Sebaceous Adenomas and Epitheliomas

Sebaceous adenomas and epitheliomas are clinically and histologically very similar. They are uncommon and may be solitary or multiple. The lesions are rounded, raised, 2 to 3 mm in diameter, yellowish nodules, which are sometimes umbilicated and may be somewhat pedunculated. They occur on the scalp, face, lid, and caruncle (Fig. 19-52). Multiple sebaceous adenomas may be associated with multiple visceral malignancies, as in the Muir–Torre syndrome.

Muir–Torre Syndrome

The Muir–Torre syndrome is probably autosomal dominant and is characterized by sebaceous adenomas or epitheliomas and malignancies of the gastrointestinal tract (usually the colon), genitourinary tract, ovary and uterus, and non-Hodgkin lymphomas.

The malignancies are often multiple. Metastases are low and survival is quite good.

The sebaceous tumors are usually multiple and are most often sebaceous adenomas, but occasionally, sebaceous carcinomas and sebaceous epitheliomas occur in the same patient.

Multiple or sometimes single keratoacanthomas are associated with squamous cell carcinoma of the larynx and lower gastrointestinal tract. Immunosuppression exacerbates the cutaneous manifestations of the syndrome.

Sebaceous Gland Carcinoma

Sebaceous gland carcinomas usually develop in women during the sixth and seventh decade. The tumor is much more common in the lid, especially the upper lid, but it may also develop in the eyebrow, caruncle, and other areas where sebaceous glands are concentrated (scalp, face, chest, and upper back). The lid tumors develop in the meibomian glands and/or the glands of Zeis.

Sebaceous gland carcinomas of the lid may present as a rubbery-feeling chalazion (Fig. 19-53), mandating that any recurrent chalazion be examined histologically. The surface may be rough or smooth. Usually, the lesions evolve slowly. Fatal metastatic disease occurs in 20% to 30% of eyelid lesions. Other times, the lesion presents as a localized yellow lid mass, a diffuse or nodular skin thickening, thickening of the tarsus, a papillomatous growth, or a fungating tumor. Not infrequently, the tumor masquerades as a chronic unilateral papillary conjunctivitis because of its tendency toward pagetoid spread. In some instances, it also involves the cornea, causing an epithelial keratitis, superficial scarring, and neovascularization. Uncommonly, it involves both upper and lower lids and, rarely, both eyes.

Sebaceous gland carcinoma of the glands of Zeis present as small, yellowish nodules that are located on the lid anterior to the gray line. Sometimes the lesions are gray-white and umbilicated, suggesting a basal cell carcinoma. Loss of lashes is common.

Sebaceous gland carcinoma of the caruncle presents as a subconjunctival, grayish-yellow mass covered by normal-appearing conjunctiva.

SWEAT GLAND TUMORS

Apocrine Gland Tumors

Apocrine Hidrocystoma (Apocrine Cystadenoma)

Apocrine hidrocystoma (apocrine cystadenoma) is a benign tumor that occurs in adults. It shows no sexual preponderance. Usually these tumors develop around the eye, especially near the medial cantus (Fig. 19-54), but they may occur in other areas of the face, ears, scalp, chest, and shoulders. They are solitary, gray or bluish, and appear as smooth, well-defined, dome-shaped, translucent cystic nodules, which contain clear or milky fluid.

Retention Cyst of a Gland of Moll

Although the retention cyst of a gland of Moll arises from occlusion of a sweat gland duct and is not a cystadenoma, its clinical appearance is similar to that of a cystadenoma. It presents as a translucent, raised, dome-shaped cystic lesion of the lid margin. Often several lesions develop on the same eyelid.

Syringocystadenoma Papilliferum (Papillary Syringadenoma)

Syringocystadenoma papilliferum (papillary syringadenoma) is a benign apocrine sweat gland tumor. It usually develops on the face and scalp in young adults. Up to 30% arise at puberty in the nevus sebaceous of Jadassohn. Clinically, the lesions present as verrucous skin-colored papules or plaques. Rarely, malignancy may occur.

Hidradenoma Papilliferum

Hidradenoma papilliferum is a benign sweat gland tumor. It is histologically similar to a syringocystadenoma and is usually found in the vulvar and perianal area, although it may occur anywhere on the skin, including the lid. It appears as a rounded, freely movable, elevated, small to medium-sized (1 to 40 mm) papule (Fig. 19-18). In some instances it ulcerates, forming a reddish-brown papillary mass.

Eccrine Sweat Gland Tumors

Eccrine Hidrocystoma

An eccrine hidrocystoma represents a mature sweat gland in which the ducts are dilated by retention of secretions. They are usually multiple and occur mainly on the cheeks and lids of middle-aged women. They appear cystic and may be bluish in color.

Eccrine Hidradenoma (Clear-Cell Hidradenoma)

Eccrine hidradenoma (clear-cell hidradenoma) is a benign sweat gland tumor that occurs in the dermis of the scalp, face, lids, and anterior trunk. It is uncommon and usually develops in women. The overlying epidermis is often thickened and sometimes ulcerated. The nodules are small (0.5 to 3 cm) and firm, have a bluish to pink-red color, and are often attached to the epidermis. Pain on pressure can be elicited in 20% of cases. Malignant eccrine hidradenomas also occur and may metastasize.

Chondroid Syringoma (Pleomorphic Adenoma; Mixed Tumor of Skin)

Chondroid syringoma (pleomorphic adenoma; mixed tumor of skin) occurs on the head, and neck, most often the nose or cheek, eyebrow, lid, and trunk. These lesions are usually very large on the trunk (5 to 10 cm), whereas on the head they usually measure 0.5 to 3 cm in diameter. They present as firm, asymptomatic, intradermal or subcutaneous nodules. Aggressive chondroid syringomas and malignant mixed tumors are more often seen on the extremities. Adenocarcinomatous metastases are usually to the viscera if they occur.

OTHER SKIN APPENDAGE TUMORS

Syringoma

Syringomas are small (1- to 2-mm), multiple translucent, pale brown to yellowish-waxy papules that occur primarily in young women, especially of Japanese extraction, at or soon after puberty. They are most often seen on the eyelids and upper cheeks (Fig. 19-55), although they also occur on the chest (Fig. 19-56), abdomen, axilla, and genital areas. They are more common in adults with Down syndrome.

Carcinomas Derived from or Differentiating Toward Eccrine Gland Structures

Virtually any of the benign tumors of the skin appendages may develop malignant changes. Their malignant behavior, however, is usually relatively benign, showing more tendency to local recurrences than to distant metastases.

Carcinomas that initially develop as cancers, on the other hand, are usually more aggressive.

Mucinous Eccrine Carcinoma (Mucinous Sweat Gland Adenocarcinoma)

Mucinous eccrine carcinomas (mucinous sweat gland adenocarcinomas) usually occur in middle-aged males. They are most common in the periorbital region and present as an elevated nodule or as a lobulated mass measuring 0.5 to 2.5 cm in diameter and varying in color from gray to bluish to pink to red.

MELANOCYTIC NEVI

Most melanocytic nevi are benign and possess little, if any, potential for malignancy. Congenital melanocytic nevi are present at birth, whereas acquired nevi develop during childhood, usually at the time of puberty. They gradually regress after the age of 30.

Freckle (Ephelis)

A freckle (ephelis) is a light-brown pigmented macule less than 5 mm in diameter. It has a poorly defined margin.

Freckles are probably autosomal dominant and usually occur in children with fair skin and red or blonde hair. They are prominent in the summer and fade during the winter.

Lentigo

A lentigo is a small brown or brown-black macule with ill-defined edges. It may be slightly raised. Single lesions are usually 2 to 3 mm in diameter; confluent lesions are sometimes more than 5 mm in diameter. They develop in childhood and increase in numbers at irregular intervals until adulthood, then fade over a period of years.

They occur anywhere on the skin, mucocutaneous border, and conjunctiva, and are often associated with various syndromes (i.e., Peutz–Jeghers syndrome, LEOPARD syndrome, Name syndrome, Lamb syndrome, centrofacial lentiginosis, and heart chamber myxomas). Lentigines increase in numbers and/or darken excessively in pregnancy, Addison disease, and other diseases with elevated melanin-stimulating hormone.

Solar Lentigo (Lentigo Senilis)

Solar lentigines are larger than simple lentigines and usually develop after the age of 20, following acute or chronic sun exposure. They occur in sun-exposed areas and usually develop rapidly following an acute sunburn. They may evolve into lichenoid keratoses or seborrheic keratoses. It is important to differentiate benign solar lentigines from lentigo maligna. (See the later section for a discussion.)

Unilateral Lentiginosis (Zosteriform Lentiginosis)

Lentigines sometimes occur only on one side of the body and often in a dermatomal-type distribution. They are occasionally associated with central nervous system abnormalities.

Eruptive Lentiginosis

Sometimes, large numbers of lentigines develop over a short period, often beginning as telangiectatic areas that quickly pigment.

Centrofacial Lentiginosis

Centrofacial lentiginosis is autosomal dominant and is characterized by small, brown or black macules that develop during the first year of life, then increase in number for 8 to 10 years. They are distributed in a horizontal band across the midface and are associated with mental retardation, epilepsy, coalescence of the eyebrows, a high-arched palate, absent upper middle incisors, sacral hypertrichosis, spina bifida, and scoliosis.

A horizontal band of hyperpigmentation also occurs in the centrofacial area of Indians living in the high Andes of Peru and Bolivia. It is probably related to intense sun exposure and develops within the first year of life.

Mucosal Melanotic Lesions

Uniform, brown, melanotic lesions occasionally develop on the lips, tongue (Fig. 19-57), genitalia (Fig. 19-58), or conjunctiva lachrymal caruncle (Fig. 19-59). It is important to differentiate these benign melanotic lesions from malignant melanomas.

CONGENITAL MELANOCYTIC NEVI

Congenital melanocytic nevi vary in size from less than 1.5 cm to more than 20 cm in diameter (Fig. 19-60) and may cover large body areas at times called *bathing trunk nevi* (Fig. 19-61). Giant congenital melanocytic nevi have a 3% to7% risk of developing malignant melanomas. Almost half of melanomas seen in young children occur in giant pigmented congenital nevi. They often become increasingly pigmented and develop coarse terminal hairs (Fig. 19-62). Giant nevi may involve the lid and face, and in some cases are associated with other abnormalities (e.g., spina bifida, meningocele, hypertrophy, or atrophy of the deeper structures of the involved extremity) or other hamartomas (von Recklinghausen disease, vascular nevi and lipomas).

Acquired Melanotic Nevi

Acquired melanotic nevi usually develop during adolescence, during pregnancy, or after administration of adrenocorticotropic hormone. They are usually less than 1.5 cm in diameter and begin as dark macules, which rapidly become thickened and develop a raised, smooth, or papillomatous surface. Junctional nevi may be flat or slightly raised, light, dark-brown, or brown-black lesions that vary from 1 to 10 mm. The surface is smooth, and the skin markings are preserved. Except on the palms, soles, and genitalia, they usually progress to form compound nevi.

Compound nevi appear as slightly raised papillomatous plaques. Clinically, they are circular or elliptical and have a smooth surface (Fig. 19-63). More advanced compound nevi may have a few dark hairs growing from their surface. After they stop growing, compound nevi become intradermal nevi.

Intradermal nevi usually develop during adult life. They appear as slightly pigmented, flesh-colored papules with a smooth surface or as sessile or pedunculated, soft, wrinkled nevi. The former are nonpigmented or only slightly pigmented and have many blood vessels on their surface, suggesting a hemangioma. The latter may be mistaken for a skin tag.

Malignant Changes

Junctional (macular) pigmented nevi are more likely to transform into melanomas than compound or intraderemal lesions. Signs that should alert the physician include recent enlargement, an irregular margin, changes in color [especially a variegate pattern with dark or brown, black or red (from increased vascularity), white (sign of regression) or blue (from deeper extension of melanocytes)]. Scaling, crusting, erosion, ulceration, bleeding, or palpable thickening suggest more advanced malignant changes. Satellite lesions indicate regional spread. Itching is an uncommon sign of malignant transformation, as is pain.

The appearance of a new, pigmented nevus in a patient older than 35 years should arouse suspicion, since about half of melanomas develop in previously normal skin, with most of the others occurring in preexisting nevi.

Spindle and Epithelioid Cell Nevus (Spitz Nevus)

Spindle and epithelioid cell nevi (Spitz nevi) are often called juvenile melanomas and are sometimes confused clinically and histologically with malignant melanomas. They rarely develop in postpubertal patients. They are common on the face (especially on the cheek) and legs. The lesion is typically rosy-red or reddish-brown. It grows rapidly at first and feels firm and rounded, and has a smooth or slightly scaly surface. Later, the surface becomes papillomatous. Sometimes it bleeds and crusts, causing confusion because of the thin overlying epidermis. Occasionally, multiple lesions develop in the same area and appear as clusters.

Dysplastic Nevus

Dysplastic (atypical) nevi may be seen in a familial setting (dysplastic nevus syndrome) or may occur sporadically. These lesions differ from common nevi both clinically and histologically. The typical dysplastic nevus measures 5 to 12 mm versus 6 mm or less for acquired nevi. It is characterized by a variegated brown, tan, and pink coloration (Fig. 19-64), irregular margination, and often a papular center, giving a so-called fried egg appearance (Fig. 19-65). In contrast to common nevi, these lesions are often seen on non–sun-exposed areas such as the scalp, breasts, and buttocks. Additionally, dysplastic nevi continue to appear over a lifetime, whereas common nevi are acquired in childhood and young adult years.

Dysplastic nevi may be clinically, and sometimes histologically, confused with melanomas. Patients with many·dysplastic nevi and a family history of melanoma are at high risk for developing malignant melanoma, not only arising in these atypical nevi, but also on normal-appearing skin. Thus these patients need to be carefully monitored.

Blue Nevus

There are two types of blue nevi, the common blue nevus of Jadassohn–Tiche and the less common cellular blue nevus. The former is a steel-blue, slowly enlarging nodule that begins in early life, most frequently found on the dorsum of the hand (Fig. 19-66) or foot and also on the forearm, shin, and at times face and buttocks. It is a benign lesion. The cellular blue nevus is larger and found on the buttocks or sacrococcygeal area. This nevus may rarely undergo malignant transformation manifest by sudden increase in size and ulceration. The dark blue appearance of these nevi is due to the deep dermal location of the melanocytes.

Halo Nevus (Sutton Nevus)

Halo nevi (Sutton nevi) frequently develop in prepubertal and early postpubertal patients. They are characterized by a sharply marginated halo of depigmentation that develops around a preexisting melanocytic nevus (Fig. 19-67). Then, over a period of several months, the nevus disappears, leaving a nonpigmented macule that over a period of years gradually repigments. In patients with halo nevi full mucocutaneous examination is indicated to rule out melanoma.

Malignant Melanoma

The incidence of melanoma has increased tenfold in the past 50 years. It is estimated that one out of every 75 persons now living in the United States will develop a melanoma. Increased exposure to ultraviolet light, perhaps partially the result of thinning of the ozone layer and the popularity of tanning parlors, is thought to be a factor.

Melanomas are most common in persons with fair skin, light eyes, blond or red hair, and freckles. The lowest incidence is in Asians. Repeated sunburns increase the risk of developing melanomas. The incidence of melanoma is low before puberty and when seen may arise in giant congenital nevi, as previously mentioned. Rarely, melanoma may be transmitted *in utero*.

Melanoma Types
Superficially Spreading Melanoma
Superficially spreading melanoma is the most common type, constituting 70% of all melanomas, with most occurring in the fourth or fifth decade. The upper back is the most common site in both sexes, with the calf a frequent location in women. Melanomas may arise in any mucocu-

taneous location, including the scalp and vagina, areas that are often overlooked. Clinical criteria for early recognition of melanoma have been widely publicized as the ABCDs (A, asymmetry; B, border irregularity; C, color; D, diameter greater than 6 mm).

Early changes include spread of pigmentation resulting in irregular margins, variegation of color producing lighter and darker shades of tan, brown, and black (Fig. 19-68). Later changes lead to pale violaceous or red coloration (due to increased vascularity), bluish areas (from deeper penetration of melanocytes), and hypopigmented sites (due to regression) (Fig. 19-69 and 19-70). Bleeding, crusting, or ulceration are late changes. Initial cutaneous metastasis may appear as a small, dark bluish macule or papule resembling a graphite tattoo (Fig. 19-71).

Later cutaneous metastasis may be manifest by rapidly appearing, firm, subcutaneous nodules that may or may not be pigmented (Fig. 19-72). Horizontal or lateral growth may continue for one to several years before invasion into the dermis occurs. Most lesions discovered and treated in this early lateral growth phase have a good prognosis.

Lentigo Maligna Melanoma
Lentigo maligna melanoma accounts for about 5% of melanomas. It is found mostly in the sixth or seventh decade, usually on chronically sun-exposed sites such as the cheek (Fig. 19-73) or nose, and occasionally the eyelid. It begins as a tan macule with gradual, uneven darkening and peripheral growth. After a period of 5 to 20 years, a melanoma, usually nodular, will develop. It is then a lentigo maligna melanoma (Fig. 19-74).

Acral Lentiginous Melanoma
About 10% of melanomas constitute this type. They are more common in blacks, Native Americans, Hispanics, and Japanese, groups in whom other kinds of melanomas are less common. An irregular enlarging macule on the palm, sole (Fig. 19-75), digit tip (Fig. 19-76), or nail fold should cause concern. Extension of pigment from the nail onto the proximal nail fold (Hutchinson sign) is highly suggestive of subungual melanoma (Fig. 19-77). Subungual melanomas can be confused with onychomycosis, warts, pyogenic granulomas, chronic paronychias, subungual hematomas, and Kaposi sarcoma.

Melanoma of the mucous membrane is rare. It may masquerade as an indolent ulcer on the lip of a polypoid tumor with or without pigment in the nose. In the mouth, a melanoma usually appears as a pigmented ulceration of the palate. In the vulva, it is usually noticed as a pruritic, bleeding ulceration after metastasis to the groin. Because of delay in recognition, most mucosal melanomas have a poor prognosis.

Nodular Melanoma

About 15% of melanomas are nodular. They are twice as common in men as in women and occur primarily on sun-exposed sites of the head (Fig. 19-78), neck, arms (Fig. 19-79), and trunk (Fig. 19-80) in the fifth or sixth decade. The typical lesion is a rapidly growing papule or nodule, reddish-brown or bluish-black, which in late stages may ulcerate and bleed. Metastasis is common (Fig. 19-81).

Amelanotic Melanoma

Rarely, melanomas may lack pigment, presenting as pale, erythematous macules or papules. Rapid growth is a clinical clue that the lesion may be malignant and should be biopsied (Fig. 19-82). These lesions are often mistaken as benign nevi or pyogenic granulomas. They are more often seen in albinos.

Secondary melanomas without evidence of a primary site sometimes arise as a metastatic focus from ocular or mucosal melanomas. They usually appear as isolated, non-pigmented, subcutaneous nodules.

Ocular Features

The early stages of malignant melanoma of the conjunctiva are sometimes difficult to distinguish from primary acquired melanosis (PAM). A clear history documenting a new, painless, brown-pigmented conjunctival lesion should lead the clinician to be suspicious of melanoma. The early malignant lesion can be clinically differentiated with bio-microscopy by the raised gray-brown pigmentation located in the center of an otherwise melanotic lesion. Excisional biopsy with examination of surgical margins is indicated in suspicious lesions, before they grow to involve the ocular adnexa and orbit (Figs. 19-83 and 19-84).

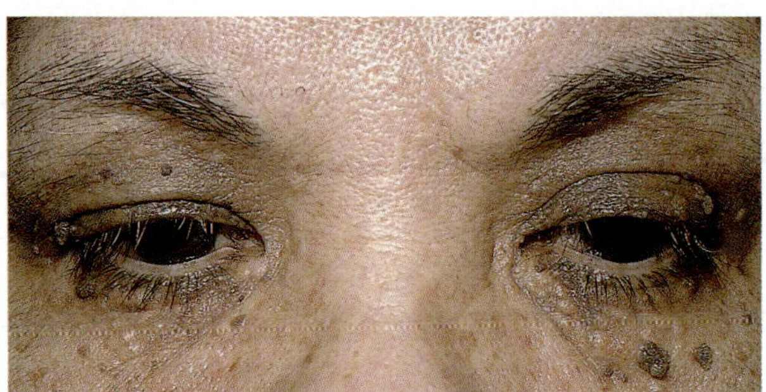

FIGURE 19-1. Seborrheic keratosis of the eyelids. In darkly pigmented persons, this is a common location and is called *dermatosis papulosa nigra*.

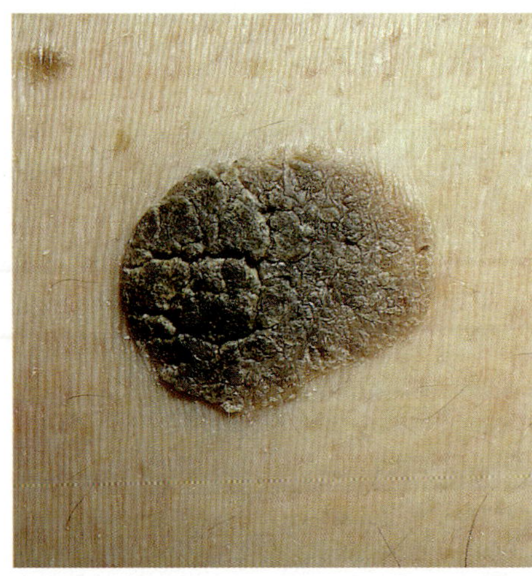

FIGURE 19-2. Seborrheic keratosis showing a sharply demarcated light to dark brown "stuck-on" appearing plaque with characteristic fissures.

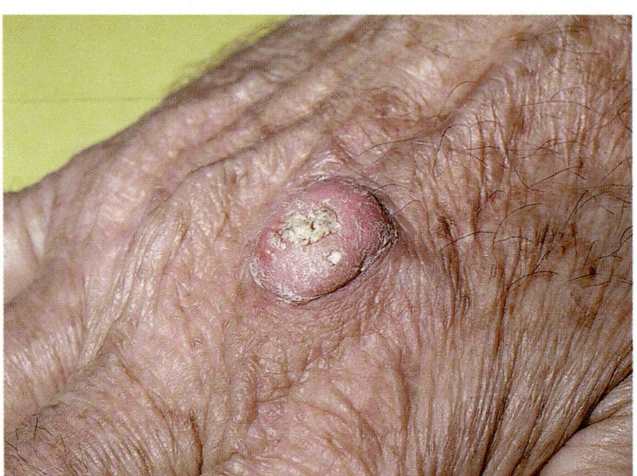

FIGURE 19-3. Keratoacanthoma on a sun-exposed site in an elderly fair-skinned man. This lesion evolved over a 3-week period. Note the characteristic central keratin plug in this dome-shaped nodule.

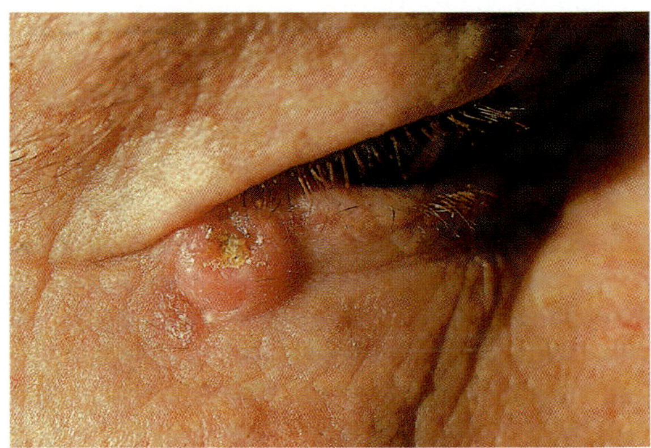

FIGURE 19-4. Keratoacanthoma of the eyelid. After an initial 4- to 6-week growth phase the lesion remained this size for 6 months, helping to differentiate it from a basal cell carcinoma. It was excised without recurrence.

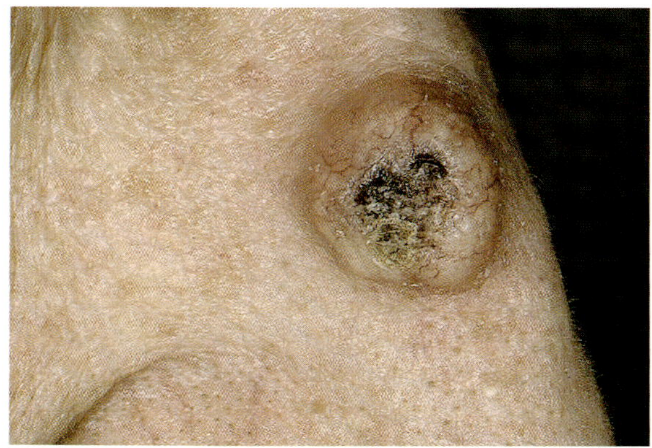

FIGURE 19-5. Giant keratoacanthoma of nose. The rolled waxy margin and telangiectasis suggest the diagnosis of a basal cell carcinoma; however, the rapid evolution over a 6-week period favored the diagnosis of keratoacanthoma.

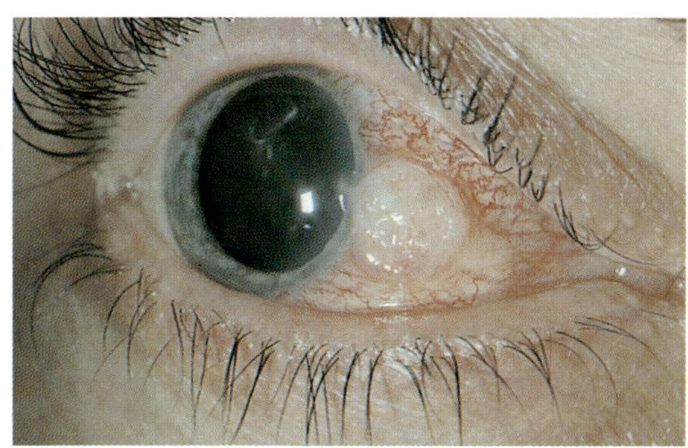

FIGURE 19-6. Conjunctival keratoacanthoma. This keratoacanthoma was present for 3 months.

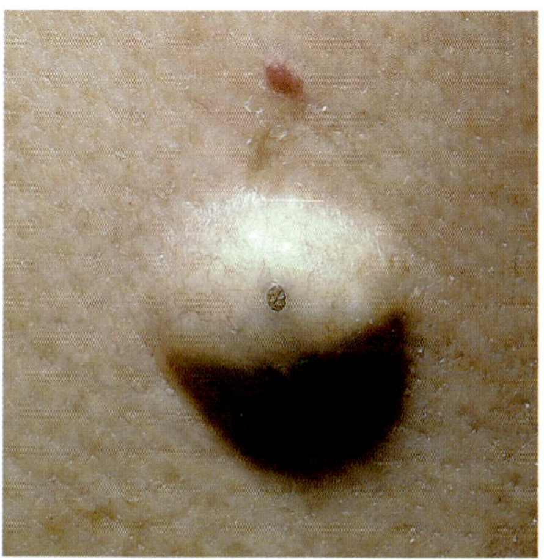

FIGURE 19-7. Epidermal inclusion cyst. Note characteristic central comedonal pore.

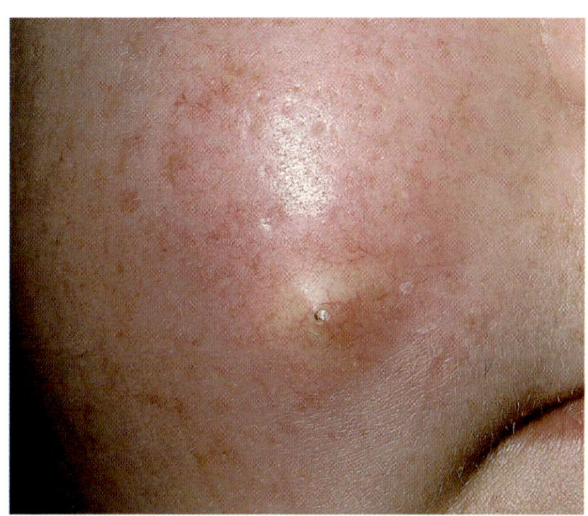

FIGURE 19-8. Painful inflamed epidermal inclusion cyst of the cheek.

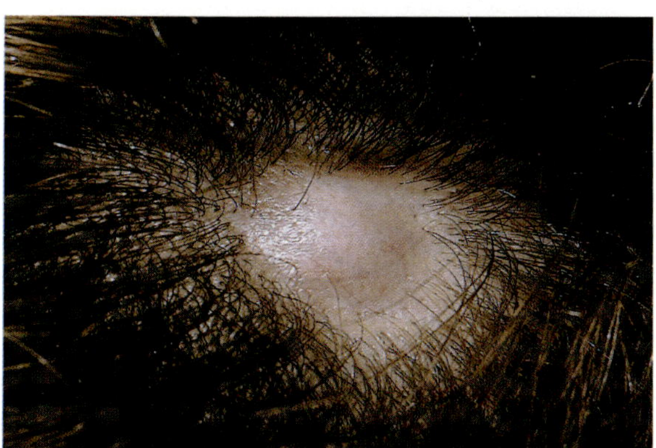

FIGURE 19-9. Trichilemmal (pilar) cyst of scalp. It is important to differentiate this lesion from alopecia neoplastica (i.e., cutaneous metastasis, especially from lymphomas).

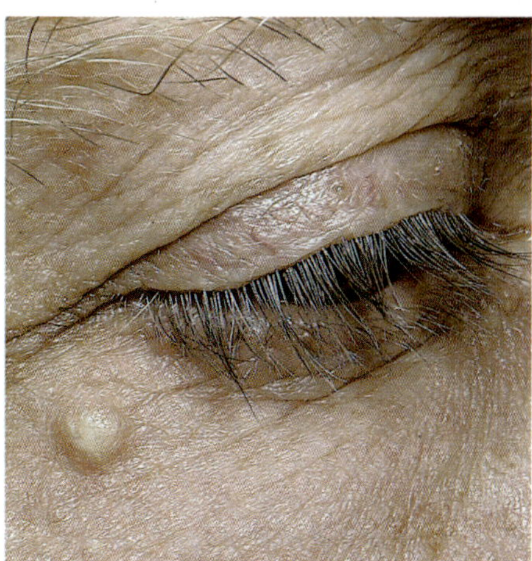

FIGURE 19-10. Milium (keratinous cyst).

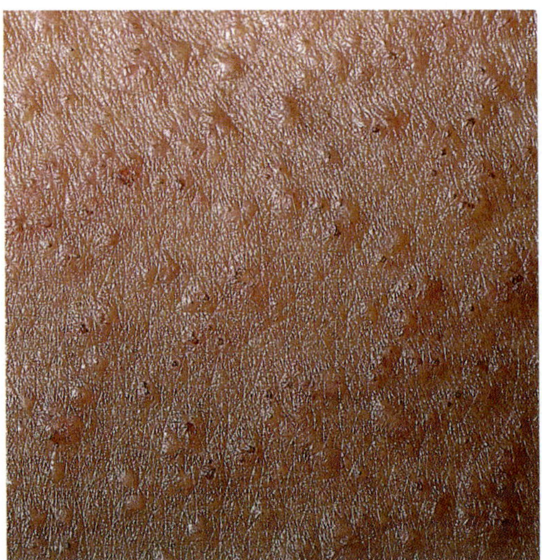

FIGURE 19-11. Miliaria rubra. Note the multiple erythematous papules with tiny central dark plugs of the eccrine ducts.

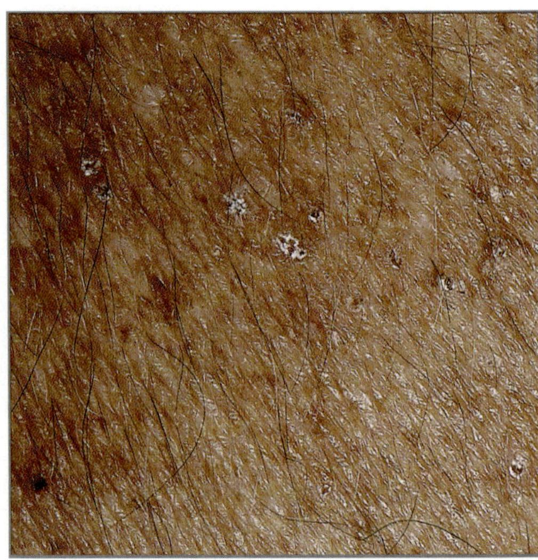

FIGURE 19-12. Miliaria ruba. Close inspection shows that the lesions, small healing crusts, spare the hair follicles differentiating miliaria (eccrine glands) from folliculitis (pilosebaceous glands).

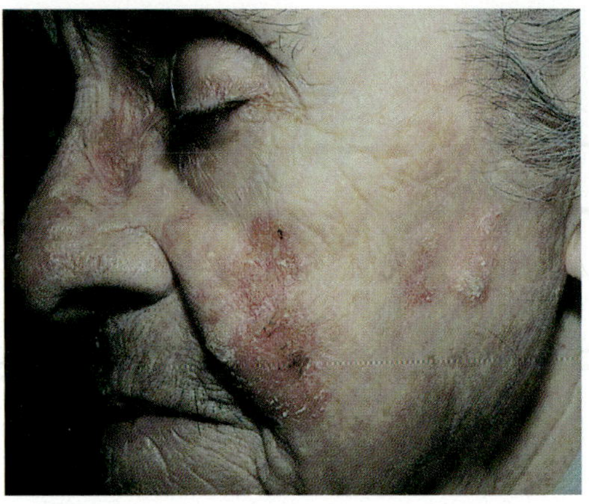

FIGURE 19-13. Multiple solar keratoses (actinic keratoses) in an 89-year-old woman.

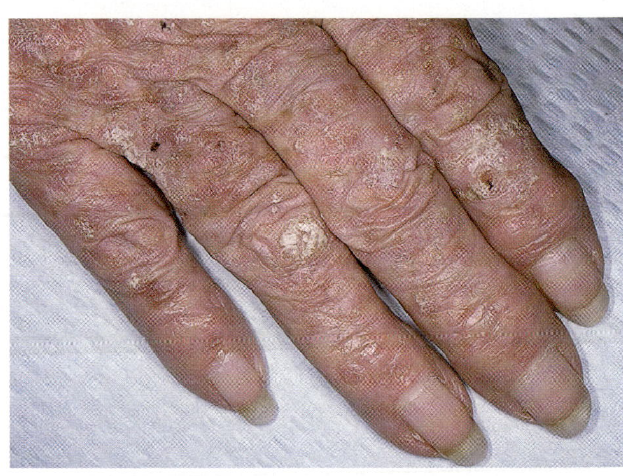

FIGURE 19-14. Hyperkeratotic actinic keratoses dorsae of fingers. Several of these lesions on excision showed early squamous cell carcinoma.

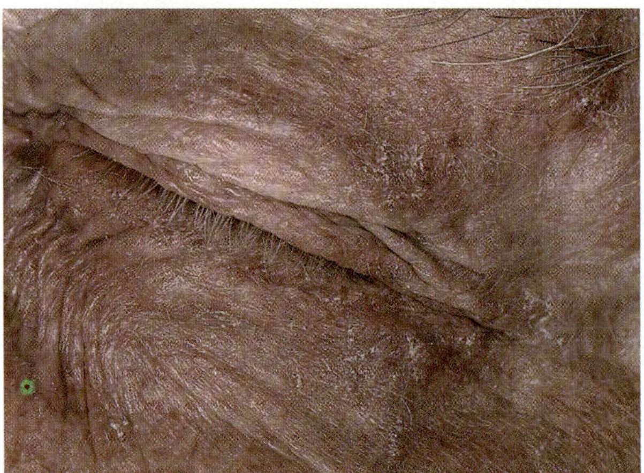

FIGURE 19-15. Actinic keratoses of eyelid. Treatment with liquid nitrogen was done very carefully to avoid injury to the eye.

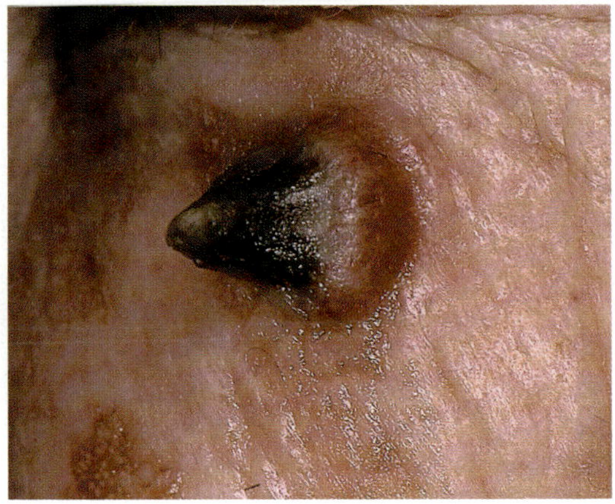

FIGURE 19-16. Cutaneous horns on upper check of elderly lady.

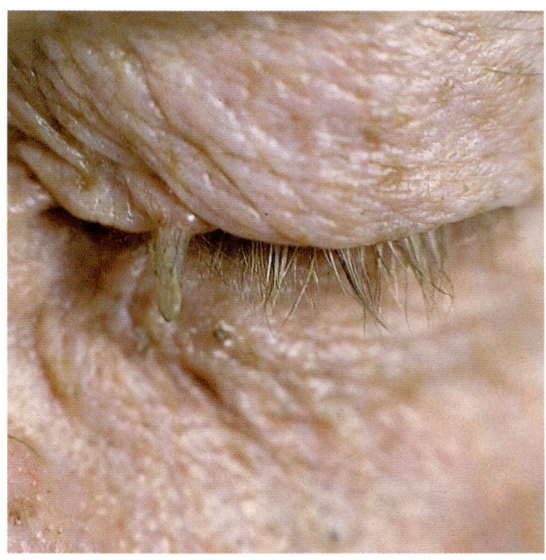

FIGURE 19-17. Cutaneous horn of eyelid.

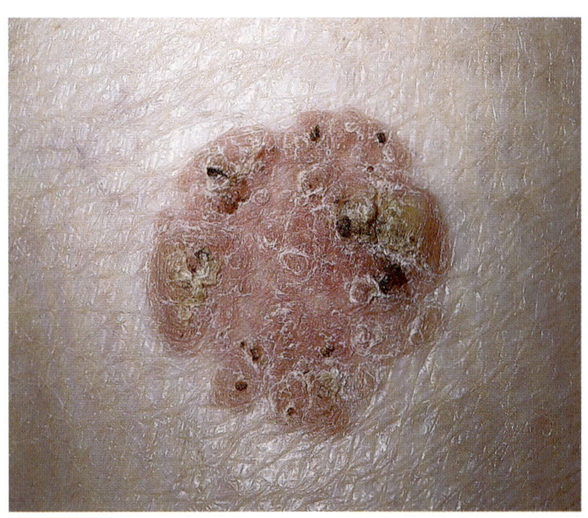

FIGURE 19-18. Bowen disease. Lesion on thigh of an elderly man. Note sharply demarcated erythematous plaque.

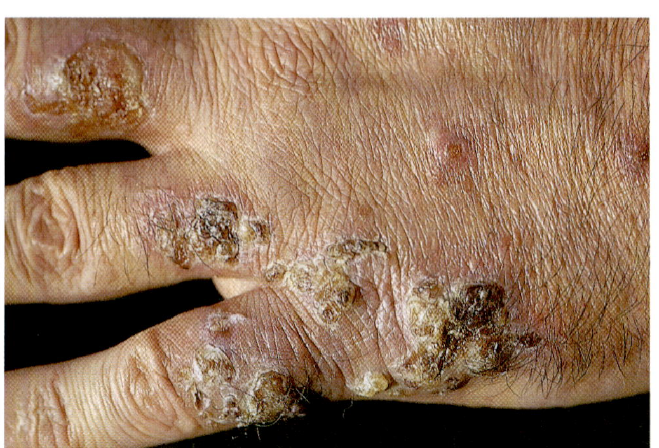

FIGURE 19-19. Multiple Bowen lesions with changes suggestive of squamous cell carcinoma. This patient wanted a refill of the oral antifungal medication that his physician had been prescribing for several years.

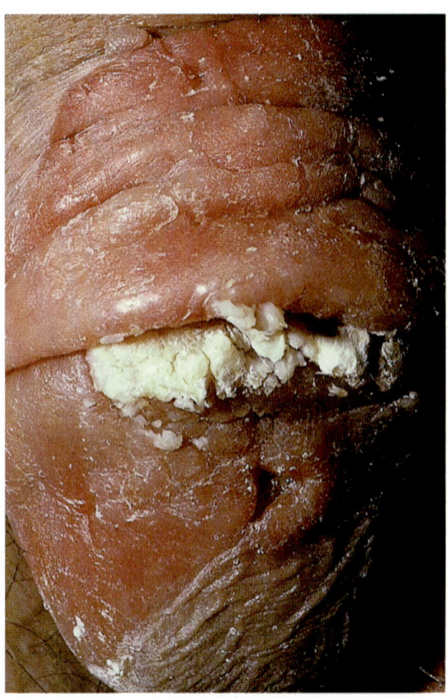

FIGURE 19-20. Bowen disease of the penis (erythroplasia of Queyrat).

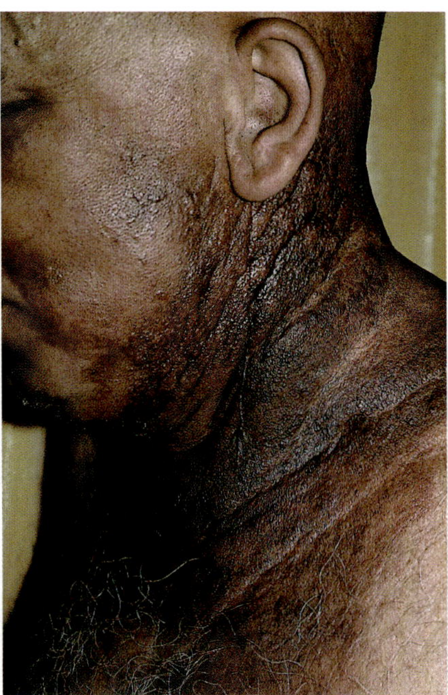

FIGURE 19-21. Acute radiodermatitis in a patient with carcinoma of parotid gland. Note dusky erythema with hyperpigmentation. The multiple discrete and confluent papules are cutaneous metastasis.

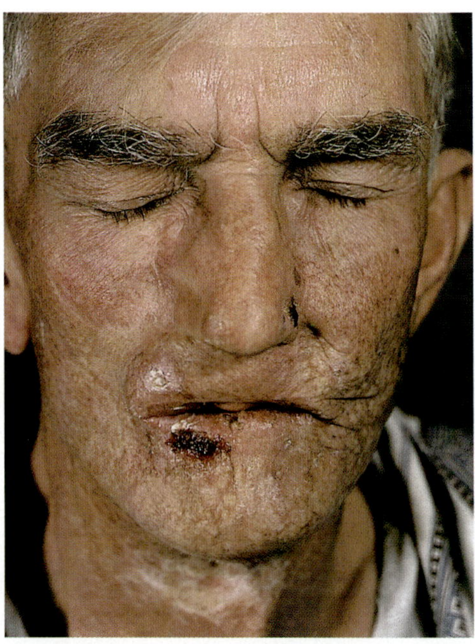

FIGURE 19-22. Chronic radio dermatitis showing atrophic skin with marked telangiectasis and several squamous cell and basal cell carcinomas around the lips and nose. Note normal skin of eyelids and forehead, which had been shielded with lead when the patient received x-ray treatment for acne as a teenager.

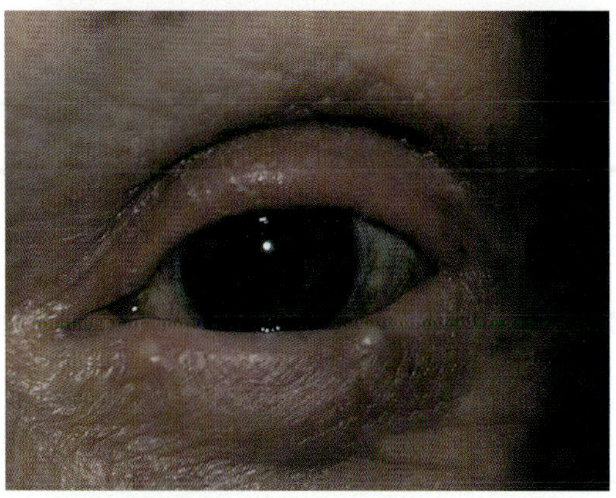

FIGURE 19-23. Postirradiation of the eyelid with loss of lashes.

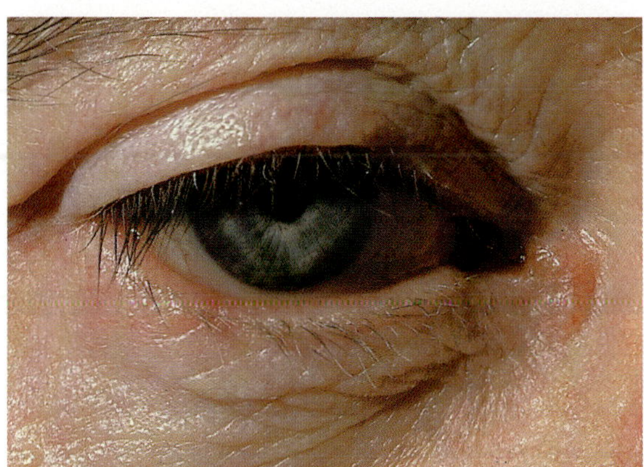

FIGURE 19-24. Nodular basal cell carcinoma of medial canthus, a common site for this tumor. This small lesion could easily be overlooked without careful inspection.

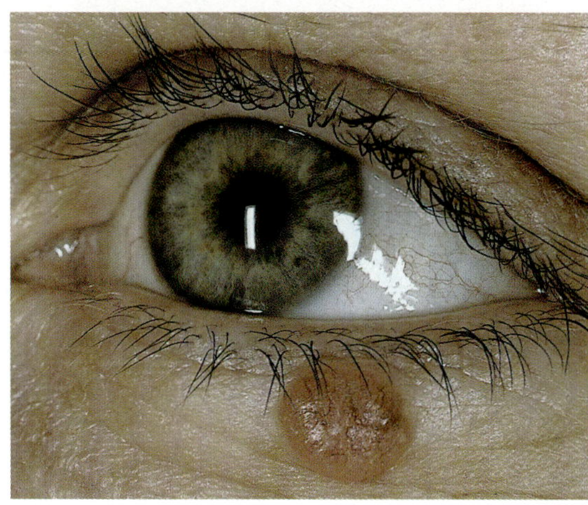

FIGURE 19-25. An obvious modular basal cell carcinoma of lower lid.

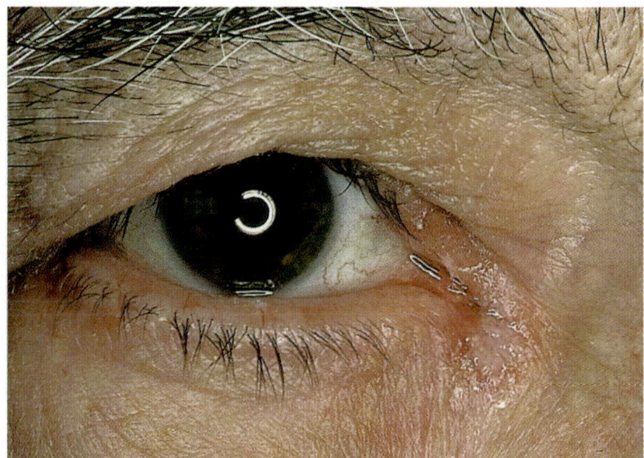

FIGURE 19-26. Subtle erosive basal cell carcinoma of medial canthus that could easily be confused with an infection.

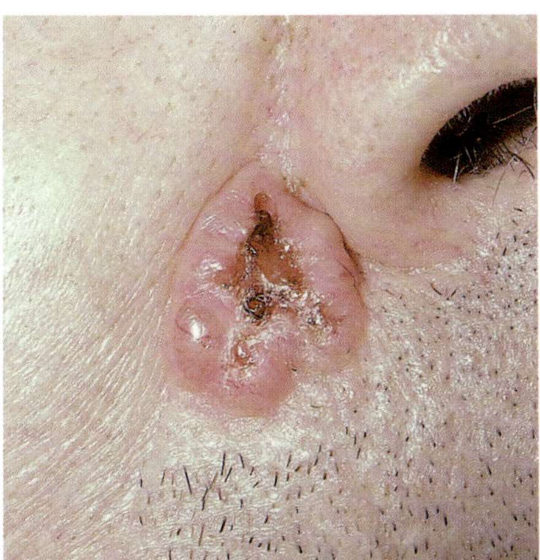

FIGURE 19-27. Basal cell carcinoma nodular type. Note characteristic rolled waxy border with a few telangiectatic vessels and central ulceration. The patient delayed seeing his physician until the tumor began to bleed.

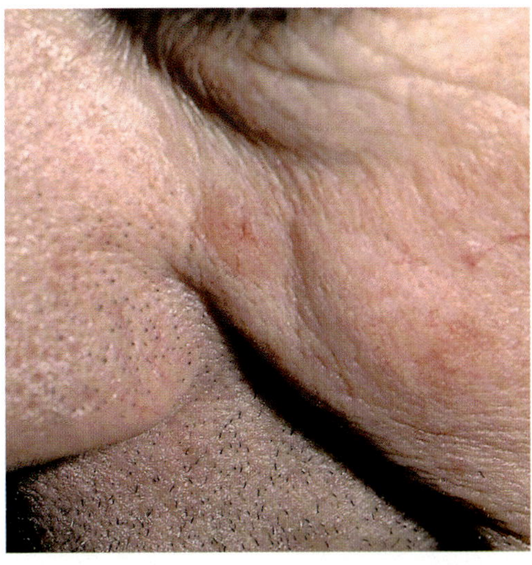

FIGURE 19-28. A basal cell carcinoma as evidenced by a somewhat subtle erythematous telangiectatic lesion just above the nasal crease.

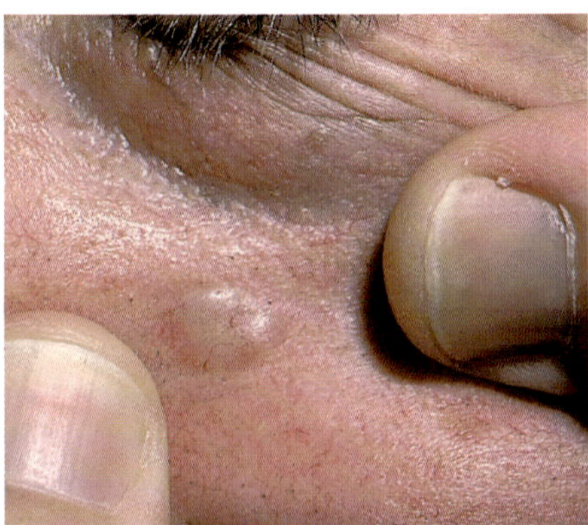

FIGURE 19-29. Same lesion as in Fig. 19-28, demonstrating obvious waxy appearance of a nodular basal cell carcinoma by stretching the area between two fingers. This is a very helpful clinical procedure.

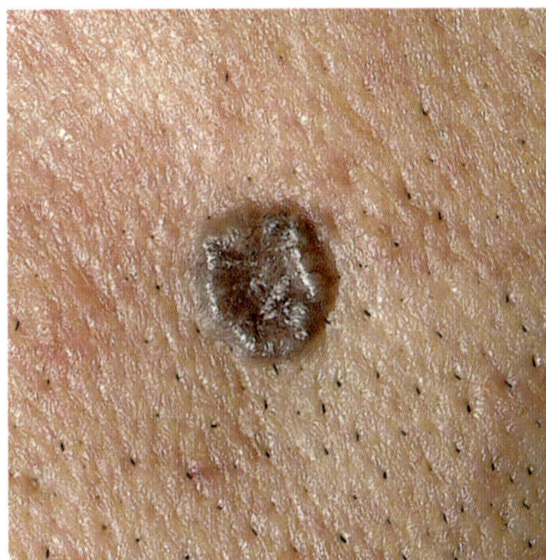

FIGURE 19-30. Pigmented basal cell carcinoma showing typical rolled pearly margin, differentiating it from a pigmented nevus.

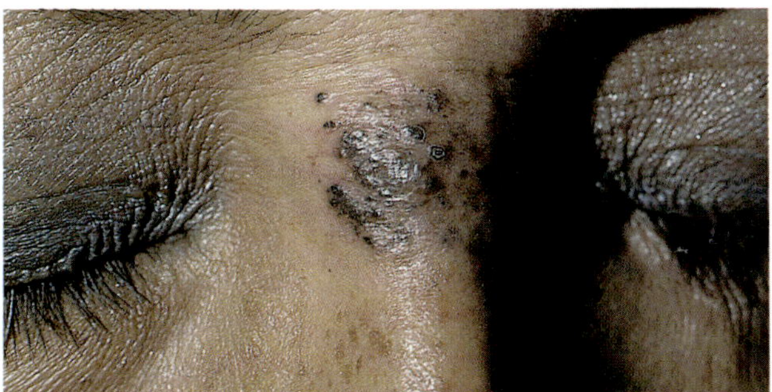

FIGURE 19-31. Atypical pigmented basal cell carcinoma resembling lentigo maligna.

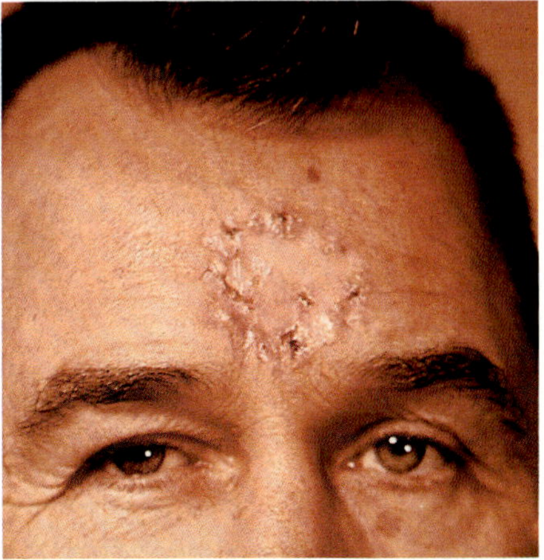

FIGURE 19-32. Morphea-like (sclerosing) basal cell carcinoma revealing central sclerotic appearance. Though rare, this type of basal cell carcinoma is aggressive and requires careful surgical removal.

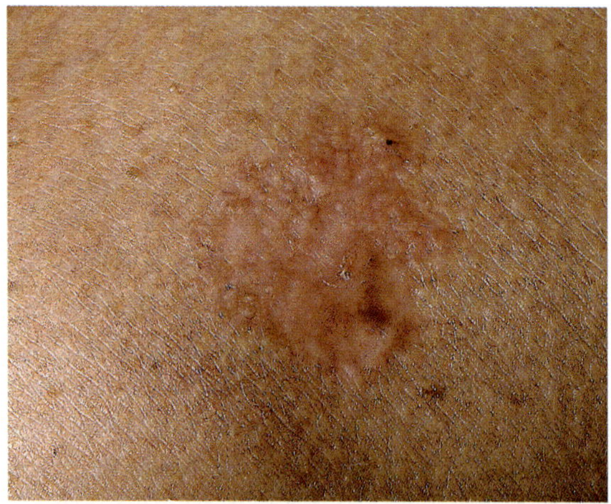

FIGURE 19-33. Sclerosing basal cell carcinoma treated as a superficial fungal infection by his nurse practitioner.

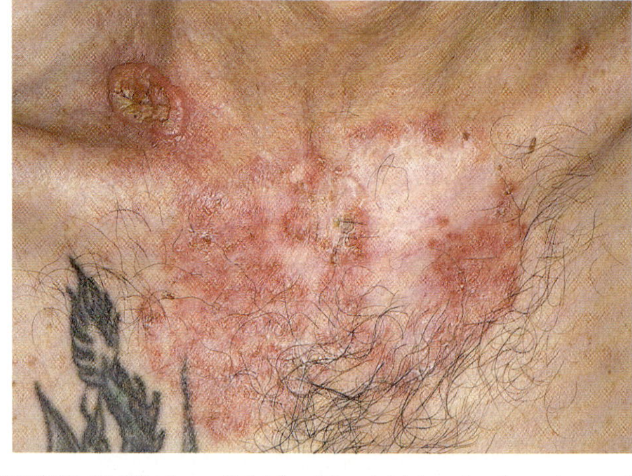

FIGURE 19-34. Superficial (multicentric) basal cell carcinoma in a welder. Note white, scarlike areas. Close inspection revealed thin, raised, thready border indicative of the diagnosis.

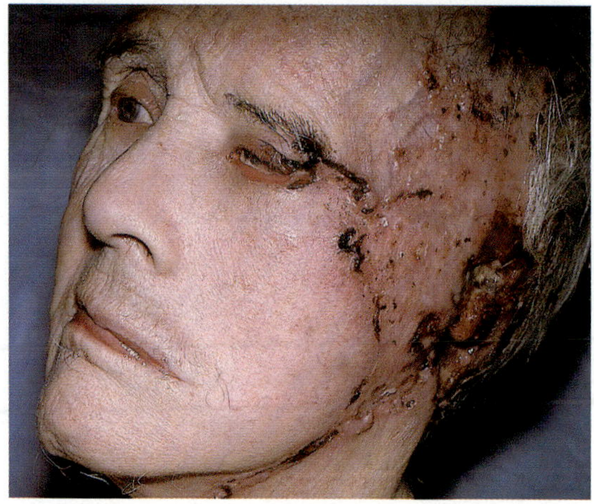

FIGURE 19-35. Extensive destructive basal cell carcinoma in an elderly depressed lady who had refused treatment for 10 years. Because the tumor had destroyed the ear, the referring physician had considered the diagnosis of leprosy. Eventually the carcinoma invaded the facial nerve, causing unilateral palsy. A computed tomography scan revealed invasion of bones around the ear. The tumor spread to the brain, with death of the patient a few weeks after this photo was taken.

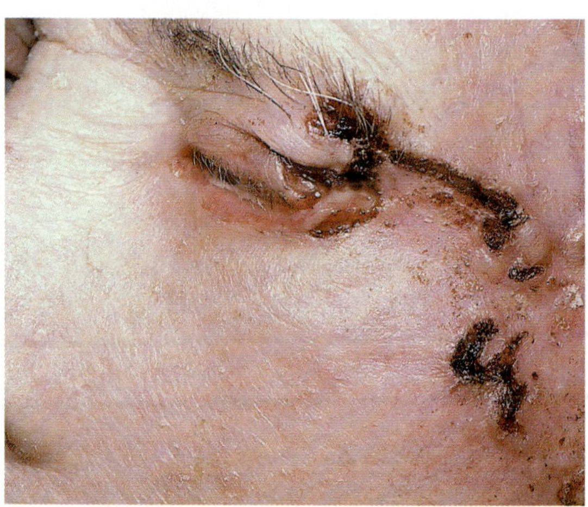

FIGURE 19-36. Close-up of patient shown in Fig. 19-35 showing invasion of eyelids and eye. The rolled pearly margin of the tumor was the diagnostic clue for the diagnosis.

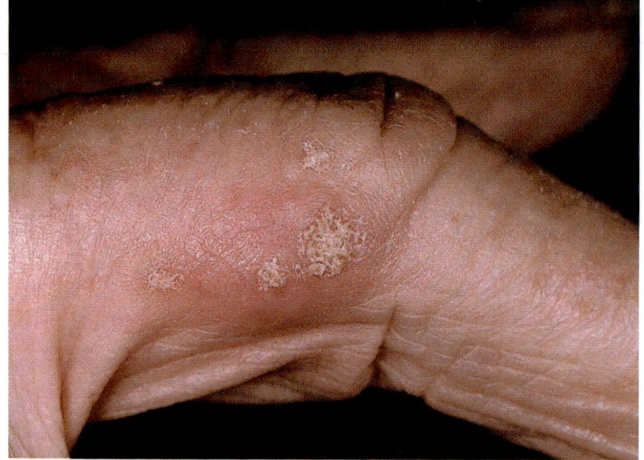

FIGURE 19-37. Early squamous cell carcinoma skin of finger. Note resemblance to actinic keratosis, but more infiltration.

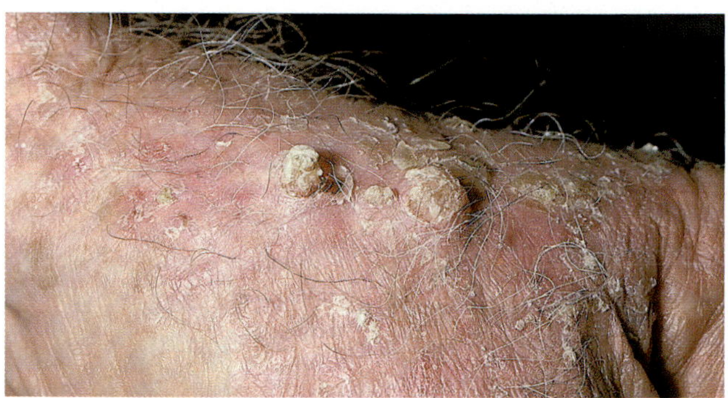

FIGURE 19-38. Squamous cell carcinomas on dorsum of hand in elderly fair-skinned gentleman at sites of multiple actinic keratoses.

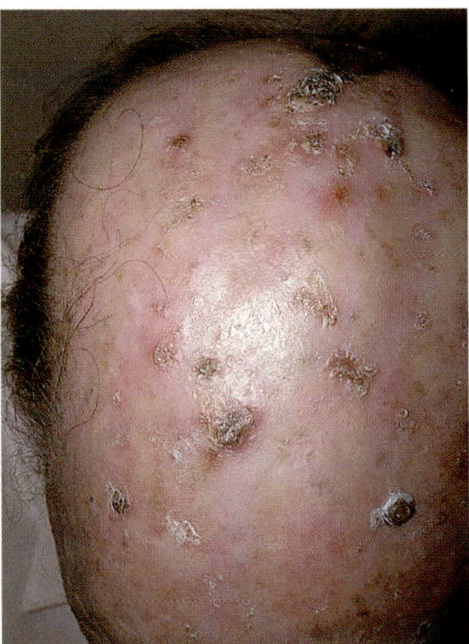

FIGURE 19-39. Multiple early squamous cell carcinomas and actinic keratoses on scalp, a common site in men.

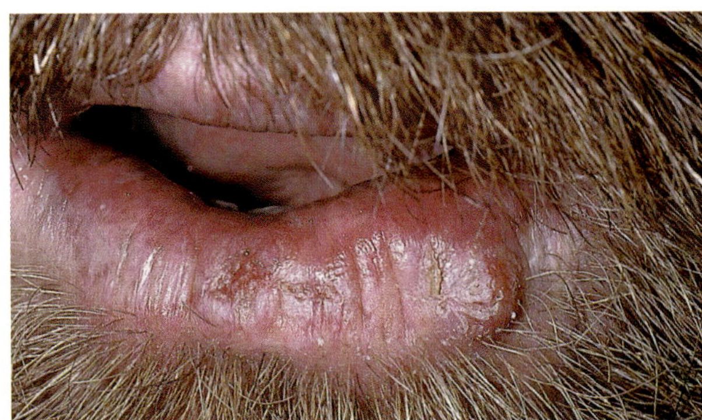

FIGURE 19-40. Squamous cell carcinoma of lower lip in a man who has smoked for many years. Tumors at these sites need to be treated aggressively, since the risk of metastasis on mucosal areas is higher than that on the skin.

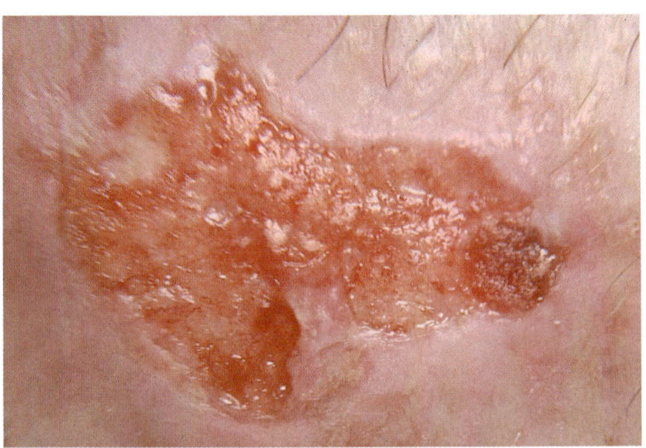

FIGURE 19-41. Squamous cell carcinomas of the skin at site of burn 20 years before. This type of tumor, also known as Marjolin ulcer, has a high risk of metastasis.

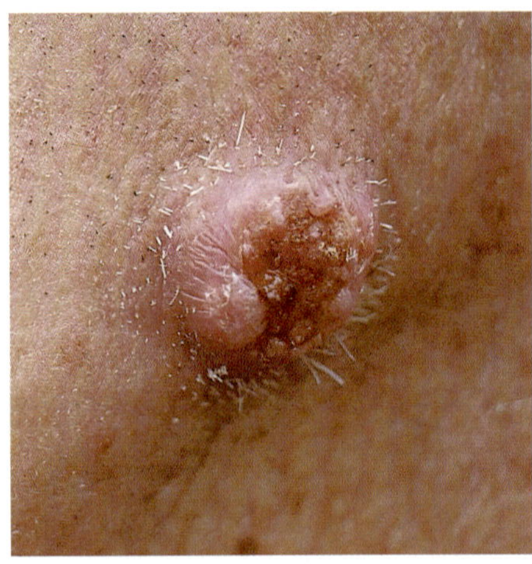

FIGURE 19-42. Squamous cell carcinoma resembling keratoacanthoma. This firm nodule with central ulceration evolved over 1 month. The diagnosis of squamous cell carcinoma was confirmed following excision.

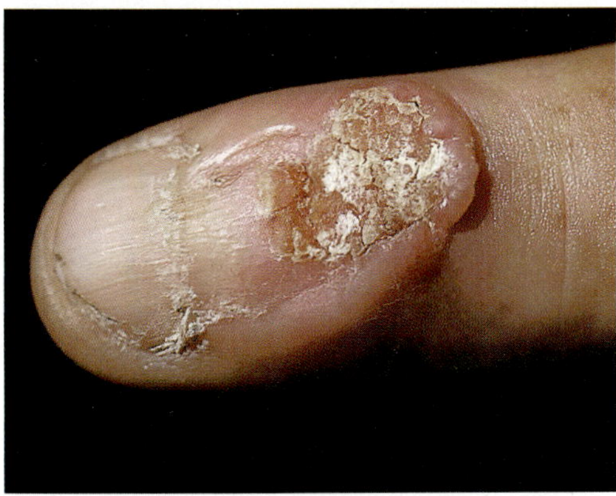

FIGURE 19-43. Squamous cell carcinoma of finger. This lesion had been treated for 10 years as a wart. It is possible that this patient originally had a human papilloma virus, which was oncogenic.

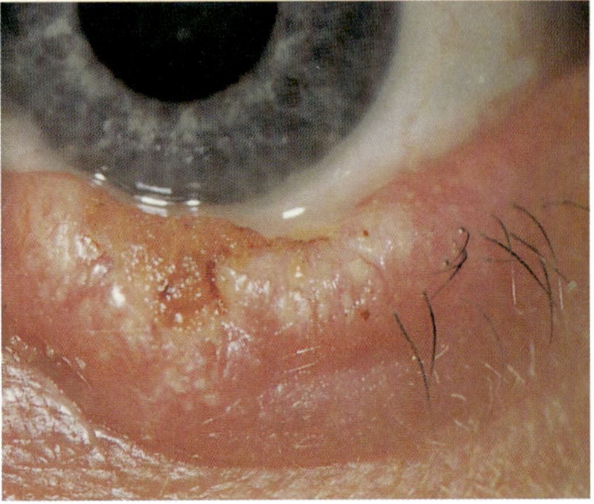

FIGURE 19-44. Squamous cell carcinoma of the lid margin.

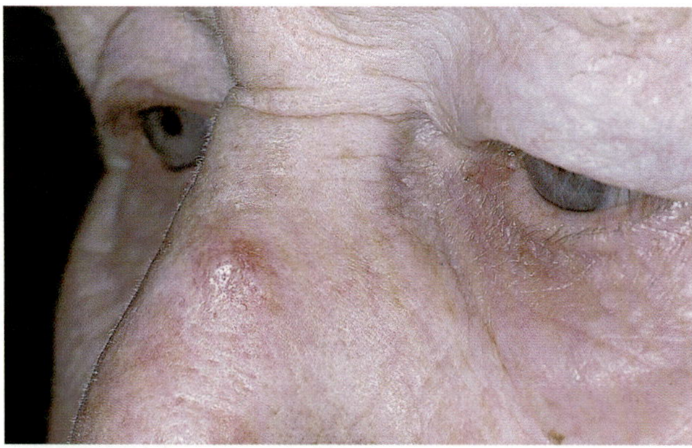

FIGURE 19-45. Merkel cell tumor. This painless, moderately firm, pale, erythematous nodule evolved over a 6-week period in this 83-year-old woman. Clinically, it was thought most likely to be a metastatic lesion to the skin.

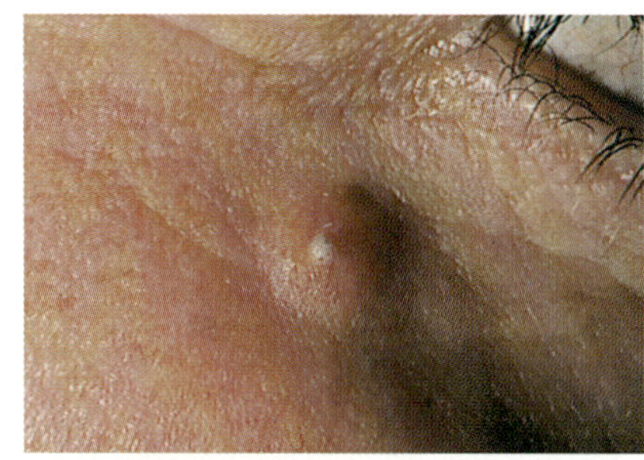

FIGURE 19-46. Trichofolliculoma.

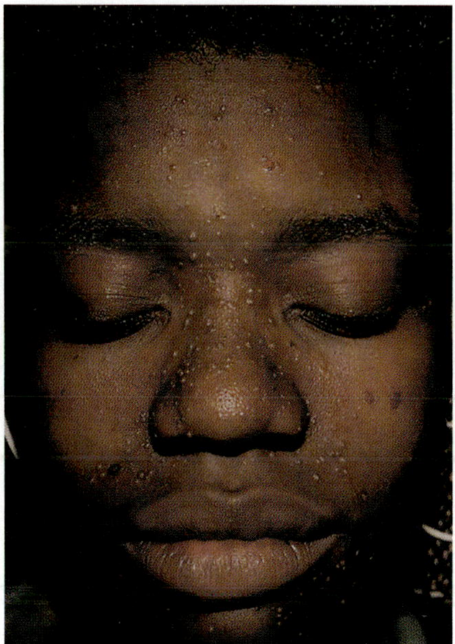

FIGURE 19-47. Trichoepithelioma of the nose, forehead, chin, and lower eyelid. (Photograph courtesy of Dr. John Reeves.)

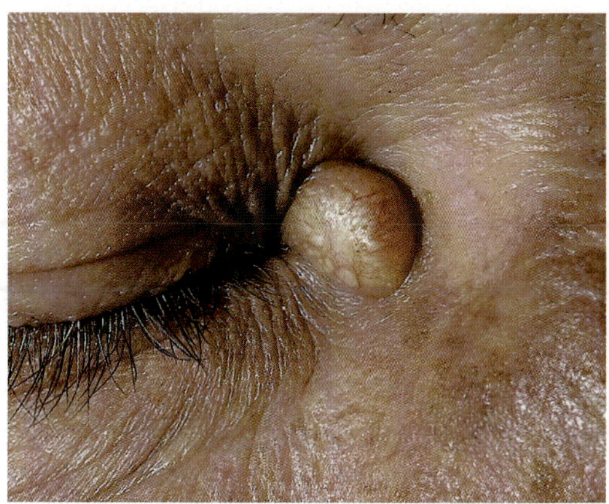

FIGURE 19-48. Sebaceous cyst of eyelid.

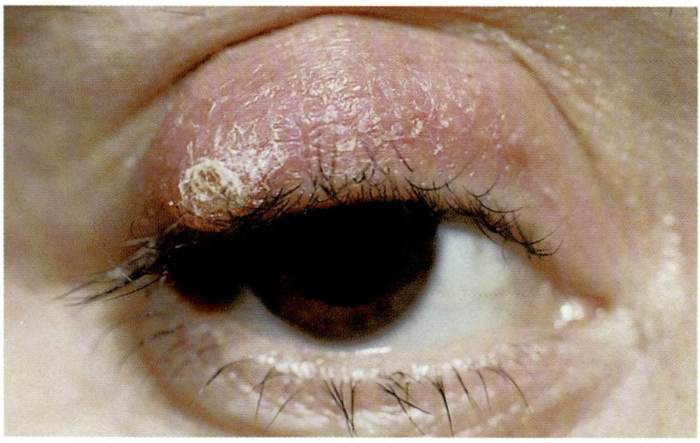

FIGURE 19-49. Chalazion. This 24-year-old woman has had a 6-month history of an upper eyelid chalazion. Although it was draining and the patient continued to use warm compresses, incision and curettage with intralesional corticosteroid injections were needed to resolve the problem.

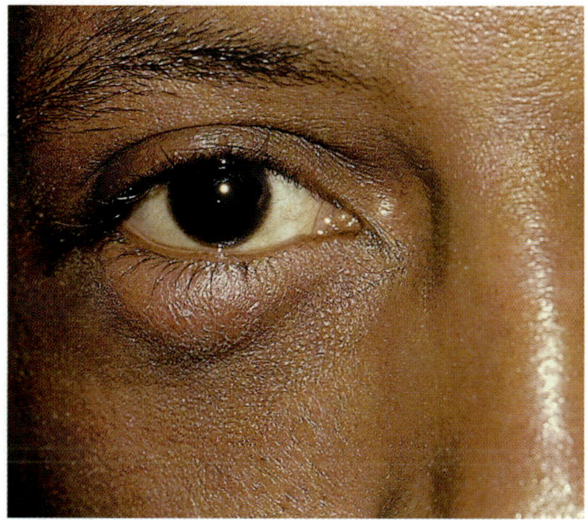

FIGURE 19-50. Chalazion. Note the localized right lower lid mass, mild skin erythema, and noninflamed bulbar conjunctiva in this 32-year-old, darkly pigmented man. The chalazion, and his symptoms of irritation, resolved after 5 days of warm compresses.

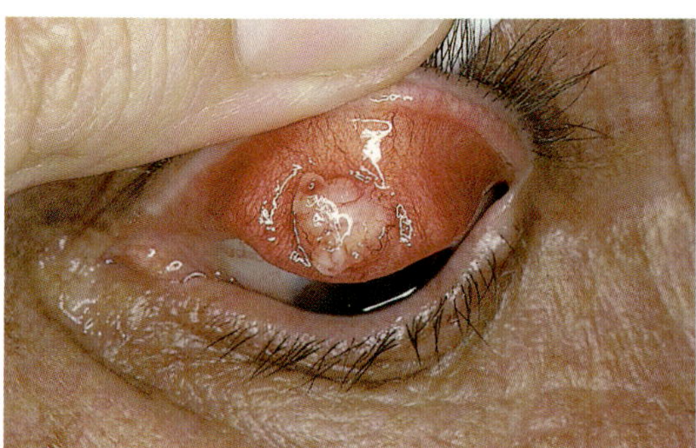

FIGURE 19-51. Carcinoma of meibomian glands. This lesion presented as an asymptomatic swelling of the eyelid and clinically was thought to be a chalazion.

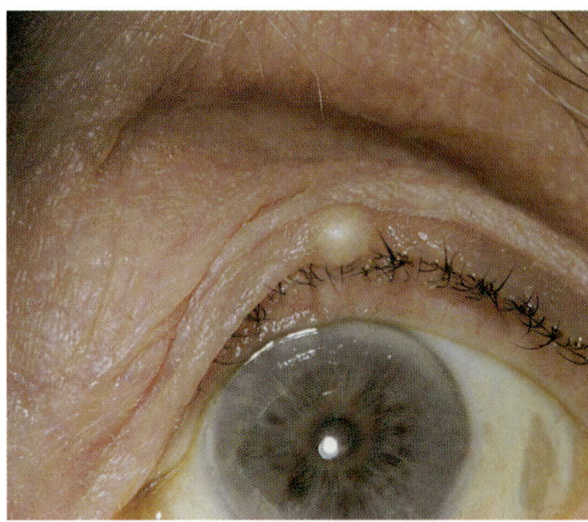

FIGURE 19-52. Sebaceous adenoma. This 74-year-old male complained of a small pimple on the upper eyelid that on excision biopsy proved to be a sebaceous adenoma. The lid skin is very loose and pendulous, and a scleral plaque is evident near the insertion of the lateral rectus muscle.

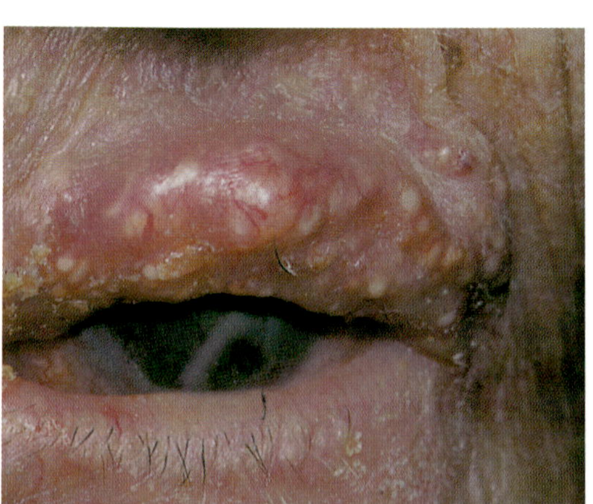

FIGURE 19-53. Sebaceous gland tumors are usually solitary, firm, somewhat raised, and yellow or orange with a translucent quality, as is seen in this patient. The surface may be rough or smooth. Fatal metastasis occurs in one-fourth of eyelid cases. Compare this photo with the chalazion in Figure 19-49.

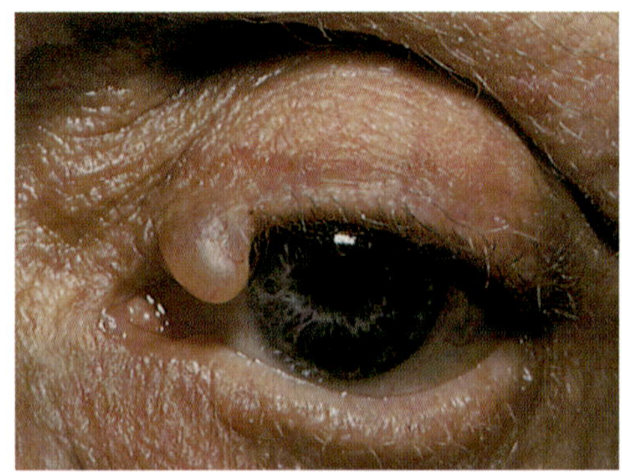

FIGURE 19-54. Apocrine hidrocystoma of eyelid.

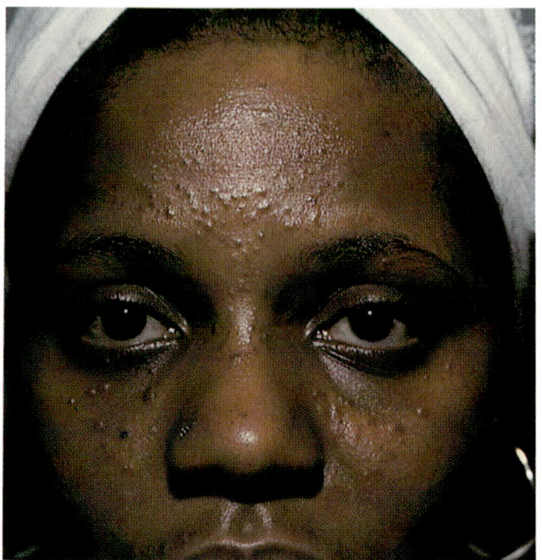

FIGURE 19-55. Syringomas of the forehead and cheeks.

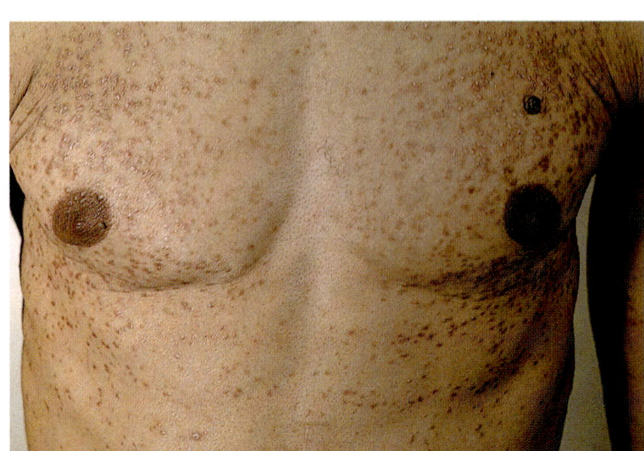

FIGURE 19-56. Syringomas—extensive lesions of trunk.

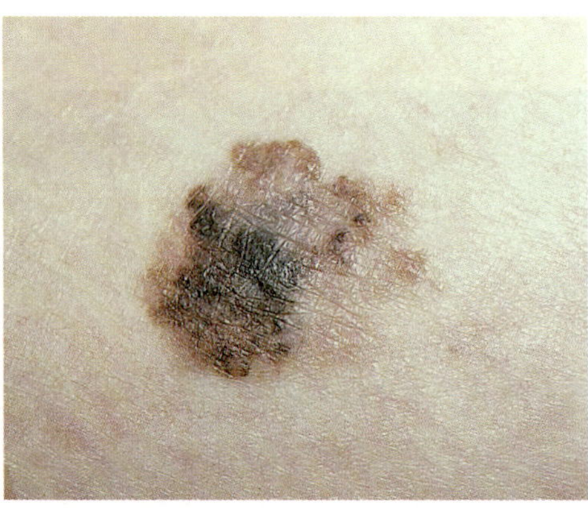

FIGURE 19-68. Superficial spreading melanoma showing variegated pigmentation.

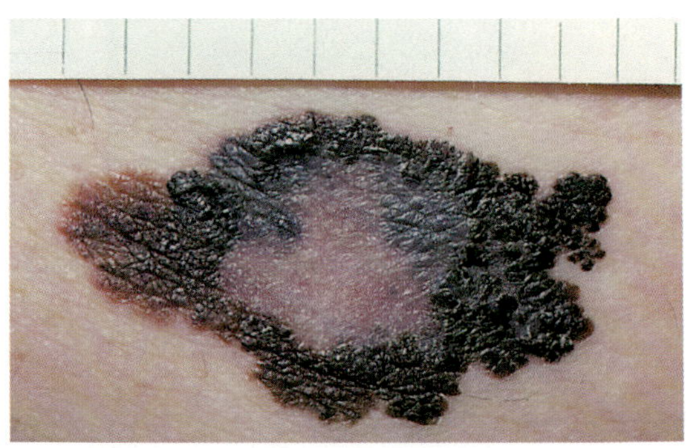

FIGURE 19-69. Superficial spreading melanoma demonstrating marked irregular notched margin and the "red, white, and blue" sign of a more advanced lesion.

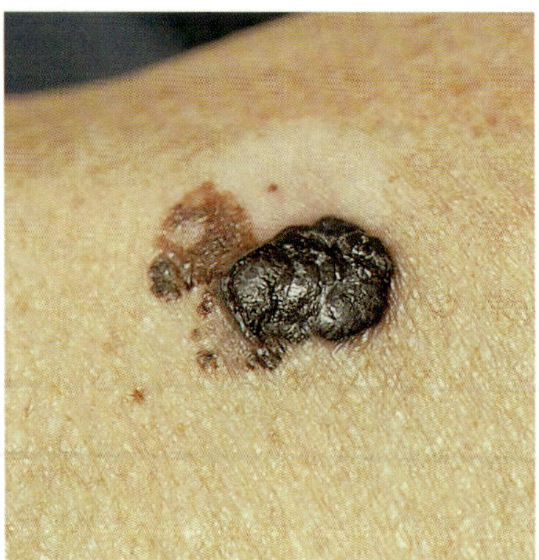

FIGURE 19-70. Nodular melanoma arising from an earlier superficial spreading melanoma. Note the hypopigmented areas of regression. The patient had positive regional lymph nodes. Although his prognosis was quite poor, he survived for 30 years with several cutaneous metastases.

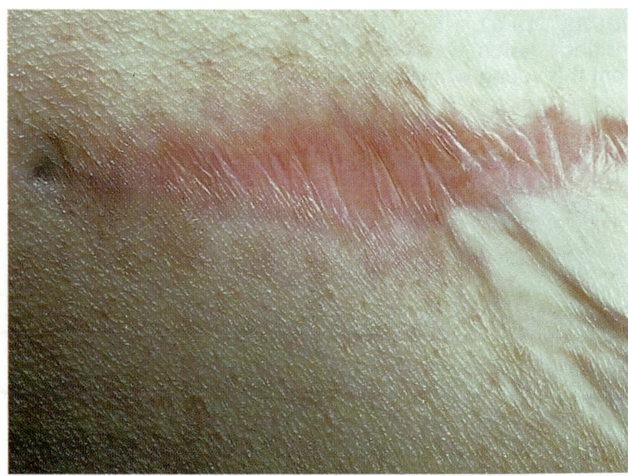

FIGURE 19-71. Cutaneous metastasis at margin of recently excised superficial spreading melanoma. Note resemblance to a graphite tattoo from a pencil lead.

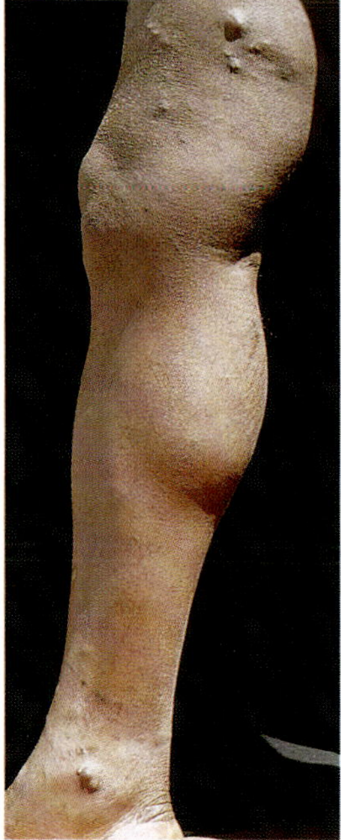

FIGURE 19-72. Late cutaneous metastases. The firm, asymptomatic, subcutaneous nodules appeared over several weeks. The initial superficial spreading malignant melanoma was of a site of injury on the instep.

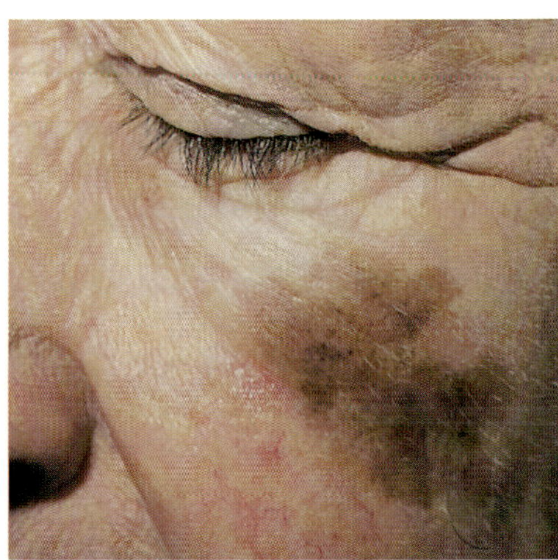

FIGURE 19-73. Lentigo maligna in a 78-year-old woman who had noticed darkening and enlargement over several years. Note the irregular margins and shades of pigmentation.

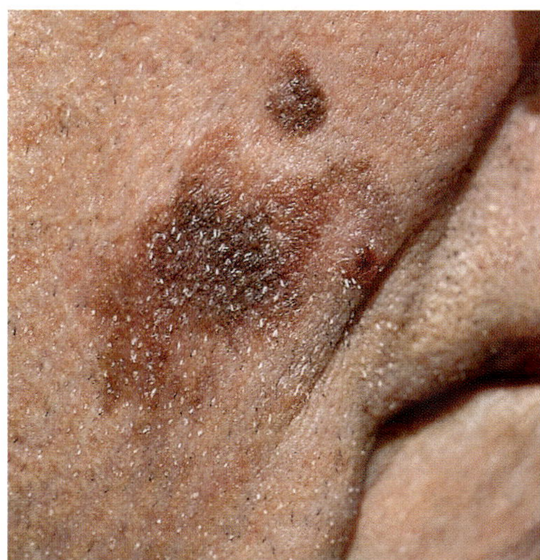

FIGURE 19-74. Lentigo maligna melanoma. The unevenly pigmented macule with the irregular scalloped margins had been slowly enlarging for the past 15 years (lentigo maligna). The small nodule near the nasolabial crease (nodular melanoma) had been noticed by the patient for only a few months.

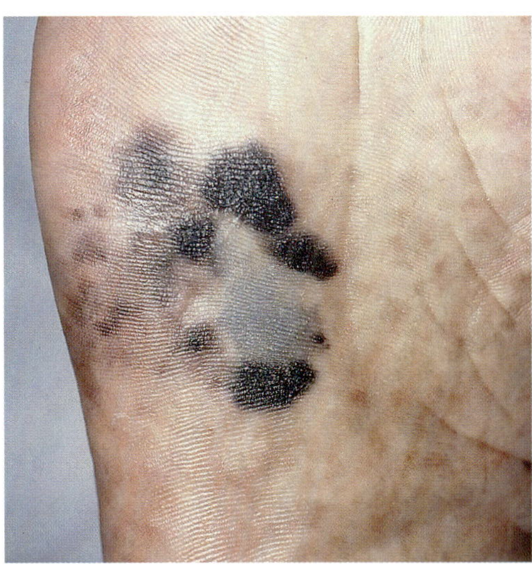

FIGURE 19-75. Acral lentiginous melanoma on the sole of an elderly lady.

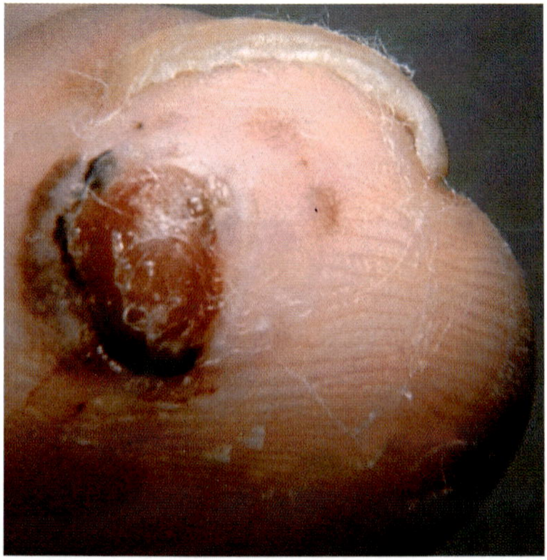

FIGURE 19-76. Acral melanoma of the big toe. The thumb and hallux are the most frequently involved.

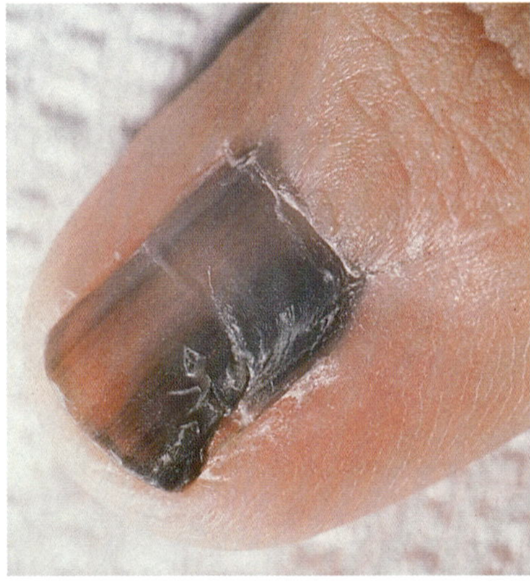

FIGURE 19-77. Subungual melanoma confirmed on biopsy of medial margin of fingernail. Note subtle extension of pigmentation past the proximal nail fold (Hutchinson sign of melanoma).

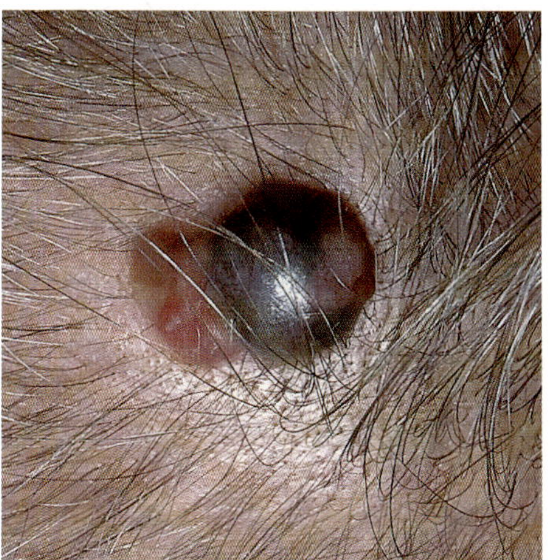

FIGURE 19-78. Nodular melanoma of the scalp. Lesions at this site have a poor prognosis because they are readily overlooked, especially in patients with dense scalp hair, and are in a vascular area.

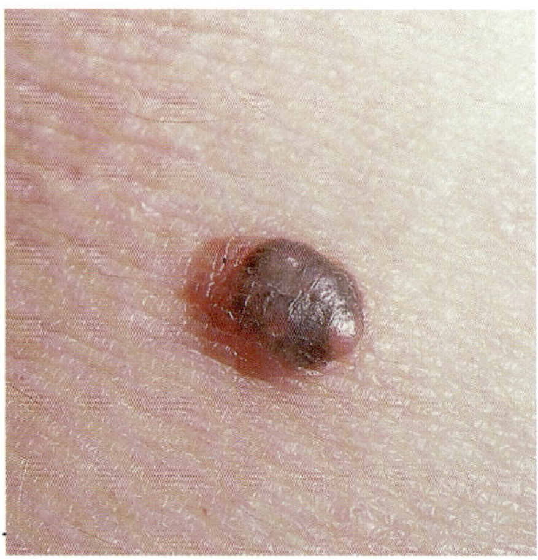

FIGURE 19-79. Nodular melanoma on the forearm of a 24-year-old woman. The lesion had evolved over several months and on initial evaluation was thought to be a pyogenic granuloma. Note the variegation of color and the erythematous base.

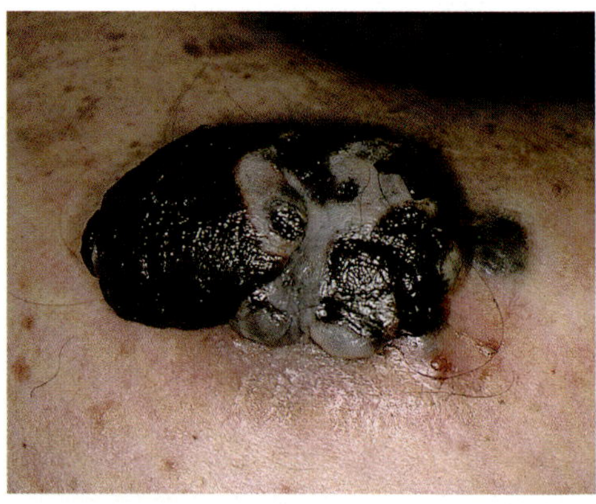

FIGURE 19-80. Nodular melanoma of back, late state showing regional cutaneous metastasis, bluish macule adjoining the large tumor. The patient had avoided physicians until he collapsed due to metastasis to the brain. He died several months after this photo was taken.

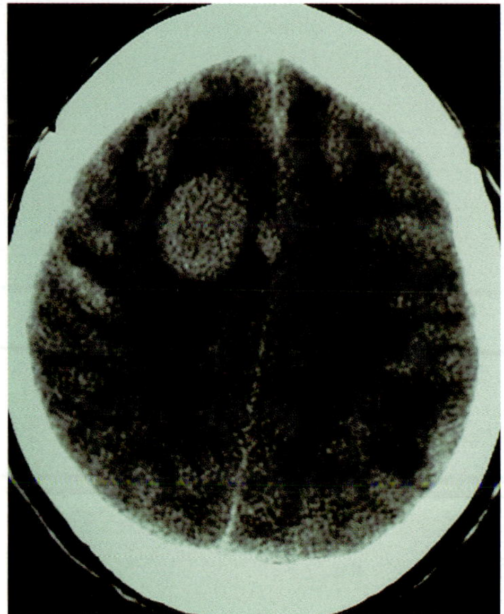

FIGURE 19-81. Computed tomography scan showing metastasis to the brain in patient pictured in Fig. 19-80.

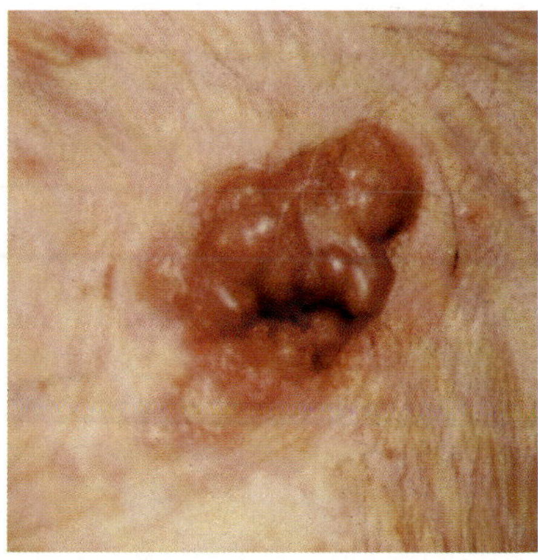

FIGURE 19-82. Amelanotic melanoma in a 90-year-old man. The lesion evolved over several months. Pulmonary metastasis was the cause of death 1 year after this photo was taken.

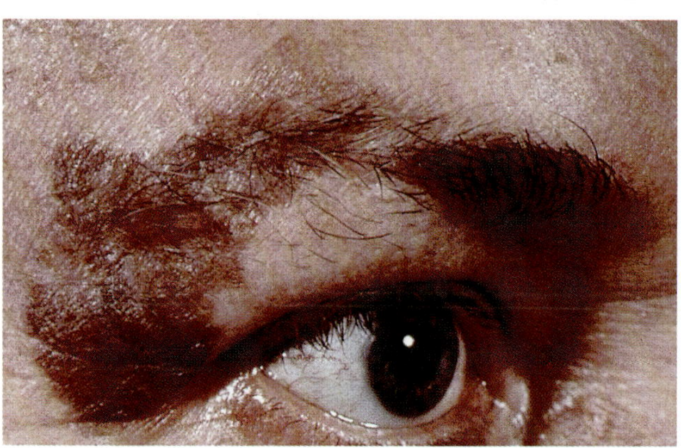

FIGURE 19-83. Superficial spreading melanoma of the eyelid. (Courtesy of Dr. Robert T. Brodell.)

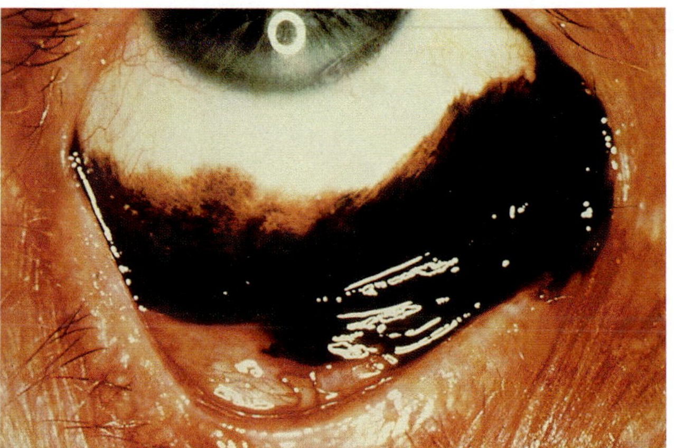

FIGURE 19-84. Malignant melanoma of the conjunctiva and eyelid. Note the extension of pigmentation from the conjunctiva onto the eyelid margin (Hutchinson sign).

20

SOFT TISSUE TUMORS

NODULAR FASCIITIS (PROLIFERATIVE FASCIITIS)

Nodular fasciitis (proliferative fasciitis) occurs at any age but is most common in young children. There is no sexual predilection. It arises from a benign reactive proliferation of fibroblasts but appears to grow rapidly, simulating a sarcoma. Lesions are most common in the forearm but occur anywhere, including the mouth and orbit. They present as rapidly growing, tender masses deep to the skin that also occasionally involve the skin.

FIBROSARCOMA

Fibrosarcomas occur at any age and are often found in scars of lupus vulgaris following treatment with intensive radiation and in tertiary syphilis, burns, and xeroderma pigmentosum. They occur anywhere on the body but are less common on the trunk. They are smooth, reddish or purple, firm, relatively slow-growing nodules that eventually ulcerate. Superficial lesions are sometimes pedunculated. Occasionally, they feel fluctuant because of hemorrhage or necrosis. Metastases are common.

EMBRYONAL RHABDOMYOSARCOMA

Most embryonal rhabdomyosarcomas occur in children but may be seen into adolescence. They present as a painless swelling, usually in the head and neck regions, but especially in the orbit, nasopharynx, or nose and occasionally in the soft part of the extremities and the retroperitoneum. Nasal lesions may cause epistaxis or difficulty breathing through the nose. Orbital involvement causes proptosis and lid swelling, and has been seen on the bulbar surface. The lesions readily metastasize to regional lymph nodes and to distant sites. Local spread is also common.

PYOGENIC GRANULOMA

Pyogenic granulomas are common and usually represent a reactive lesion to an injury. Their color varies from bright red to brownish-red or blue-black. They are highly vascular and bleed readily after minor trauma. The surface is smooth and intact in early lesions, whereas in older lesions, it becomes eroded, and crusted. They may be pedunculated or verrucous in appearance. Often there is a collarette at the base of the lesion (Fig. 20-1).

Pyogenic granulomas are more common in children and during pregnancy (Fig. 20-2). They are most often seen on fingers (Fig. 20-1), hands, lips, and upper trunk but may also occur in the mouth, conjunctiva (Fig. 20-3), eyelid (Fig. 20-4), and perianal area. The lesions often develop within a few days to weeks. There are no symptoms other than recurrent bleeding. Palpebral lesions are not uncommon following spontaneous drainage of a chalazion, and bulbar lesions may be seen after any conjunctival surgery, but especially after pterygium removal. Corneal involvement has been described following penetrating keratoplasty.

KAPOSI SARCOMA

Since its original description by Moritz Kaposi in 1872, Kaposi sarcoma has been divided into five subtypes.

Classic Kaposi Sarcoma

Seen mainly in middle-aged to elderly men of southern and eastern European extraction and (in New York City) in Galician Jews. This type usually presents with reddish or violaceous macules or patches on the feet (Fig. 20-5). The course is indolent with coalescence of lesions and rarely is the cause of death.

African Cutaneous Kaposi Sarcoma

African cutaneous Kaposi sarcoma, an endemic form of Kaposi sarcoma, is seen primarily in young to middle-aged men in tropical Africa. It presents as nodules and vascular infiltrates primarily on the extremities, and though locally aggressive, pursues an indolent course.

African Lymphadenopathic Kaposi Sarcoma

African lymphadenopathic Kaposi sarcoma is an aggressive form of Kaposi sarcoma often resulting in death within several years. Lymph nodes are frequently involved with or without skin lesions. It may be seen in Banta children with markedly enlarged lymph nodes, especially cervical. Massive hemorrhagic tissue may hang down from eyelids with swelling of the lacrimal, parotid, and submandibular glands.

AIDS-Associated Kaposi Sarcoma

About 29% of patients with AIDS may develop or present with Kaposi sarcoma. Skin lesions begin as small, pale, erythematous macules most often on the trunk (Fig. 20-6), head, neck, or extremities; they rapidly progress to firm, violaceous papules (Fig. 20-7) and nodules (Fig. 20-8). Kaposi sarcoma lesions at times follow skin lines (Fig. 20-9) and may have a bruiselike or contusiform appearance (Fig. 20-9). Mucosal lesions are common and may be the initial and only Kaposi sarcoma lesions found. The palate (Fig. 20-10), gums (Fig. 20-11), and tongue (Fig. 20-12) may be involved. Late lesions of Kaposi sarcoma may be extensive, with lymphatic obstruction leading to edema of feet and legs (Fig. 20-13) and scrotum (Fig. 20-14).

The course of AIDS-related Kaposi sarcoma before the advent of highly active retroviral therapy (HART) was often rapidly progressive with systemic involvement, especially of the gastrointestinal tract as well as the lungs, liver, heart, adrenal glands, abdominal lymph nodes, and conjunctivae. Bone involvement suggests a poor prognosis.

Both AIDS-related and classic Kaposi sarcomas have been linked to the presence of human herpes virus 8.

Immunosuppression-Related Kaposi Sarcoma

Skin lesions seen in immunosuppression-related Kaposi sarcoma, a less common form of Kaposi sarcoma, are similar to those seen in classic Kaposi sarcoma.

Ocular Features

Kaposi sarcoma may involve the skin of the entire eyelid (Fig. 20-15). Occasionally, the lesion ulcerates and becomes secondarily infected, causing a severe blepharoconjunctivitis. Infrequently, it causes massive lid swelling with entropion and trichiasis. It involves the conjunctiva in about 10% of patients. The lesion usually begins in the conjunctival fornix and resembles a subconjunctival hemorrhage (Fig. 20-16). As it enlarges, the tumor gains in bulk and may then cause discomfort.

GRANULAR CELL MYOBLASTOMA (ABRIKOSSOFF TUMOR)

A granular cell myoblastoma (Abrikossoff tumor) is an uncommon, slow-growing, reactive lesion. It usually occurs during the third to fifth decade. The lesion is usually solitary and involves the skin, tongue, and deeper areas of the body, such as the bronchus.

Skin Features

The skin lesions are deep, firm, and rounded, and have indistinct margins. They are sometimes pedunculated. The color varies from pink to grayish-brown. The overlying epithelium is occasionally thickened or ulcerated.

Ocular Features

Ocular areas of involvement include the lacrimal sac and orbit.

BENIGN LYMPHOCYTIC INFILTRATION OF JESSNER-KANOF

Benign lymphocytic infiltration of Jessner-Kanof is an uncommon benign condition that represents a chronic T-cell infiltrative skin disorder. It is characterized by smooth, red, raised, firm nodules or plaques on the face or exposed areas of skin. The lesions sometimes resolve spontaneously but more commonly persist and gradually increase in numbers, especially during the winter months. They occasionally burn or itch but are usually asymptomatic.

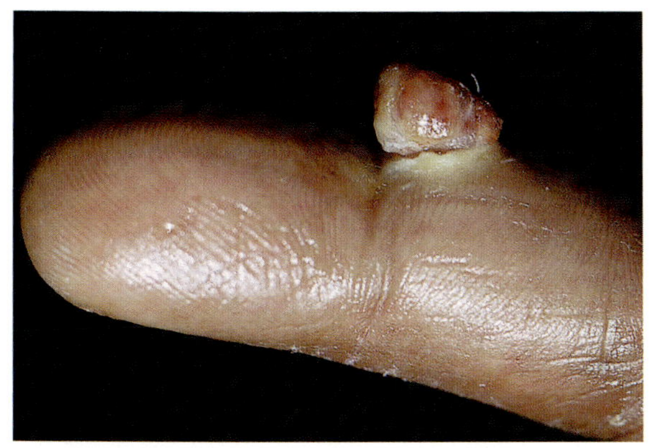

FIGURE 20-1. Pyogenic granuloma of finger. Note typical collarette at base.

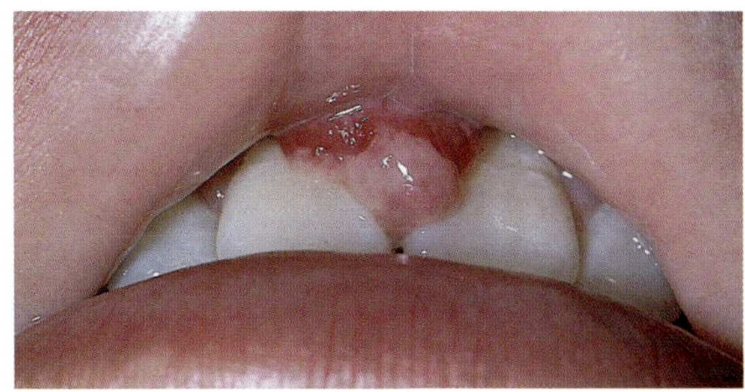

FIGURE 20-2. Pyogenic granuloma of the gingival occurring during pregnancy (also called *granuloma gravidarum* or *epulis*). The patient developed this lesion during the second trimester of her pregnancy.

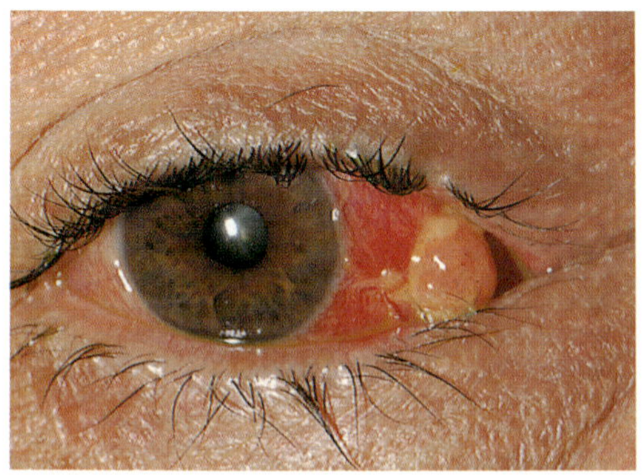

FIGURE 20-3. Pyogenic granuloma of the conjunctiva.

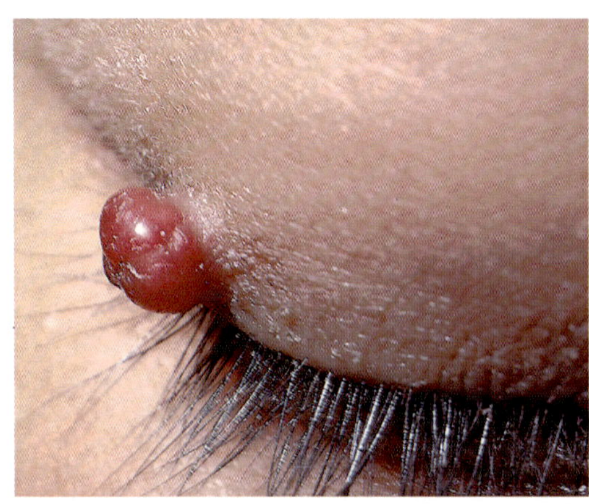

FIGURE 20-4. Pyogenic granuloma of the eyelid.

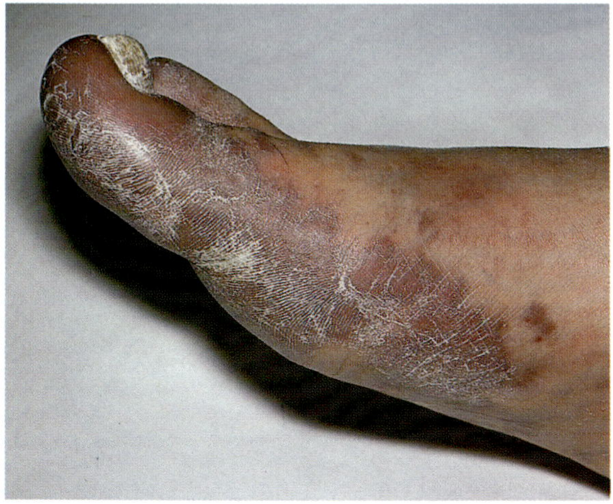

FIGURE 20-5. Kaposi hemorrhagic sarcoma of the foot. A 75-year-old man without evidence of AIDS.

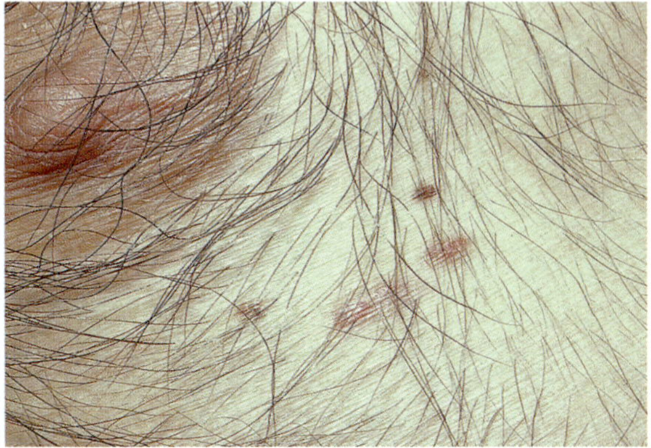

FIGURE 20-6. Early cutaneous lesions of AIDS-related Kaposi sarcoma showing small, pale, erythematous macules.

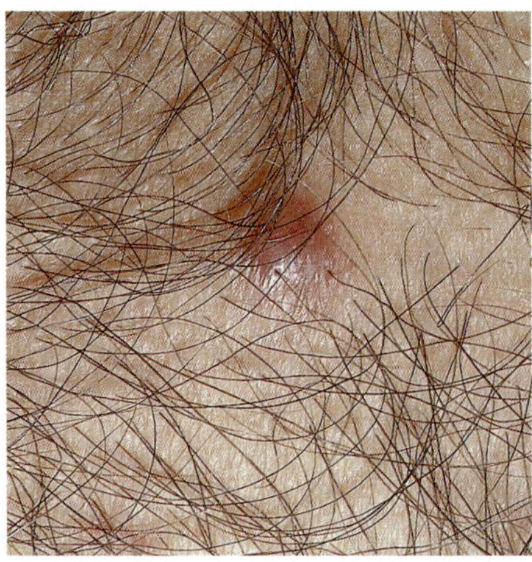

FIGURE 20-7. Small, solitary, pale, erythematoviolaceous papule of Kaposi sarcoma. This insignificant-appearing lesion could easily be overlooked or dismissed as a benign nevus.

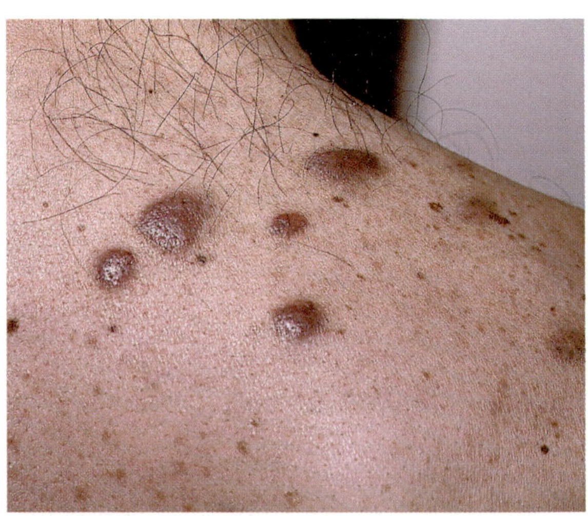

FIGURE 20-8. Firm, violaceous nodules of Kaposi sarcoma.

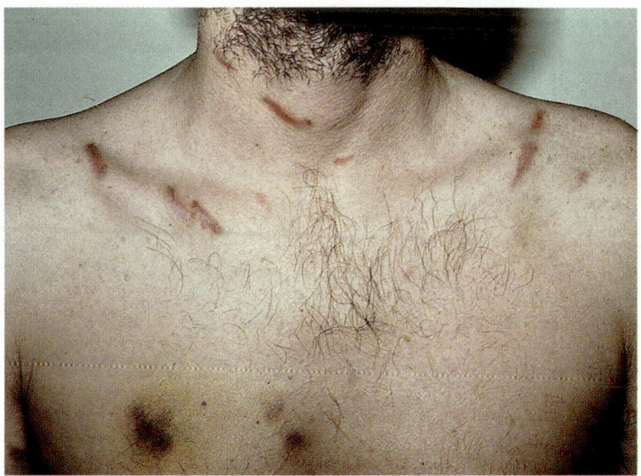

FIGURE 20-9. Kaposi sarcoma lesions showing the often noted pattern following skin lines as well as the contusiform appearance.

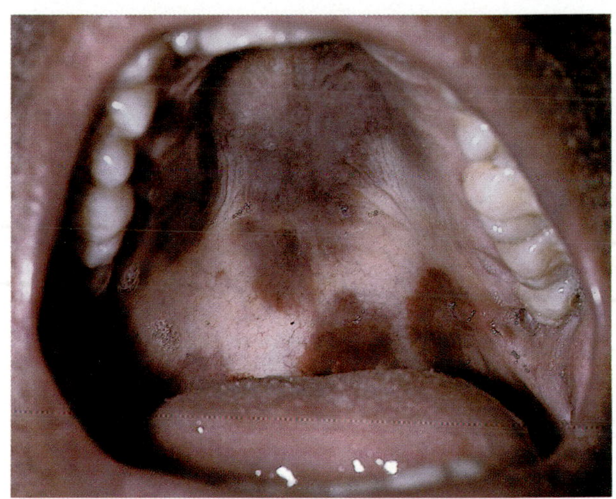

FIGURE 20-10. Kaposi sarcoma of palate. A frequent and early site.

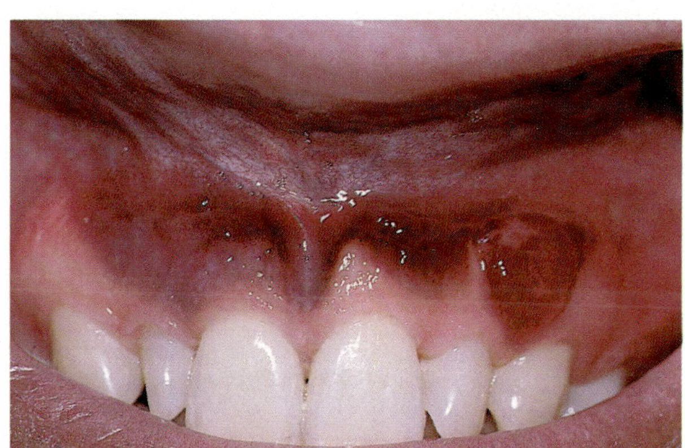

FIGURE 20-11. Kaposi sarcoma of gums. (Courtesy of Sol Silverman, D.D.S., School of Dentistry, University of California, San Francisco.)

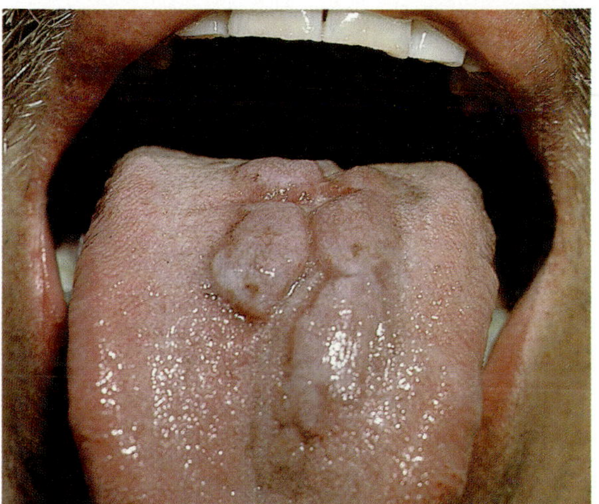

FIGURE 20-12. Kaposi sarcoma of tongue.

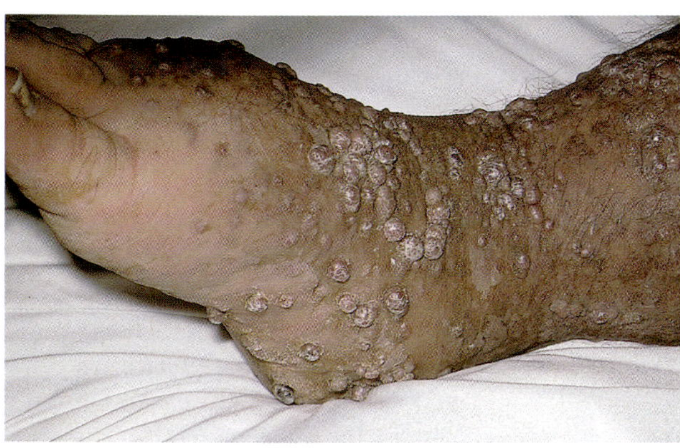

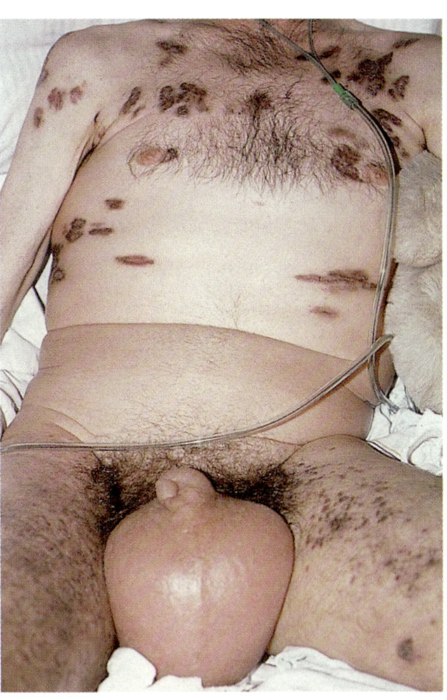

FIGURE 20-13. Lymphedema and multiple modules of late Kaposi sarcoma. Differential diagnosis was bacillary angiomatosis in this patient with AIDS.

FIGURE 20-14. Multiple Kaposi sarcoma lesions in a patient with advanced AIDS. Lymphatic obstruction led to painful lymphedema of legs and scrotum. Partial temporary improvement followed treatment with vincristine.

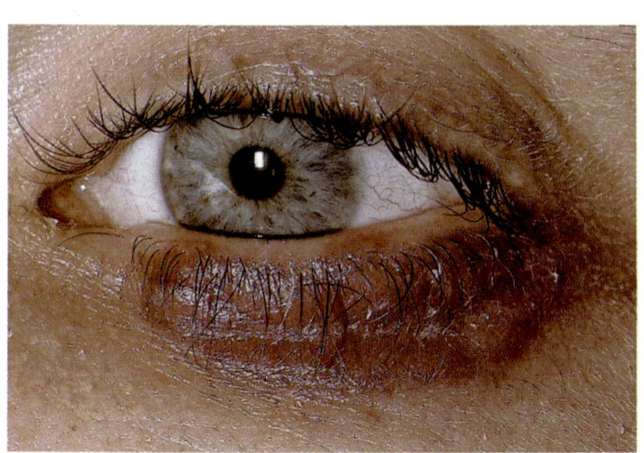

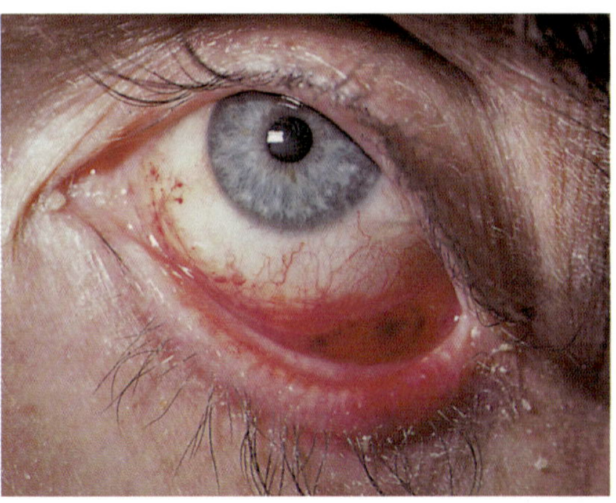

FIGURE 20-15. Kaposi sarcoma of eyelid in a patient with AIDS.

FIGURE 20-16. Kaposi sarcoma of conjunctiva and lid margin in a patient with AIDS.

21

HEMATOLOGIC DISORDERS

DISSEMINATED INTRAVASCULAR COAGULATION

Disseminated intravascular coagulation (DIC), a complex acquired syndrome, is caused by formation of fibrin thrombi throughout the body, but especially in the skin, brain, lungs, heart, spleen, liver, kidneys, and adrenal glands. The thrombi are triggered by production or release of procoagulant substances (e.g., amniotic fluid, tissue thromboplastin) into the bloodstream. It arises following abortion attempts, bacterial septicemia, massive tissue injury, and reactions to various drugs and snake venom.

The procoagulant substances induce a cascade of reactions, which leads to a hypocoagulative state. The reactions include the following:

1. Intravascular thrombus formation leads to thrombocytopenia through consumption of platelets.
2. Plasminogen binds to fibrin to form the active enzyme plasmin.
3. Plasmin consumes various clotting factors and degrades fibrinogen and fibrin to form fibrinogen–fibrin split products.
4. Plasmin has a fibrinolytic action.

The disease develops suddenly, causing the following:

1. Hemorrhage, especially gastrointestinal bleeding from mucosal ulceration.
2. Shock, which is often much more severe than expected from the amount of blood loss.
3. Skin hemorrhages with patches of hemorrhagic necrosis (Fig. 21-1).
4. Central nervous system damage characterized by convulsions or coma.
5. Pulmonary damage from interstitial hemorrhage with findings of an acute respiratory distress syndrome.
6. Renal damage with hematuria, oliguria, or anuria.
7. Hemorrhagic necrosis of the adrenal cortex with findings of Waterhouse–Friderichsen syndrome.

Ocular Features

The ocular features include bleeding into the conjunctiva, iris, anterior chamber, and vitreous; choroidal vessel occlusion with patchy loss of the choroidal pattern (presenting as gray, yellow, or reddish-brown areas); and, rarely, serous retinal detachment.

THE LEUKEMIAS

The leukemias represent proliferation of abnormal hematopoietic cells that are unresponsive or poorly responsive to normal regulation, have a decreased ability to differentiate normally, and possess the ability to proliferate at the expense of normal cell lines. They are classified according to the stem cells (i.e., myeloid leukemias arise from myeloid stem cells, and lymphocytic leukemias arise from lymphocytic stem cells) and according to their presentation and behavior (i.e., acute or chronic). The diagnosis of the type of leukemia depends on the findings in the peripheral blood and bone marrow.

Acute Leukemia

Clinical Manifestations

Untreated acute leukemia leads to death within a short period of time (Fig. 21-2). In the acute leukemias, thrombocytopenic purpura of the skin or mucous membranes is common.

Anemia

The pallor, asthenia, headache, tinnitus, dyspepsia, angina, edema, and congestive heart failure that these patients often exhibit arise from the anemia.

Hemorrhage

Coagulation disorders are often the initial manifestation of acute leukemia. Epistaxis, oozing gums, prolonged bleeding following tooth extraction, ecchymosis, petechiae, melena, and gross hematuria may occur.

Infections

Prolonged upper respiratory infections, sinusitis, bronchitis, dental infections, urinary tract infections, skin infections, and paronychia are common early manifestations. Acute leukemia also causes fever of unknown origin.

Infiltration

Lymphadenopathy, splenomegaly, and hepatomegaly develop from cellular infiltration. Other manifestations include bulging interdental papillae and bone tumefaction.

Myelocytic Leukemia

Clinical Manifestations

Patients with chronic myelocytic leukemia usually experience an insidious onset of fatigue, anorexia, and weight loss. Sometimes there is a feeling of heaviness or fullness in the right upper quadrant of the abdomen. Infrequently, there are symptoms of anemia, hemorrhage, thrombosis, gout, or abdominal pain.

Infiltration

Splenomegaly is common, and frequently the spleen is very large.

Chronic Lymphocytic Leukemia

Clinical Manifestations

About one-fourth of patients with chronic lymphocytic leukemia have no symptoms. Other patients experience malaise, easy fatigability, complicating infections, bleeding diathesis, and unexplained fever.

Skin Features of Leukemia

The skin lesions in leukemia are usually nonspecific and are caused by the associated anemia, thrombocytopenia, infections, or drugs. They include generalized pruritus; prurigo-like papules; erythroderma; marked thickening of the skin, especially over the face; disseminated herpes zoster infections; bullous lesions; and anhidrosis.

Specific skin lesions (leukemia cutis) are uncommon but occasionally occur in monocytic leukemia and rarely in other forms of leukemia. They appear as asymptomatic, small, firm, light red, brown, or violaceous macules and nodules. Sometimes they develop rapidly and spontaneously regress. The gums are infiltrated in about one-fourth to one-half of the patients.

In chronic lymphatic leukemia, skin ulcerations around the ankles are occasionally found. Leukemids in the form of scattered papules or vesicles may be found, and herpes zoster infections are more frequent than in normal patients.

Ocular Features

The ocular features of the various leukemias are similar. They are more common in the acute form and may persist until death. In chronic leukemias, the ocular findings frequently resolve before death. They include the following:

1. Infiltrates and hemorrhages in the lids and conjunctiva. The limbal epibulbar tissue infrequently becomes slightly thickened, then develops gelatinous yellow or flesh-colored nodules.
2. Peripheral corneal ulcers (acute myelogenous leukemia) and peripheral corneal infiltrates and corneal edema (chronic myelomonocytic leukemia).
3. Gelatinous yellow or flesh-colored nodules near the emissary vessels of the sclera.
4. Proptosis, extraocular muscle palsy, and an orbital mass (acute leukemias).
5. Iritis is uncommon, although tumor necrosis in the posterior segment may cause a cell and flare.
6. Choroidal thickening that is often unrecognized during life.
7. Retinal changes (Fig. 21-3). The retinal findings in both acute and chronic leukemia include retinal hemorrhages (flame-shaped, striate, round, preretinal, white-centered, and subretinal); periphlebitis; abnormal color changes in the retinal vessels reflecting increased white cells; vascular sheathing; tortuous, dilated, and irregular veins; soft cotton-wool and hard, yellow exudates in the posterior pole; proliferative retinopathy and retinal detachment.
8. Massive vitreous hemorrhages.
9. Other findings, including glaucoma, papilledema, and involvement of the 3rd, 4th, 6th, 7th, and occasionally the 5th cranial nerves.

Hodgkin Disease

Hodgkin disease is a malignant neoplasm that primarily affects the lymph nodes and spleen.

Skin Features

Specific skin lesions of Hodgkin disease are uncommon but usually appear as small scalp nodules or ulcerative lesions. Nonspecific skin lesions occur in up to 50% of cases and include the following:

1. Increased melanin pigmentation that is generalized or may appear in the axilla, groin, or around the nipples.
2. Pruritus, which may be the presenting symptom and usually begins in the legs and then spreads upward (Fig. 21-4).
3. Prurigo, which usually occurs on the trunk and often leads to excoriations with bleeding and crusting.
4. Ichthyosiform atrophy, characterized by thin, dry scales along with red streaks that are found on the legs or may be generalized. Erythroderma and exfoliative dermatitis may also be seen and are probably part of ichthyosiform atrophy.
5. Alopecia resulting from itching and scratching, endocrine changes, specific scalp infiltration, or occurring as part of the ichthyosiform atrophy.

6. Herpes zoster that sometimes generalizes (Fig. 21-5).

B-Cell Lymphoma

Skin Features

B-cell lymphomas develop at any skin site but are most common on the legs. They appear as multiple cutaneous, deep-seated nodules and sometimes ulcerate. The nodules may be associated with lymph node, spleen, or liver involvement.

DYSPROTEINEMIA

Multiple Myeloma (Plasmacytoma)

Multiple myeloma (plasmacytoma) or plasma cell myeloma represents a malignant neoplasm caused by unchecked growth of a single clone of plasma cells. It usually occurs after the age of 30. The manifestations include the following:

1. Increased susceptibility to infection.
2. Hyperviscosity that often causes widespread circulatory disturbances (following exposure to cold because of erythrocyte aggregation in the presence of cold agglutinins) and obstruction of vessels of the hands and feet in the presence of cryoglobulinemia.
3. Renal findings of glomerulonephritis, tubular atrophy, and glomerulosclerosis.
4. Peripheral neuropathy.
5. Osteolytic lesions of the skull, vertebrae, and ribs with severe bone pain and pathologic fractures.
6. Hypercalcemia, which may lead to nausea, vomiting, somnolence, thirst, and polyuria.

Skin Features

Multiple myeloma skin lesions present as small, red tumors (Fig. 21-6). Acral cyanosis, livedo reticularis, or purpura may occur in patients with cryoglobulinemia. Cutaneous necrosis of the acral regions may occur in the presence of cold agglutinins.

Ocular Features

Sludging of red blood cells in the conjunctival vessels occasionally occurs and arises from hyperviscosity. It is intensified by application of an ice bag over the eyelids for a few minutes before examination. Conjunctival and corneal crystals (Fig. 21-7). Numerous delicate, scintillating crystals may sometimes be seen in the conjunctiva and cornea representing immunoglobulin deposition. The crystals in the cornea are concentrated in the anterior stroma or are interspersed throughout the corneal stroma. Band keratopathy may occur from hypercalcemia.

Proptosis, diplopia, and visual loss occasionally occur early in the disease process from orbital bone and orbital cavity involvement. Osteolytic lesions of the orbital bones may also occur.

Other findings include scintillating crystals in the lens; choroidal tumors and infiltrates; retinal vascular tortuosity, engorgement, exudates, hemorrhages, and venous thrombosis; and secondary glaucoma.

Waldenström Macroglobulinemia

Waldenström macroglobulinemia is a chronic neoplastic disease of the reticuloendothelial system. It usually occurs in males over the age of 50, is characterized by excessive IgM production, and usually involves the lymph nodes, bone marrow, liver, and spleen.

Most of the clinical manifestations are caused by blood hyperviscosity. Nonspecific symptoms include weakness, fatigability, malaise, anorexia, fever, weight loss, and recurrent infections.

Clinical Manifestations

Manifestations include recurrent epistaxis, bleeding from the oral mucosa, hematuria, hematemesis, melena, a history of prolonged postoperative bleeding, hemolytic anemia, and hepatosplenomegaly.

The cardiovascular findings include recurrent episodes of congestive heart failure, dyspnea, and hypervolemia.

Renal abnormalities occur in about one-third of patients.

Neurologic findings are seen in about one-fourth of patients and comprise headaches, paresthesias, dizziness, vertigo, somnolence, stupor, nystagmus, generalized seizures, and coma.

Skin Features

Acral cyanosis, livedo reticularis, or purpura may occur from the cryoglobulins. Lymphadenopathy and pallor are common.

Ocular Features

The ocular findings include the following:

1. Nonspecific sludging of blood in the conjunctival vessels and iridescent crystals scattered throughout the superficial epithelial layers of the bulbar conjunctiva.
2. Discrete iridescent crystals in the superficial layers of the corneal stroma and widespread amorphous deposits in the deeper corneal stroma. The deposits are both peripheral and central.
3. Retinal findings of bilateral tortuous segmented veins, flame-shaped hemorrhages, beading of the retinal veins,

cotton-wool exudates, venous occlusions, low-grade papilledema, microaneurysms, neovascularization, macular degeneration, retinal detachment, and vitreous hemorrhages.

4. Cellular infiltration and enlargement of the lacrimal glands and a hemianopsia may occur from lymphocytic and plasma cell infiltration into the occipital lobe.

T-CELL LYMPHOMAS

Mycosis Fungoides

Mycosis fungoides (MF) has a variable rate of progression and is characterized by formation of skin papules, plaques, nodules, ulcerated tumors, and infrequently, disseminated disease with symptoms of fever, fatigue, and weight loss. In some patients, the disease presents as an erythroderma (Figs. 21-8 and 21-9) or arcuate plaques (Fig. 21-10), which may ulcerate, whereas indurated tumors usually occur late in the disease (Fig. 21-11). Most patients develop erythematous oval or circular plaques, which are covered with fine scales in covered areas, such as the buttocks. The plaques usually gradually enlarge to cover large areas of skin; occasionally, they partially involute, leading to polycyclic plaques; other times, they remain stationary or occasionally disappear.

Infrequently, patients develop poikiloderma, instead of plaques or nodules, that is characterized by alternating increased and decreased pigmentation and epidermal atrophy. It is usually widespread and such lesions may precede MF by many years (Fig. 21-12).

Follicular mucinosis (alopecia mucinosa) may occur anywhere on the skin, but usually develops on the scalp and face. It is characterized by a boggy swelling, a sticky discharge from the hair follicles, loss of hair, and hair follicle atrophy (Fig. 21-13).

Lymph node involvement is common, and in some instances there is peripheral blood involvement.

Ocular Features

Ocular lesions may appear as solitary or multiple lid tumors, single tumors of the conjunctiva, caruncle, cornea, or orbit. Small iris tumors have been seen, and involvement of the choroid, vitreous, and retina with retinal hemorrhage and edema may occur. Mycoses fungoides develops rapidly in some patients, producing erythroderma. Pruritus, burning, and pain are common symptoms (Fig. 21-14).

Sézary Syndrome

Sézary syndrome usually occurs in elderly males and is characterized by generalized erythroderma, lymphadenopathy (Fig. 21-15), and hyperkeratosis of the palms and soles. Pruritus is often very severe and constant. The peripheral

blood contains at least 10% atypical mononuclear cells. Sézary syndrome has a more fulminating course than ordinary mycosis fungoides, with death in 5 to 7 years. The skin lesions in Sézary syndrome often meet the criterion of mycosis fungoides histologically and clinically before development of erythroderma.

THE HISTIOCYTOSES

The Histiocytic Society suggests dividing the histiocytoses into three classes based on the predominant cell and the presence of malignancy.

Class I = Langerhans cell histiocytosis, which includes histiocytosis X, eosinophilic granuloma, Letterer–Siwe disease, Hand–Schüller–Christian syndrome, and Hashimoto–Pritzker disease.

Class II = Histiocytoses of mononuclear phagocytes other than Langerhans cells.

Class III = Malignant histiocytic diseases that includes all the malignant histiocytic diseases.

Class I Histiocytosis

Langerhans Cell Histiocytosis

Patients with Langerhans cell histiocytosis (LCD) often have single organ involvement, including bone and skin, whereas others have multisystem disease. The disease is therefore variable in presentation. The etiology of LCD is unknown, but it appears to represent a reactive condition.

Many patients complain of fever, malaise, and weight loss, and children usually fail to thrive and may not develop physically, mentally, or sexually.

The most frequent manifestation of LCD is swelling of a bone, especially the calvaria, ribs, vertebrae, pelvis, scapula, or long bones. The lesions are osteolytic, solitary, or multiple and may be painful or tender. Soft-tissue swelling often develops in areas of bone destruction of the skull and may be completely painless. In some instances bone marrow involvement causes pancytopenia.

Focal involvement at the base of the skull may involve the cranial nerves with loss of taste or cause symptoms of a brain tumor or diabetes insipidus. Focal cerebellar lesions or lesions of the temporal lobe and occipital lobe may also occur.

Less common findings include cough, dyspnea, chest pain, hepatomegaly, ascites, and cholestatic jaundice.

Skin Features

The scalp skin is often erythematous and has greasy scales, suggesting seborrheic dermatitis (Fig. 21-16). Trunk lesions appear as discrete yellow-brown scaly papules often associated with purpura (Fig. 21-17). Sometimes the lesions become nodular, crusted, and eroded. In adults, the flexural creases, groin, and perianal area may ulcerate.

The Hashimoto–Pritzker variant of LCD occurs in the neonate and is characterized by a generalized eruption of nodular lesions resembling chickenpox. The eruption includes the palms and soles.

Skin involvement of the external auditory canal causes persistent discharge or polypoid formation. Gum infiltration may cause destruction of the alveolar ridge and loosening of the teeth. In children, the infiltrate may cause premature tooth eruption; in adults a palpable tender mass may develop in the mandibular arc.

Ocular Features

The ocular features include the following:

1. Focal involvement of the optic nerve or orbit, causing blindness.
2. Lid findings of xanthomatous deposits, especially in adults; a papular eruption in infants; and a yellow or bronze color of the skin of the lid, edema, ecchymosis, and blepharitis.
3. Lipogranulomatous infiltrations appearing as yellow masses in the bulbar and palpebral conjunctiva and cornea.
4. Yellow scleral plaques and a diffuse scleritis in infants.
5. Unilateral or bilateral proptosis from focal orbital deposits. The proptosis is usually downward and may be pulsatile.
6. Limitation of ocular movement from paralysis of the 3rd, 4th, or 6th cranial nerves.
7. Other ocular findings include choroidal infiltrates, retinal hemorrhages and exudates, papilledema or optic atrophy, nystagmus, and internal ophthalmoplegia.

Class II Histiocytosis

Class II histiocytosis comprises a number of heterogeneous diseases that may involve the eye and skin, such as juvenile xanthogranuloma, multicentric reticulohistiocytic granuloma, benign cephalic histiocytosis, familial sea-blue histiocytosis, necrobiotic xanthogranuloma, and xanthoma disseminatum.

Juvenile Xanthogranuloma (Nevoxanthoendothelioma)

Juvenile xanthogranuloma (JXG) (nevoxanthoendothelioma) is a benign histiocytic tumor that usually occurs in white infants and young children (Fig. 21-18). JXG is characterized by rapidly developing single or multiple skin tumors that after a few months or years spontaneously involute, leaving small atrophic scars. They are usually located on the scalp and head, are occasionally located on the neck and upper trunk, or are widely scattered over the body. The lesions begin as small, pinkish papules that gradually become yellow-brown plaques or macules and often have some surface telangiectasis. Satellite lesions may also occur. They feel firm and rubbery and occasionally ulcerate.

Lesions infrequently develop in the deeper soft tissue and visceral organs such as the lung, pericardium, spleen, gastrointestinal tract, liver, testes, and kidney.

Ocular Features

Ocular lesions occur in about 10% of cases and sometimes precede skin involvement. They include the following:

1. Lid lesions (similar to other skin lesions).
2. Corneal xanthogranuloma.
3. Iris lesions (salmon-colored or darkly pigmented solitary lesions or, occasionally, heterochromia). Spontaneous hyphemas frequently accompany iris lesions.
4. Orbital infiltration with sudden proptosis.
5. Episcleral tumors.
6. Secondary glaucoma caused by intraocular hemorrhage or exfoliation of cells from the iris or ciliary body.

Multicentric Reticulohistiocytosis (Giant Cell Histiocytoma)

Multicentric reticulohistiocytosis (giant cell histiocytoma) is a rare reactive histiocytosis of unknown cause that usually occurs in middle-aged women (Fig 21-19). Many patients complain of fever and weight loss. It usually involves the joints, skin, and mucous membranes; typically, arthritis occurs first. It is usually symmetric, erythematous, and deforming, and involves the interphalangeal joints of the hands, leading to shortening and mutilation of the fingers. Other joint involvement includes the temporomandibular joint, vertebrae, shoulders, elbows, wrists, hips, ankles, and feet.

Skin Features
The skin lesions usually develop on the extensor surfaces of the hands and forearms; less frequently, on the scalp, face, and ear; uncommonly, on the trunk and legs. In the 20% to 30% of patients who have an associated internal malignancy, the skin lesions usually precede the diagnosis of malignancy (Fig. 21-19). Pruritus occurs in about one-fourth of patients. The lesions are firm brown or yellow papules and plaques of variable size that seldom ulcerate. Xanthomas also occur in about 30% of patients. Paronychia may develop from the coral beadlike arrangements of the nodules around the nail fold. More than 50% of patients have mucous membrane lesions of the mouth, gingiva, pharynx, or larynx. Other organ involvement includes the bone marrow, lymph nodes, skeletal muscle, heart, lungs, liver, and kidney. Carcinoma of the stomach, ovary, breast, and uterus and lymphomas have been observed in about 30% of patients with multicentric reticulocytosis.

Ocular Features

As many as 30% of patients have xanthelasma of the lid. Sjögren syndrome and scleral involvement may also be found.

Benign Cephalic Histocytosis (Papular Histiocytosis of the Head)

Benign cephalic histiocytosis (papular histiocytosis of the head) is uncommon. It usually develops about the end of the first year of life, beginning as asymptomatic erythematosus macules, papules, or nodules on the cheeks that spread to involve the forehead, ear lobes, and neck. Occasionally, they spread onto the upper extremities, the trunk, and, rarely, the buttocks. Gradually, the lesions become reddish-brown and are self-limited, resolving after a few years.

Diffuse Plane Xanthomatosis (Atypical Xanthoma Disseminatum)

Diffuse plane xanthomatosis (atypical xanthoma disseminatum) is usually associated with paraproteinemia arising from multiple myeloma or a granulocytic or lymphocytic leukemia. It is extremely uncommon and presents with large, flat, plaquelike xanthomatous lesions of the skin of the eyelids, neck, upper trunk, flexures, and buttocks.

Familial Sea-Blue Histocytosis

Familial sea-blue histiocytosis is a rare autosomal recessive disorder and usually becomes manifest in young adults with hepatosplenomegaly and thrombocytopenia. It probably represents a storage disease. Skin lesions appear as irregular, brownish-gray patches on the face, upper chest, and shoulders. Sometimes they are associated with swelling of the eyelids.

Other involved organs include the lungs, gastrointestinal tract, and the central nervous system. Central nervous system involvement causes ataxia, epilepsy, and dementia. White, stippled deposits may be found at the margins of the macula or fovea, and discoloration of the macula may occur. Associated panuveitis has been seen.

Necrobiotic Xanthogranuloma

Necrobiotic xanthogranuloma occurs in older patients and is characterized by reddish-yellow xanthomatous-like lesions of the periocular area, subcutaneous nodules, and xanthomatous plaques on the trunk and extremities, and a paraproteinemia. The lesions usually progress to atrophy and ulceration. Patients frequently have symptoms of fatigue, nausea, vomiting, epistaxis, back pain, and Raynaud phenomenon. Subcutaneous lid nodules may occur and have been observed to extend into the orbit, causing proptosis. Conjunctivitis and uveitis have also been observed.

Xanthoma Disseminatum (Disseminated Anthosiderohistiocytosis)

Xanthoma disseminatum (disseminated anthosiderohistiocytosis) is a rare, histiocytic proliferative disease with lipid deposition occurring secondarily. It is more common in males and is usually found in children and young adults. It is self-limiting.

The skin lesions are discrete, multiple, papular, red-yellow or mahogany-brown papules and nodules that later become confluent. They are distributed symmetrically and occur on the face, trunk, and flexor surfaces of the upper extremities.

Mucous membrane involvement of the pharynx, larynx, and bronchi occurs in about 30% of patients. Meningeal involvement may lead to diabetes insipidus, growth retardation, and epilepsy. Ocular involvement includes the typical skin eruption on the eyelids and conjunctiva. Corneal involvement and yellow scleral plaques are occasionally seen.

Class III Histiocytosis

Class III histiocytosis includes monocytic leukemia (see earlier), malignant histiocytosis, and true histiocytic lymphoma.

SICKLE CELL DISEASE

Sickle cell is an inherited disease, comprising a group of erythrocytic function abnormalities caused by production of abnormal hemoglobin (hemoglobin S and C). The presence of hemoglobin S in red cells—especially if there is anoxia—causes the cell to assume a rigid sickle shape instead of the normally pliable biconcave disk shape. The rigidity of the red cells in turn causes obstruction of small vessels, resulting in further anoxia and more rigidity of the cells.

Patients who are homozygous for hemoglobin S develop sickle cell anemia; patients who are doubly heterozygous for hemoglobin S and hemoglobin C develop sickle-C or -SC disease. Patients carrying a gene for hemoglobin S and a gene for normal hemoglobin develop the sickle trait AS disease.

Systemic Manifestations

Patients with sickle cell anemia have the most severe manifestations. The disease causes a chronic compensated hemolytic anemia, vasoocclusive phenomenon, acute vasoocclusive complications, and chronic organ damage.

Cold, dehydration, infections, and other factors precipitate the vasoocclusive phenomena, which is manifested by acute, often excruciating, pain in the back, chest, extremities, or occasionally, other body areas. The acute vaso-occlusive complications include cerebrovascular accidents, acute chest syndrome, hepatic crisis, acute renal papillary infarction, and priapism.

Sickle cell disease also causes damage to many organ systems, including the skin (chronic ulcers of the lower extremities) (Fig. 21-20), bones (acute infarcts), joints (aseptic necrosis of the head of the femur), kidney (microinfarction of the medulla), and spleen (scarring and loss of function). Other manifestations include increased infections, cholelithiasis, and abnormal growth and development.

Ocular Features

The ocular manifestations are caused by the vaso-occlusion and are most common in the heterozygous state (SC), less common in the homozygous state (SS), and rare in the heterozygous state (AS). They include lid edema arising during the period of crisis, sickling in the conjunctival vessels (conjunctival sickling sign), localized iris atrophy and neovascularization, angioid streaks, and retinal changes, including silver wiring, salmon patch hemorrhages, black sunbursts or black chorioretinal scars, peripheral neovascularization, and peripheral sickle cell retinopathy.

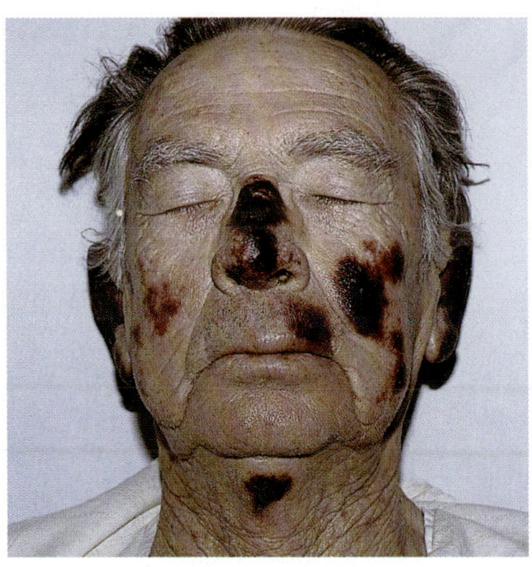

FIGURE 21-1. Disseminated intravascular coagulation (DIC) arising in a patient with carcinoma of the lung. DIC can occasionally be a cutaneous marker of internal malignancy.

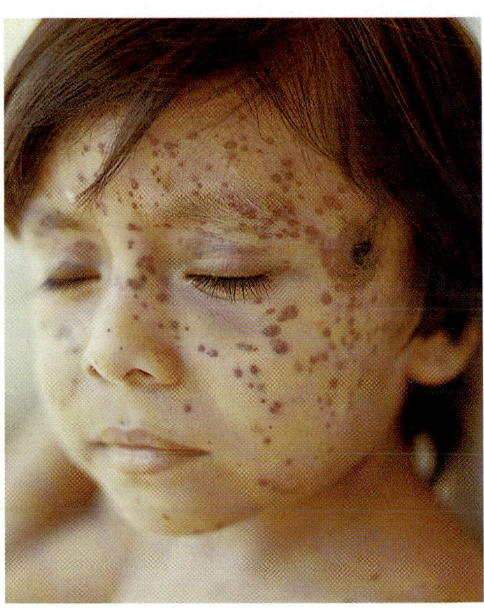

FIGURE 21-2. Thrombocytopenic purpura in a child with acute myelogenous leukemia.

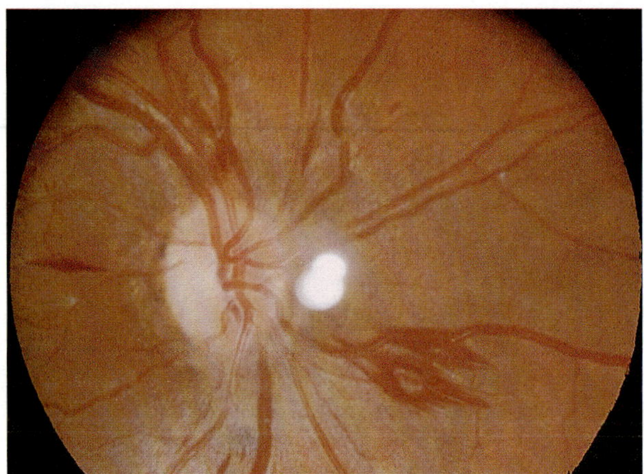

FIGURE 21-3. Retinal findings in acute and chronic leukemia. Retinal hemorrhages with white centers are visible in this fundus photograph of a 30-year-old man with acute myeloblastic leukemia.

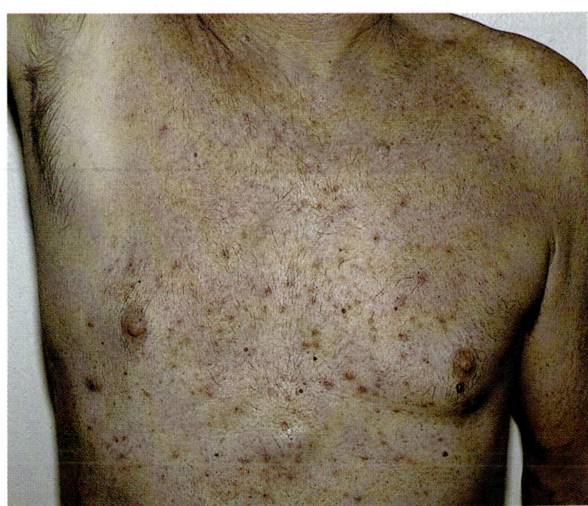

FIGURE 21-4. Hodgkin lymphoma in a 40-year-old man. He had experienced severe generalized itching for 3 or 4 months unresponsive to the usual topical and systemic antipruritics. Note the small excoriated papules that the patient was convinced were due to ectoparasites. Chest x-rays and CT scans were normal, but an abdominal CT scan showed enlarged lymph nodes.

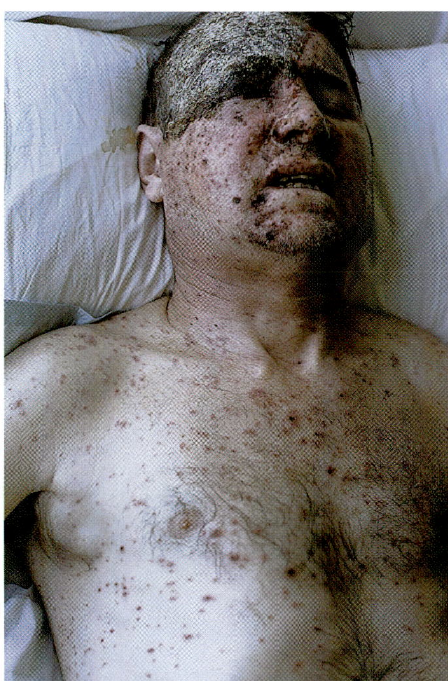

FIGURE 21-5. Severe herpes zoster ophthalmicus with generalized zoster lesions in a patient with terminal Hodgkin lymphoma. Zoster is usually a late manifestation of lymphomas and other malignancies and not a helpful early cutaneous clue of such an illness. Note large right axillary lymph node.

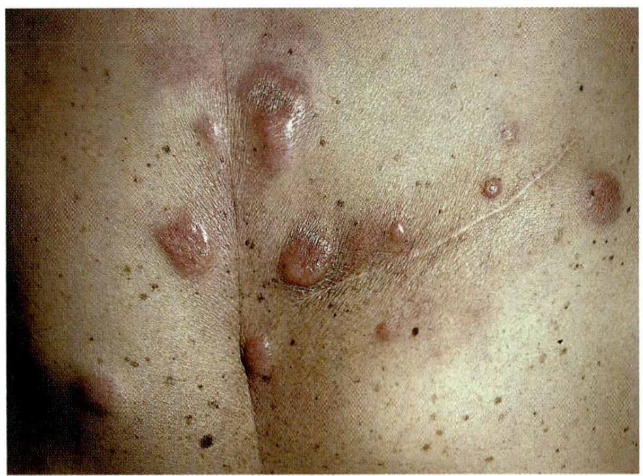

FIGURE 21-6. Cutaneous plasmacytomas appearing by direct spread from underlying multiple myeloma of the bones.

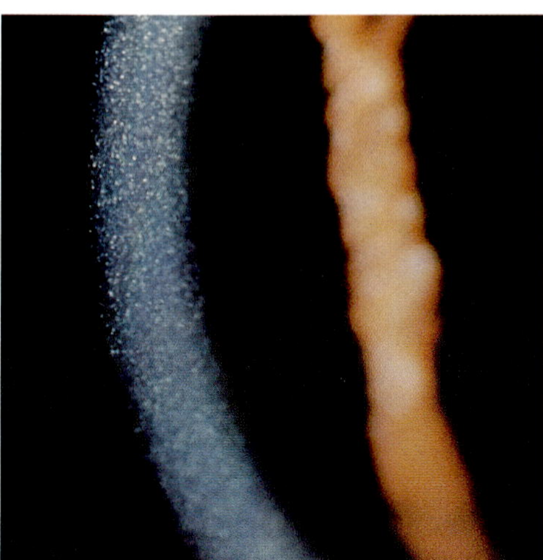

FIGURE 21-7. Scintillating crystals of the cornea in multiple myeloma. The crystals are evident in the parallelepiped produced by the slit lamp. (Courtesy of Dr. Jonathan Belmont.)

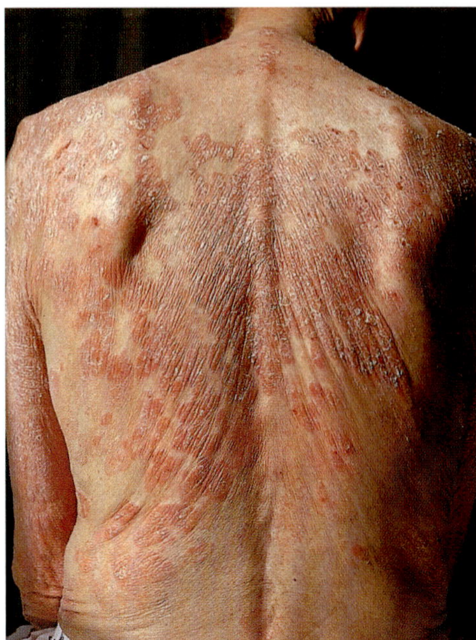

FIGURE 21-8. Mycosis fungoides presenting as pruritic erythematous scaly patches. The patient thought he had psoriasis.

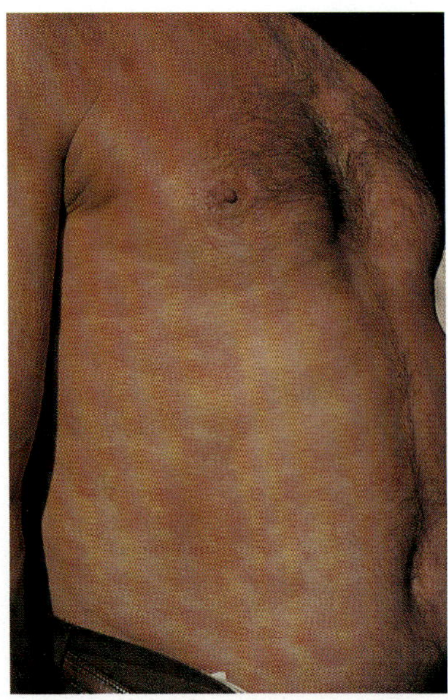

FIGURE 21-9. Mycosis fungoides of the trunk, plaque stage. These indurated erythematous maculopapular lesions were very pruritic. Severe pruritus is an early and common symptom.

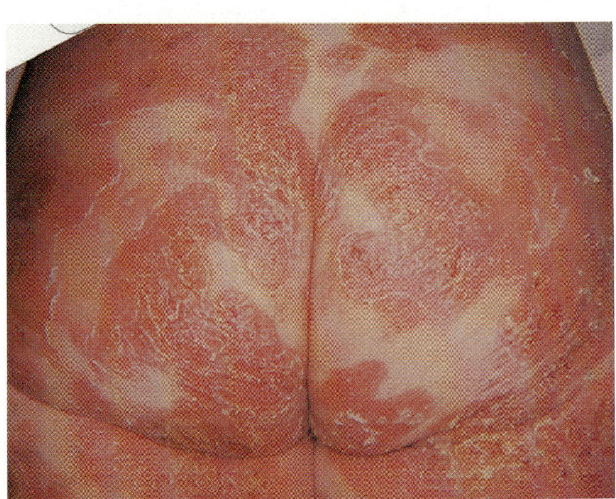

FIGURE 21-10. Erythematous plaques with scaling in mycosis fungoides. The arcuate patterns are highly suggestive of the disease.

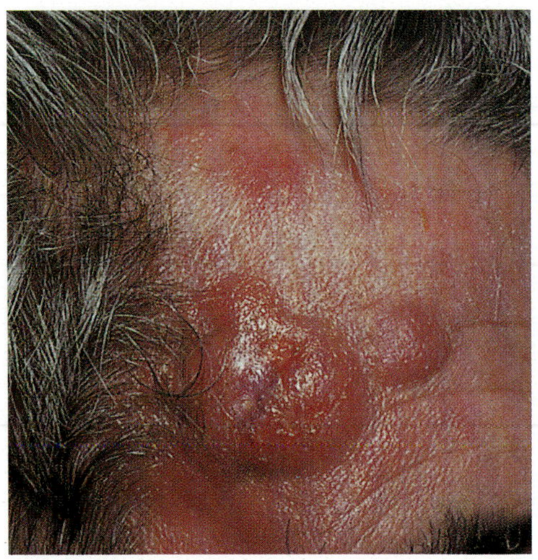

FIGURE 21-11. Mycosis fungoides tumor stage.

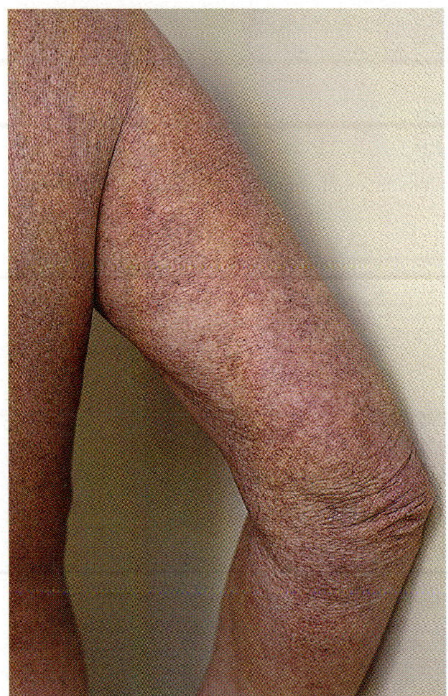

FIGURE 21-12. Poikiloderma characterized by variegated hypopigmentation, atrophy, and telangiectasia may precede mycosis fungoides by many years.

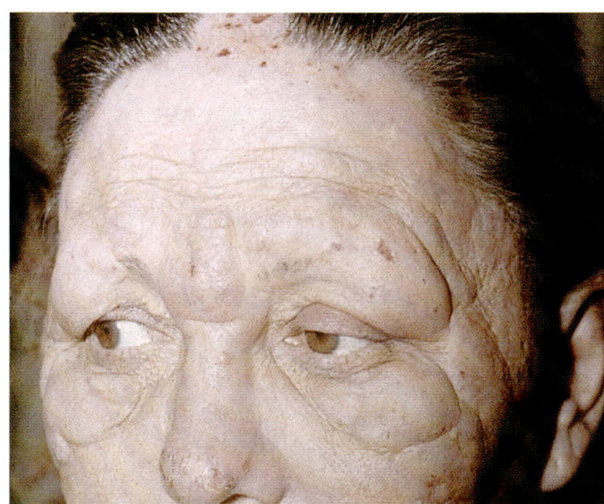

FIGURE 21-13. Alopecia mucinosa. Note boggy infiltration of eyebrows with alopecia. Approximately 30% of adult patients have associated mycosis fungoides. (Courtesy of Dr. Lewis Shapiro.)

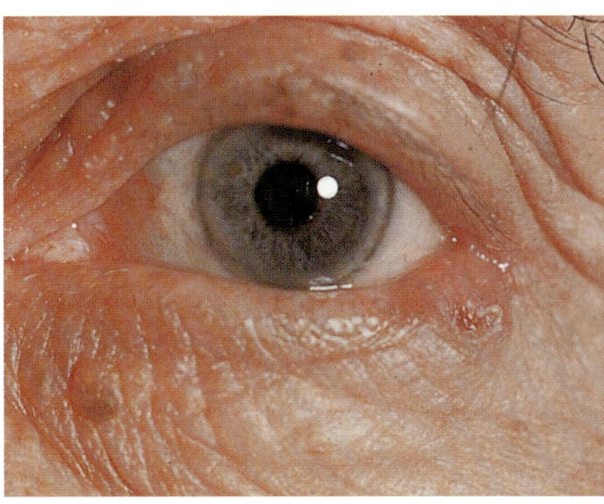

FIGURE 21-14. Mycosis fungoides tumors of eyelid.

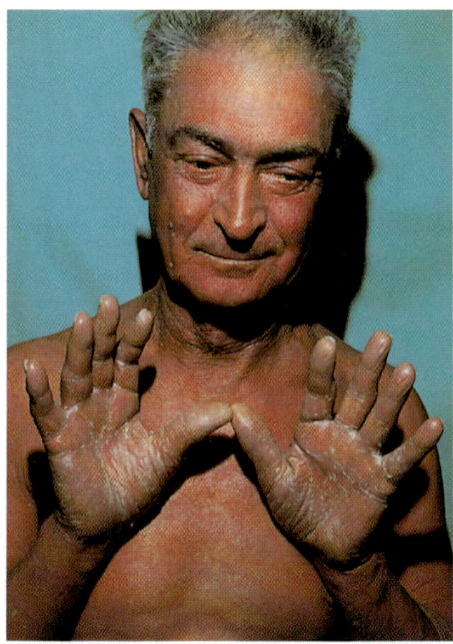

FIGURE 21-15. Erythroderma in Sézary syndrome. Note generalized scaly exfoliative erythroderma and hyperkeratosis of the palms. Years of unrelenting pruritus refractory to multiple therapeutic trials became so unbearable that this patient committed suicide.

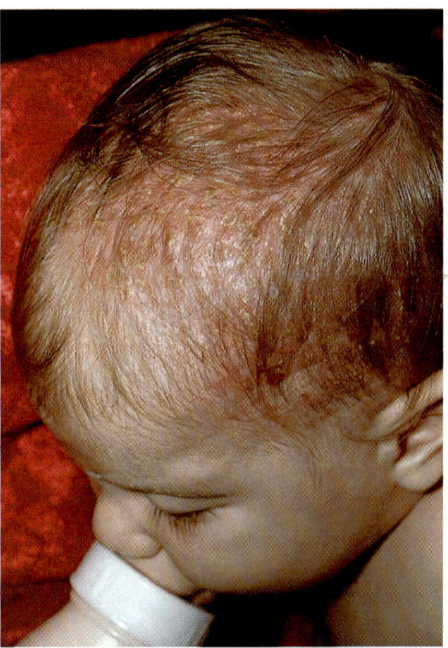

FIGURE 21-16. Letterer–Siwe type of Langerhans cell histiocytosis. This is the most common skin presentation, especially in children, and may be involved with multisystem disease, especially bone. Note the resemblance to seborrheic dermatitis. Careful inspection, however, reveals tiny papules and a slight hemorrhagic component not seen in seborrheic dermatitis. (Courtesy of Dr. Ted van Ravensway.)

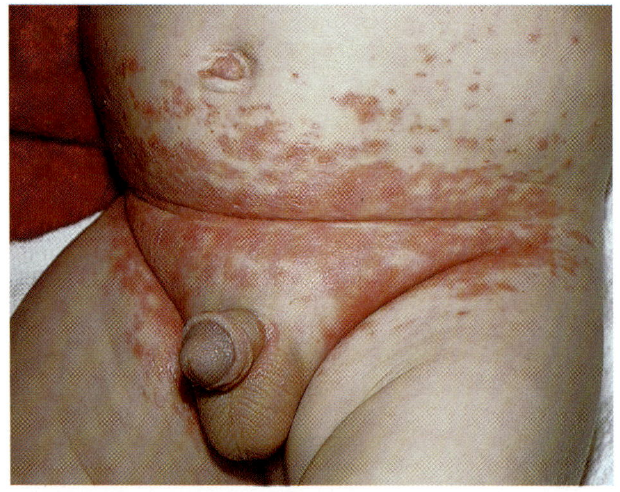

FIGURE 21-17. Letterer–Siwe type of Langerhans cell histiocytosis resembling seborrheic dermatitis. Same patient as shown in Fig. 21-16. (Courtesy of Dr. Ted van Ravensway.)

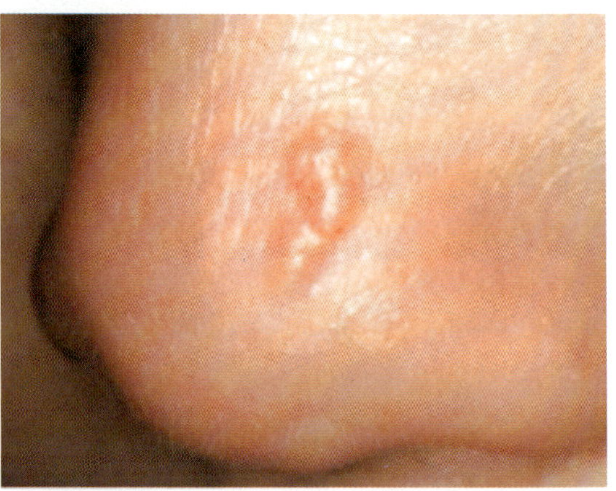

FIGURE 21-18. Nevoxanthoendothelioma of the nose.

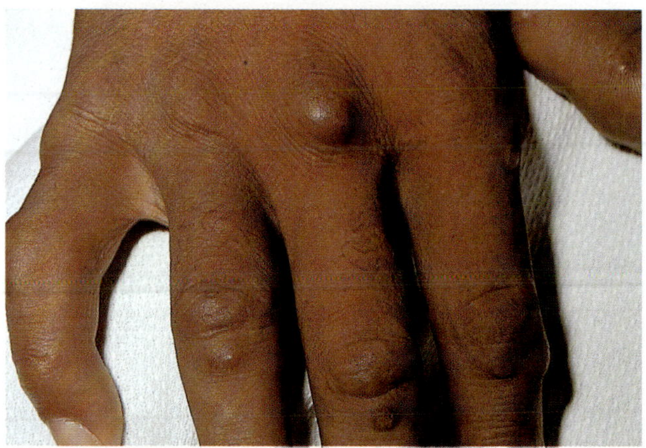

FIGURE 21-19. Multicentric reticulohistiocytosis with flesh-colored, firm cutaneous nodules and moderately severe arthropathy. The previously frequently seen severe arthropathy with telescoping deformities of the digits has been largely prevented by early aggressive treatment.

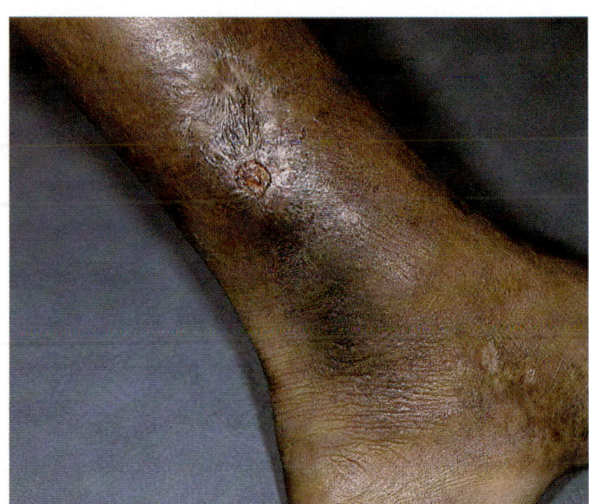

FIGURE 21-20. Chronic painful recurrent ulcers of the lower leg in young teenage Afro-American girls with sickle cell disease.

JOINT DISEASES

RHEUMATOID ARTHRITIS

Rheumatoid arthritis is a chronic systemic disease that primarily affects the synovium of joints but also produces a wide range of clinical findings. During the acute phase, symmetric joint inflammations and effusions often predominate. During the acute and chronic stages, there is soft-tissue inflammation, particularly around joints. In the late stage, fibrous ankylosis occurs. The cause is unknown.

It affects females three times more frequently than males and usually begins between the ages of 20 and 40.

Clinical Manifestations

The onset is usually insidious, with anorexia, weight loss, malaise, fatigue, vasomotor disturbances, low-grade fever, weakness, and equivocal joint findings of stiffness and pain. Occasionally, it begins acutely following stress (e.g., infection, surgery, trauma).

Rheumatoid arthritis may involve any joint (Fig. 22-1). Rheumatoid arthritis characteristically causes symmetric joint involvement manifested by pain, stiffness, and warmth. The stiffness is especially apparent in the morning or following inactivity, then it subsides during the day. Any joint may become inflamed, but the most common are the interphalangeal and metacarpophalangeal finger joints, wrists, knees, ankles, and toes. Early in the disease process, it involves only single joints.

Vasculitis occurs in less than 1% of patients and is of the small-vessel obliterative type, leading to peripheral neuropathy, subcutaneous vasculitis leading to ischemic skin ulceration, or necrotizing vasculitis of the medium and large vessels, similar to that found in polyarteritis nodosa. Neurologic involvement is usually peripheral and is caused by vasculitis or nerve entrapment.

Other organ involvement includes splenomegaly and enlargement of the lymph nodes, nonspecific pericarditis, pleural involvement, and rheumatoid nodules of the myocardium, pericardium, heart valves, lungs, dura mater, larynx, and synovium.

Skin Features

Skin findings include the following:

1. Palmar erythema and tiny hemorrhagic infarcts of the finger pulps and nail folds from vasculitis. The infarcts are characterized by painful hemorrhagic maculopapular lesions. Nail fold involvement is characterized by small, painless, reddish-brown infarcts.
2. Subcutaneous nodules (Fig. 22-2). Subcutaneous nodules occur in about 20% of patients. They are usually located over bony prominences such as the elbow, extensor surface of the forearm, back of the hands, knees, ears, and occasionally, other areas. They are nontender and round or oval. The nodules tend to ulcerate with trauma.
3. Generalized hyperpigmentation.
4. Pyoderma gangrenosum.
5. Mucous membrane involvement is characterized by dryness.

Ocular Features

About 50% of patients have eye involvement. Findings include the following:

1. Keratoconjunctivitis sicca (Fig. 22-3). Keratoconjunctivitis sicca (Sjögren syndrome) is not uncommon in rheumatoid arthritis.
2. Marginal corneal furrows (Fig. 22-4A,B). Corneal furrows are typically located 1 to 2 mm inside of the limbus and usually occur inferiorly.
3. Central areas of corneal thinning and keratolysis.
4. Peripheral corneal infiltrates and neovascularization associated with a necrotizing scleritis.
5. Rheumatoid nodules at the limbus.
6. Less common corneal changes include granular opacities in the deep stroma and a band-shaped keratopathy.
7. Simple or nodular episcleritis (Figs. 22-5 and 22-6). A simple or nodular episcleritis may occur in rheumatoid arthritis. It is sometimes bilateral and recurrent.
8. Scleritis, sclerokeratitis, and necrotizing scleritis (Figs. 22-7 to 22-9) of the anterior or posterior sclera.

Rheumatoid arthritis may be associated with scleritis, sclerokeratitis, necrotizing scleritis with or without inflammation (scleromalacia perforans), and a massive granulomatous reaction of the anterior or posterior sclera.

 9. Scleral rheumatoid nodules (Fig. 22-10).
10. Nongranulomatous iridocyclitis and choroidal effusion associated with the scleritis.
11. Retinal cotton-wool patches.
12. Chronic orbital myositis or tenonitis with lid edema, proptosis, and diplopia.
13. Complicated cataracts.
14. An optic neuritis associated with posterior scleritis.
15. Other ocular findings include transient extraocular muscle paralysis, glaucoma, vitreous opacities, and, sometimes phthisis bulbi.

Felty Syndrome

Felty syndrome (rheumatoid arthritis, splenomegaly, and neutropenia) occurs most frequently in patients with rheumatoid nodules and high levels of rheumatoid factor. Although the arthritis is often inactive, the other features may be found. These patients are more prone to develop bacterial infections and often have hyperpigmentation and chronic leg ulcers.

JUVENILE RHEUMATOID ARTHRITIS

Juvenile rheumatoid arthritis (JRA) is classified into five subgroups, although two of these are very similar and may be the same process. This classification system is based on the age of onset, number of joints involved, serology, and associated symptoms. Occasionally, it is associated with generalized hyperpigmentation.

Still Disease

Still disease accounts for approximately 10% of patients with JRA, and these patients usually have high fever, lymphadenopathy, hepatosplenomegaly, leukocytosis, and anemia. This presentation may occur at any pediatric age, although it tends to occur at less than 5 years of age and may be slightly more common in boys. This syndrome does not always have arthritis, but the arthritis is usually polyarticular when it occurs. Anti-nuclear antibody (ANA) and rheumatoid factor (RF) are usually negative.

Most patients develop a salmon-colored evanescent maculopapular rash on the trunk, extremities, and occasionally, face and neck, characterized by small, nonitching macules or papules with slightly irregular margins. Larger lesions (5 cm or so) have central pallor. The rash lasts only a few hours, appearing at midday or evening, and is associated with increased environmental temperature or fever.

Ocular involvement in this subgroup is uncommon to rare.

Polyarticular Disease—RF Positive

The disease begins at any age and is associated with low-grade fever, malaise, mild anemia, and often growth retardation. Polyarticular disease is defined by the involvement of five or more joints during the first 6 months of the disease and is much more common in girls. The RF is positive and the disease resembles rheumatoid arthritis. The arthritis is usually symmetric, deforming, and persistent. Polyarticular disease accounts for 40% of patients with JRA.

Skin and ocular involvement in this subgroup is uncommon.

Polyarticular Disease—RF Negative

Children with polyarticular disease who are RF negative are generally in more than 10 years of age. Although RF negative, these patients have a severe deforming form of arthritis. There is a characteristic fusion of C2 and C3 vertebrae associated with sacroiliitis and/or spondylitis. This is probably a variant of ankylosing spondylitis (AS), because these patients are HLA-B27 positive. The disease may be associated with HLA-DR4, which is also associated with adult rheumatoid arthritis. These patients have an acute recurrent iridocyclitis in approximately 25% of cases. Skin disease is rare.

Pauciarticular Disease—Young Children

In young children, pauciarticular disease usually begins before the age of 5, with a mean of 3, and is much more common in girls. Patient complaints are minimal and only a few of the larger joints (except the hips and sacroiliac joints) are involved, and usually the pain resolves on its own. Skin findings are uncommon.

The ANA is positive in 80% of these patients, and ocular findings occur in 50% or more (Fig. 22-11) and include low-grade iridocyclitis. This is often not recognized until the patient's vision is checked on routine examination or the patient is noted to have a white pupil from cataract or band keratopathy. This disease is frequently associated with HLA-DR5 and DR8. Glaucoma is common in these patients.

Pauciarticular Disease—Older Children

In older children the pauciarticular disease usually has a mean age of onset of 12. This syndrome involves boys much more frequently than girls. There are minimal constitutional symptoms. Joint involvement is usually restricted to a few of the larger joints, especially the hip and sacroiliac joints. Skin findings are uncommon. The sacroiliitis often progresses to ankylosing spondylitis (AS), and this form of the disease is probably also a variant of AS because 90% of these patients are HLA-B27 positive.

An acute iridocyclitis occurs in about 25% of patients and is characterized by photophobia, tearing, redness, and pain, typical for AS.

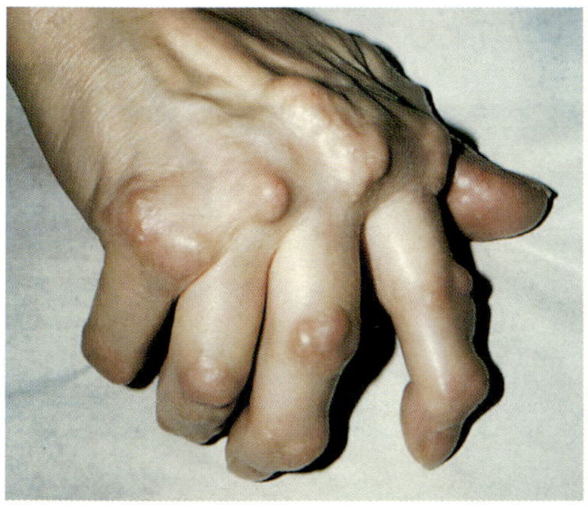

FIGURE 22-1. Finger joint involvement in rheumatoid arthritis. (Courtesy of Dr. John Reeves.)

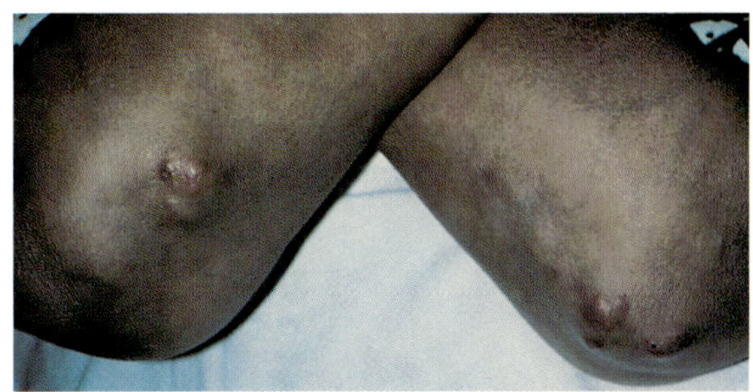

FIGURE 22-2. Rheumatoid nodules of the elbows.

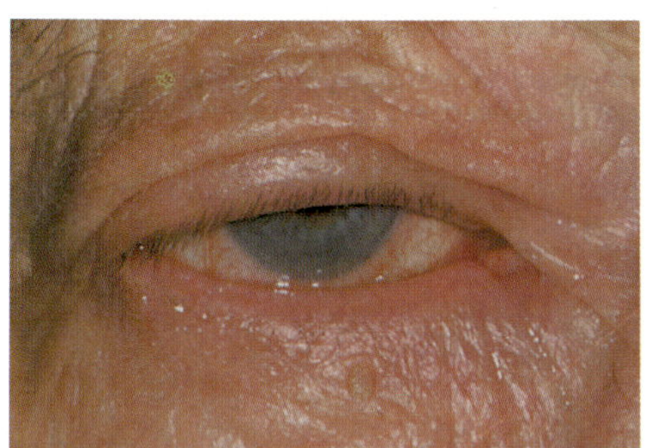

FIGURE 22-3. Keratoconjunctivitis sicca in a patient with rheumatoid arthritis. A deficient tear film containing some mucus can be seen medially.

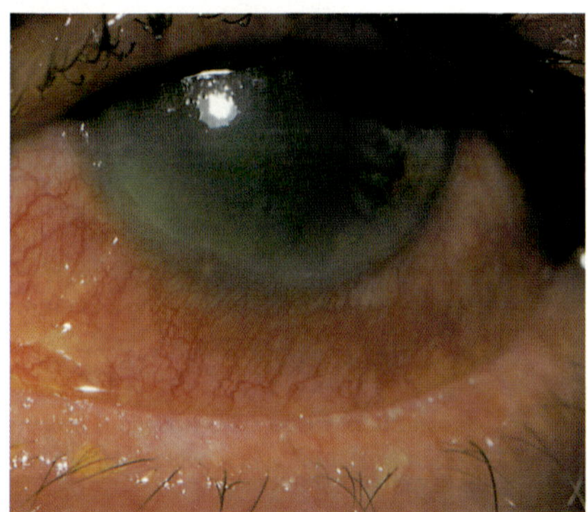

A

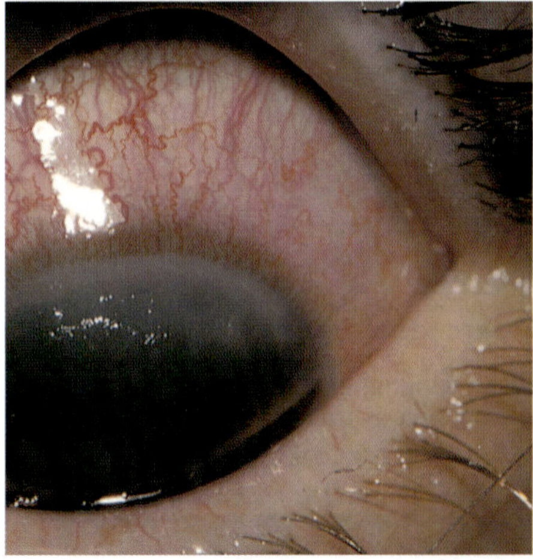

B

FIGURE 22-4. A: Marginal corneal furrow in rheumatoid arthritis. **B:** Peripheral corneal thinning is evident in each of these photographs.

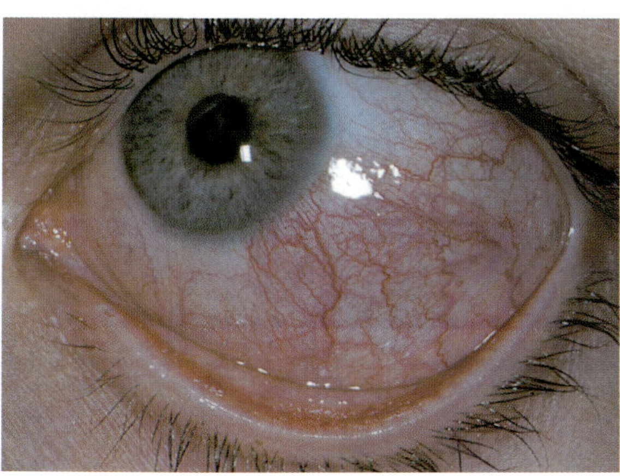

FIGURE 22-5. Diffuse episcleritis in rheumatoid arthritis. A typical bluish discoloration is evident, arising from episcleral involvement.

rhea and primarily left colon involvement. Fever, weight loss, and toxemia are usually present in severe disease.

Diarrhea with blood and mucus is a characteristic complaint. Although cramping may be mild, rectal tenesmus may be present. Perforation occasionally occurs.

Skin Features

About 20% of patients with Crohn disease have skin involvement. Skin findings may arise by extension of the intestinal disease with perineal abscesses, fistulas, and sinus formation of the abdominal wall, groin, or even submammary folds. Other skin changes include the following:

1. Erythema nodosum or pyoderma gangrenosum.
2. Pyoderma gangrenosum (Fig. 23-1).
3. Livido.
4. Nodules of cutaneous vasculitis and joint pain in the lower extremities.
5. Epidermolysis bullosa acquisita.
6. Acne fulminans and recurrent facial abscesses.
7. Recurrent aphthous stomatitis and glossitis that may follow the course of the bowel disease.

The skin changes associated with ulcerative colitis are similar, but they occur in only about 10% of patients. Nonspecific skin eruptions include urticaria, angioedema, erythema, and purpura.

Specific skin eruptions include the following:

1. Pyoderma gangrenosum found (1% to 10% of patients). Its severity is directly proportional to the severity of ulcerative colitis. It begins as a papule or pustule and then develops vegetating epithelial proliferations leading to ulceration with an undermined border.

2. Pyostomatitis vegetans characterized by oral lesions with pustules, erosions, and plaques. The erosions have been likened to a snail's track.
3. Nodular vasculitis associated with fever, malaise, joint swelling, and pain. They are red, indurated nodules that occur on the shin or occasionally elsewhere. Sometimes they ulcerate, forming persistent pyodermal lesions.

Ocular Features

As many as 10% of patients with Crohn disease develop ocular symptoms, whereas ocular symptoms are much less common in ulcerative colitis patients. The ocular changes include the following:

1. Marginal corneal infiltrates/ulcerations and anterior stromal opacities in Crohn disease. (Marginal corneal infiltrates/ulcerations are much less common in ulcerative colitis.)
2. Episcleritis (the most common ocular manifestation of Crohn disease). Its presence suggests disease activity. (It is not seen in ulcerative colitis.)
3. Posterior scleritis in Crohn disease. The scleritis that occurs in Crohn disease is often posterior and may be associated with marked scleral thinning, exophthalmos, exudative retinal detachments, and edema of the optic nerve head (Figs. 23-2 to 23-5).
4. Orbital inflammation that represents an orbital pseudotumor.
5. Uveal tract involvement in Crohn disease includes an acute iritis, a chronic iridocyclitis, or a panuveitis. (A chronic iridocyclitis occasionally occurs in ulcerative colitis.)
6. Fundus manifestations of Crohn disease include central serous retinopathy, macular edema, and optic neuropathy.

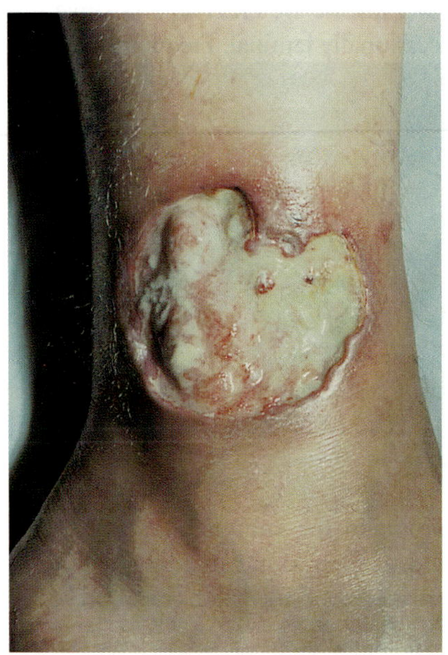

FIGURE 23-1. Pyoderma gangrenosum in Crohn disease. Note characteristic sharply marginated, undermined, rolled border with a dusky hue. The ulcer was very painful. Differential diagnoses would include spider bite, factitious ulcers, and infections such as deep fungal, mycobacterial, amebiasis, and gummatous syphilis.

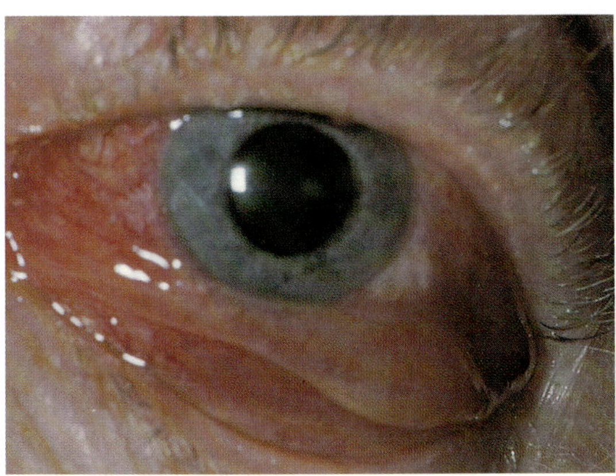

FIGURE 23-2. Posterior scleritis in Crohn disease. Chemosis and severe injection of the globe are evident in this patient.

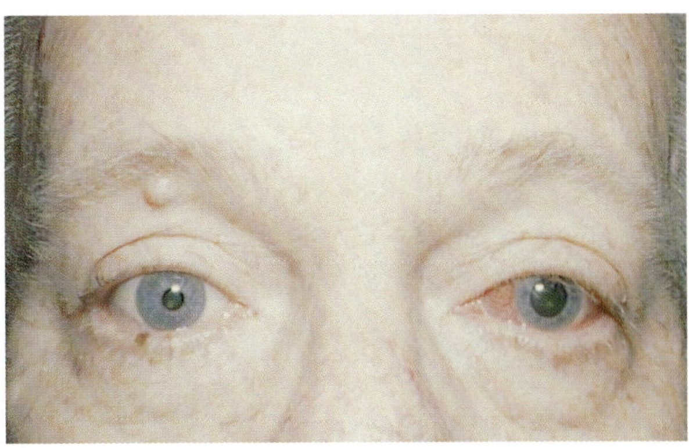

FIGURE 23-3. Proptosis of the left eye in Crohn disease arising from posterior scleritis.

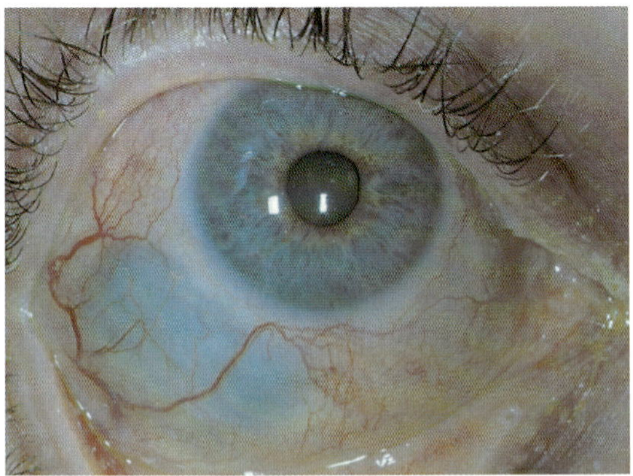

FIGURE 23-4. Scleromalacia in Crohn disease. The bluish discoloration in this photograph is caused by the scleral thinning.

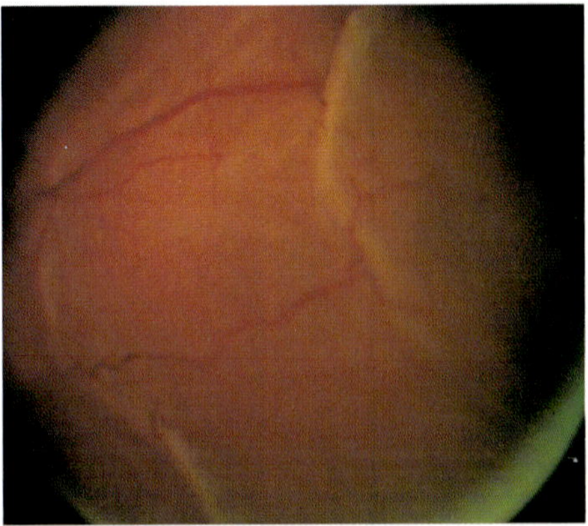

FIGURE 23-5. Exudative retinal detachment in Crohn disease. This is the same patient as is shown in Fig. 23-3. The retinal detachment is readily evident.

24

MISCELLANEOUS SYSTEMIC DISEASES

REITER DISEASE

Reiter disease is a symptom complex of recurring nonbacterial urethritis, conjunctivitis or iridocyclitis, and polyarthritis. Other manifestations include plantar fasciitis, Achilles tendonitis, keratoderma blennorrhagica, and balanitis. The cause is unknown, but the syndrome may follow an attack of nonspecific urethritis or an attack of bacillary dysentery. It appears to be closely related to genital infection with *Chlamydia trachomatis*. The role of mycoplasma is unknown. The disease occurs worldwide. Most cases occur during the third and fourth decade of life. The disease occurs more frequently in males than in females. Approximately 80% of these patients will be HLA-B27 positive.

The epidemic "dysenteric" form of Reiter syndrome, more often seen in young children, typically occurs following an enteric infection with *Shigella flexneri*, *Salmonella* spp., *Campylobacter jejuni*, *Clostridium* spp., or *Yersinia* spp.

Clinical Manifestations

It is uncommon for all the major manifestations of Reiter syndrome to occur at onset. In about 85% of patients, a nongonococcal urethritis is the initial manifestation, followed within 2 to 6 weeks by the remainder of the triad (usually conjunctivitis, followed by arthritis). The arthritis is usually polyarticular and asymmetric at first; later, it becomes oligoarticular. It usually involves the large peripheral weight-bearing joints and typically begins in the knees, ankles, or proximal interphalangeal joints of the feet. The arthritic symptoms vary from a slight arthralgia to marked tenderness and exquisite pain. A moderate fever may accompany the arthritis and persist for 1 to 4 weeks. The signs vary from no visible signs to severe erythema, effusions, and complete immobility of the involved joint. The arthritis may persist for many weeks or months. Sacroiliitis is common; during the early period, it is usually unilateral and asymptomatic except for morning stiffness or low backache.

Tendonitis, especially of the Achilles tendon, the plantar fascia, and the tendons of the chest wall (particularly the scapular region), is common. Plantar fasciitis occurs in approximately 20% of patients. A fasciitis with calcaneal spurs is very suggestive of Reiter syndrome.

The urethritis in males (endemic and epidemic forms) is clinically indistinguishable from uncomplicated nongonococcal urethritis and is often associated with a balanitis (Figs. 24-1 to 24-3). The urethritis causes mild to moderate dysuria, a mucoid or mucopurulent discharge, and occasionally, hematuria. Occasionally, there is marked purulent discharge, severe dysuria, and meatal inflammation. The urethritis is usually short-lived and lasts only several weeks. Prostatitis (usually low-grade), acute epididymitis, orchitis, and hemorrhagic cystitis occur in fewer than one-fifth of patients. The spectrum in females is unknown, although cervicitis is common and vaginitis, bartholinitis, or cystitis may occur.

Skin Features

Keratoderma blennorrhagica develops in more than 50% of patients, usually 1 to 2 months after onset of arthritis and conjunctivitis. It is characterized by thickened, heaped-up, crusted, and yellowish scaling lesions of the acral regions, especially the soles of the feet (Fig. 24-1 to 24-3). The extensor surfaces of the legs and the dorsal aspects of the toes, feet, hands, fingers, nails, and scalp also may be involved. The lesions begin as erythematous macules with a vesicular component that gradually enlarge and thicken to form hyperkeratotic papules. In some instances, the lesions are diffuse or pustular. In flexural areas, the lesions may form confluent circinate erosions or appear as greasy, brown maculopapules.

Circinate balanitis occurs in as many as 85% of males and is diagnostic for Reiter syndrome. It is painless and, in uncircumcised males, begins as red, moist erosions (Fig. 24-2), that coalesce to form a large erosion with a geographic shape. In circumcised males, hyperkeratotic papules may also develop that closely resemble the hyperkeratotic skin lesions (keratoderma blennorrhagica).

Nail involvement (Figs. 24-1 and 24-5) presents as brownish-yellow thickening of the nails due to subungual accumulation of hyperkeratotic material. Painless red swelling at the base of the nail fold may be seen. The nail plate may be severely distorted, and the nail plate may be shed.

Painless shallow ulcerations of the palate, tongue, buccal mucosa, tonsillar pillars, pharynx, or lips occur in about 25% to 30% of patients. The lesions appear as nonspecific erosions or elevated erythematous areas with circinate, whitish borders. Reddened papillae or erosions may occur on the tongue and, in some instances, may develop into geographic lesions.

Systemic Involvement

Malaise, fever, anorexia, and weight loss occur during the acute attack. Other findings include the following:

1. Cardiovascular involvement (<10%) is usually transient and is manifested by electrocardiographic abnormalities, myocarditis, pericarditis, acute aortitis, aortic valve incompetence, and associated congestive failure.
2. Neurologic complications (1%) include peripheral neuropathy, various cranial nerve palsies, hemiplegia, organic brain syndrome, epilepsy, neuralgic amyotrophy, polyradiculitis, and meningoencephalitis.
3. Other systemic complications include pleuritis, pneumonitis, lymphadenopathy, thrombophlebitis, and amyloidosis.

Ocular Features

Ocular involvement may occur at onset of the disease or develop weeks or months later. The findings include the following:

1. Conjunctivitis (Fig. 24-6). Papillary conjunctivitis (Fig. 24-7) occurs in about 50% of cases during the initial episode. It is usually bilateral and causes minimal symptoms except for a mucopurulent discharge. It is occasionally recurrent.
2. Keratitis (Figs. 24-8 and 24-9). Keratitis occasionally occurs with the conjunctivitis or iridocyclitis. It presents as a fine epithelial keratitis, a central loss of epithelium, or round subepithelial infiltrates in the peripheral cornea. The keratitis clears as the conjunctivitis or iridocyclitis improves, although the subepithelial opacities may persist.
3. Nongranulomatous iridocyclitis with fine to medium-sized white nongranulomatous keratic precipitates, anterior chamber cells and flare, and sometimes posterior synechiae. It is usually unilateral and usually occurs during recurrences.
4. Other ocular manifestations include a simple episcleritis, optic neuritis, papilledema, and macular edema.

ERYTHRODERMA

Erythroderma represents any inflammatory skin disease with generalized erythema. It is usually accompanied by mild to severe exfoliation. Most cases occur after the age of 45; males are more commonly involved than females. Erythroderma has many causes, including ichthyosiform erythroderma (Chapter 5) pityriasis rubra pilaris (Chapter 5); atopic dermatitis (Chapter 2); psoriasis (Chapter 7); an untoward reaction to drugs, such as organic arsenicals, gold, mercury, penicillin, and barbiturates (Chapter 2); pemphigus foliaceus (Chapter 8); lymphomas (Chapter 21); leukemia (Chapter 21); toxic shock syndrome (Chapter 26); lupus erythematosus (Chapter 13); and some unknown causes (idiopathic or Wilson disease).

The overall picture of erythroderma as it develops and progresses is modified by the underlying disease. Erythroderma arising in association with eczema and lymphomas, for example, has an acute onset beginning with patchy erythema that quickly generalizes.

Erythroderma is usually associated with fever, shivering, malaise, and, sometimes hypothermia. After several days, exfoliation begins, which at first is more marked in the flexural areas; also at this time, there is marked redness, and the skin feels hot and thickened. Patients may complain of a tight feeling or irritation.

After several weeks the body and scalp hair may be shed; the fingernails become ridged and thickened, and are sometimes shed. Patchy or widespread areas of depigmentation may occur in dark-skinned races. A generalized lymphadenopathy that is usually moderate (but sometimes grossly evident) may accompany the erythroderma. High output failure due to marked vascular shunting to the skin is sometimes seen.

The periorbital skin is edematous, causing ectropion with resultant conjunctival and sometimes corneal exposure with epiphora.

ENDOCARDITIS

Nonbacterial thrombotic endocarditis arises from endothelial damage, usually in the setting of an underlying cardiac defect, allowing deposition of platelets and fibrin. Some of the various cardiac defects include congenital heart defects (patent ductus arteriosus and ventricular septal defects); acquired heart defects (mitral valve defects from rheumatic fever and mitral valve prolapse); deposition of foreign substances, such as occurs with IV drug abusers; and deposition of immune complexes, as is seen in systemic lupus erythematosus (Libman–Sacks endocarditis).

Infective endocarditis arises from blood-borne bacterial or fungal organisms adhering to the platelet-fibrin plaques present in nonbacterial thrombotic endocarditis. Here the organisms proliferate and induce further deposition of platelets and fibrin; eventually, the plaques become quite large. Most infective endocarditis is caused by alpha-hemolytic streptococci.

Clinical Manifestations

Manifestations that arise directly from the cardiac abnormalities include arrhythmia and heart failure with dyspnea, pain, palpitation, and fatigue.

Manifestations of disease at distant sites are caused by emboli during the acute stage of the disease and may lead to arterial occlusion, infarction, abscess formation, and mycotic aneurysms. An immune complex vasculitis of the kidneys and skin is usually seen during the more chronic phase of disease and arises from the circulation of immune complexes.

The musculoskeletal features generally arise from immune complex disease and include myalgia, back pain, arthralgia, arthritis, and osteomyelitis. Renal infarction and abscess formation generally arise from embolization. A focal or diffuse glomerulonephritis is usually caused by immune complex disease. The embolic phenomenon may cause a stroke, suppurative meningitis, brain abscess, or mycotic aneurysm.

Skin Features

Skin involvement arises from embolic or immune complex disease. The mucocutaneous lesions include widespread petechial hemorrhages (Fig. 24-10); linear splinter hemorrhages in the bed of the fingernails (Fig. 24-11) and toenails; tender, small, red or purple nodules (Osler nodes) (Fig. 24-12); and nontender, red macules (Janeway lesions) (Fig. 24-13).

Ocular Features

The petechial hemorrhages of the bulbar and palpebral conjunctiva are similar to those of the skin (Fig. 24-14). Uveal involvement includes uveitis and choroiditis, and in some instances of infective endocarditis, the uveitis is the presenting feature of the disease.

Retinal changes include single or multiple superficial hemorrhages, Roth spot (white-centered retinal hemorrhages), branch or central retinal artery occlusion, cotton-wool spots arising from small vessel occlusion, and focal retinitis. Vitreitis may also be seen.

In acute infective endocarditis, the patient may experience acute endophthalmitis.

Neuroophthalmic manifestations often arise from central nervous system involvement and include visual field defects, 3rd, 4th, or 6th cranial nerve involvement with diplopia, nystagmus, and papilledema.

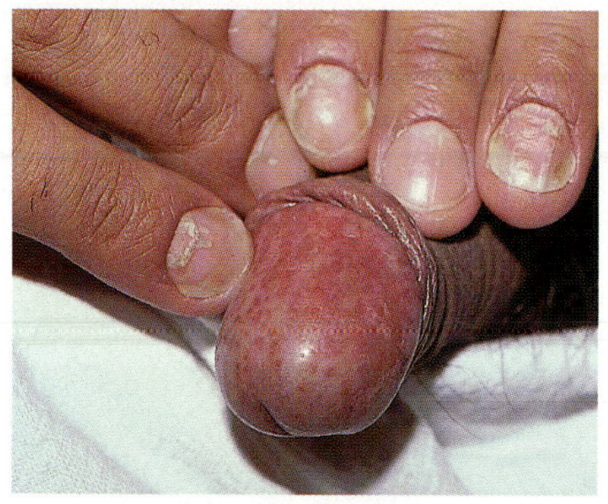

FIGURE 24-1. Arthritis, nail dystrophy, and balanitis in Reiter syndrome.

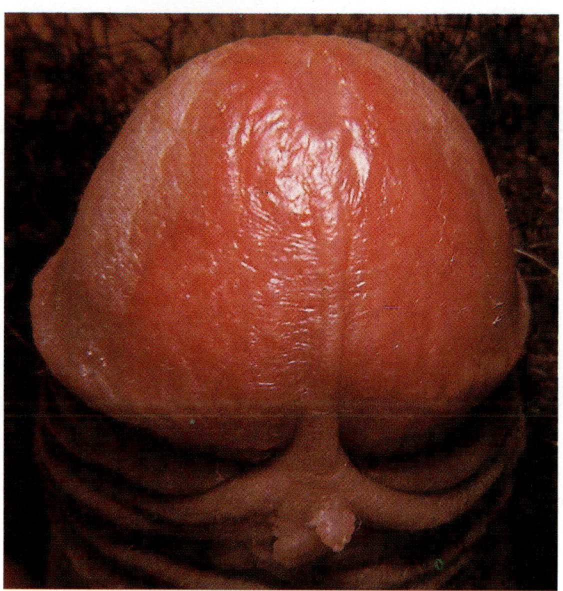

FIGURE 24-2. Balanitis in Reiter syndrome.

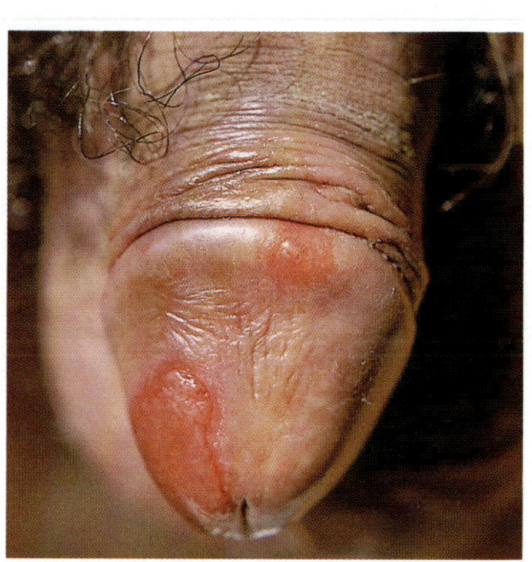

FIGURE 24-3. Circinate and perimeatal balanitis. Reiter balanitis often begins as meatitis, as in this patient.

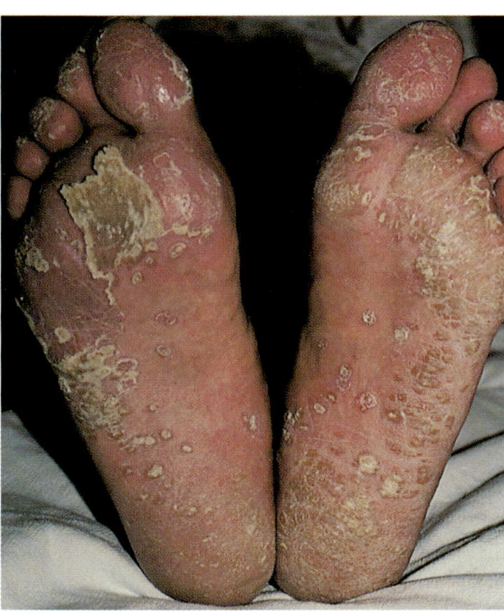

FIGURE 24-4. Keratoderma blennorrhagicum in Reiter syndrome. Lesions began as small pustules, eventuating in keratotic crusted papules. Note similarity to psoriasis and late secondary syphilis.

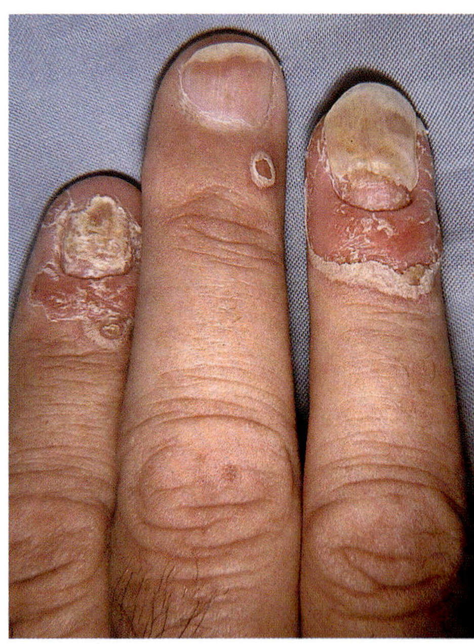

FIGURE 24-5. Nail involvement in Reiter syndrome. Note periungual erythema, scaling, and crusting as well as nail dystrophy resembling severe nail lesions in psoriasis.

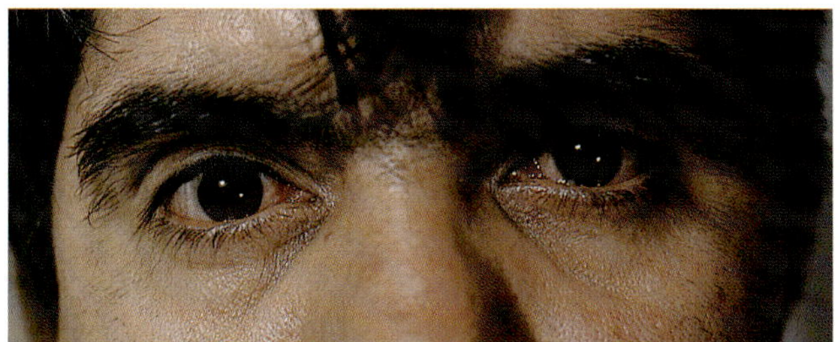

FIGURE 24-6. Conjunctivitis in Reiter syndrome.

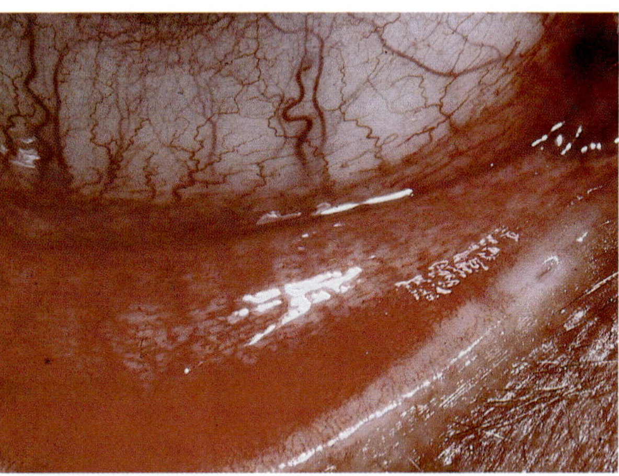

FIGURE 24-7. Papillary conjunctivitis in Reiter syndrome.

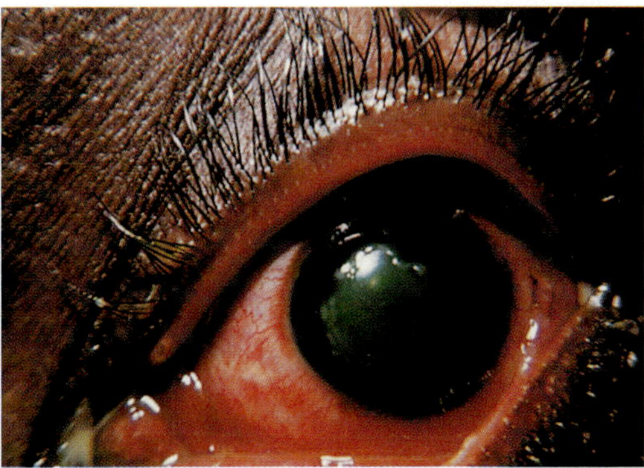

FIGURE 24-8. Loss of central corneal epithelium in Reiter syndrome together with a nongranulomatous iridocyclitis. (Courtesy of Dr. Robert Sexton.)

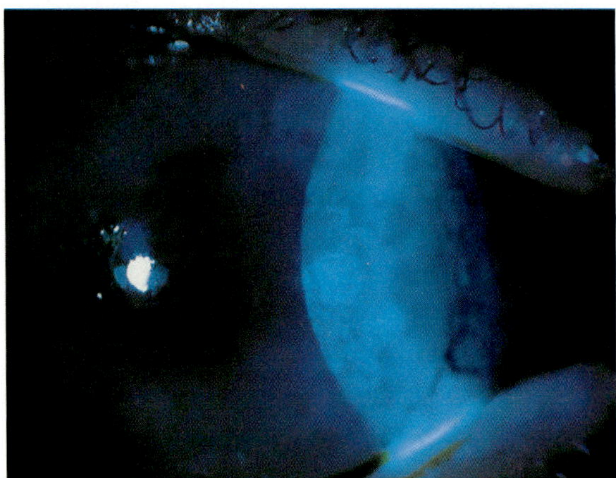

FIGURE 24-9. Fine epithelial keratitis in Reiter syndrome.

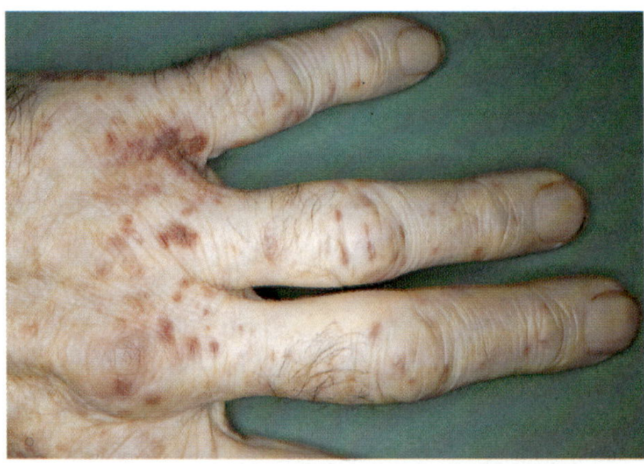

FIGURE 24-10. Petechial hemorrhages of the skin of the hand in subacute bacterial endocarditis.

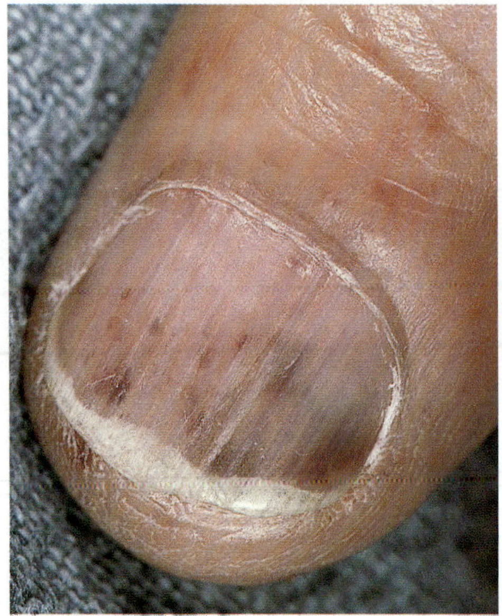

FIGURE 24-11. Splinter hemorrhages of thumbnail in a patient with subacute bacterial endocarditis due to staphylococcal septicemia. Infarcts to the brain caused visual loss in this man.

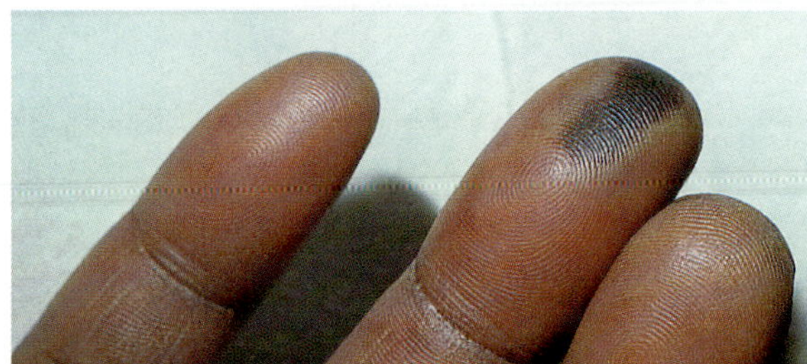

FIGURE 24-12. Osler node on finger pad (a classic site) in a patient with acute endocarditis as a complication of intravenous drug abuse.

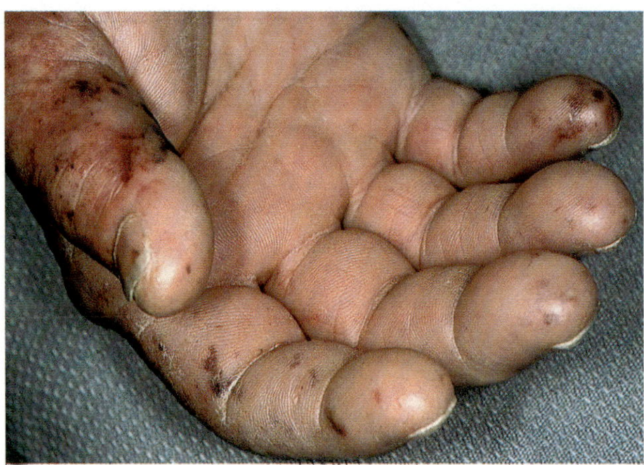

FIGURE 24-13. Janeway lesions in a patient with subacute bacterial endocarditis. This is the patient shown in Fig. 24-11.

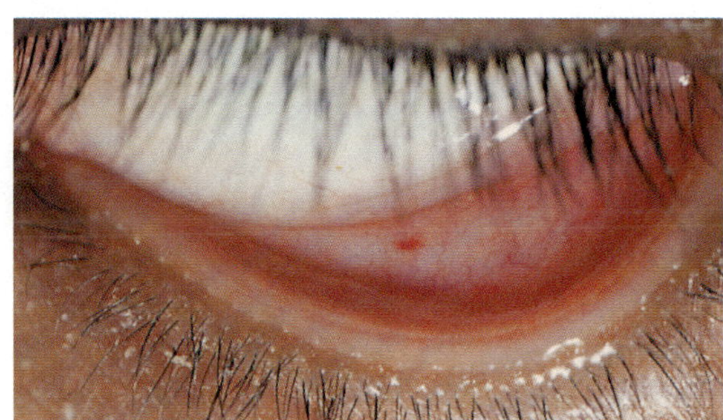

FIGURE 24-14. Petechial hemorrhage of the conjunctiva in subacute bacterial endocarditis.

DISEASES OF THE HAIR

There are three types of hair, namely: lanugo, vellus hair, and terminal hair. Lanugo hair is the fine hair found on the fetus.

Vellus hair, replaces the lanugo in all areas of the body except the scalp before birth or in early infancy. It is soft, fine, occasionally pigmented, and less than 2 cm in length.

Terminal hair includes the hair of the scalp, eyebrows, lashes, and, after puberty, the hair of the beard, axilla, and pubic regions. This hair is coarse, pigmented, thick, and somewhat longer than 2 cm. It varies in color, texture, curl, and cross section from patient to patient.

Hair growth is cyclic and has three stages, namely:

1. Anagen (growth) stage, lasts for 2 to 6 years in the scalp and for shorter periods on the arm. Its root is dark, soft, and moist.
2. Catagen (transition) stage, lasts for 1 to 2 weeks and is characterized by a small, relatively stiff bulb at the proximal end of the hair shaft.
3. Telogen (resting) stage, occurs before shedding and lasts 3 to 4 months. It is characterized by a small, white knob at the proximal end of the shaft (club hair) that represents keratinization of the hair matrix. The telogen hairs are pushed out by a new hair produced by the same follicle.

At any one time, growing and resting hairs are randomly distributed, and each follicle's activity is independent of its neighbor. The duration of each phase varies from region to region, and the cycle phase is influenced by circulating hormones (androgens, glucocorticoids, and thyroxine) and the season of the year. Hair other than scalp hair (axillary, pubic, chest, and other body hair) is clearly dependent upon androgen production.

Overall, about 85% of the hair of the head is in a growing (anagen) stage; 13%, in a resting (telogen) stage; and about 2%, in a transitional (catagen) stage. The hair of the eyebrow and eyelid has a high proportion of telogen stage hairs at any one time.

Dystrophic hair is characterized by the tapering of the shaft at its narrowest point and the breakage of the root. Dysplastic hair is often deformed, with the root sheath missing or loose; it has a small-diameter matrix.

HYPERTRICHOSIS

The term *hypertrichosis* is used for excessive hair growth other than the hair growth patterns related to androgen secretion.

Congenital Hypertrichosis Lanuginosa (Hypertrichosis Universalis Congenita)

Congenital hypertrichosis lanuginosa (hypertrichosis universalis congenita) is a rare form of hypertrichosis. It is autosomal dominant and is characterized by persistence of lanugo hair (fine, soft, nonmedullated, and usually, unpigmented hair) after birth. At birth, excessive lanugo hair covers most of the body except for the palms and soles. The lanugo hair grows to more than 10 cm in length and persists throughout life. These unfortunate people were often exhibited at the circus as "dog-faced boy" or "human werewolf." The eyebrows and lashes are long, and the brows are thick. Associated anomalies include ear deformity and hypo- or anodontia and gingival fibromatosis. Photophobia, severe visual impairment, and absence of night blindness with slight macular pigment epithelial changes were described in two cousins who also had trichomegaly and excessive facial and body hair.

Forehead hypertrichosis, lid agenesis, macrostomia, and psychomotor retardation have also been observed in one child. Epilation with lasers has proven useful in these patients.

Acquired Hypertrichosis

A number of rare syndromes may be accompanied by increased hair growth. Among these are Cornelia de Lange syndrome, Rubenstein–Taybi syndrome, Hurler syndrome, Laband syndrome, Morgogu syndrome, Winchester syndrome, Schynzel–Giedier syndrome, stiff skin syndrome, leprechaunism, and lipoatrophic diabetes.

Drugs that may cause hypertrichosis include cyclosporin, minoxidil (now used primarily as a topical agent for increasing hair growth on the scalp), diphenylhydantoin, topical androgens, and topical steroids. The use of topical prostaglandins in the management of glaucoma often causes lengthening and darkening of eyelashes.

Localized hypertrichosis may be seen in some melanocytic nevi (e.g., Becker's nevi), as a result of repeated rubbing or sucking of skin (as often seen in mentally retarded patients). Porphyrid cutanea tanda often shows hirsutism over the malar areas.

Acquired Hypertrichosis Lanuginosa

There are several types and patterns of acquired hypertrichosis lanuginosa. One of the most important, though rare, is known as "malignant down," in which one sees a sudden appearance of profuse soft nonpigmented hair on the face. This is a paraneoplastic syndrome associated with carcinoma of the lung and, at times the colon, gallbladder, and uterus.

ALOPECIA

Alopecia is characterized by abnormal loss of hair on any part of the body (scalp, face, brows, lashes, axillae, trunk). Alopecia can be divided into nonscarring forms, such as alopecia areata, and scarring, or cicatricial, forms (Table 25-1).

TABLE 25-1. CAUSES OF ALOPECIA

Congenital
Total alopecia (usually autosomal recessive)
Congenital circumscribed alopecia
Hidrotic ectodermal dysplasia
Moynahan syndrome
Baraitser syndrome
Progeria
Oculocerebrocutaneous syndrome
Bitemporal aplasia cutis congenita
Focal facial dermal dysplasia
Conradi syndrome
Incontinentia pigmenti
Hallermann–Streiff syndrome
Down syndrome
Inflammatory, infectious, or neoplastic conditions
Vogt–Koyanagi–Harada syndrome
Staphylococcal folliculitis
Candida folliculitis
Herpes zoster
Irradiation
Syphilis
Tinea capitis
Alopecia neoplastica (metastasis)
Nevus sebaceous of Jadassohn
Dissecting cellulites of the scalp
Follicular mucinosis
Burns
Endocrine induced
Hypopituitarism (Sheehan syndrome)
Hypothyroidism
Hyperthyroidism
Hypoparathyroidism
Diabetes mellitus
Pregnancy (post partum)
Medication induced
Long-term high-dose corticosteroids
Excess vitamin A
Anticoagulants–heparin and warfarin
Thyroid antagonists–thiouracil and iodine
Oral contraceptives
Lithium carbonate
Propanol
Levodopa
Cimetidine
Ibuprofen
Nutritional/metabolic induced
Marasmus
Kwashiorkor
Zinc deficiencies
Homocystinuria
Thyroiditis
Autoimmune associated
Systemic lupus erythematosus
Myasthenia gravis
Atopic dermatitis
Thyroiditis
Alopecia areata
Alopecia totalis
Alopecia universalis
Vitiligo
Unknown or psychiatric associated
Trichotillomania
Stress related
Traumatic alopecia
Fever
Surgery
Cicatricial
Pseudopelade
Folliculitis decalvans
Discoid and systemic lupus erythematosus
Post radiation
Scleroderma (morphea)
Facial hemiatrophy (Rhomberg disease)
Ichthyosis
Lichen sclerosis
Lichen plano pilaris
Graham Little syndrome
Hypotrichosis
Congenital hypotrichosis
Keratosis pilaris
Keratosis lentiginosis
Hypomania, hypotrichosis, facial hemangioma syndrome
Marie–Umma type hypotrichosis
Phenylketonuria
Hallermann–Streiff syndrome
Werner syndrome
Marinesco-Sjögren syndrome
Keratosis pilaris–associated monilethrix
Pili torti
Menkes kinky hair syndrome
Anhidrotic ectodermal dysplasia
Rothmund-Thomson syndrome
Netherton syndrome
Ankyloblepharon–ectodermal defects–cleft lip and palate
Ectrodactyly–ectodermal dysplasia–cleft lip/palate
Conradi syndrome
Progeria

Widespread alopecia may be seen as part of a number of rare congenital syndromes, including the following:

Hidrotic ectodermal dysplasia (Chapter 10).

Moynahan syndrome (alopecia of scalp, mental retardation, and epilepsy).

Baraitser syndrome, an autosomal recessive disorder characterized by almost total alopecia (including brows and lashes following loss of downy hair at birth). Physical and mental retardation are also present.

Progeria (Chapter 12).

Congenital Alopecia

Congenital alopecia is a rare heterogeneous group of disorders with alopecia at birth and having no other abnormalities (Fig. 25-1). When total congenital alopecia occurs as an isolated phenomenon, it is usually autosomal recessive. The scalp hair is absent at birth or disappears within the first 6 months of life. The eyebrows, eyelashes, and other body hair are also absent or sparse. There is no further hair growth.

Congenital Circumscribed Alopecia

Those conditions in which congenital circumscribed alopecia has ocular significance include the following:

Epidermal nevi involving the brow or lashes (Chapter 9).

Syndromes with congenital absence of skin (oculo-cerebro-cutaneous syndrome, bitemporal aplasia cutis congenita, and focal facial dermal dysplasia (Chapter 9).

Pseudopelade characterized by irregular areas of cicatricial alopecia without preceding inflammatory changes seen in Conradi syndrome (Chapter 5) and incontinentia pigmenti (Chapter 6).

Circumscribed noncicatricial alopecia caused by aplasia or hypoplasia of a circumscribed area of hair follicles in the Hallermann–Streiff syndrome (Chapter 9).

Telogen Effluvium

Telogen effluvium represents a rapid increase in the number of hairs in the telogen phase that results in rapid shedding of hair. Telogen effluvium may occur spontaneously; it may occur with fever or surgery; appear in the early postpartum period; be precipitated by stress, malnutrition, crash dieting, iron deficiency; or be provoked by hormonal contraceptives. It is not uncommon in children.

Diffuse Alopecia Induced by Endocrine Abnormalities

Alopecia is often associated with endocrine abnormalities such as the following:

1. Hypopituitarism. Total alopecia is found in patients with hypopituitarism occurring before puberty. In Sheehan syndrome, the scalp hair is very sparse; both the axillary hair and pubic hair are absent; and the skin lacks turgidity and appears yellow and dry.
2. Hypothyroidism. Diffuse loss of scalp and body hair and loss of the outer aspect of the eyebrows or diffuse thinning is common. Loss of axillary hair occurs in about 50% of patients.
3. Hyperthyroidism. Diffuse alopecia of moderate degree, alopecia areata, and vitiligo are each more prevalent in hyperthyroidism than in the normal population.
4. Hypoparathyroidism. In both hypoparathyroidism and pseudohypoparathyroidism, there is often a patchy alopecia of the scalp, the hair being coarse, dry, sparse, and easily shed.
5. Diabetes mellitus. Diffuse alopecia may rarely occur in some diabetics who are under poor control.
6. Pregnancy. A transient hair loss occurs about 4 to 6 months following delivery arising from the marked increase in numbers of hairs in telogen during pregnancy.

Chemically Induced Alopecia

A few of the drugs known to induce alopecia include the following:

Most of the chemotherapeutic agents. (Telogen effluvium occurs weeks to months after the start of therapy, and with higher dosage direct toxic damage may result in anogen effluvium.)

Long-term high-dose corticosteroids.

Excess vitamin A (more than 50,000 IU/day over a period of several months).

Thyroid antagonists, such as thiouracil and iodine.

Anticoagulants, such as heparin and warfarin.

Miscellaneous drugs such as trimethadione, oral contraceptives, lithium carbonate, propanol, levodopa, cimetidine, and ibuprofen.

Nutritional and Metabolically Induced Alopecia

Alopecia occurs in marasmus and kwashiorkor (Chapter 33), zinc deficiency (Chapter 33), and possibly iron deficiency. The metabolic error in homocystinuria results in deficiency of methionine and marked thinning of the hair (Chapter 17). Some inflammatory conditions such as Vogt–Koyanagi–Harada syndrome (Chapter 6) will cause alopecia as well as poliosis, which will be discussed later.

Alopecia Areata

Alopecia areata (AA) is a common condition of patchy hair loss most often seen on the scalp (Fig. 25-2) though it sometimes involves the bearded area (Fig. 25-3), brows (Fig. 25-

4), lashes (Fig. 25-5), or trunk (Fig. 25-6). At the periphery of the patch one may find short stumps of hairs that, when pulled out, show a tapered attenuated bulb as a result of atrophy, giving the appearance of an "exclamation point" hair. This finding along with the absence of scarring helps to differentiate AA from tinea capitis, syphilis, trichotillomania, lupus erythematosus, and alopecia neoplastica (Fig. 25-7). New bald patches may appear at times, resulting in total loss of scalp hair (alopecia totalis) (Fig. 25-8). Hair loss not only of the scalp but of the entire body is called *alopecia universalis* (Fig. 25-9). The earlier the onset of AA, the poorer is the prognosis for regrowth. Usually, there are no associated diseases with AA, but one sees a higher prevalence in patients with Down syndrome atopic dermatitis and autoimmune diseases such as thyroiditis, vitiligo, systemic lupus erythematosus, and myasthenia gravis.

The causative factor of alopecia areata is unknown but is most likely autoimmune, in addition to genetic susceptibility. In 25% of the patients there is a positive family history of AA (Fig. 25-10).

Traumatic Alopecia

Traction alopecia is common in women who wear their hair tightly braided, producing prolonged tension on the hair (Fig. 25-11).

Trichotillomania is a fairly common psychoneurosis in which the patient experiences an irresistible urge to pull out his or her hair. It is more common in children than in adults and often occurs in a setting of psychosocial stress in the family. The scalp (Fig. 25-12) as well as the eyebrows (Fig. 25-13) and eyelashes (Fig. 25-14) are frequent sites. Broken hairs of varying length as well as the microscopic appearance of broken or twisted ends are helpful in diagnosis.

Cicatricial Alopecia

Cicatricial alopecia has many causes. We list some of the causes along with other causes of alopecia in Table 25-1. The pattern of hair loss and the presence or absence of cicatrization offer valuable clues in helping to elicit the cause (Fig. 25-15).

Pseudopelade

Pseudopelade is characterized by follicle destruction with permanent patchy baldness, which is not accompanied by clinical evidence of inflammatory pathology.

Folliculitis Decalvans

Folliculitis decalvans represents a cicatricial alopecia in which there is evidence of a pustular folliculitis of the advancing margin of the involved area.

HYPOTRICHOSIS

Congenital hypotrichosis occurs as an isolated abnormality or, in some of the hereditary disorders, is associated with other ectodermal defects. The hair is sparse and often brittle and poorly pigmented. Hypotrichosis occurring as an isolated abnormality is characterized by normal-appearing hair that is shed before 5 years of age and is never fully replaced. The eyebrows, lashes, and vellus hair may also be shed.

Some hereditary disorders associated with hypotrichosis include the following:

Hypotrichosis of the lashes and eyebrows appearing as an autosomal dominant condition.

Keratosis pilaris (Chapter 5); keratosis pilaris and lentiginosis (Chapter 6).

Hypomelia, hypotrichosis, facial hemangioma syndrome (Robert syndrome) (Chapter 9).

Hypotrichosis (Marie–Unna type) characterized by sparse lashes, brows, and body hair at birth and absence of scalp hair at birth or soon thereafter, followed by regrowth of scalp hair for a short period, then progressive cicatricial alopecia.

Phenylketonuria.

Hallermann–Streiff syndrome (Chapter 9).

Werner syndrome (Chapter 12).

Marinesco–Sjögren syndrome (Chapter 10).

Monilethrix associated with keratosis pilaris and loss of hair on the scalp, eyebrows, or lashes. In some instances, the hair appears normal at first and then becomes brittle, appears beaded, and is only 1 to 2 cm in length.

Pili torti (twisting of hair) as is seen in Menkes kinky hair syndrome (Chapter 33).

Hypohidrotic ectodermal dysplasia (Chapter 10).

Rothmund–Thomson syndrome (Chapter 14).

Netherton syndrome (bamboo hair) characterized by fine, dry scales in a polycyclic fashion on the trunk, eczema, and dry, lusterless, brittle hair. The lashes and brows are usually sparse or absent.

The ankyloblepharon–ectodermal defects/cleft lip and palate syndrome (AEC), and ectrodactyly–ectodermal dysplasia/cleft lip and palate syndrome (EEC) (Chapter 10).

CHANGES IN HAIR COLOR

In general, the eyebrows, eyelashes, and hair of the pubic region and axilla are darker than the scalp hair in patients with blond or red hair, and the lashes are usually the darkest hair in all patients. Eyelashes may darken with the use of topical prostaglandins in the treatment of glaucoma. These agents, including Xalatan™ and Lumigan™, may also cause eyelashes to lengthen as well as darken.

Heterochromia

Heterochromia indicates the presence of hair of two different colors in the same patient. Patches of different-colored hair are found in the following:

1. Hair growing from melanocytic nevi.
2. Autosomal dominant heterochromia characterized by a patch of black hair or tufts of red hair surrounded by blond scalp hair.

3. Piebaldism (Chapter 6).
4. Kwashiorkor (Chapter 33).
5. Methotrexate therapy in childhood leukemia, which may produce altered bands of pigmentation ("flag sign").
6. Eyelashes may be heterochromic with the unilateral use of topical prostaglandins for the treatment of glaucoma.

Canities (Graying of the Hair)

Canities usually occurs from aging and is manifested by graying of the hair shaft and failure of tyrosine production in the hair bulb. It is usually progressive and permanent.

Premature canities occurs in pernicious anemia, hyperthyroidism, hypothyroidism (Chapter 18), progeria, Werner syndrome (Chapter 21), dystrophia myotonia, and Rothmund–Thomson syndrome (Chapter 14).

Poliosis

Poliosis represents a patch of white hair caused by deficiency of melanin in a group of adjacent hair follicles. It occurs in

1. Piebaldism (Chapter 6).
2. Waardenburg syndrome (Chapter 6).
3. Tiez syndrome characterized by deaf mutism, generalized areas of white spots of the skin and hair, and hypoplasia of the eyebrows.
4. Vitiligo (Chapter 6).
5. Vogt–Koyanagi–Harada syndrome (Chapter 6).
6. Alezzandrini syndrome (Chapter 6).
7. Von Recklinghausen disease (Chapter 11).
8. Tuberous sclerosis (Chapter 11).

Poliosis is also caused by inflammatory processes:

1. Staphylococcal blepharitis (Chapter 26).
2. Herpes zoster (Chapter 29).
3. Irradiation (Chapter 19).

Albinism

The hair is white, yellowish-brown, or yellowish-red in albinism (Chapter 6), kwashiorkor (Chapter 33), Menkes kinky hair syndrome (Chapter 33), phenylketonuria, and homocystinuria (Chapter 17).

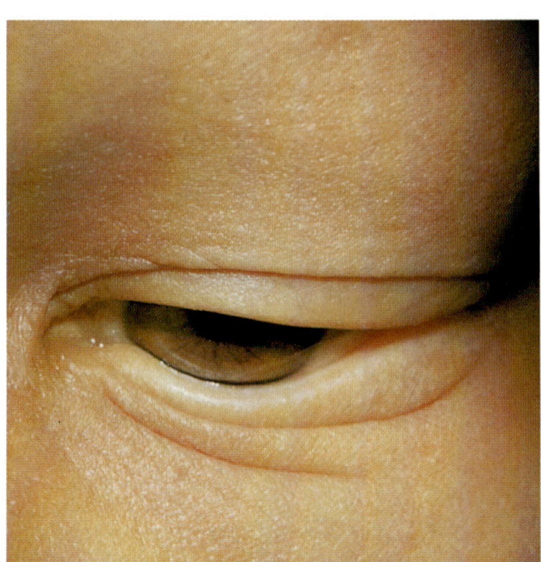

FIGURE 25-1. Congenital total alopecia in a child who had no eyebrows or lashes since birth.

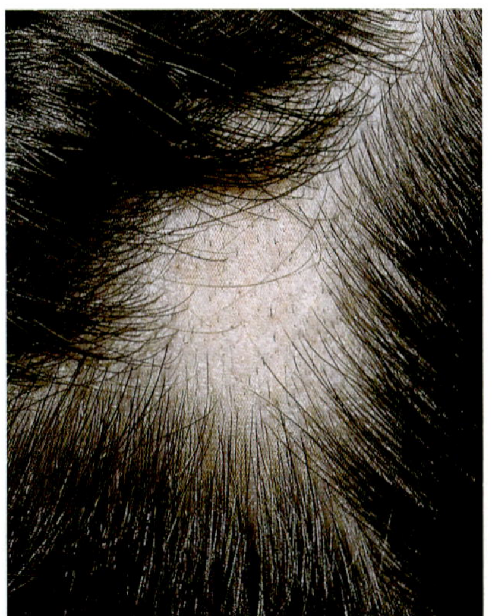

FIGURE 25-2. Alopecia areata of the scalp. Note small, stable hairs at peripheral margin that when epilated may show "exclamation point" thinning towards the base, a helpful diagnostic feature.

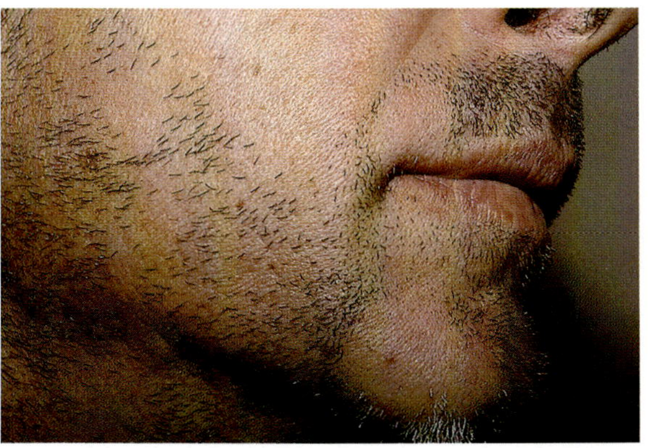

FIGURE 25-3. Alopecia areata of bearded area, a fairly frequent site.

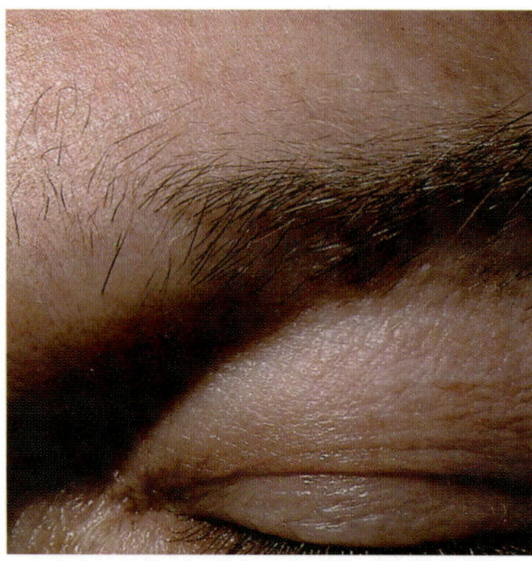

FIGURE 25-4. Alopecia areata of eyebrow, an uncommon finding. Differential diagnosis would include "moth eaten" alopecia in secondary syphilis.

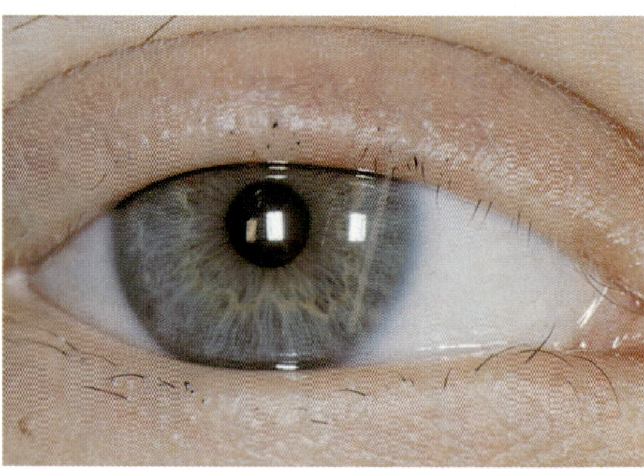

FIGURE 25-5. Alopecia areata of eyelashes. This must be differentiated from trichotillomania.

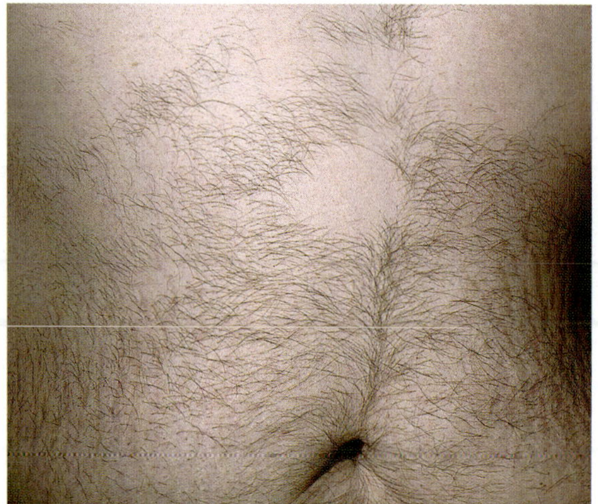

FIGURE 25-6. Alopecia areata of trunk.

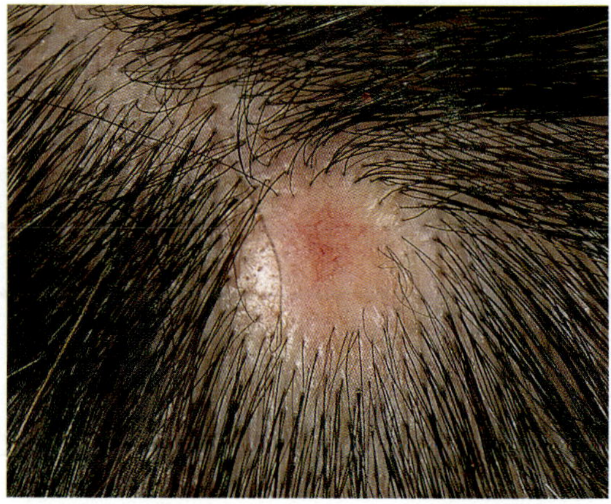

FIGURE 25-7. Alopecia neoplastica in a 40-year-old woman with metastasis to the scalp from carcinoma of the breast. The presence of a firm asymptomatic subcutaneous nodule fixed to the underlying galea helped differentiate this lesion from more common cysts of the scalp.

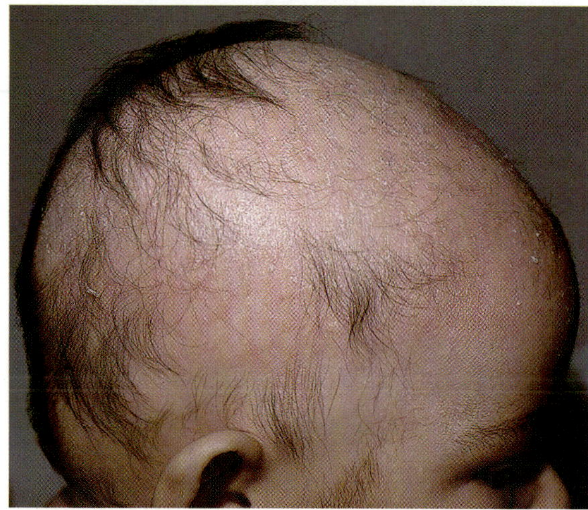

FIGURE 25-8. Alopecia areata in a 3-month-old child with progressive scalp hair loss leading to total loss of scalp hair (alopecia totalis).

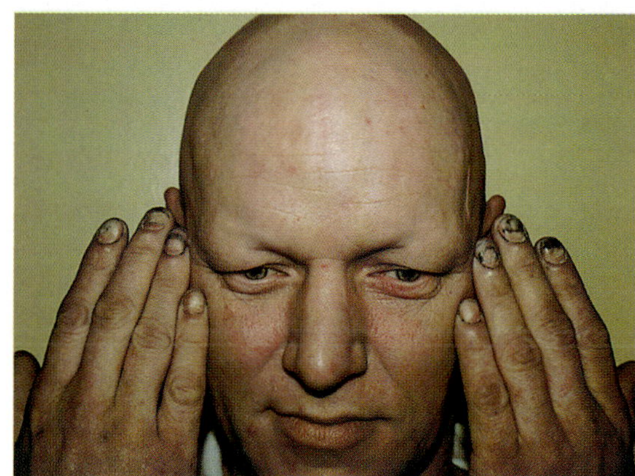

FIGURE 25-9. Alopecia universalis (total loss of all body hair). The beau's lines (horizontal linear depressions of the nails) were due to recent severe illness.

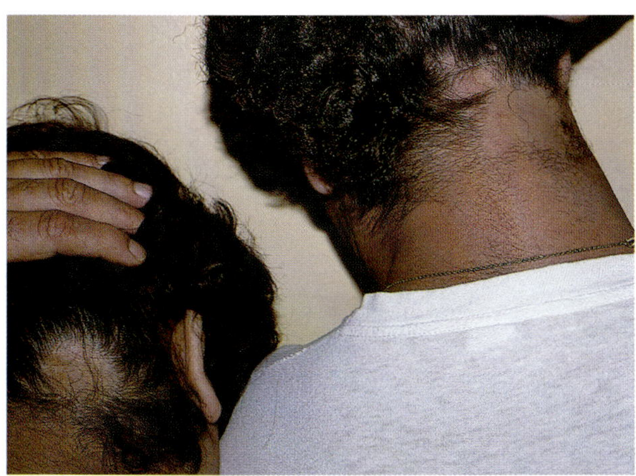

FIGURE 25-10. Alopecia areata in siblings. Twenty-five percent of patients with alopecia areata have a positive family history, as in these sisters.

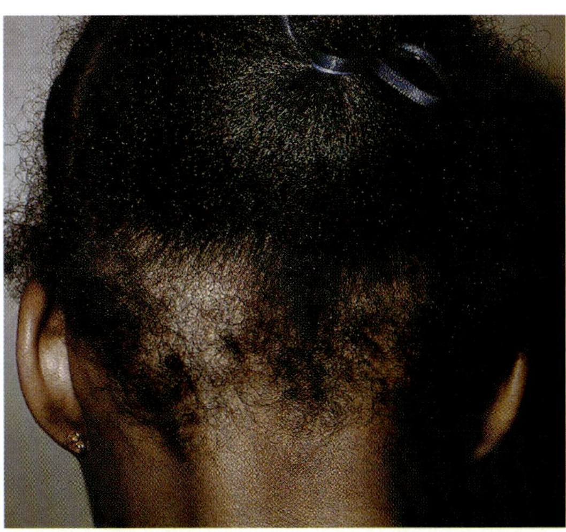

FIGURE 25-11. Traction alopecia due to constant pulling of scalp hair because of hair style as seen in this young woman.

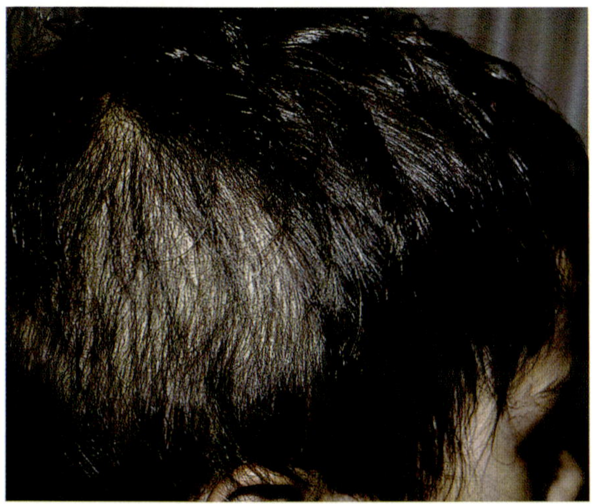

FIGURE 25-12. Trichotillomania in a 4-year-old boy. The cause of his hair loss was initially thought to be due to tinea capitis until further interview revealed that the child was very unhappy with his new stepfather.

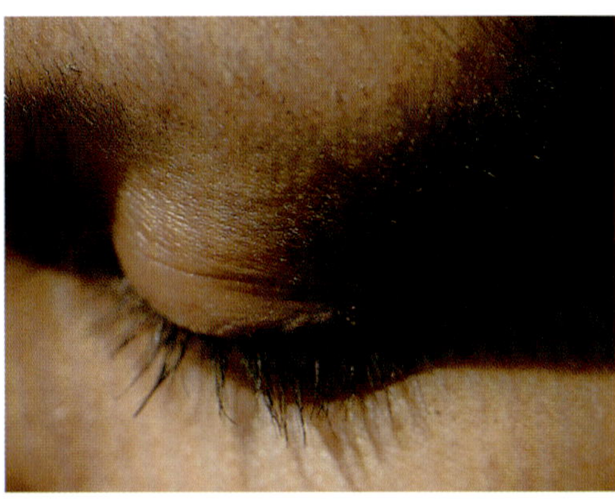

FIGURE 25-13. Trichotillomania of eyebrows in a young depressed girl.

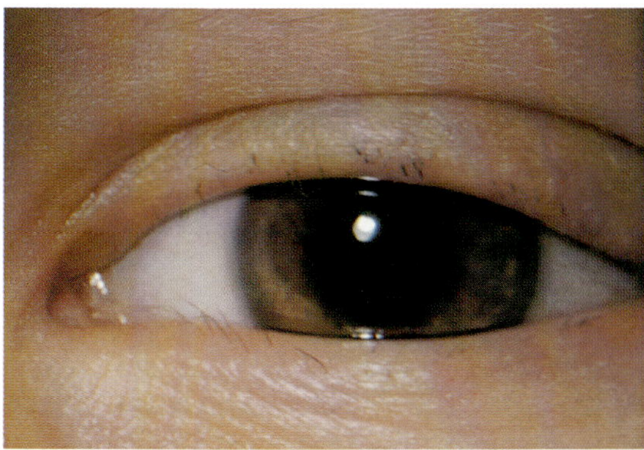

FIGURE 25-14. Trichotillomania of eyelashes in a child. It is often helpful to speak with the child without the parent's presence to obtain a more reliable history.

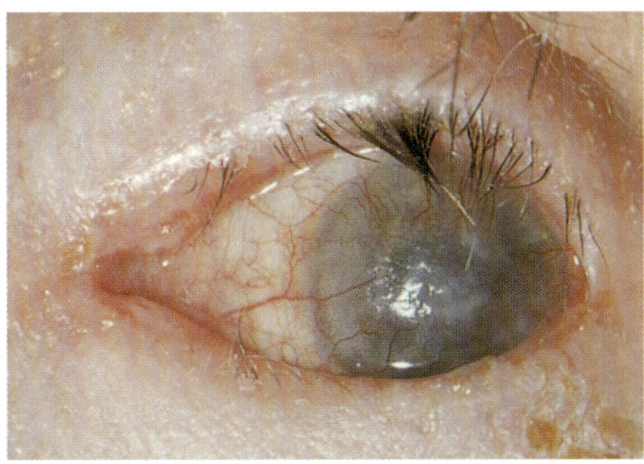

FIGURE 25-15. Alopecia of lower eyelashes as a result of radiation therapy for sebaceous gland carcinoma. Note corneal vascularization and scarring.

BACTERIAL INFECTIONS

STAPHYLOCOCCAL INFECTIONS

Staphylococcal Toxin–Associated Skin and Eye Diseases

Staphylococcal Scalded Skin Syndrome

Staphylococcal scalded skin syndrome is caused by the action of an epidermolytic exotoxin produced by certain strains of staphylococcus. Staphylococcal scalded skin syndrome occurs in the newborn, occasionally in older children, and infrequently in renal compromised or immunosuppressed adults. The infection source is often the nose, conjunctiva, middle ear, pharynx, or umbilical stump.

The syndrome is characterized by tender skin and a widespread erythematous eruption that develops and becomes deep red and erythematous over a 24 to 48 hour period followed by epidermal splitting immediately below the granular layer, leading to flaccid bullae and a positive Nikolsky. Favored eruption sites are the central face, axilla, and groin. Healing occurs after 1 to 2 weeks.

Ocular Features

The ocular features include lid skin involvement and a moderate papillary conjunctivitis that occasionally leads to scarring.

Toxic Shock Syndrome

Toxic shock syndrome (TSS), when originally described, was traced to toxin producing strains of *Staphylococcus aureus* found on the cervix in menstruating women using superabsorbent tampons. Most cases currently have resulted from infections in wounds, contraceptive diaphragms, nasal packings, and catheters. TSS caused by group A streptococci producing pyrogenic exotoxin A has recently been described. Though similar to staphylococcal TSS, its course is more rapid and destructive of soft tissue, at times resulting in necrotizing fasciitis.

The syndrome usually begins acutely with fever and, sometimes, vomiting, diarrhea, severe circulatory shock, edema of the hands and feet, and muscle, liver, kidney, and central nervous system disease.

Patients develop early a diffuse, itchy, macular, erythematous, scarlatiniform or papulopustular rash, followed within 1 to 2 weeks by mild desquamation, especially of the palms (Fig. 26-1) and soles. Sometimes the rash is purpuric. Other skin features include reversible patchy alopecia; telogen effluvium; transverse ridging of the nails; partial nail loss; and erythema, ulceration, or occasionally, vesicles and bullae of the oral, esophageal, vaginal, or bladder mucosa.

Ocular Features

The ocular features include a rash of the lid skin, conjunctival hyperemia, and subconjunctival hemorrhages.

Clinical Manifestations of Direct Staphylococcal Skin Infections

Impetigo

Impetigo is a pyogenic superficial skin infection, which may be bullous (caused by *Staphylococcus aureus*) or nonbullous (caused by *S. aureus, S. pyogenes,* or synergism between both organisms). It usually involves the face, especially perioral areas (Figs. 26-2 and 26-3) and sites of skin inflammation [e.g., eczema (Fig. 26-4) or parasitic infections]. Regional lymphadenopathy is uncommon.

Nonbullous Impetigo

Nonbullous impetigo usually affects children under the age of 6. It is more common in temperate climates. Predisposing conditions include overcrowding, poor hygiene, and preexisting skin conditions. It begins as a vesicle on an erythematous base; the vesicle quickly ruptures, leaving a thin crust (Fig. 26-5). The lesion gradually extends and may become confluent with other lesions. Healing causes temporary hypopigmentation, but otherwise the lesion heals without scarring.

Bullous Impetigo

Bullous impetigo is usually sporadic, is most common in summer, and affects both children and adults. Minor skin abrasions or other conditions may predispose to infection.

Impetigo neonatorum (neonatal bullous impetigo) is highly contagious and potentially very serious. The infection often becomes manifest about the second week of life, although the infection is usually acquired during or soon after hospital delivery. It is characterized by bullae several centimeters in diameter that often persist for several days. The bullae at first contain clear fluid that later becomes cloudy. They eventually rupture, leaving a thin, flat, brownish (varnish-like) crust, with an underlying moist surface.

Impetigo neonatorum usually affects the perineum, periumbilical area, or neck creases; often it is widespread. The bullae are usually massive and associated with generalized toxicity. The infection may lead to pneumonia, lung abscess, osteomyelitis, and death.

Ocular Features

Both forms of impetigo affect the lid, and the clinical manifestations are similar. Impetigo may lead to gangrene in the presence of measles or scarlet fever.

Infectious Eczematoid Dermatitis (see Chapter 3)

Ecthyma

Ecthyma is a pyogenic skin infection characterized by adherent skin crusts overlying an actively ulcerating area. It is more common in children. Usually, *S. aureus* and *S. pyogenes* act synergistically to cause ecthyma. Minor skin abrasions and parasitic infections, such as scabies, often determine the site of the lesion. Multiple lesions usually occur by autoinoculation.

Small vesicles or bullae develop on an erythematous base, leading to exudation and a hard crust (Fig. 26-6). The crusted area gradually enlarges and later covers a purulent, irregular, indurated ulcer. The lesion heals by scarring.

Folliculitis

Superficial pustular folliculitis (Bockhart impetigo). *Staphylococcus aureus* is the most frequent cause of these thin-walled, small, white to yellowish follicular pustules (Fig. 26-7), which may be surrounded by an erythematous margin (Fig. 26-8). These fragile pustules develop in crops and heal in a few days. They can be differentiated from miliaria (heat rash) by their follicular location as opposed the to nonfollicular location (sweat gland sites) of the former. Superficial folliculitis of the eyelashes is common.

Sycosis Vulgaris (Sycosis Barbae)

Sycosis barbae is a chronic, recurrent staphylococcal folliculitis of the bearded region, which is aggravated by shaving. Burning or itching precedes the appearance of follicular erythema and pustules (Fig. 26-9). Marginal blepharitis and conjunctivitis often accompany severe cases.

Pseudo-folliculitis barbae is caused by ingrowing beard hairs and is most commonly seen in African-American patients (Fig. 26-10). The resultant multiple, often painful pustules are best treated by removal of the offending hairs.

Pyogenic Paronychia

Paronychia is an acute or chronic inflammation of the nail folds, usually as a result of minor trauma and/or excessive exposure to moisture. Yeast paronychia are most often seen in dishwashers or bartenders, and in patients with diabetes. Secondary bacterial infection usually ensues changing the initially white purulent discharge to yellow (staph) (Fig. 26-11) or green (*Pseudomonas*).

Furuncles (Boils)

A furuncle represents an acute staphylococcal hair follicle infection that leads to abscess formation and necrosis. It usually occurs on the face, neck, arms, wrists, fingers, buttocks, and anogenital region. Sometimes furuncles occur in crops.

A furuncle begins as a small inflammatory follicular nodule, which quickly pustulates and becomes necrotic. Eventually, a necrotic core is discharged, following which, healing occurs with scarring. The lesions may cause fever; tenderness and pain are common, especially when the nose or external ear is involved.

Cellulitis

Cellulitis represents an acute, subacute, or chronic inflammation of the skin and loose subcutaneous connective tissue. It occurs in any location and is characterized by pain, tenderness, erythema, heat, swelling (Fig. 26-12), bullae, and dermal necrosis. Lymphangitis (Fig. 26-13) and, in some instances, lymphadenitis accompany the cellulitis.

Preseptal cellulitis is limited anteriorly by the skin of the lids and orbital rim, and posteriorly by the orbital septum. It is characterized by lid erythema and edema with minimal conjunctival chemosis and minimal restricted ocular movements.

Orbital cellulitis represents infection of the loose orbital connective tissue. It is manifested by pain, lid erythema and edema, conjunctival chemosis, limited ocular motility, proptosis, and sometimes, marked reduction in visual acuity (Fig. 26-14).

Pyoderma

Chancriform pyoderma is uncommon but usually occurs in children, where it may involve the lid, the perioral skin, or genitalia. It is characterized by a well-defined 1 cm or larger ulcer and an indurated base surrounded by a red areola. Usually, there is a tender regional lymphadenopathy. Blastomycosis-like pyoderma (dermatitis vegetans) is a form of chancriform pyoderma that may affect multiple sites, including the lid (see later).

Ocular Features of Staphylococcal Skin Infections

Staphylococcal Blepharitis

Staphylococcal blepharitis may cause pain, photophobia, tearing, redness, blurred vision, and discharge. Prominent features include lid hyperemia (Fig. 26-15), yellow crusts, collarettes, folliculitis, perifolliculitis, poliosis, pustules, external and internal hordeola, abscesses, and ulcerative blepharitis.

A collarette is almost pathognomonic for staphylococcal blepharitis. It is a fibrinous crust that is pierced by an eyelash and resembles a piece of paper impaled upon a stick. The crust arises from exudation of fibrin at the time of ulceration. Because the ulceration occurs in the orifice of a lash follicle, the fibrin surrounds a lash; then, as the lash grows, the fibrin is carried away from the skin surface while surrounding the lash, giving the appearance of a small collar (i.e., a collarette) (Fig. 26-16).

Folliculitis embodies a small pustule of a lash follicle that leads to crusting. The inflammation subsides or progresses to a perifolliculitis characterized by erythema and tenderness.

Folliculitis frequently leads to a small ulcer of a lash orifice, which is frequently masked by crusting. Healing occurs by primary intention but may lead to scarring, trichiasis, and lash loss (Fig. 26-17).

Localized poliosis (whitening of individual lashes) is common in staphylococcal blepharitis and is caused by damage to the pilosebaceous unit while the lash itself is retained (Fig. 26-18). (Generalized poliosis is only rarely caused by staphylococcal infections.)

An external hordeolum (sty) is common in staphylococcal lid infections. It represents infection of a sebaceous gland of the lash follicle (gland of Zeis) and causes localized pain, redness, and edema; the pain intensity is proportional to the degree of edema. The abscess involves the lumen and points to the skin surface. Once the pus is evacuated, the symptoms rapidly subside. Sequelae include a small depression in the lid margin and trichiasis. An internal hordeolum represents a meibomian gland abscess. It causes marked swelling, occasionally results in pain, and usually points toward the skin or conjunctival surface (Figs. 26-19 to 26-21).

Other findings include short and broken lashes, lash misdirection, madarosis, chalazia, verrucous excrescence of the lid margin, tylosis, granulomas, angular blepharitis (Fig. 26-22), and gangrene. Staphylococcal angular blepharitis is more severe than in *Moraxella* infections. Angular staphylococcal blepharitis involves only the outer or inner canthal region and is usually associated with an angular conjunctivitis. It causes a sensation of the skin splitting whenever the lids are opened. The canthal skin is macerated, erythematous, and often covered by secretions.

Staphylococcal Conjunctivitis

Staphylococcal blepharitis may lead to subacute catarrhal, chronic catarrhal, angular, or less commonly, purulent or a pseudomembranous conjunctivitis.

Staphylococcal Keratitis

Staphylococcal exotoxins arising in staphylococcal blepharitis frequently cause epithelial keratitis, epithelial erosions, catarrhal infiltrates and ulcers (Fig. 26-23), and phlyctenules (Figs. 26-24 and 26-25). Catarrhal infiltrates usually occur at the 2, 4, 8, or 10 o'clock areas. They are arc-shaped, located 1 or 2 mm inside the limbus, and are separated from the limbus by a lucid interval. They cause photophobia, pain, redness, and tearing. The overlying epithelium often breaks down to form an ulcer. Healing occurs by scarring and often leads to peripheral neovascularization. A limbal phlyctenule straddles the limbus and affects both cornea and conjunctiva. It causes corneal scarring only, leading to a limbal-based triangular scar that is almost pathognomonic for previous phlyctenulosis.

A corneal phlyctenule begins as a white or yellow superficial infiltrate; it ulcerates and heals in about 10 to 14 days. The necrosis leads to scarring and usually attracts a leash of superficial blood vessels and may eventually lead to a fascicular keratitis.

STREPTOCOCCAL INFECTIONS

Streptococci may infect any tissue, and both skin and eye may be affected by circulating toxins or allergic hypersensitivity reactions. The group A streptococcus is the major streptococcal pathogen, and group A streptococcal skin infections may be followed by glomerulonephritis. Groups B, C, D, F, G, and L streptococci also cause skin and eye infections. Anaerobic and microaerophilic streptococci may play a role in progressive bacterial synergistic gangrene and necrotizing fasciitis.

Skin Diseases Caused by Circulating Streptococcal Toxins

Scarlet Fever

Scarlet fever is caused by an erythrogenic exotoxin that produce group A streptococci. It usually affects children between the ages of 1 and 10, and most frequently arises from streptococcal pharyngitis; but it may follow infection of surgical or other wounds.

Skin Features

Scarlet fever is characterized by a diffuse erythematous exanthem with tiny papules, giving the skin a rough sandpaper feel (Fig. 26-26). The rash blanches on pressure and is often accentuated in the antecubital and axillary folds, producing a linear petechial eruption known as Pastia lines. Initially, the tongue has a white coating through which reddened papillae project, producing the so-called white strawberry appearance (Fig. 26-27). Within a few days, the coating disappears, leaving a bright red tongue, the red strawberry tongue (Fig. 26-28). The skin eruption usually begins on the neck and rapidly spreads to the trunk and finally the extremities. The face is flushed except for circumoral pallor (Fig. 26-28). As the eruption fades, it leaves a superficial desquamation with peeling of the palms (Fig. 26-29) and soles about 2 weeks after the onset of the illness.

Ocular Features

The rash may involve the lids and may be associated with a catarrhal conjunctivitis during the exanthematous phase or desquamative phase of the rash. The conjunctiva is diffusely injected, and there is moderate chemosis.

Direct Streptococcal Skin and Subcutaneous Infections

Impetigo

The streptococcus alone or acting in synergism with staphylococcal infections may cause nonbullous impetigo (Figs. 26-30 and 26-31). Poststreptococcal glomerulonephritis may be associated with the impetigo.

Ecthyma

Ecthyma caused by *Staphylococcus pyogenes* or by a synergistic infection with *S. aureus* is similar to that caused by *S. aureus.*

Erysipelas

Erysipelas comprises a streptococcal infection of the skin and upper subcutaneous tissue, and usually involves the cheek. The skin lesions are warm, red, tense, swollen, and erythematous. They have a sharp, raised, indurated border (Fig. 26-32) that characteristically appears to advance daily. Frequently, it causes vesicles or bullae containing seropurulent material or sometimes blood. Chills, high fever, headache, malaise, and joint pains often precede the onset of skin manifestations by a few hours. Erysipelas heals without scarring and occasionally leads to acute glomerulonephritis.

Facial erysipelas frequently involves the lid (Fig. 26-33) and occasionally is associated with a pseudomembranous or membranous conjunctivitis. Rarely, acute dacryoadenitis, orbital infection, cavernous sinus thrombosis, or lid gangrene is found.

Necrotizing hemorrhagic streptococcal cellulitis (Fig. 26-34) is an especially challenging cutaneous manifestation associated with infection with this organism.

Infectious Eczematoid Dermatitis

Streptococcal infections occasionally cause infectious eczematoid dermatitis (Fig. 26-35). The lesions are similar to those caused by staphylococci.

Ocular Features of Streptococcal Infections

Streptococcal ocular infections may cause a pseudomembranous conjunctivitis, corneal ulcer, and infectious crystalline keratopathy.

Clostridia Spp.

Gas gangrene organisms (e.g., *Clostridium perfringens*) and the tetanus organism, *Clostridium tetani,* may affect the skin and eye. Usually, they require dirty, contaminated wounds and tissue necrosis to cause infection.

Gas Gangrene (Myonecrosis)

Gas gangrene (myonecrosis) begins suddenly. Hemolysis, jaundice, and acute renal failure leading to uremia are the hallmarks of gas gangrene sepsis. The temperature is only mildly elevated, but tachycardia and hypotension followed by prostration, stupor, coma, and delirium occur. Vomiting and diarrhea that is sometimes bloody may also occur.

Skin Features

Pain develops at the infection site and rapidly increases in intensity; the tissue is swollen; the surrounding skin is pale; a foul-smelling, brown, occasionally blood-tinged, serous fluid drains from the wound. As the infection progresses, the surrounding tissue becomes dusky, deeply discolored; red, fluid-filled vesicles develop, which coalesce. Crepitation can often be palpated in the affected tissues.

Ocular Features

Gas gangrene of the lid and inner canthus may follow trauma. The cornea is sometimes involved in the same process and is manifested by profound corneal edema and small gas bubbles in the corneal stroma.

Tetanus

Generalized Tetanus

The infection usually develops in a puncture wound, burn, laceration, or in newborns whose umbilical stump is treated with ashes (Fig. 26-36). At onset, there is pain and tingling of the infection site, followed by spasticity of the surrounding groups of muscles, and eventually, stiffness of the jaw and neck, dysphagia, and irritability. Later, hyperreflexia and spasms of the jaw and/or facial muscles occur, followed by descending paralysis. The abdominal, neck, and back muscles become rigid due to spasm (Fig. 26-36), and painful tonic convulsions are induced by even minor auditory, tactile, or visual stimuli. The spasms are at first widely separated in time; later, they become more frequent, often occurring every few days; during recovery they become spaced further apart. The patient remains alert, and there is only mild fever during the entire illness.

Cephalic Tetanus

Cephalic tetanus is characterized by cranial nerve palsies during the uncontrolled tetanic spasms. It arises from head, face, neck, and occasionally eye infections. Sometimes the involved cranial nerve is permanently paretic.

Local Tetanus

Local tetanus usually progresses to generalized tetanus but occasionally remains localized.

Ocular Features

Ocular adnexal wounds may cause tetanic symptoms, while intraocular infections rarely do. Tetanic corneal ulcers usually cause moderate to severe pain. Extraocular muscle palsies may occur during the acute generalized or cephalic stage of tetanus.

Actinomycosis

Although uncommon, actinomycosis may involve most body areas, including the eye.

The various forms of actinomycosis (cervicofacial or lumpy jaw, disseminated, primary cutaneous, and ocular) may all involve the skin and eye. They are characterized by a chronic, slowly progressive granulomatous inflammation with deep excavations and chronic draining sinus tracts that spread without regard to tissue planes. "Sulfur granules" (small white or yellow aggregates) can be found in the discharge and contain the organism.

Cervicofacial Actinomycosis

Cervicofacial actinomycosis develops following dental work, gum infections, or oral trauma. The infection begins with induration, reddish or bluish discoloration, and irregularity of the overlying skin, which slowly progresses to an abscess and chronic draining fistulas (Fig. 26-37). Muscle spasm may occur, but pain, fever, and inflammation are minimal unless there is secondary infection. It occasionally causes periostitis and osteomyelitis, and sometimes extends to the lacrimal gland, orbit, skull bones, or brain.

Disseminated Actinomycosis

Disseminated actinomycosis occurs by hematogenous spread from pulmonary infection and may cause soft tissue, bone, visceral, brain, or eye infection, resulting in abscesses, draining sinus tracts, and evidence of mass lesions.

Primary Cutaneous Actinomycosis

Primary skin involvement is rare and usually involves exposed skin. It causes subcutaneous nodules that slowly enlarge, extend, and break down to form chronic draining sinuses. Regional lymphadenopathy may also occur.

Ocular Features

Lid involvement is similar to that seen in primary cutaneous actinomycosis. Secondary bacterial infection is common. Orbital infection is caused by spread of infection from the mouth, nose, paranasal sinuses, or infrequently, lid, conjunctiva, or canaliculus. It is typified by painless, gradually increasing proptosis, redness, and conjunctival edema. The ocular motility is decreased early, suggesting a retrobulbar tumor or abscess. Later, nodular infiltration of the skin of the lid(s) develops, followed by a chronic draining fistula, or the infection extends posteriorly to the sphenoidal sinus or cranial cavity.

DIPHTHERIA

Diphtheria represents an acute bacterial infection of the pharynx, larynx, nose, skin, conjunctiva, cornea, lacrimal system, or orbit. The eyelid may be involved primarily or secondary to a membranous conjunctivitis.

Diphtherial toxins induce local necrotic lesions and systemic effects. The severity of toxic manifestations varies according to the extent of membrane formation and toxin production. Toxin produced by nasal, cutaneous, or ocular diphtheria alone is usually insufficient to cause major systemic effects.

Toxemic manifestations include rapid pulse, myocarditis with arteriovenous (A-V) conduction abnormalities, congestive heart failure, cardiogenic shock, peripheral neuritis, and restlessness.

Pharyngeal Diphtheria

Pharyngeal diphtheria causes fever, malaise, a mild sore throat, toxemia, and prostration. It begins as a mild pharyngitis with a thin pharyngeal exudate, which progresses to a thick, light gray, or black membrane that is fused to the underlying tissue. Removal of the membrane causes bleeding. The pharynx becomes markedly swollen, causing dyspnea and thick speech. The patient is weak and lethargic. Cervical and submandibular lymphadenopathy and edema of the neck give the appearance of a bull neck.

Nasal Diphtheria

Nasal diphtheria usually accompanies pharyngeal involvement and is characterized by a serosanguineous discharge, a gray membrane, and occasionally, ulcerations that are covered by a thin exudate.

Cutaneous Diphtheria

Cutaneous diphtheria may be primary or occur in a preexisting wound and is usually associated with regional adenopathy. It is more common in the tropics, where the lesions usually involve the lower extremities. In temperate regions, the lesions are usually behind the ears and around the umbilicus, genitocrural flexures, toe clefts, fingers, or toes. Cutaneous diphtheria begins as a pustule that evolves into a superficial, clearly defined, punched-out ulcer, covered by a gray or grayish-brown adherent membrane. Later, the ulcer deepens, and the edge appears rolled, raised, and avascular. Infection of a preexisting wound, insect bite, or eczema causes erythema, a purulent exudate, and membrane.

Neurologic Features

Diphtheria mainly affects the motor nerves and causes paralysis in the following order:

1. Palatine paralysis (nasal voice and regurgitation of fluid through the nose).
2. Pharyngeal and laryngeal paralysis usually associated with palatine paralysis (hoarseness and difficulty swallowing).
3. Accommodative paralysis, usually in young children, which is usually bilateral. Pupillary reaction to light and nearness (accommodation) is usually retained. Rarely, it causes an "inverse" light–nearness dissociation.
4. Extraocular muscle paralysis (usually of the 6th cranial nerve and occasionally bilateral). Bilateral ptosis and a superior oblique palsy may accompany the lateral rectus palsy.
5. Optic nerve involvement (probably represents an untoward reaction to antidiphtherial serum).
6. Nerves to intercostal muscles or muscles of the extremities.

The nerve function returns in the order in which the paresis appeared.

Ocular Features

In diphtheritic membranous and pseudomembranous conjunctivitis the lids are red, tender, and markedly edematous, and have a boardlike hardness. Uncommonly, meibomitis occurs in association with the conjunctivitis.

Primary diphtheritic blepharitis without mucous membrane involvement may follow an abrasion. The lesion is moist and has eczematoid areas interspersed with hypertrophic areas of inflammation, or it begins as a clear vesicle surrounded by erythema, which quickly breaks down to form a central grayish slough and then persists as an indolent ulcer. Lid gangrene or entropion may eventuate.

Conjunctival diphtheria is membranous, pseudomembranous, purulent, or occasionally, catarrhal. The preauricular lymph nodes are usually enlarged. Healing often occurs, with extensive scarring, symblepharons, entropion, trichiasis, and xerophthalmia.

The conjunctivitis may lead to marginal or central corneal ulceration, corneal perforation, and loss of the eye.

Metastatic diphtherial inflammation rarely causes unilateral dacryoadenitis, and dacryocystitis may occur from diphtheritic spread from nasal cavity or conjunctiva. Healing occurs by secondary intention, producing a disfiguring scar.

PROPIONIBACTERIUM SPP.

Propionibacterium acnes and *P. granulosum* may cause infection in many organs, including the skin and eye. *P. acnes* may cause lipolysis of sebum, which probably contributes to the lesions of acne. The lipolytic activity of the organism contributes to meibomitis by producing irritating free fatty acids. It may also cause inflammatory pustules and cysts of the skin of the lid and face. The organism has also been implicated in chronic endophthalmitis cases following cataract extraction.

Anthrax

Human anthrax usually occurs in individuals working with animal byproducts but occasionally is mediated through insect bites, although recently it has been used in bioterrorism. When encountered as a naturally occurring disease in the United States, it is most frequently seen in those working with wool, hence the common name *wool-sorter's disease*. The organism can be inhaled, resulting in pneumonia, or ingested, causing gastrointestinal disease.

It usually does not cause septicemia, but infrequently, there are mild general symptoms or, rarely, high fever, headache, toxemia, tachycardia, hypotension, and meningitis, resulting from local spread to the lymphatics. Death rarely occurs but can occur in the cutaneous form or the gastrointestinal form, although it results more commonly from the pneumonic form.

Skin Features

The cutaneous infection is characterized by a malignant pustule of the face, neck, hands, or arms at the site of an infected abrasion. Multiple lesions are common. It is a painless, circumscribed, carbuncle-like lesion that begins as a small, pruritic, reddish macule that within a day progresses to a red, indurated papule that quickly becomes bullous in character. It is surrounded by a zone of brawny, nonpitting, gelatinous edema and erythema, and within this zone, several vesicles may be evident. The lesion contains sanguineous fluid from which the organism can be readily recovered. Rupture of the bulla leaves a red base that dries, blackens, and forms the typical eschar surrounded by a vesicular zone. The surrounding edematous area gradually extends and becomes more red in appearance. Nontender regional lymphadenopathy may occur. The lesions heal after 2 to 3 weeks.

Ocular Features

Anthrax of the lid represents a form of cutaneous anthrax (Fig. 26-38). Lid infection usually arises from rubbing or scratching. It is manifested by severe upper and lower lid swelling and occasionally involves the face, neck, and chest, and even impinges on the tongue, throat, and trachea. Exophthalmos and bilateral optic atrophy have been recorded. Ectropion occasionally occurs as a late sequela.

Occasionally, the infection causes severe lid edema without evidence of a primary pustule because of laxity of the tissues of the lids. The edema becomes so severe that vesicles filled with the bacilli develop within the edematous skin.

Orbital anthrax, although rare, may occur from hematogenous dissemination or from a malignant pustule of the forehead, nose, lip, or chin. It progresses to an orbital thrombophlebitis with severe lid edema and acute proptosis and is frequently complicated by cavernous sinus thrombosis.

NEISSERIA SPECIES

Neisseria gonorrhoeae

Gonorrhea (GC) is usually transmitted venereally and is characterized by purulent discharge (Fig. 26-39). Occasionally, the primary lesion may be intraoral (Fig. 26-40).

Primary Skin Infections

Primary skin infections occur from skin contamination by urethral, vaginal, or rectal discharge. Lesions are characterized by multiple, nonindurated erosions with sharply marginated, red, oval, rounded, or ragged margins and a light red base. Pustules occasionally occur on the coronal sulcus or the fingers, especially if there are preexisting skin abrasions. Healing occurs when the discharge stops.

Features of Dissemination

Skin lesions are common in the fulminant form of dissemination and represent a septic vasculitis. The dissemination may be fulminant and lead to death through endocarditis, whereas the benign form may persist for months. It is associated with chills, high fever, migratory polyneuralgias, and polyarthritis, myocarditis, pericarditis, and toxic hepatitis.

Successive crops of hemorrhagic or vesiculopustular skin lesions, usually numbering from three to 20, occur on the distal extremities during the bacteremia. They begin as punctate erythematous lesions, usually of the palms and soles, which gradually enlarge to form purpuric areas. Vesiculopustular lesions (Figs. 26-41 and 26-42) begin as erythematous macules, papules or, rarely, bullae that become necrotic (Fig. 26-43). The lesions persist 1 to 2 weeks, then they reappear in smaller numbers at the time of the menstrual period.

Ocular Features

Gonorrheal ophthalmia usually causes copious secretion of pus, severe lid edema, occasionally a lid abscess and, exceptionally, lid gangrene and sloughing (Figs. 26-44 to 26-47). There is severe bulbar chemosis, marked papillary hypertrophy, and occasionally, pseudomembrane. Healing often occurs with scarring. Marginal or central corneal ulceration may occur if treatment is not started promptly.

GC ophthalmia neonatorum (Fig. 26-48) unfortunately is still seen when adequate preventive care is unavailable.

Meningococcal Infections

Systemic meningococcal infections may present as:

1. Fulminant meningococcemia without signs of meningitis.
2. Acute meningococcemia with signs of meningitis.
3. Chronic meningitis.
4. Chronic basilar meningitis.

Patients with fulminant meningococcemia usually die within 24 hours from Waterhouse–Friderichsen syndrome and often before signs of meningeal involvement become evident.

Cases of acute meningococcemia with signs of meningitis are less severe than the fulminant cases, but death often occurs within 3 days. Signs of meningeal involvement are pronounced.

Chronic meningitis cases usually begin with acute signs, but the disease then becomes chronic and lasts for weeks.

Chronic basilar meningitis usually occurs in infants, causing hydrocephalus from basilar meningeal involvement.

Specific central nervous system findings include confusion, delirium, coma, twitching, frank convulsions, stiff neck, opisthotonos, positive Kernig and Brudzinski signs, squint, pupillary changes, hydrocephalus, deafness, blindness, papilledema, and spinal cord syndromes.

During meningococcemia, the organism occasionally localizes in various sites, including the meninges, joints, skin, ears, lungs, and adrenal glands.

Skin Features

Half to two-thirds of patients develop petechial eruptions most often on the trunk and lower extremities (Figs. 26-49 and 26-50). The lesions may progress to ecchymoses and necrosis. Occasionally, a blanchable morbilliform eruption may be the only cutaneous finding.

Hemorrhages also involve the mucous membranes. Infrequently, there is a vasculitis that causes nodules or bullae and sometimes ulcerations. It begins 5 to 9 days following onset of infection.

Ocular Features

The preauricular nodes are usually tender and enlarged when there is hyperacute conjunctivitis. Severe lid edema is a common early sign of both the meningitis and hyperacute conjunctivitis. Petechial hemorrhages may involve the lid.

Sometimes the conjunctivitis is the presenting sign of meningococcal infection; rarely, it is the only sign of infection. It is usually hyperacute with purulent discharge, papillary hypertrophy, chemosis, and often, subconjunctival hemorrhages. In some cases, the conjunctivitis is pseudomembranous; occasionally, it is catarrhal.

Corneal involvement associated with the hyperacute conjunctivitis begins as a gray peripheral haze that progresses to ulceration, scarring, and neovascularization. Other ocular findings include episcleritis; iridocyclitis retinal detachment, retinal inflammation, and retinal vein thrombosis; and endophthalmitis and panophthalmitis.

MORAXELLA SPP. INFECTIONS

The *Moraxella* organism causes a gonococcemia-like systemic infection, arthritis with skin lesions, angular blepharoconjunctivitis (Fig. 26-51), marginal or central corneal ulcer, subacute or chronic dacryocystitis, and endophthalmitis. The angular blepharitis is usually bilateral and commonly associated with angular conjunctivitis. It causes itching, smarting or pain, erythema, scaling, fissuring, maceration and crusting of the outer or inner canthal region, and mild mucoid discharge that adheres to the eyelashes.

Moraxella conjunctivitis is more marked in the lateral or medial canthal region and usually is associated with an angular blepharitis (see earlier). Occasionally, *Moraxella* causes follicular conjunctivitis in children and adults. Moraxella marginal corneal ulcers are similar to the marginal corneal ulcers in staphylococcal disease.

Cat-Scratch Disease (*Bartonella henselae*)

Cat-scratch disease (*Bartonella henselae*) is a benign systemic infection characterized by malaise, mild fever, anorexia, lassitude, weakness, headache, local area of skin or conjunctival involvement that represents the site of inoculation, and regional lymphadenopathy that may progress to suppuration. The infection is usually indolent.

Skin Features

Most of the skin lesions occur on the hands or arm, and some are found on the head and neck. A single papule or multiple papules initially develop at the site of inoculation and progress to vesiculation, ulceration, and crusting before healing by superficial scarring. Occasionally, there is a maculopapular rash, urticaria, thrombocytopenia, purpura, erythema nodosum, erythema multiforme, or erythema marginatum. The regional lymph nodes are often tender or painful and may suppurate and spontaneously drain (Fig. 26-52).

Ocular Features

In about 10% of patients, the conjunctiva represents the primary inoculation site. Conjunctival involvement is manifested by a conjunctival granuloma with a grossly enlarged preauricular node (Fig. 26-53) and usually no exudate. The granuloma is usually located in the bulbar conjunctiva or the superior palpebral conjunctiva (Fig. 26-54). It is nontender, is seldom larger than 2 cm in size, and has a whitishyellow appearance and an erythematous margin. Smaller granulomata may also be seen. The surrounding conjunctiva is usually erythematous. The granulomata subside without scarring after 4 to 6 weeks, and may be treated with appropriate antibiotics.

The organism may cause neuroretinitis with optic nerve edema and a macular star (Fig. 26-55). Although the infection is usually self-limited, visual loss secondary to optic nerve damage or retinal damage may result. Prompt antibiotic treatment probably prevents visual damage.

Rhinoscleroma (Scleroma)

Rhinoscleroma (scleroma) is a chronic, slowly progressive granulomatous disease caused by *Klebsiella rhinoscleromatis*. Rhinoscleroma is mildly contagious and, at first, localized to the nasal fossa area (Fig. 26-56); later, it spreads to the upper respiratory tract and occasionally to the lacrimal system, lids, and orbit.

The rhinitis stage is characterized by symptoms of a common cold, with headache, nasal stuffiness, rhinorrhea, crusting, epistaxis, foul odor, and hypertrophy of the nasal mucous membranes, especially of the septum.

The infiltrative period begins soon after the cold symptoms subside and causes nasal obstruction from granulomatous infiltration of the nasal fossa, as well as crusting and friability of the lower part of the nasal septum (Fig. 26-57). Later, it also involves the pharynx and larynx, leading to a change in modulation of the voice and to anesthesia of the soft palate. Occasionally, the scleromatous mass spreads to the cervical lymph nodes.

During the nodular period, the contiguous nasal areas (e.g., upper lip, nasolacrimal duct, lacrimal sac, lids, and orbit) become infiltrated, leading to the Hebra nose, loss of smell and taste, epistaxis, and respiratory tract obstruction. The overlying skin becomes brownish-red in color with telangiectatic vessels and scales.

During the fibrotic stage, the inflammatory mass is replaced by fibrotic tissue that results in anatomic distortion and obstruction.

Ocular Features

The lids are often involved in the nasal process. Conjunctival infection occurs by direct extension from the lower lid or lacrimal passages to the medial aspect of the conjunctiva. A dacryocystitis is quite common and arises from direct infection or from nasolacrimal duct occlusion. Unilateral or, occasionally, bilateral exophthalmos occurs from extension into the orbit from the lacrimal passages.

PSEUDOMONAS INFECTIONS

Pseudomonas occasionally infects the skin and the external eye. It not infrequently causes relatively minor, localized skin infections of the trunk (Fig. 26-58), external ear canal, toe webs, and nails. Umbilical infection in the neonate leads to a foul-smelling, bluish-green discharge, and spreading erythema. Occasionally, systemic pseudomonas infections involve the skin. *P. aeruginosa* has been linked to a distinct folliculitis associated with the use of hot tubs and swimming pools. Numerous discrete pruritic follicular papules develop in covered areas (e.g., buttocks and hips) and quickly evolve into erythematous papules with a fine central pustule. The lesions drain spontaneously and heal with fine, desquamative, red-brown macules. Recurrences are common.

Pseudomonas toe web infections are characterized by pruritic, foul-smelling, thick, hyperkeratotic, greenish plaques. Nail infection may cause the toenail or a portion of the nail to become greenish (Fig. 26-59). A nontender paronychia may also occur.

Infection of the lips or cheeks may result in progressive gangrene.

Pseudomonas bacteremia usually occurs in neutropenic patients. It is life-threatening and often associated with ecthyma gangrenosum (Fig. 26-34). The skin lesions are painless, well-delineated edematous areas that rapidly evolve (often within several hours) into round, erythematous macules; hemorrhagic vesicles; bullae; and gangrenous ulcers covered by gray-brown eschars and delineated by an indurated, erythematous rim. Single or multiple lesions usually occur in the axilla, groin, buttocks, or extremities. Other skin lesions in pseudomonas bacteremia include petechiae, ecchymosis, and erythematous macules.

Ocular Features: Ecthyma Gangrenosum of the Lid

The pseudomonas organism occasionally causes a severe pseudomembranous or purulent conjunctivitis in neonates, premature infants, immunosuppressed patients, or normal patients following injudicious use of an ocular dressing (Figs. 26-60 and 26-61).

A mild papillary conjunctivitis occasionally occurs in pseudomonas folliculitis.

Pseudomonas bacteremia in the debilitated infant may lead to central corneal involvement associated with ecthyma gangrenosum; in the adult, it may lead to an acute ring abscess followed by necrosis, sloughing, and loss of the eye. Rarely, ecthyma gangrenosum involves the lid, causing severe lid edema and sloughing.

Other ocular findings include central corneal ulcers (Fig. 26-62) and scleral ulceration (Fig. 26-63). Pseudomonas central corneal ulcers are characterized by sudden onset with pain, photophobia, tearing, and mild discharge. The central cornea is infiltrated and ulcerated, and there is a hypopyon. Corneal perforation and loss of the eye are common. Pseudomonas scleral infection and ulceration occurs from spread of infection from the cornea or following retinal detachment surgery.

Tularemia

Tularemia begins suddenly with headache, fever, nausea, and often severe pain from local lesions. The spleen may be tender and enlarged; a generalized rash, generalized aches and pains, and exhaustion often occur. The toxemic phase of infection is often associated with erythema multiforme, a maculopapular eruption, or profuse crops of nodules that usually involve the extremities.

The skin and eye are involved in the ulceroglandular and oculoglandular forms of tularemia.

Ulceroglandular Tularemia

Ulceroglandular tularemia arises from transcutaneous inoculation from contact with tissues or body fluids of infected animals (e.g., rabbits), or from tick bites or other vectors, such as deer flies. It develops about 2 to 5 days following inoculation and begins with an erythematous macule at the site of inoculation that evolves over several days into a pruritic papule and finally into an ulcer with raised borders. It is associated with marked regional, painful lymphadenitis that may eventually suppurate and drain.

Oculoglandular Tularemia

Oculoglandular tularemia may occur from transconjunctival infection, such as rubbing the eyes with contaminated fingers (Figs. 26-64 to 26-66). It is usually unilateral and causes pain, itching, photophobia, and a mucoid or purulent discharge.

Infrequently, the primary lesion develops on the lid, causing gross edema and preauricular and submaxillary lymphadenopathy. Periorbital edema also occurs with conjunctival involvement. Invasion of the tarsal plate during conjunctival infection produces small, indurated areas, which simulate multiple chalazia.

Conjunctival granulomata appear as small, yellow nodules on the lower palpebral conjunctiva; occasionally, on the upper palpebral conjunctiva; or rarely, on the bulbar conjunctiva. The nodules quickly ulcerate to form discrete ulcers measuring 1 to 5 mm and are covered by a gray, necrotic membrane. The surrounding conjunctiva is severely injected and chemotic. The discharge is usually scanty and mucoid. Healing occurs without scarring, although prolonged infiltration and erythema are common. Sometimes the lymph nodes suppurate and require drainage, which yields thick, white pus.

Other findings may include peripheral corneal infiltrates that are preceded by recurrent limbal nodules, peripheral opacity with a fascicular pannus, corneal edema, intense circumcorneal injection and corneal ulceration, nonspecific purulent dacryocystitis, bilateral optic neuritis, and endophthalmitis.

Chancroid

Chancroid (soft chancre) is an infectious, sexually transmitted disease caused by the Gram-negative bacillus *Haemophilus ducreyi*. It is seen more often in men than in women.

Skin Features

Chancroid appears as one or more small, painful, purulent ulcerations with erythematous margins several days to a week after infectious sexual contact. The most frequent locations in the male are on the distal penis, especially the coronal sulcus (Fig. 26-67) and the frenulum (Figs. 26-68 and 26-69). Chancroid is seen less often in women, in whom the ulcerations are found on the vulva, labia (Fig. 26-70), cervix, perineum (Fig. 26-71), and perianal areas. Extragenital lesions on the fingers, lips, breasts, and eyelids are occasionally reported. Autoinoculation frequently produces "Kissing ulcers" (Fig. 26-72). In about half of the patients, painful, usually unilateral inguinal lymphadenitis will accompany the ulcers (Fig. 26-73). Paraphimosis (Fig. 26-74) and phimosis (Fig. 26-75) are occasional complications. Mixed infections may lead to phagedenic ulcerations and gangrenous balanitis.

The diagnosis of chancroid, which at one time was one of exclusion, can now be confirmed by culture with special media. A new combined polymerase chain reaction (PCR) test allows differentiation from syphilis and herpes simplex, which may mimic or be co-infectious with chancroid.

Ocular Features

Soft chancres occasionally involve the lid and are similar to genital lesions. There is gross enlargement of the preauricular and cervical lymph nodes. Conjunctival lesions are similar to the skin lesion. The ulcer base is covered by a dirty gray membrane.

Glanders

Glanders is a rare, usually fatal, specific acute or chronic lung infection that frequently progresses to widespread suppuration of many body regions. It occurs from contact with diseased horses, mules, or donkeys. The causative organism is *Pseudomonas mallei*.

Clinical Manifestations

Most patients develop subclinical disease and probably develop evidence of active infection only if their immune system wanes. Glanders presents as an acute or subacute pneumonitis or a septicemia associated with multiple abscesses. The septicemic form is frequently fatal. The acute manifestations include markedly indurated vesicular or carbuncular skin and subcutaneous lesions that later slough, a regional adenopathy leading to chronic draining fistulas (farcy buds) and occasionally, large gangrenous patches. Primary nasal (Fig. 26-76) or oral infection leads to extensive nasal septal and palatal necrosis; a profuse, purulent nasal discharge; and chills and fever. After several days, metastatic ulcerative lesions, which often coalesce, develop on the face and near the joints. Deep abscesses with multiple sinuses may occur. Death often supervenes. Chronic glanders is characterized by one or two small focal abscesses and ulcerations, and minimal systemic signs. It may relapse at any time, however, causing acute symptoms and death.

Melioidosis

Melioidosis is an infection caused by a glanders-like bacillus, *Burkholderia* (previously known as *Pseudomonas pseudomallei*). Most frequently, it occurs as an acute pulmonary and septic illness with multiple miliary abscesses resulting in early death. A chronic course with subcutaneous abscesses and multiple draining sinuses of the soft tissues is encountered less often (Fig. 26-77). Melioidosis has been endemic in Southeast Asia.

Ocular Features

The vesicular and carbuncular lesions in glanders may occur on the lids and may then spread progressively through the entire lid substance to involve the globe, producing a panophthalmitis. It causes regional lymphadenopathy with chronic draining sinuses (farcy buds) and signs of septicemia. Occasionally, the infection is more chronic and milder.

Primary conjunctival infection is unusual but is severe and has a violent onset. It is associated with preauricular lymphadenopathy, septicemia, and nasal and oral involvement. Usually, the conjunctiva is involved during systemic infection and is ulcerative or granulomatous in type.

Orbital glanders begins acutely, arising from lid or conjunctival infection, and causes proptosis, severe lid edema, conjunctival chemosis, and limited extraocular movement.

Granuloma Inguinale (Donovanosis)

Granuloma inguinale (donovanosis) is a chronic, mildly contagious, granulomatous disease characterized by indolent progressive ulcerations of the genitalia, groin, anus, and pubic area. It is caused by the Gram-negative bacterium *Calymmatobacterium granulomatosis.*

Skin Features

The infection begins as subcutaneous nodules that slowly evolve into painless or mildly painful vegetative granulation tissue. The early lesions have a characteristic beefy-red appearance and are friable (Fig. 26-78). Some lesions have a rolled margin (Fig. 26-79), suggestive of cutaneous carcinoma. Most lesions involve the genitalia and remain limited to that area. The prepuce, or glans, in men and the labia, in women, are the most frequent sites. The inguinal region is involved in about 10% of patients (Fig. 26-80), with less frequent occurrence in the pubic (Fig. 26-81), anal, and more distant areas. The lesions enlarge by autoinoculation with serpiginous ulcerations gradually undermining adjacent tissue. Persisting sinuses and hypertrophic scars may block lymphatics, producing pseudoelephantiasis of the genitals. Rarely, squamous cell carcinoma may occur. Dissemination by lymphatic or hematogenous channels to the liver, other organs, distant cutaneous sites, lips, eyes, and bones has been reported.

Ocular Features

Lid lesions are uncommon. They begin as a nontender, reddish papule that resembles an acute hordeolum but without pain or tenderness. They form a progressive destructive ulcer with a diffuse dirty gray slough that progresses to severe lid and tarsal destruction.

Tuberculosis

Tuberculosis, which had been on the decline since the introduction of effective drugs over the past 50 years, is again becoming a significant problem, both in the United States and worldwide, primarily because of the AIDS epidemic and because of increasing resistance to medications.

Cutaneous and ocular tuberculosis are uncommon. They occur by primary inoculation and contiguous spread, as from draining lymph nodes or hematogenous dissemination.

Tuberculous Chancre

A tuberculous chancre usually represents a primary skin infection, beginning as a red or brownish papule that becomes indurated, then forming a chronic, nonhealing, painless ulcer with undermined edges and a granular hemorrhagic base. Regional lymphadenopathy occurs, and the nodes sometimes break down, forming chronic draining sinuses.

Congenital Tuberculosis

Congenital tuberculosis develops *in utero* and presents with small, discrete, umbilicated, erythematous papules measuring about 4 mm in diameter.

Tuberculosis Verrucosa Cutis

Tuberculosis verrucosa cutis occurs from exogenous inoculation in a previously sensitized person with reasonable immunity against *Mycobacterium tuberculosis.* Exposed areas such as fingers (Fig. 26-82), hands, arms (Fig. 26-83), feet, legs, and buttocks (Figs. 26-84 and 26-85) are the most commonly affected. The infection begins as a solitary indolent warty papule (Fig. 26-84) that slowly enlarges with or without central clearing. Arcuate configurations with reddish-brown or plum colors and scarring may ensue (Fig. 26-85).

Scrofuloderma

Scrofuloderma is characterized by indurated, skin-colored, or erythematous nodules (Fig. 26-86) that ulcerate, forming chronic draining sinus tracts (Fig. 26-87). It occurs by spread of infection from underlying infected lymph nodes, bone, or other tissue and is often associated with exudate, edema, and secondary infection. Healing leads to puckered scars.

Lupus Vulgaris

Lupus vulgaris usually occurs on the head, face, and neck; sometimes on the extremities; and only rarely on the trunk. It is chronic, slowly progressive, and characterized by soft "apple-jelly"-colored nodules evident on diascopy. There are five general patterns:

1. A red or brown plaque that heals with peripheral scarring.
2. An ulcerative or mutilating type that involves deep tissue and underlying cartilage (Fig. 26-88).

3. A vegetating form characterized by infiltration, necrosis, phagedena, and minimal scarring.
4. A tumor-like form with elevated, soft, smooth nodules or a soft, reddish-yellow plaque that slowly evolves without scarring.
5. A papular or nodular form.

Miliary Tuberculosis

Miliary tuberculosis usually affects infants and children. The skin lesions present as bluish papules, erythematous nodules or vesicles, pustules, or purpuric lesions that may later ulcerate.

Tuberculous Gummata

Tuberculous gummata are extremely unusual and arise by hematogenous dissemination from a primary focus. They present as firm, subcutaneous nodules that gradually break down to form an ulcer with undermined edges and sinus tracts. The surrounding skin has a bluish appearance.

Tuberculid (see Chapter 3)

Mucocutaneous Infections

Oral mucocutaneous lesions usually occur in males with poor general health and long-standing tuberculosis (Fig. 26-89). They develop by direct extension from the skin or nose and begin as a small, firm, red nodule of the tongue (Fig. 26-90), tooth socket, or gum that enlarges and ulcerates. Ulcerating nodules of the nose sometimes destroy the septal cartilage.

Ocular Features

Tuberculous lid infections usually occur by local extension from the face, conjunctiva, underlying bone, lymph nodes, or lacrimal sac; by hematogenous dissemination; or rarely, by primary inoculation. They are similar to other skin lesions and may lead to ectropion, lid destruction, and thinning or loss of the brows or tarsus. Tuberculous tarsitis causes tarsal thickening and destruction, and may simulate recurrent chalazia.

Conjunctiva

The conjunctiva is usually infected by direct extension from the face, nose, sclera, lacrimal sac, or orbit. Infection by exogenous conjunctival inoculation is extremely uncommon. Such conjunctival inoculation is nearly always unilateral.

Primary conjunctival tuberculosis usually presents as a localized tuberculoma or conjunctival lupus vulgaris. A conjunctival tuberculoma begins insidiously and is associated with a grossly visible preauricular and/or submandibular lymph node that may later suppurate and drain. Alternatively, it begins as an acute purulent or pseudomembranous conjunctivitis that progresses to a granuloma with a grossly visible preauricular node. Fever and malaise usually occur at the onset of the conjunctivitis.

Primary conjunctival granulomas are ulcerative, nodular, hyperplastic, or polypoid, and may be single or multiple. The ulcerative form is chronic and indolent and may eventually spread to the lid, sclera, or cornea.

Nodular conjunctival granulomas appear as small, yellow, or gray subconjunctival nodules of the bulbar conjunctiva and upper fornix, and gradually develop into large, cauliflower-like growths that ulcerate centrally. The associated follicles, granulation tissue, and superior corneal infiltration may be confused with trachoma.

The hypertrophic papillary (Fig. 26-91) form of tuberculous granuloma develops in the fornix and, occasionally, on the tarsus. It begins with severe conjunctival and lid edema, followed by a granuloma (or granulomas) that gradually enlarges, becomes pedunculated, and eventually assumes a jelly-like character or, occasionally, ulcerates.

The polypoid form occurs on the tarsus and is pedunculated.

Conjunctival lupus vulgaris usually develops by extension from the skin and, rarely, as an isolated conjunctival lesion. It causes mild photophobia, tearing, itching, and mucoid discharge and has an "apple-jelly" appearance encircled by an erythematous zone. The lesion slowly enlarges peripherally while the central area ulcerates or scars—often repeatedly breaking down. It sometimes leads to stromal keratitis or phthisis bulbi.

Secondary tuberculous conjunctival manifestations appear as tuberculids (Chapter 3) or phlyctenules (Fig. 26-92) and occur in immune patients, especially in those with a prominent delayed hypersensitivity. Tuberculous phlyctenulosis represents a hypersensitivity reaction to tuberculoprotein. The phlyctenules usually occur at the limbus and occasionally appear on the bulbar and tarsal conjunctiva, cornea, or lid margin. Corneal and limbal phlyctenules cause scarring.

A conjunctival phlyctenule begins as a small, reddish conjunctival elevation surrounded by a zone of hyperemia. It increases in size, then, after a few days, ulcerates and heals without scarring. Limbal phlyctenules straddle the limbus and heal with a triangular corneal scar with the base of the triangle directed toward the limbus.

Cornea

Phlyctenulosis

Corneal phlyctenules are commonly associated with and usually arise from limbal phlyctenules. They are marginal, miliary, or fascicular and cause intense photophobia, pain, irritation, tearing, and severe blepharospasm. They usually evolve over 8 to 12 days, but new phlyctenules often develop as others are healing. They usually cause superficial scarring and neovascularization.

Marginal phlyctenules develop adjacent to the limbus and have a linear shape, with the long axis directed toward the visual axis. Miliary phlyctenules appear as slightly opaque, minute elevations of the superficial cornea that progress to form small ulcers before healing. They cause minimal or no scarring.

A fascicular phlyctenule begins as a gray, superficial infiltrate that ulcerates and heals with minimal scarring. The infiltrate attracts superficial blood vessels that actively advance toward the gray infiltrate. Often a new infiltrate develops central to the previous infiltrate, causing the vessels to advance further and further into the cornea. This phenomenon leads to a fascicular lesion in which a leash of superficial vessels appears to wander aimlessly toward the visual axis. Sometimes multiple phlyctenules develop near the limbus, resulting in a sectorial or circumferential phlyctenular pannus.

Interstitial Keratitis

Tuberculous interstitial keratitis is characterized by infiltration and neovascularization of the middle and deep corneal stroma (Figs. 26-93 and 26-94). It is often confined to a sector of the cornea and sometimes causes patchy scarring.

Sclerosing Keratitis

Tuberculous sclerosing keratitis occasionally accompanies tubercular scleritis and is manifested by scleralization of the deep peripheral cornea adjacent to the scleritis (Fig. 26-95). It is gray or grayish-yellow at onset and later becomes bluish-white or dense-white. There is minimal vascularization. Individual opacities are often triangular or tongue shaped, with the base directed toward the limbus.

Infiltrative Lesions

Corneal suppuration usually arises by organismal spread from the conjunctiva, sclera, or uveal tract. The ulcers are indolent, have very little tendency to heal, and may perforate. Corneal neovascularization and recurrences are common.

Infiltrative corneal lesions are uncommon. The lesions are superficial; spread toward the visual axis as a gray, tonguelike opacity; or are located centrally in the deep stroma (keratitis pustuliformis).

A posterior tuberculous corneal abscess probably arises secondary to tuberculous iritis. It begins in the deep stroma and causes intense corneal edema and a large hypopyon.

Sclera

Ulcerative scleritis is not uncommon in primary tuberculosis and usually arises from a nodular scleritis that caseates the ulcerates (Fig. 26-96).

Lacrimal System Infections

The lacrimal system is sometimes involved in the form of an acute tuberculous dacryoadenitis, a chronic dacryadenitis, or a dacryocystitis. An associated regional lymphadenopathy is an important diagnostic feature, especially in tuberculous dacryocystitis.

Orbital Infections

Tuberculous orbital involvement develops by hematogenous or contiguous spread to the orbital bones from surrounding areas. Tuberculous orbital periostitis almost always occurs at the outer orbital margin.

A tuberculoma of the orbital soft tissues develops from hematogenous spread, usually in the superior orbit, and may involve the extraocular muscles and lacrimal gland, causing pain, tearing, and gradual increasing proptosis.

Uveal Tract

Uveal tract infection occurs from hematogenous dissemination (Fig. 26-97). There are several forms, including proliferative tuberculous lesions that are miliary or granulomatous in type and diffuse inflammations that arise from a delayed hypersensitivity response.

Choroidal tubercles may also develop without evidence of miliary meningitis. Gray, raised lesions are found during the active stage, and white, flat lesions occur during the inactive stage. The granulomatous nodules appear as small, yellow nodules located deep to the retina.

Retina

Retinal involvement occurs from hematogenous dissemination or by spread from the choroid, ciliary body, or optic nerve. It usually causes a perivasculitis (usually a periphlebitis and occasionally a periarteritis) that may lead to retinal vein occlusion (Figs. 26-98 and 26-99). Hemorrhages, miliary tubercles, and conglomerate retinal tubercles may also occur but are rare.

MYCOBACTERIUM FORTUITUM/CHELONEI COMPLEX INFECTIONS

The *Mycobacterium fortuitum/chelonei* complex group of organisms consists of atypical mycobacteria that may cause cutaneous and ocular infections. Skin infections usually occur in diabetics, arising from injections (e.g., infection of the peroneal tendons) or from superficial injuries (granulomatous skin abscesses).

Ocular Features

Ocular manifestations include a chronic granulomatous lid ulcer following a dacryocystitis, indolent corneal ulcers, orbital infections, and endophthalmitis. The indolent corneal ulcers are similar in many respects to mycotic and nocardial corneal ulcers. The ulcer base is infiltrated and often has the appearance of a cracked windshield with radiating lines. Satellite lesions composed of white, fluffy infiltrates with fuzzy edges are often present in all layers of the stroma. An immune ring, an endothelial plaque, and moderate to marked anterior chamber reaction with hypopyon often occur.

Other manifestations include an orbital granuloma and a low-grade postoperative endophthalmitis.

Hansen Disease (Leprosy)

Hansen disease (leprosy) is a chronic granulomatous disease with a wide spectrum of manifestations governed by the immunologic status of the host. It is characterized by infiltration, anesthesia, hypopigmentation of the skin, involvement of the oral and upper respiratory tract mucous membranes, and involvement of the testis and eye. Infection probably occurs through the skin or the nasal or oral mucous membranes.

Clinical Manifestations

There are two distinct forms—tuberculoid (TT) and lepromatous (LL)—and many patients present with features of both types (borderline–borderline or dimorphous). Some have features favoring the tuberculoid side (borderline tuberculoid), and others have features favoring the lepromatous side (borderline lepromatous). There is also an indeterminate type in which the full immunologic response has not developed, and the disease type has not been fully expressed at that time.

Lepromatous leprosy has a malignant, progressive course; tuberculoid leprosy has a benign, progressive course.

Nerve Involvement

The early manifestations of leprosy are caused by peripheral nerve invasion and the resultant dermal sensory and autonomic nerve fiber destruction; most major deformities arise from trauma or infection of anesthetic areas.

Nerve damage in tuberculoid leprosy is usually asymmetric, limited, and localized to one or only a few nerves, especially the ulnar and lateral perineal nerves (Fig. 26-100).

Peripheral nerve damage in lepromatous leprosy occurs late and is symmetric and diffuse. Occasionally, it involves all the major nerve trunks. At first, the sensory disturbances affect the hands and feet, then spread centripetally to involve the trunk and face. Early manifestations of peripheral sensory nerve involvement include loss of (discrimination of) heat from cold (Fig. 26-101) and local paresthesias and dysesthesias. Later manifestations include loss of sensation to touch and, eventually, true anesthesia, leading to trophic ulcers of sole (malum perforans pedis) (Figs. 26-102 and 26-103). Absorption of the digits may occur as a result of loss of sensation (Fig. 26-103).

Motor nerve involvement is manifested by weakness, paralysis, and muscle atrophy. Motor nerve involvement often causes early atrophy of the interosseous hand muscles, followed by atrophy of the thenar, hypothenar, and forearm muscles, producing a claw hand (Fig. 26-104).

The involved nerves are usually enlarged, thickened, and sometimes painful. Chiefly affected are the superficial nerve trunks, which are also most easily observed. These include the ulnar, median radial, peroneal, posterior tibial, fifth and seventh cranial and especially the greater auricular (Fig. 26-105).

In approximate order of frequency, the enlarged nerves include the following:

1. Ulnar nerve—enlarged near and up to several inches above the olecranon process.
2. Posterior tibial—enlarged between the heel and the medial malleolus.
3. Superficial peroneal nerve—enlarged as it winds around the neck of the fibula.
4. Greater auricular nerve—enlarged as it crosses the sternocleidomastoid muscle.
5. Median nerve—enlarged in the antecubital fossa or just proximal to the carpel tunnel.
6. Radial nerve—thickened as it winds around the radius at the wrist.
7. Facial nerve—thickened as it crosses the zygoma or at the area near the stylomastoid foramen.
8. Trigeminal nerve—enlarged as its branches emerge from their respective foramina.
9. Supraorbital nerve—enlarged as it emerges above the orbital rim.

Skin Features of Indeterminate Leprosy

The skin changes in indeterminate leprosy develop on the face, trunk, buttocks, and upper extremities and consist of poorly defined, slightly hypopigmented macules, with varying degrees of edema. They measure several centimeters in diameter. Many eventually disappear. There are minimal sensory changes.

Skin Features of Tuberculoid Leprosy

The skin changes in tuberculoid leprosy (TT) consist of erythematous, often hyper- or hypopigmented plaques with sharp outer margins measuring 3 to 30 cm in diameter, usually on the extremities (Fig. 26-106), back (Fig. 26-107), and buttocks. Healing begins centrally, leaving a flattened, rough, hairless, hypopigmented, anhidrotic and anesthetic, clear zone. The lesions are typically asymmetric and limited to one or two dermatomes.

Skin Features of Lepromatous Leprosy

Early skin lesions in lepromatous leprosy (LL) appear as multiple, bilateral, symmetric, erythematous, ill-defined macules and papules that ultimately form plaques and nodules. (The macules are usually not anesthetic.) Sites of predilection include the ear lobes (Fig. 26-108), nose, brows, eyelids (Fig. 26-109), forehead [resulting in leonine features (Fig. 26-110)], cheeks, lips, extensor surfaces of the extremities, fingers, and elbows. The affected skin is usually dry from loss of sebaceous and sweat gland function. Alopecia of the brows, lashes, and body hair is common, but the scalp hair is usually unaffected.

Mucous membrane involvement may occur in early lepromatous leprosy. Nasal mucous membrane involvement in early lepromatous leprosy causes nasal stuffiness, coryza, epistaxis (Fig. 26-111), and, late in the disease process, septal perforation, and collapse of the nasal bridge (Fig. 26-112). Oropharyngeal infiltration causes loss of teeth and ulceration of the uvula and tonsils. Laryngeal infiltration occasionally causes hoarseness, stridor, and even asphyxia.

Skin Features of Borderline Leprosy

The cutaneous manifestations of borderline or dimorphous leprosy are similar to those of tuberculoid leprosy, except that the lesions are smaller, more numerous, and less sharply marginated (Figs. 26-113 and 26-114). They are asymmetric and macular or plaquelike, and often dome-shaped instead of crater-like. Bandlike lesions with a sharply punched-out center are not uncommon. Sensory changes occur in the involved areas.

Lepra Reactions (Reversal and Downgrading)

Occasionally, leprosy lesions become acutely reactive, caused by changes in cell-mediate immunity. (Increased immunity causes reversal; decreased immunity, downgrading.) The clinical manifestations are similar in both forms, and the skin lesions rapidly evolve.

The reactive state in tuberculoid leprosy may cause an acute neuritis, which, when it involves a major nerve trunk, causes severe pain and severe nerve damage, if not treated promptly and vigorously.

Reversal and downgrading reactions may cause edema and erythema of the face and/or extremities (Figs. 26-115 and 26-116). Reversal and downgrading reactions in patients with dimorphous leprosy are extremely severe. The symptoms include swelling, erythema, and ulceration of the skin; pain and tenderness of the involved skin and nerves; and swelling and widespread damage of the involved nerves. Constitutional symptoms of fever, malaise, and edema (especially of the hands and face) are common.

In downgrading reactions of borderline lepromatous leprosy patients, there is bacillary invasion of previously spared skin areas. The skin lesions rapidly increase in size and become less distinct. Erythema multiforme–type skin lesions also occur. Systemic manifestations include fever, arthralgia, malaise, and occasionally, severe prostration. Other manifestations include iritis, orchitis, inflammation of the digits, epistaxis, and laryngeal edema.

Erythema Nodosum Leprosum

Erythema nodosum leprosum (ENL) occurs only in patients with lepromatous leprosy or, occasionally, in patients with borderline lepromatous leprosy, and especially in patients who are on and responding to chemotherapy. The reaction tends to recur and to persist; it usually does not develop until several months after therapy is started. Crops of tender, red, warm skin nodules develop on the face, trunk, and extremities. In rare instances, they are restricted to the pretibial area. In severe ENL reactions, the skin nodules become hemorrhagic or, more commonly, bulbous (Figs. 26-117 and 26-118) or frankly suppurative with the purulent exudate containing many acid-fast bacilli. Other manifestations include malaise, fever, arthralgia, polyneuralgia, lymphadenopathy, orchitis, bone pain, edema, albuminuria from increased vascular permeability, glottal inflammation, glomerulonephritis, and rarely, hemolytic anemia, episcleritis, and acute iridocyclitis.

The Lucio Phenomenon

The Lucio phenomenon [erythema necroticans (Fig. 26-119)] represents an unusual variety of ENL. It occurs in patients from western Mexico or Costa Rica with diffuse lepromatous leprosy and is characterized by a necrotizing vasculitis that results in crops of large polygonal ulcerating and sloughing lesions (Fig. 26-120).

Ocular Features

Leprosy, especially lepromatous leprosy, commonly involves the eye.

Lids in Tuberculoid Leprosy

Paralytic ectropion (especially of the lower lid), epiphora and lagophthalmos (Figs. 26-121 to 26-123) with corneal exposure, and a tendency for corneal ulceration may occur from facial nerve paralysis.

Tuberculoid leprosy occasionally causes tarsitis, which leads to absorption of the tarsal plate, lid shrinkage, entropion, and trichiasis. Keratinization and drying of the exposed conjunctiva occur from lagophthalmos and paralytic ectropion. A nonspecific conjunctival inflammation and corneal ulceration may also occur (Fig. 26-124).

Lids in Lepromatous Leprosy

Lepromatous leprosy commonly involves the lids and brow. Early signs include brow loss (usually beginning temporally), thickening of the supraciliary ridge and skin, induration of the skin extending through the entire substance of the eyelid, and pain and facial neuralgia. Loss of brow and lashes is often associated with the typical skin lesions of lepromatous leprosy. The outer one-third of the brow, since these hairs are held less firmly, is usually lost; occasionally, the entire brow is lost. Lash loss usually begins at the temporal and nasal areas of the lower lid and is preceded by canities and splintering of the hair. The lid margin eventually becomes markedly thickened and has a rolled appearance of nodular thickening, resembling multiple chalazia. Blepharochalasis arises from skin infiltration and stretching. Other lid changes include ptosis and pachyblepharon.

Conjunctiva in Tuberculoid Leprosy

Keratinization and drying of the exposed conjunctiva occur from lagophthalmos and paralytic ectropion. A nonspecific conjunctival inflammation and corneal ulceration may also occur.

Conjunctiva in Lepromatous Leprosy

Lid margin lesions, skin lesions, or episcleral nodules occasionally extend into the conjunctiva, producing yellow-colored, limbal, subconjunctival nodules. They are often associated with a punctate stromal or interstitial keratitis.

Yellow or white isolated limbal lepromas, which gradually break down to form an ulcer with a raised indurated border and a dirty necrotic base, may also occur. They are usually located in the upper temporal quadrant and are occasionally bilaterally symmetric. The lesions spread posteriorly over the sclera, anteriorly into the cornea, or circumferentially around the limbus. In the cornea, they replace the superficial corneal layers and represent a giant leproma.

Cornea

The corneal sensation may be decreased in all forms of leprosy.

A punctate keratitis is the most common corneal change in lepromatous leprosy and is pathognomonic (Fig. 26-125). A punctate keratitis is the most common corneal change in lepromatous leprosy and is pathognomonic. It usually begins in the upper temporal quadrant at the limbus, then it gradually extends centrally to involve the upper one-half of the cornea. Nearest the limbus, the lesions frequently involve the entire thickness of the corneal stroma. Near the central cornea, they are more superficial, which imparts a wedge-shaped pattern to the entire process. Central lesions cause blurred vision. Individual lesions appear as minute white spots with an irregular outline resembling a grain of chalk. They occur in the epithelium, subepithelium, or anterior stroma. They do not stain with fluorescein but are sometimes surrounded by a gray, milky stromal opacity. Unlike other lepromatous corneal lesions, punctate keratitis regresses and can even completely disappear with therapy. Occasionally, punctate keratitis is complicated by pannus or vascularization of the middle stroma, and sometimes the infiltrates progress to miliary corneal lepromata.

An avascular interstitial keratitis may develop in the superficial, middle, or deep stroma, usually in response to ciliary body involvement or by extension of inflammation from a limbal nodule. Early, it causes mild photophobia and circumcorneal injection. Blurred vision occurs when the keratitis is far advanced. The inflammation is seen in the superior temporal quadrant at the limbus and extends to the superior nasal, then the inferior temporal, and finally, the inferior nasal quadrant. Eventually, it involves the central cornea. The infiltrates are small and rounded at first and are located just posterior to Bowman layer. There is also edema and corneal thickening. Usually, a punctate keratitis (see earlier) accompanies the interstitial keratitis. Late in its course, a few stromal vessels may be seen in the upper temporal quadrants.

Corneal nerve beading develops early in lepromatous leprosy and is pathognomonic. Sometimes it is the earliest sign of infection but is often transitory. Usually there is some degree of corneal anesthesia associated with the beading. The individual lesions are about the size of the corneal nerve but vary in size from minute white dots to obvious beadlike swellings. They usually occur in the superior cornea near the limbus.

Occasionally, a giant corneal leproma develops in the superficial cornea. At onset, it may resemble a highly vascularized pterygium with periodic episodes of hyperemia, swelling, tenderness, and pain. The leproma may be seen as a raised, mass lesion and may involve the visual axis.

Other Ocular Findings

Lepromatous leprosy may involve the sclera (Fig. 26-126), lacrimal system (dacryoadenitis or dacryocystitis), and uvea (Fig. 26-127). Scleral and episcleral involvement in lepromatous leprosy includes a simple or nodular episcleritis or a nodular scleritis. The episcleritis is usually bilateral, involves the superior temporal limbus symmetrically, and is transient and often nodular in type. It begins acutely with pain, tenderness, and circumcorneal injection and is often associated with erythema nodosum leprosum.

Nodular scleritis usually begins with multiple fine dots and sheathing of the limbal vessels followed by development of large, shiny gelatinous nodules with a yellow center. It usually becomes chronic, gradually enlarges over a period of years, and often leads to a staphyloma. Iridocyclitis is common in lepromatous leprosy. It is often chronic, low-grade, granulomatous in type and is manifested by iris pearls, large mutton-fat KPs, or solitary lepromata. Sometimes it begins acutely and presents as a severe plastic iridocyclitis.

Leprotic pearls are pathognomonic for Hansen disease. They are often multiple and have the appearance of grains of white sand lying on the surface of the iris or protruding from its interstices. Iris nodules also occur in the iris stroma.

Isolated iris lepromata are uncommon. They begin in the ciliary body, then encroach on the anterior chamber angle, are usually associated with a keratitis, and may involve the anterior choroid and sclera, and lead to phthisis bulbi.

Syphilis

Syphilis is transmitted by intimate person-to-person contact. Less commonly, it is transmitted by blood transfusions, accidental inoculation, or transplacentally after the tenth week of pregnancy (prenatal syphilis). Not uncommonly, it occurs with AIDS and other venereally transmitted diseases.

The manifestations of syphilis are almost legion, and any indolent, indurated genital or anal lesion accompanied by unilateral adenopathy should arouse the suspicion of syphilis.

Clinical Manifestations

Acquired Syphilis

Acquired syphilis is characterized by

1. An incubation period of about 3 weeks (9 to 90 days).
2. A primary stage, manifested by a chancre at the inoculation site and regional lymphadenopathy.
3. A secondary stage, manifested by cutaneous and systemic signs. It is occasionally recurrent.
4. A latent stage, manifested by only a positive serology.
5. A late stage, characterized by serious complications that can lead to crippling and death.

About two-thirds of patients with untreated syphilis fail to develop clinical manifestations, and many have negative nontreponemal tests.

Primary Syphilis

A classic chancre is painless, measures up to 1 cm in diameter, and evolves slowly. It begins as a small, red papule that gradually enlarges, and then erodes centrally. The ulcer base is smooth and covered by a thin, grayish, slightly hemorrhagic crust. The surrounding tissue is raised, indurated, and surrounded by a few millimeters of red areola; it has a constancy of cartilage—hence the name *hard chancre* (Figs. 26-128 and 26-129). It heals with a slightly depressed, depigmented, atrophic scar. Chancres occur anywhere on the body. Extragenital chancres are often less indurated but are larger, are more painful and erythematous, and run a more chronic course. Most are found on the anal area (Fig. 26-130) and mouth (Fig. 26-131).

Regional, painless, nonsuppurative lymphadenopathy develops 1 to 2 weeks following development of the chancre. The nodes are usually small, firm, discrete, rubbery, and freely movable.

Secondary Syphilis

Secondary syphilis occurs 6 to 8 weeks after the chancre. Skin lesions appear most often as symptomatic pale erythematous macules of the trunk and/or palms and soles (Figs. 26-132 to 26-137).

Temporary, random, "moth-eaten" alopecia of the scalp hair, beard, or the brows or lashes (Figs. 26-138 and 26-139) may be found. Condyloma lata may be seen on moist sites such as ano-genital area (Fig. 26-140). The "split papule" at the corner of the lip is highly suggestive of secondary syphilis (Fig. 26-141). A sore throat is common.

Mucous patches of buccal mucosa, tongue (Fig. 26-142), lip, palate, throat, cervix, and conjunctiva are distinctive and highly infectious. They appear as dull, erythematous patches or erosions covered by a grayish white exudate.

Lymphadenopathy

There is usually a generalized nontender lymphadenopathy. The nodes are discrete, rubbery, and most readily detected in the posterior triangle of the neck, occipital, auricular, axillary, and epitrochlear regions.

Systemic Involvement

The constitutional symptoms are usually mild and more pronounced at night. They include fever, chilliness, malaise, headache, anorexia, arthralgias, body pains, weight loss, anemia, hepatitis, transient myocarditis, myositis, periostitis (Fig. 26-143), epididymitis, and nephritis.

Neurologic Involvement

Neurologic involvement is manifested by headache, meningismus, acute aseptic or acute basilar meningitis, nerve deafness, transverse myelitis, cranial nerve palsies (Fig. 26-144), thrombosis of the cerebrospinal arteries, and meningomyelitis with paraplegia.

Latent Syphilis

Patients with latent syphilis have only a positive serology and are not infectious. Early latent syphilis represents latent syphilis of less than 4 years duration. It sometimes relapses into secondary syphilis, especially during the first year, and may then become infectious. Late latent syphilis does not relapse.

Late (Tertiary) Syphilis

Late (tertiary) syphilis is divided into late benign syphilis (gummatous syphilis), cardiovascular syphilis, and neurosyphilis. It is noninfectious.

Late Benign Syphilis

Gummata are the hallmark of late benign syphilis. They are painless and develop in skin, bone, subcutaneous tissue, mucous membrane, muscle, and internal organs. Those that develop in skin, bone, subcutaneous tissue, and muscle tend to ulcerate. Gummata may appear 3 to 5 years after infection as

1. Solitary nodular lesions of the extensor surfaces of the arms (Fig. 26-145), legs, scalp, face, back, and sternum. They are firm, are coppery-red, and extend peripherally as they heal centrally, leading to a ring-shaped or a multiple ring-shaped appearance (Fig. 26-146). Sometimes they have waxy scales.
2. Noduloulcerative lesions. They begin as nodules that later ulcerate and lead to destruction of the deeper layers of the skin. They are typically painless. The walls are ver-

tical and indurated, and the base is composed of clean, wet granulation tissue. Spontaneous, incomplete healing occurs either centrally or on one side of the lesion. The lesions heal with thin atrophic scars that fail to contract and are often hyperpigmented at their border.

Mucous membrane gummata frequently ulcerate and scar. They involve the nasal septum, palate, pharynx, and larynx. Nasal septal and palatal perforation is common (Fig. 26-147). Leukoplakia also occurs and is precancerous.

Ocular Features of Primary Acquired Syphilis
Lids
Lid chancres usually develop on the lower lid margin, inner canthus, or occasionally, upper lid. They cause permanent madarosis, mild lid deformity, and infiltrative conjunctivitis. They are associated with preauricular lymphadenopathy.

Conjunctiva
Conjunctival chancres are found on the bulbar or upper tarsal conjunctiva; less frequently, on the limbus, lower tarsus, or caruncle; rarely, in the fornix. They begin as a hard, indolent, painless papule that increases in size, then they ulcerate to form a "punched-out" spreading, superficially or deeply indurated ulcer covered by a pseudomembrane. Sometimes the disease causes a superior pannus or interstitial keratitis. The lymph nodes are grossly enlarged.

Cornea
A unilateral interstitial keratitis similar to that seen in prenatal syphilis may arise from a lid or conjunctival chancre.

Other
Other ocular features include lacrimal sac involvement, episcleritis, and scleritis.

Ocular Features of Secondary Acquired Syphilis
The generalized macular or papular eruption often involves the lids. Other lid findings include ulcerative blepharitis, lid cicatrization, deformity, and madarosis, or sometimes, a temporary patchy (moth-eaten) or generalized hair loss. Condyloma lata, similar to other condyloma lata, occasionally occur at the inner canthus. Conjunctival mucous patches may cause lid margin distortion and ectropion (see later).

Conjunctiva
Conjunctival involvement in secondary syphilis presents as simple, severe papillary or granular conjunctivitis; scleroconjunctivitis; or mucous patches similar to other mucous patches. The granular conjunctivitis causes a rose-colored thickening of the bulbar conjunctiva and upper fornix with superior pannus and almost transparent follicle-like lesions of the tarsus, simulating trachoma. The tarsus develops an almost cartilaginous consistency.

Cornea
The interstitial keratitis of late secondary syphilis is usually unilateral and sectorial in nature but is otherwise similar to that which occurs in prenatal syphilis. Other corneal findings include a nummular keratitis and marginal corneal infiltrates similar to catarrhal corneal infiltrates.

Sclera
Scleral involvement is in the form of acute diffuse episcleritis, anterior diffuse scleritis with insidious onset, nodular or annular scleritis, diffuse intercalary scleritis leading to ectasia, or, in rare instances, posterior scleritis.

Lacrimal System
Occasionally, secondary syphilis causes dacryoadenitis or dacryocystitis.

Uvea
Uveal tract involvement may present as:

1. Roseola of the iris (Fig. 26-148). Roseola of the iris is characterized by transient dilation of the superficial vascular iris loops, which causes reddish spots on the lesser circle of the iris.
2. Acute, nonspecific, severe iridocyclitis and occasionally, hyphema.
3. Nongranulomatous iritis with sclerokeratoconjunctivitis.
4. Disseminated syphilitic chorioretinitis (Fig. 26-149). Disseminated syphilitic chorioretinitis occurs late in secondary and, occasionally, tertiary syphilis and may be bilateral. It involves the posterior pole and circumpapillary region, causing a hazy vitreous, decreased vision, variable field defects, micropsia, metamorphopsia, photopsia, and circumscribed gray-yellow areas in the posterior fundus, flame-shaped hemorrhages, and edema of the nerve head and retina. The lesions are usually large and confluent, and have a polymorphous shape. Fresh lesions may develop as other lesions become dormant. The disease causes prominent pigmentation around the inflammatory margins and along the vessels as well as sheets of fibrous tissue deep in the retina, simulating retinitis pigmentosa.
5. Disseminated chorioretinitis of the posterior pole (Fig. 26-150). Disseminated chorioretinitis involving the posterior pole causes severe visual loss and "salt and pepper" changes, with occasional macular involvement. Discrete, rounded, and ringed areas may also be seen.
6. Bilateral areolar choroiditis begins as disseminated choroiditis of the macular region, which eventually involves the peripheral retina as the macula heals. The lesions are at first black, but eventually the center and finally the entire area develops into an atrophic white scar.
7. Diffuse choroiditis that appears gray but, as healing occurs, assumes a fleck-form of superficial choroidal atrophy.

8. Central chorioretinitis, causing severe unilateral visual loss, diffuse leakage in the posterior pole, and multifocal areas of staining along the retinal vessels.
9. Localized chorioretinitis similar in appearance to the chorioretinitis of other diseases. It often involves the macula and the area adjacent to the nerve head but may occur anywhere in the fundus.

Other: Papillitis
Papillitis is common in secondary syphilis (Fig. 26-151). The optic neuritis, retrobulbar neuritis, and papilledema that sometimes occur are discussed under late syphilis. Orbital changes include a marginal periostitis and a chronic orbital myositis. Frontal bossing is common.

Ocular Features of Late Benign Syphilis
Lids
Lid gummata are uncommon and are usually solitary but may be bilateral, multiple, and symmetric (Fig. 26-147). Subcutaneous lid gummata may simulate a chalazion at first. Tarsitis causes diffuse lid swelling, severe ptosis, and the lid feels cartilaginous and may be marginal, nodular, vegetative (polypoid), or diffuse. A regional lymphadenopathy usually accompanies the tarsitis.

Conjunctiva
Conjunctival gummata (noduloulcerative syphilids) usually occur on the bulbar conjunctiva near the limbus. They measure up to 4 mm, cause minimal inflammation, and eventually ulcerate, forming a ragged yellow defect.

Cornea
Peripheral corneal gummata are usually elevated. The deeper corneal layers and uveal tract appear normal.

Posterior corneal gummatous abscesses usually occur in the peripheral cornea (keratitis pustuliformis profunda) but may also occur in the central cornea and communicate with the anterior chamber.

Keratitis punctata profunda (focal avascular interstitial keratitis) occurs in late acquired syphilis and late prenatal syphilis. It is characterized by discrete, gray, well-defined (discoid), punctate opacities in the posterior stroma and associated iritis. The cornea does not vascularize.

Sclera
Late benign syphilis involves the sclera in the form of a nodular episcleritis or scleritis and scleral gummata. Scleral gummata eventually ulcerate and may lead to perforation.

Lacrimal System
Lacrimal system involvement in late benign syphilis includes a dacryoadenitis and gummatous involvement of the lacrimal sac.

Orbit
Orbital gummata are sometimes multiple, and bony absorption is often considerable. Orbital periostitis may lead to paresis of the 3rd, 4th, 5th, and 6th cranial nerves and to an optic perineuritis.

Uvea
The uveal tract is involved in tertiary syphilis in various forms: severe acute iridocyclitis (iritis papulosa); acute iritis associated with keratitis punctata profunda (see earlier); disseminated syphilitic chorioretinitis; unilateral neuritis papulosa, characterized by multiple dense vitreous opacities and an irregular white mass covering the nerve head; and other uveal and retinal lesions, such as juxtapapillary chorioretinitis, circumscribed elevated retinal mass, hemorrhagic areas in the retina, and choroidal and retinal gummata.

Optic Nerve
Optic nerve involvement includes optic neuritis and neuroretinitis, axial or retrobulbar neuritis, optic perineuritis, bilateral papilledema, simple progressive primary optic atrophy, and gummata of the nerve head.

Pupillary Reaction
Abnormal pupillary reactions are the most important early ocular signs of symptomatic neurosyphilis. The Argyll–Robertson pupil is virtually pathognomonic for neurosyphilis.

Lens
The lens is sometimes dislocated or becomes cataractous from inflammation or a ciliary body gumma.

Clinical Features of Prenatal (Congenital) Syphilis
Early prenatal (congenital) syphilis occurs before the age of 2 (often during the first 10 weeks of life). Early prenatal syphilis is usually infectious. (Syphilis acquired during the newborn period should be considered as such, and the manifestations are usually those of acquired syphilis.)

The manifestations usually develop after the first 3 weeks of life.

Skin Features in Early Prenatal Syphilis
Cutaneous lesions develop between the second and eighth week of life and are highly infectious. They are usually maculopapular and occur on the buttocks, back, thighs, soles, palms, and perioral area. Initially, they are pink or red but subsequently become coppery brown in color. A fine desquamation develops as the lesions change color (Fig. 26-152). Occasionally, they appear annular, iridic, or circinate.

About 3% of infants develop vesicular and bullous eruptions of the palms, soles, and anogenital region. The bullae contain a cloudy or hemorrhagic fluid and, following rupture, leave a denuded area. Petechial lesions, jaundice, and paronychia may also be seen.

Condyloma lata of the perioral, perianal, and occasionally, intertriginous areas develop after the first 2 to 3 months. They are single or multiple, moist, flat-topped, wartlike papules; deep fissures that eventually form fine scars (rhagades) (Fig. 26-153) often radiate from the affected orifices.

The skin eruption in secondary syphilis is usually asymptomatic, symmetric, polymorphous, and involves the palms and soles. It heals without scarring, except for occasional residual hyper- or hypopigmentation of the hands and neck (necklace of Venus).

The lesions present as:

1. Macular syphilid or syphilitic roseola with erythematous macules of the abdomen, chest, extensor surfaces of the arms, and brown areas on the palms and soles.
2. Papular syphilids, appearing as copper-colored, grouped papular lesions of the face and trunk and resembling acne. Sometimes they scale (papulosquamous or squamous syphilid) or are associated with hyperkeratotic palmar lesions (lues cornea).
3. Annular and arciform lesions, small follicular papules resembling pityriasis rosea (corymbiform syphilid), and necrotic and deep ulcerations of pustular lesions (malignant syphilis or lues maligna).
4. Condyloma latum (large, pale, flat-topped, eroded, hypertrophied papules or plaques) of moist skin areas (e.g., perineum, genitalia, corners of the mouth, behind the ear, under the breast, axilla, and between the toes) (see Fig. 30-19).

Rhinitis and nasal discharge (snuffles) (Fig. 26-154) develop between 1 to 12 weeks of life and may eventually lead to a saddle nose (Fig. 26-155). Frontal bossing, saddle nose, and a relative protuberance of the mandible occur from failure of proper bony development or prolonged inflammation. Other bony changes include periostitis of the long bones, especially the tibia (leading to saber shins) (Fig. 26-156); unilateral thickening of the sternoclavicular portion of the clavicle with resultant sternoclavicular swelling (Higoumenakia sign) (Fig. 26-157); Clutton joints (hydrarthrosis of the knee or other large joints); and scaphoid scapulae.

Rhinitis and nasal discharge (snuffles) (Fig. 26-154) develop between 1 and 12 weeks of life. The discharge is often profuse, purulent, and even blood-tinged and is highly infectious. Nasal ulcerations may also occur and can lead to osteitis, nasal cartilage inflammation, and a saddle nose. The mucous patches of the lips, tongue, nasal mucosa, and conjunctiva are similar to those of acquired syphilis.

Clinical Manifestations of Late Prenatal Syphilis

Late prenatal syphilis develops after the age of 2 and is not infectious. The major findings include Hutchinson triad (Hutchinson teeth, interstitial keratitis, and eight nerve deafness); mulberry molars; Clutton joints; and frontal bossing.

Hutchinson teeth (Fig. 26-158) are specific for late prenatal syphilis and are characterized by central notching or a peg shape of the permanent upper central incisors and, occasionally, the lower central incisors. The teeth are widely spaced, thickened in the anterior posterior direction, and narrower at the cutting edge than at the gum margin. The enamel of the notched area is markedly thinned and discolored. Mulberry molars (Moon or Fournier molars) (Fig. 26-158) are the first molars and possess many small cusps instead of the usual four well-developed cusps. The grinding surface is narrower than at the gum margin, and the enamel is poorly developed.

About 3% of patients with late prenatal syphilis develop 8th nerve deafness about the age of puberty, occasionally as late as the third or fourth decade. The high tones are affected first; the lower tones are affected later.

Bony Changes

Gummata of the palate or vomer occasionally occur and may lead to perforation (Fig. 26-147).

Central nervous system involvement in late prenatal syphilis is manifested by mental retardation, arrested hydrocephalus, convulsive disorders, juvenile general paresis, and cranial nerve palsies, including optic atrophy.

Ocular Manifestations: Prenatal Syphilis

Lid involvement in early prenatal syphilis includes a papular or vesiculobullous eruption, ulceration, lid margin deformity, permanent lash loss, rhagades of the lateral canthal region (clefts or skin excoriations), obliteration of the upper or lower lacrimal punctum, and ectropion. Lid gummata that may ulcerate and lead to severe lid deformities are occasionally observed in late prenatal syphilis.

Conjunctiva

Conjunctival mucous patches are similar to those in acquired syphilis (see earlier).

Cornea

Interstitial keratitis (IK) in late prenatal syphilis is usually bilateral and accompanied by other stigmata. It is characterized by chronic edema, cellular infiltration, and vascularization of the deeper corneal layers, and is often associated with anterior uveitis. It causes severe pain, photophobia, tearing, blepharospasm, and severe visual loss. It begins with knobby endothelial excrescences (usually in the periphery of the upper cornea); fine, droplike nebulae in the region of Descemet membrane; small, discrete, faint gray nebulae in the middle and deep stroma; and discrete keratic precipitates. The nebulae progressively enlarge and coalesce. Deep and superficial neovascularization begins soon after the generalized haziness develops, with the vessels preferentially invading the areas of most intense inflammation. The superficial vessels form an epaulet (Fig. 26-159). The superficial vessels are located just under the epithelium and often form an epaulet (a prominent crescentic swelling at the superior margin of the cornea). The deep vessels are variable in size, brushlike in appearance, and proliferate radially to invade the cornea at the level of Descemet membrane. Because of the vessel's depth and the overlying inflammation, the area (especially the superior cornea) assumes the appearance of a dull, reddish-pink patch (salmon patch). As the vessels advance centrally, they are preceded by a dense corneal haze; at the same time, the peripheral infiltrates are partially absorbed, leaving areas of clearing. Resorption usually leads to opacities (Fig. 26-160) and ghost vessels (Fig. 26-161). Resorption of the interstitial keratitis usually leads to corneal thinning. Usually, some opacities and deep "ghost" vessels remain. The superficial vessels usually disappear.

Other forms of keratitis include a dense central inflammatory reaction with relative sparing of the periphery; a peripheral form of interstitial keratitis; a sectoral form of IK, keratitis punctata profunda; posterior corneal abscess; central, marginal, or posterior corneal ulcer; and superficial, isolated, gummata-like lesion.

Sclera

The scleral changes in late prenatal syphilis are limited to anterior or posterior scleritis.

Lacrimal System

The dacryoadenitis in late prenatal syphilis is similar in all respects to that seen in late benign syphilis.

Orbit

Marginal orbital periostitis, although uncommon, causes severe destruction of much of the orbital and facial bones.

Uvea

Uveal tract involvement includes acute iridocyclitis; chorioretinitis, especially a "pepper and salt fundus" most marked near the periphery (Fig. 26-150); larger pigmented black masses located in circumscribed areas but scattered throughout the entire periphery or in the midzone; white, atrophic areas scattered over the fundus and forming confluent areas of white scars in the central or peripheral fundus; pigmented macular lesions; and perivasculitis (Fig. 26-162). Optic atrophy, narrowing and sheathing of the retinal vasculature, perivasculitis, and vessel obliteration often accompany the chorioretinitis of syphilis.

Other

Optic nerve inflammation occasionally occurs. Lens involvement includes dislocation and cataracts.

Pinta

Pinta usually occurs in remote, primitive tropical areas and is more common in Indians of the Americas but affects all races living in close proximity. Congenital infection does not occur.

It has an early stage with primary and secondary skin lesions, an early and a late latent stage lasting up to 3 years, and a late stage. The lesions of the early and late stages are often present at the same time.

Early Stage

The primary lesion develops at the inoculation site and is characterized by erythematous, indurated, somewhat scaly red to violaceous-colored papules. In infants, the lesion is found on the buttocks, posterior thighs, and trunk; in older children, on the wrists, forearms, ankles, and dorsum of the foot. It begins as a papule, which gradually enlarges to form psoriasiform plaques that persist for several months to years. Healing occurs with occasional depigmentation.

Secondary skin lesions (Fig. 26-163) of the early stage usually develop within 1 year of infection. They are similar to the primary lesions but occur in sun-exposed areas (face, neck, arms, and legs) and are varying shades of slate blue, gray, yellow-brown, dark brown, black, or they are hypochromic. Occasionally, they appear as erythematous squamous growths. They heal spontaneously, producing depigmented atrophic areas. Hyperkeratotic lesions of the palms and soles may also occur and resemble the hyperkeratotic lesions of yaws ("crab" yaws).

Generalized lymphadenopathy occurs during the latter part of the infection. In the exceptional case, central nervous system and cardiovascular disease occur in the early stage of pinta.

Latent Stage

The latent stage lasts up to 3 years, during which time no new lesions develop.

Late Stage

The late stage is characterized by depigmented skin areas over bony prominences (inner aspects of the wrists, elbows, and ankles) that are often interspersed with hyperpigmented lesions, giving a peculiar grayish, ashy, or bluish color to the skin. Hyperkeratotic lesions also develop on the legs, forearms, elbows, knees, ankles, palms, and soles.

Skin atrophy with thinning, wrinkling, dryness, loss of sweating, and sebaceous secretions occurs in areas near the larger joints.

Ocular Features

The lid may be involved with the primary and secondary skin lesions of the early stage and late stage.

Yaws

Yaws is largely limited to tropical regions of Africa, Asia, the Pacific Islands, Australia, and Central and South America. (Heat and humidity favor its transmission.) It causes granulomatous skin, mucous membrane and bone lesions, and is transmitted by nonsexual contact. The infection is limited to descendants of the African race. Infection occurs early in life (age 2 or 3).

Clinical Features

The early stage of yaws corresponds to the primary and secondary stages of syphilis; the late stage, to late syphilis. There is no prenatal form of infection. The central nervous system and cardiovascular system are not affected.

Early Stage

Infection occurs through the skin. The initial lesion begins as a painless, nonindurated, moist, erythematous papule at the inoculation site (usually the leg or foot) that later ulcerates and is covered by a yellow crust. Other papules develop adjacent to the initial papule and coalesce to form a large, elevated, warty papilloma (resembling a raspberry) that bleeds easily (mother yaw). The lesion heals spontaneously after several months, leaving a large, depigmented scar that may be surrounded by a dark halo. A regional lymphadenopathy or sometimes, a regional adenitis occurs. Constitutional disturbances are uncommon.

Secondary Stage

After several months, a widespread papular eruption occurs, which is often concentrated around the mouth, nose, anus, and vulva (Fig. 26-164). Many of the papules heal spontaneously, whereas others enlarge to form individual, large, raised lesions similar to the mother yaw. Some may extend to form circinate papillomas (tinea yaws), which are reddish-yellow, often having a granular surface from which serum tends to exude. Eventually, they are covered with a black eschar. Successive crops of skin lesions usually occur, and the soles and palms often develop hyperkeratotic plaques (crab yaws). Spontaneous healing occurs with little scarring and only temporary hypopigmentation.

Headache, fever, joint and bone pain, generalized lymphadenopathy, and malaise often occur before the skin eruption.

Late Stage

Papillomatous, nodular, and tuberous lesions of the hands and feet herald the onset of the late stage. They usually develop after an asymptomatic period of 3 or more years. The lesions are usually single and break down to form small, superficial or large, deep, destructive ulcers that heal with skin depigmentation and extensive scarring, sometimes with extensive contractures. Hyperkeratosis of the palms and soles with painful fissures often develop, making walking difficult.

Bony lesions include a gummatous periostitis, hypertrophic periostitis, osteitis, and osteomyelitis. Single bone lesions are the rule and often lead to ulceration of the overlying skin. Other bony changes include digital inflammation and goundou (a bilateral swelling and enlargement of the frontal processes of the maxilla that is extremely disfiguring and may encroach on the eyelids and orbit).

Synovitis and tendinous synovitis of the knee, ankle, or elbow cause marked swelling, severe pain, and disability. Occasionally, synovial cysts develop along the tendons, resulting in a painless swelling that resembles a ganglion.

Gangosa is a severe, destructive form of late-stage yaws. It begins as an ulcerative lesion in the pharynx and soft palate, then it progressively spreads to involve the nose, face, and eyelids.

Ocular Features

The primary lesion of yaws occasionally occurs on the lid and resembles other primary lesions.

The widespread skin eruption of secondary yaws may involve the lid and lid margin and be associated with chronic catarrhal conjunctivitis.

Gangosa of the lids is uncommon but may lead to cicatricial ectropion and lagophthalmos.

Conjunctival changes include catarrhal conjunctivitis associated with papillomatous lesions of the lid margin and conjunctival drying, thickening, and scarring from conjunctival exposure during the late stage of yaws.

Interstitial keratitis with mild iridocyclitis rarely occurs during the late stage of yaws. Corneal exposure and gross corneal changes may be seen in gangosa.

Infrequently, bony tumors of goundou gradually encroach on the orbit, displacing the globe.

Lyme Disease

Lyme disease represents a multisystemic infection that is transmitted by ticks, deer flies, and mosquitoes.

Clinical Features

Early Phase

The early phase of Lyme disease is characterized by an erythematous, flat (or slightly elevated) skin lesion that expands several centimeters a week while clearing centrally [erythema chronicum migrans (Fig. 26-165)]. It is usually single and often occurs at the inoculation site (groin, axilla, or thigh). The erythema may be intense, and sometimes slight scaling occurs. Vesiculation at the edge of the lesion and central necrosis may occur. It may persist for months and is occasionally associated with regional lymphadenopathy, fever, chills, headache, malaise, fatigue, and myalgia.

Second Stage

The second stage begins several weeks to months later and is characterized by fatigue, lethargy, sore throat, nonproductive cough, severe headache, arthritis; neurologic complications [relapsing meningoencephalitis or meningitis, Bell palsy, and peripheral radiculopathy]; and heart disease [myocarditis, conduction defects, and occasionally, cardiomegaly]. Lymphadenopathy, splenomegaly, testicular swelling, and laboratory findings suggestive of a hepatitis and nephritis may also occur.

The skin lesions include ones that are similar to but smaller and less migratory than the original lesion; a diffuse maculopapular rash; localized or generalized urticaria; and septal panniculitis.

Third Stage

The third stage of infection occurs several weeks to 2 years after inoculation and is manifested by pain in and about the larger joints with or without signs of arthritis and chronic synovitis (up to 50%); neurologic signs (encephalomyelitis, demyelinating and psychiatric syndromes); and skin involvement (localized scleroderma-type lesions or acrodermatitis chronica atrophicans).

The arthritic findings are usually chronic and recurrent but gradually subside. Synovitis often leads to permanent disability.

Acrodermatitis chronica atrophicans presents as single or multiple painless, dull-red, or bluish-red nodules or plaques on the extremities that slowly extend centrifugally. The scleroderma-type lesions may be accompanied by ulceration. They occur on the lower one-third of the legs and on the trunk.

Ocular Features

Transient blurred vision and photophobia have been observed.

Conjunctiva

A transient, infiltrative conjunctivitis is perhaps the most common ocular manifestation and is occasionally hemorrhagic.

Cornea

A dendritiform keratitis and a focal avascular interstitial keratitis may occur in the late stages of Lyme disease. The interstitial lesions occur at all levels and locations in the cornea and have hazy borders. Sometimes the opacities involve the full thickness of the stroma.

Uvea and Retina

Iritis, endophthalmitis, and loss of the eye have been reported. In the early phase of infection, there may be an iridocyclitis. Bilateral diffuse choroiditis manifested by choroidal thickening with exudative retinal detachment and paracentral scotomas have also been observed.

Retinal vasculitis, hemorrhages, exudative retinal detachment, and cystoid macular edema may occur in the early stages of Lyme disease.

Neuroophthalmic Findings

Edema, retrobulbar neuritis, ischemic optic neuropathy, pseudotumor cerebri, and diplopia arising from 3rd or 4th cranial nerve paralysis have all been observed in the late stages of infection.

Leptospirosis

Leptospirosis represents an acute systemic illness. Weil disease represents one part of the spectrum of leptospirosis. Infection occurs by contact with infected urine or contact with tissue. The portal of entry is the gastrointestinal tract; other mucous membranes, including the conjunctiva; and occasionally, abraded skin.

Clinical Features

Leptospirosis is a biphasic disease; both phases are characterized by fever. The initial phase is a bacteremic phase; the second phase is immunologic.

The initial phase lasts 4 to 7 days and simulates a viral illness with spiking fever, chills, malaise, prostration, and prominent myalgia. The patient then becomes afebrile and asymptomatic for several days before the onset of the immunologic phase of the illness. The immunologic phase lasts several days to several weeks and is manifested by fever, malaise, prostration, and myalgia.

Skin Features

A maculopapular, petechial, or purpuric rash of the trunk is sometimes seen.

In Fort Bragg fever (pretibial fever), erythema nodosum develops on the shins during the fourth or fifth day of the initial phase of infection.

Ocular Manifestations

Photophobia is common during the second stage of illness.

Conjunctival suffusion without discharge occurs on the third or fourth day of the initial phase of the illness. Icterus is sometimes seen in Weil disease.

An iritis often occurs during the immunologic stage, and roseola may be found on the iris together with small glassy or crystal appearing keratic precipitates, many cells, moderate anterior chamber flare, and posterior synechiae.

Relapsing (Recurrent) Fever

There are two forms of relapsing fever: an acute tropical form and a milder, sporadic form. The acute tropical form occurs in North Africa and the Far East. The organism is harbored by a rodent and is deposited on the host's skin by the louse; infection occurs through a scratch or abrasion.

The milder, sporadic form occurs worldwide and is harbored by rodents, with a tick serving as the vector.

Clinical Features

The infection is characterized by relapsing fever, dizziness, and mental confusion. Signs of extracellular fluid deficit and calf muscle tenderness are common. Headache and pains in the long bones occur at onset and persist for 1 or 2 days, followed by chills, a rapid rise in temperature, prostration, tachycardia, nausea, vomiting, and constipation or diarrhea. The temperature returns to normal 4 to 7 days later, and the patient feels well. Recurrent but less severe symptoms of fever then occur 4 to 18 days later, and the cycle repeats itself three or more times, occasionally as many as 10 times.

Chronic headaches may be a prominent sign and suggest neurologic involvement. Occasionally, there is meningitis, mental derangement, and paralysis. Other findings include aphasia, hemiplegia, paraplegia, incontinence, and epileptiform seizures.

Skin Features

Jaundice and petechial hemorrhages of the skin and mucous membranes occur during attacks.

Ocular Features

Ocular manifestations usually develop only during relapses. They include the following:

1. Lid edema and a unilateral or bilateral facial paralysis. Ptosis from 3rd nerve involvement.
2. A benign, self-limited conjunctivitis; subconjunctival hemorrhages; and icterus.
3. Superficial keratitis that usually involves the superior cornea; band-shaped keratitis; and a mild, superficial, interstitial keratitis with only mild neovascularization.
4. Bilateral uveitis with a fibrinous anterior chamber reaction, hypopyon, and grossly visible vitreous exudates. Chronic cyclitis with vitreous exudates. Occasionally, it is complicated by a secondary glaucoma.
5. Retinal hemorrhages and engorged retinal veins.
6. Transient optic neuritis or retrobulbar neuritis leading to optic atrophy and 6th and 7th cranial nerve paralysis.

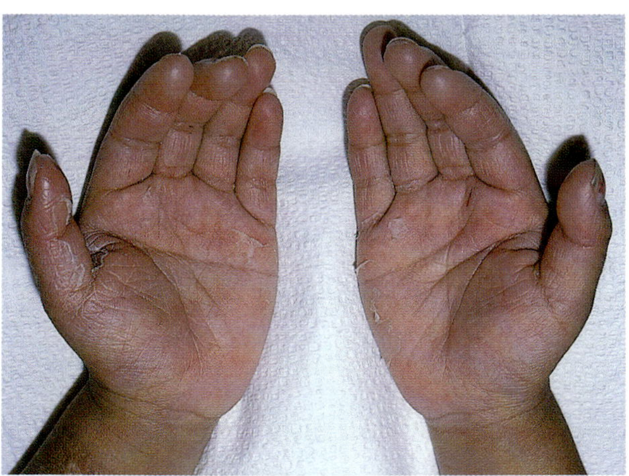

FIGURE 26-1. Desquamation of palms following toxic shock syndrome in women.

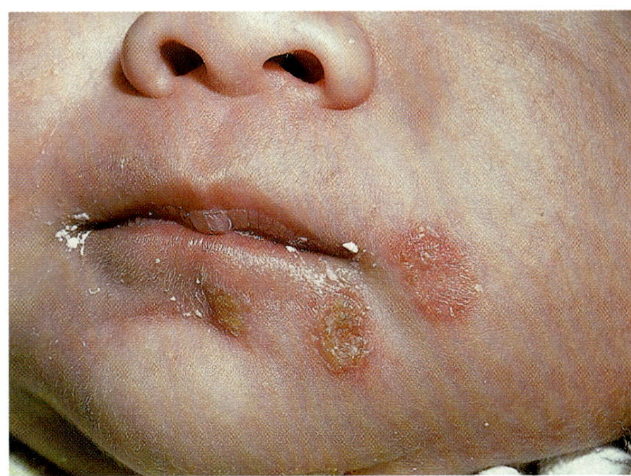

FIGURE 26-2. Impetigo in an infant. Note characteristic "honeycomb" crusting.

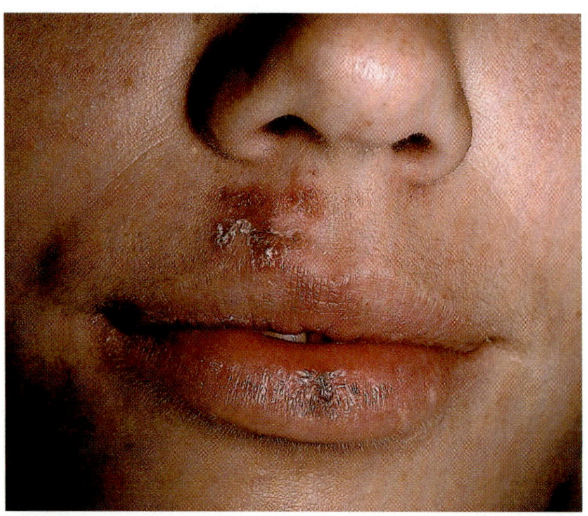

FIGURE 26-3. Impetigo in a child. Paranasal location is common and usually indicates staph nasal carriage.

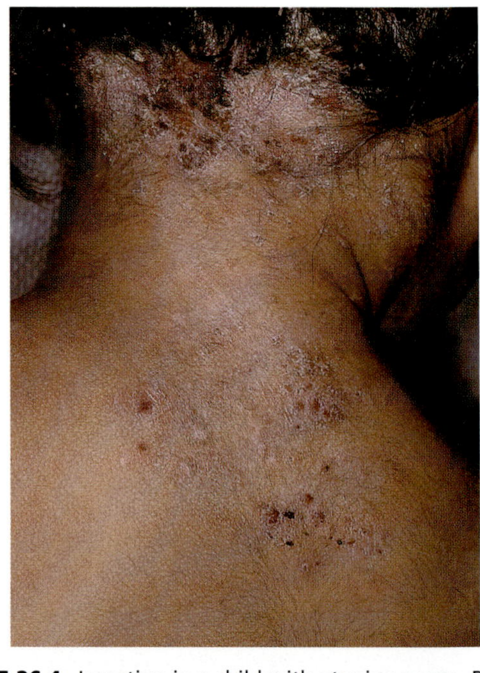

FIGURE 26-4. Impetigo in a child with atopic eczema. Differential diagnosis should include infected tinea capitis and pediculosis capitis.

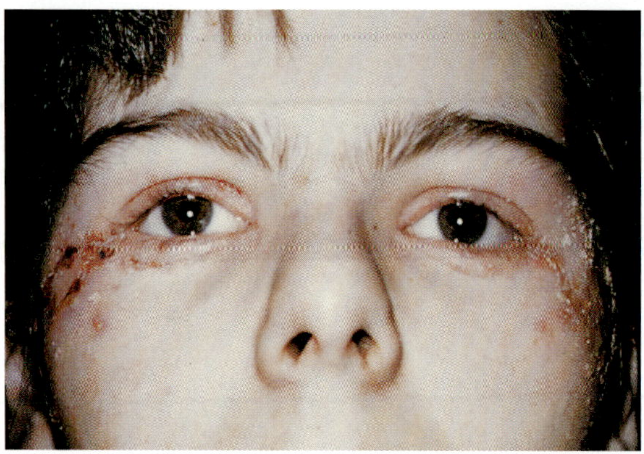

FIGURE 26-5. Impetigo (nonbullous staphylococcal) extending to eyelids. (Courtesy of Dr. Phillips Thygeson.)

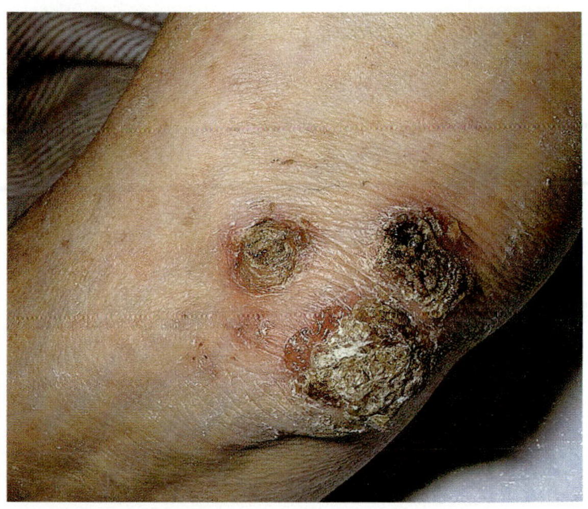

FIGURE 26-6. Erythema following abrasion of the elbow.

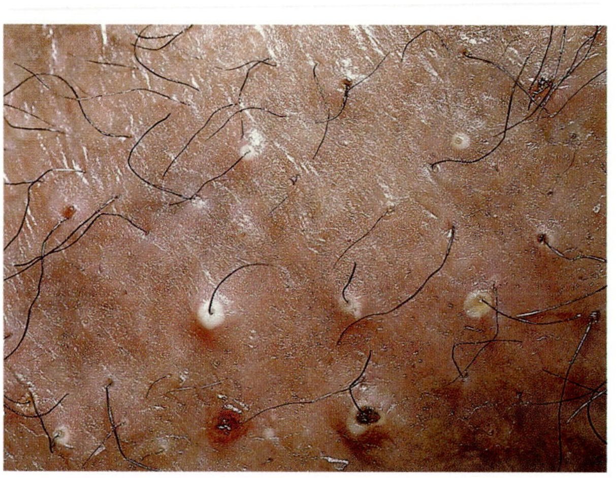

FIGURE 26-7. Superficial pustular folliculitis.

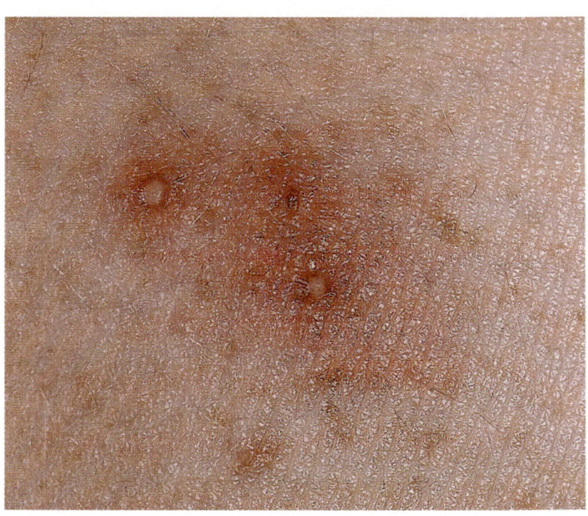

FIGURE 26-8. Pustular folliculitis showing erythematous aureola.

262

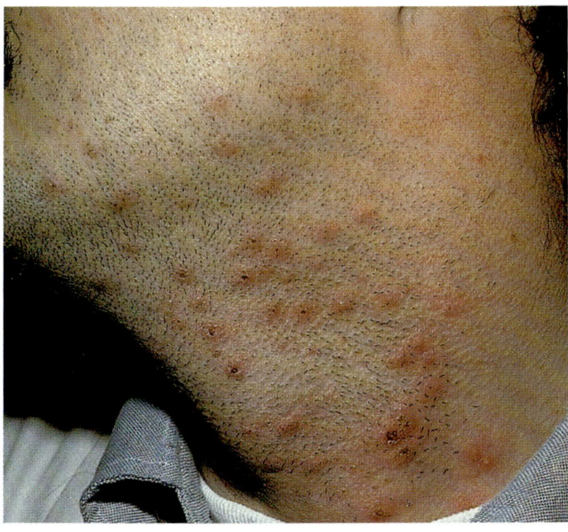

FIGURE 26-9. Sycosis barbae. Note multiple follicular pustules and erythema. *Staphylococcus aureus* is the most frequent causative organism.

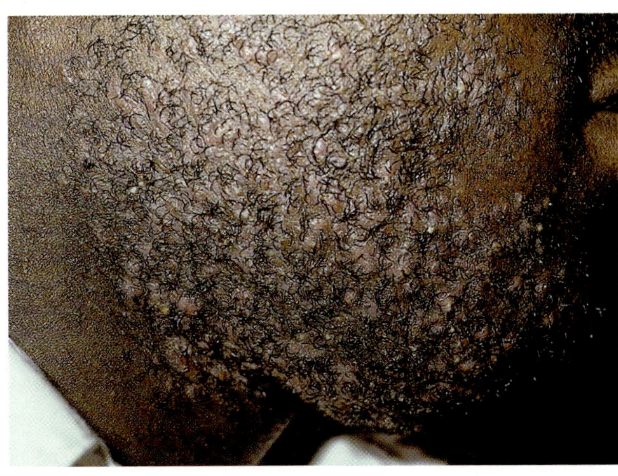

FIGURE 26-10. Pseudo-folliculitis barbae. A frequent problem in African-American patients, these stubborn infections are caused by the sharply pointed beard hairs piercing the skin.

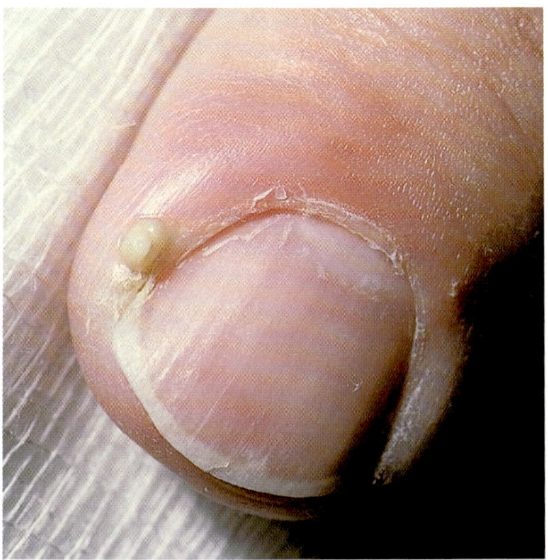

FIGURE 26-11. Acute pyogenic paronychia. Note the yellow purulence due to *Staphylococcus aureus.*

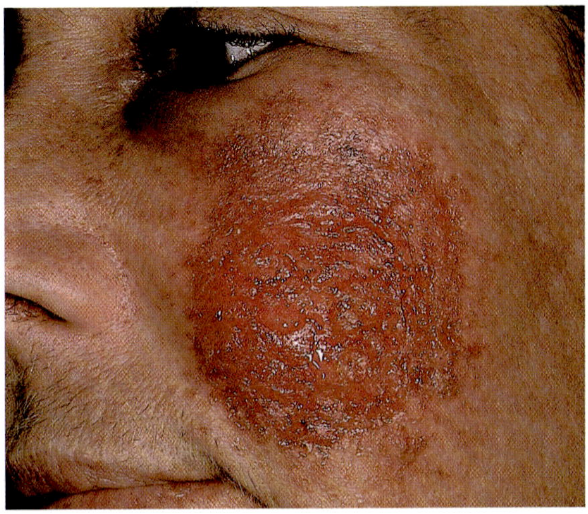

FIGURE 26-12. Cellulitis resulting from squeezing a pimple on the cheek.

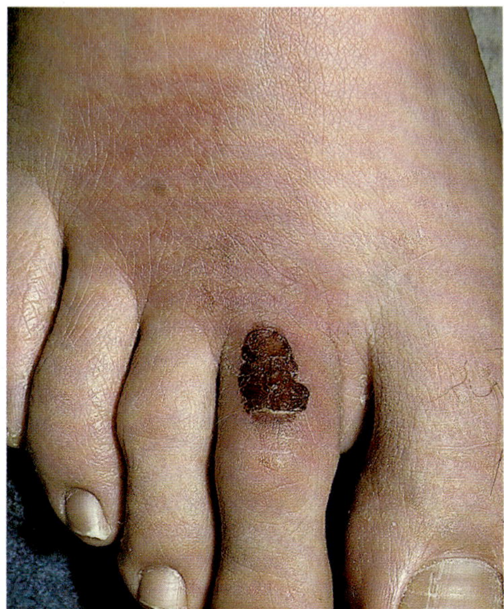

FIGURE 26-13. Cellulitis with lymphangitis. The patient had taken a long hike with poorly fitting shoes.

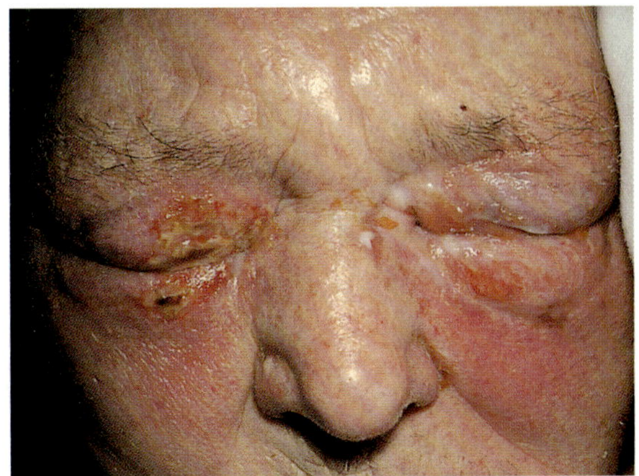

FIGURE 26-14. Orbital cellulitis due to staphylococcal infection.

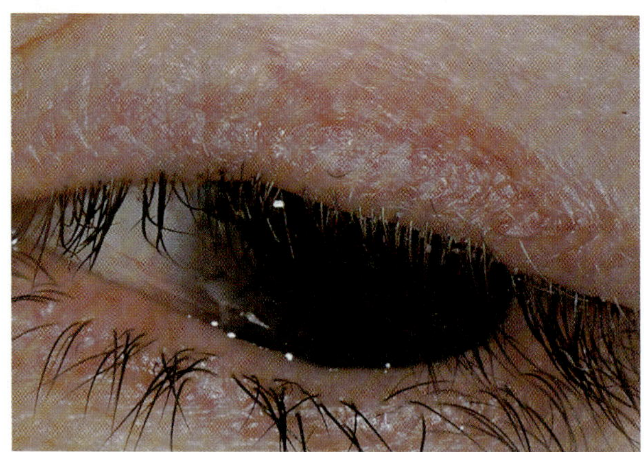

FIGURE 26-15. Staphylococcal blepharitis with hyperemia. Hyperemia of the lid with moderate crusting and misdirection of the lashes is evident in this patient.

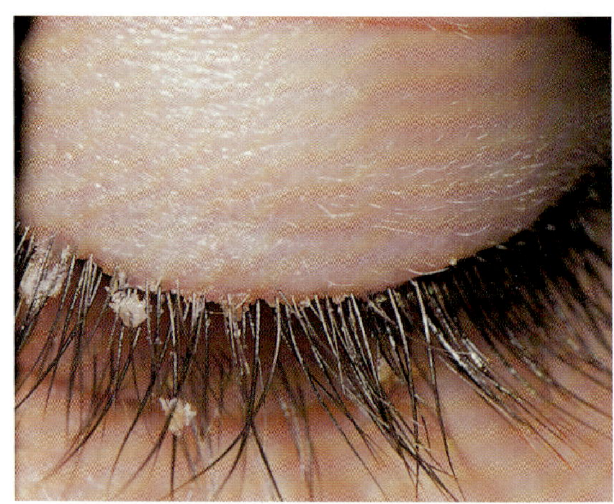

FIGURE 26-16. Collarettes in staphylococcal blepharitis. Be certain to differentiate this from pediculosis palpebrum.

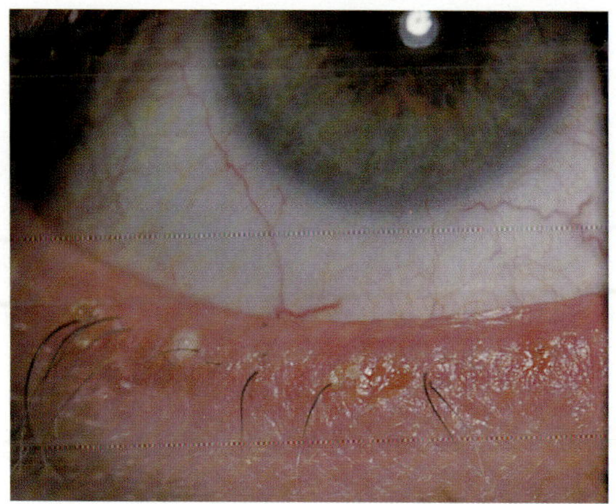

FIGURE 26-17. Folliculitis in staphylococcal blepharitis.

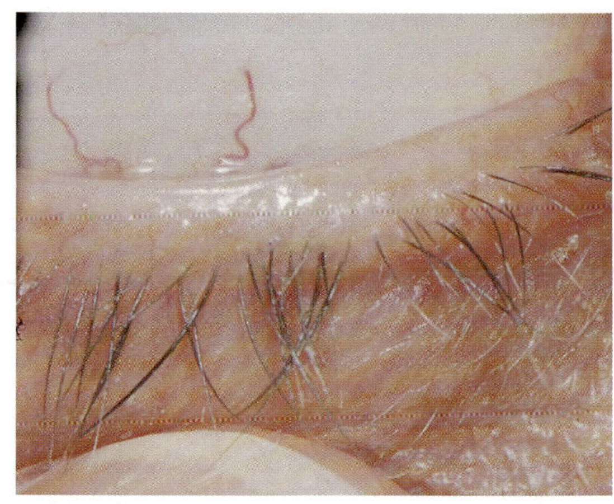

FIGURE 26-18. Partial poliosis in staphylococcal blepharitis.

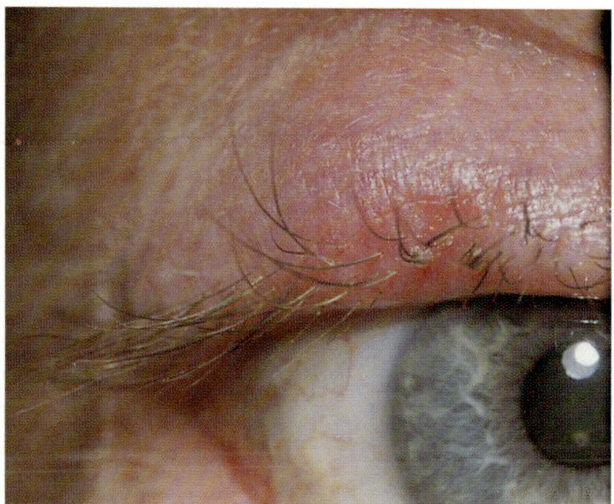

FIGURE 26-19. Early external hordeolum in staphylococcal blepharitis.

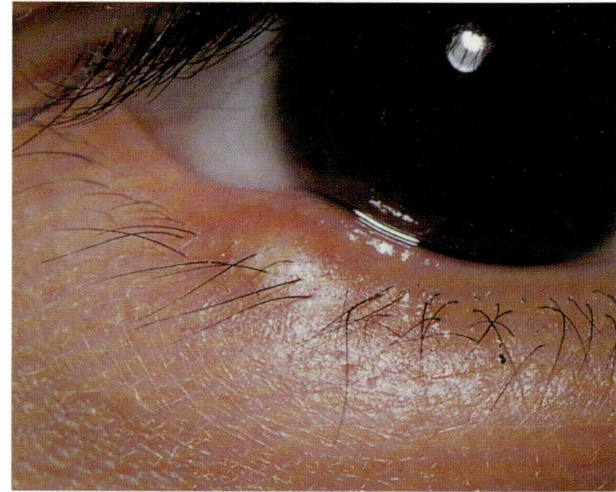

FIGURE 26-20. The external hordeolum is more advanced in this patient.

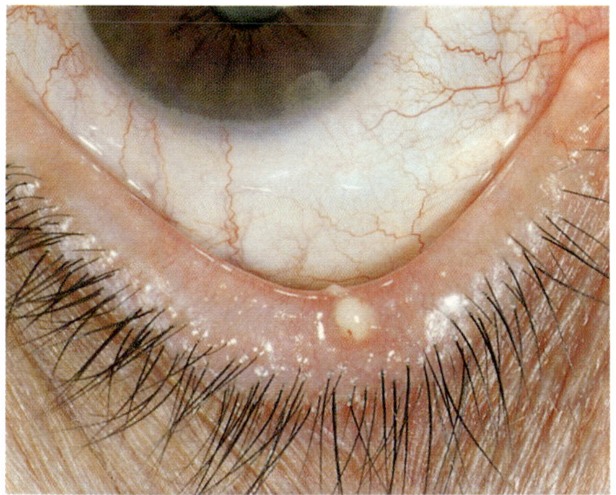

FIGURE 26-21. Early drainage of an internal hordeolum.

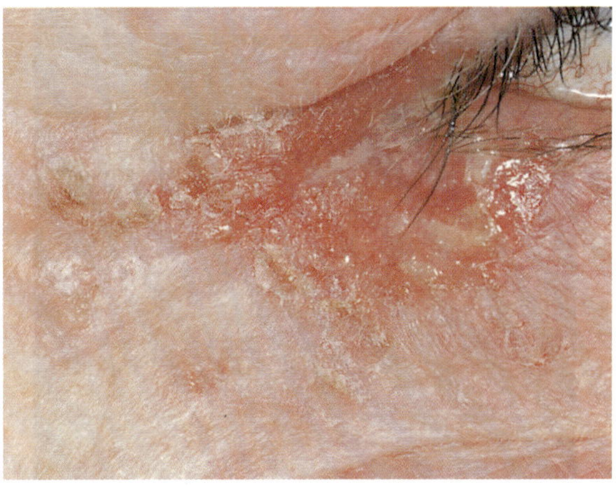

FIGURE 26-22. Angular staphylococcal blepharitis. (This photograph should be contrasted with Fig. 26-51.)

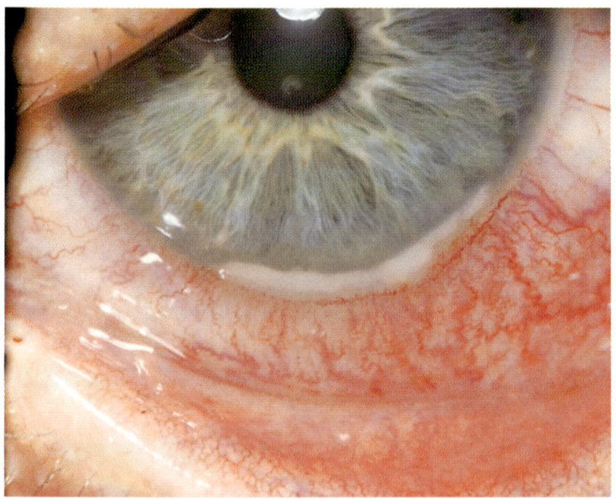

FIGURE 26-23. Staphylococcal catarrhal infiltrate. The catarrhal infiltrate, in this patient, started at the 8 o'clock limbus and extended to the 6 o'clock region. Prominent corneal infiltration is evident together with moderate injection of the limbus.

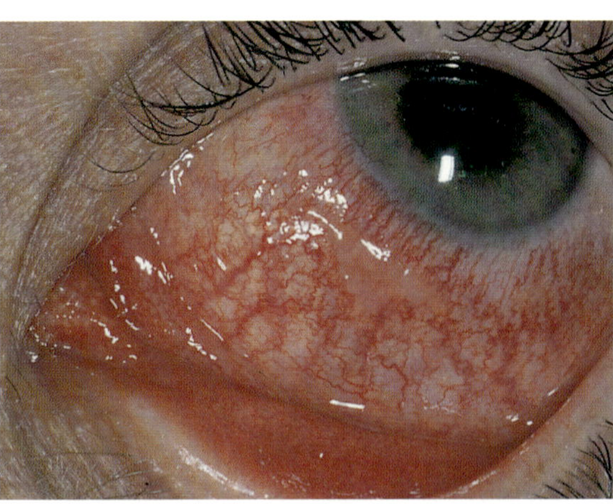

FIGURE 26-24. Resolving conjunctival phlyctenule. The elevated conjunctiva at the 8 o'clock position represents the phlyctenule's site just before ulceration.

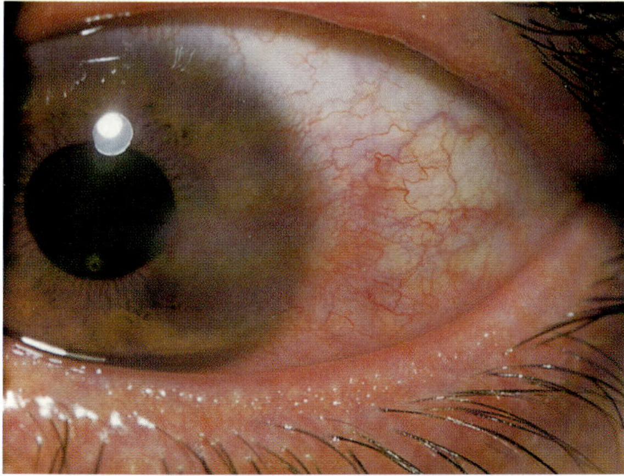

FIGURE 26-25. A fascicular keratitis in which two separate leashes of vessels have invaded the cornea. A resolving infiltrate is evident at the 4 o'clock margin of the pupil.

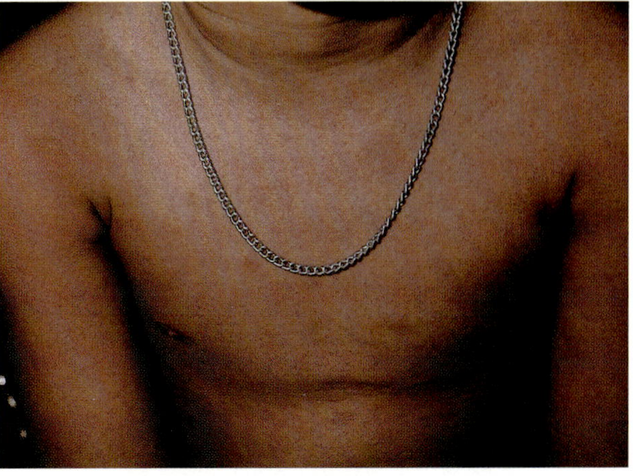

FIGURE 26-26. Rash of scarlet fever. Tiny papules give the skin the feel of sandpaper.

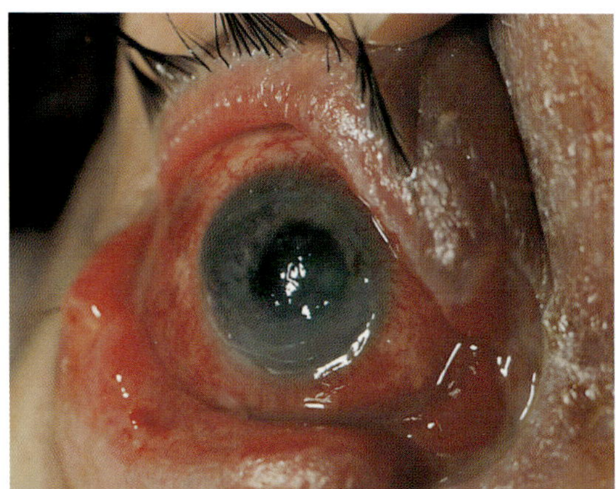

FIGURE 26-61. Ecthyma gangrenosum of the lid 3 days later.

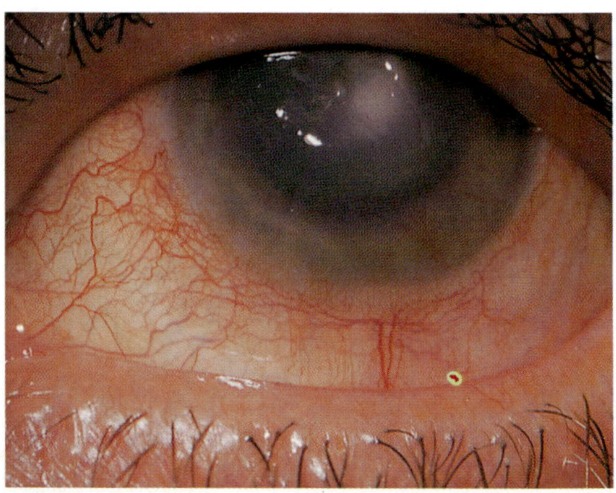

FIGURE 26-62. Pseudomonas corneal ulcer. This patient developed a central corneal ulcer following a scratch with a hair brush.

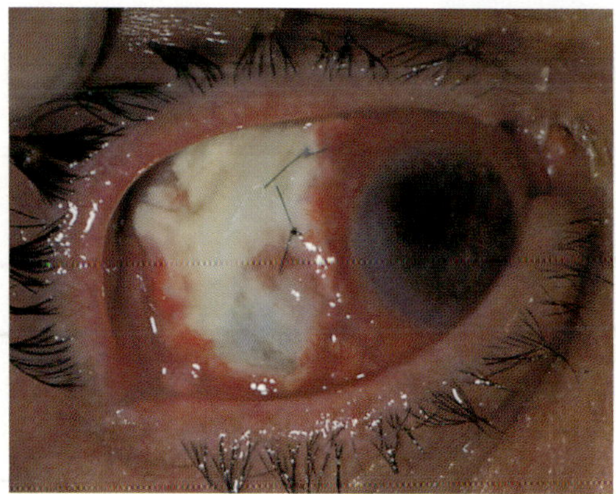

FIGURE 26-63. Pseudomonas scleral ulceration following retinal detachment surgery.

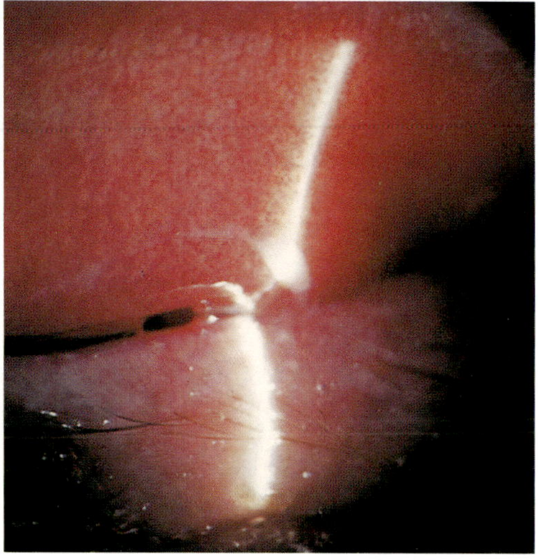

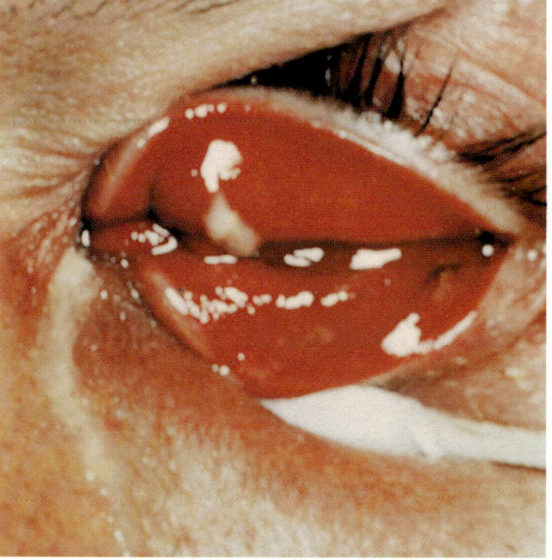

FIGURES 26-64 AND 26-65. Oculoglandular tularemia with severe papillary hypertrophy. The conjunctiva is severely injected and chemotic. Each fine dot represents a papilla. (Courtesy of Dr. Alson Braley.)

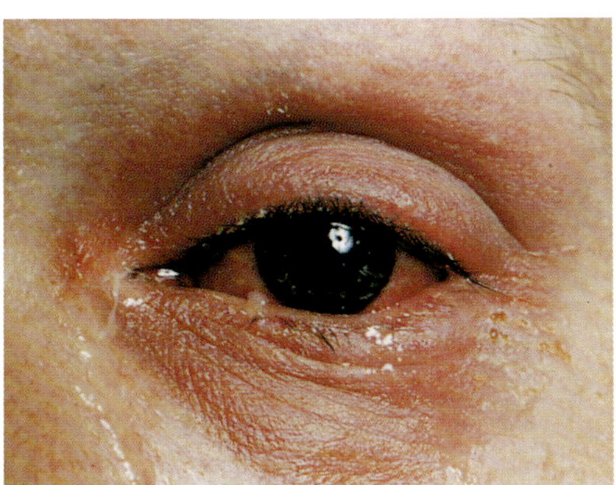

FIGURE 26-66. The lids in oculoglandular tularemia. Severe lid and conjunctival injection, lid edema, and mucoid discharge are evident. (Courtesy of Dr. Alson Braley.)

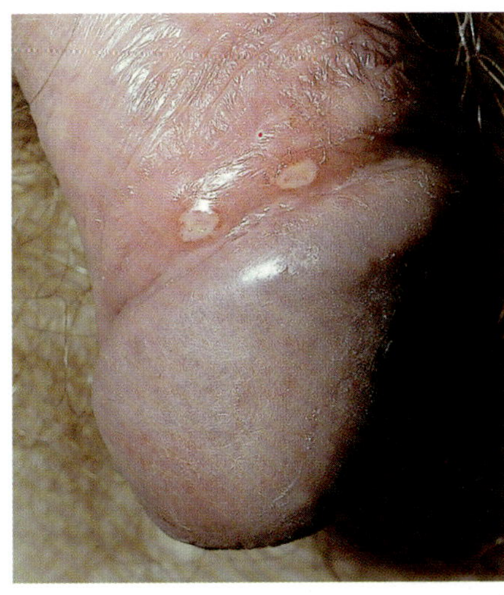

FIGURE 26-67. Chancroid, early lesions showing two small painful, purulent ulcerations on a nonindurated edematous base.

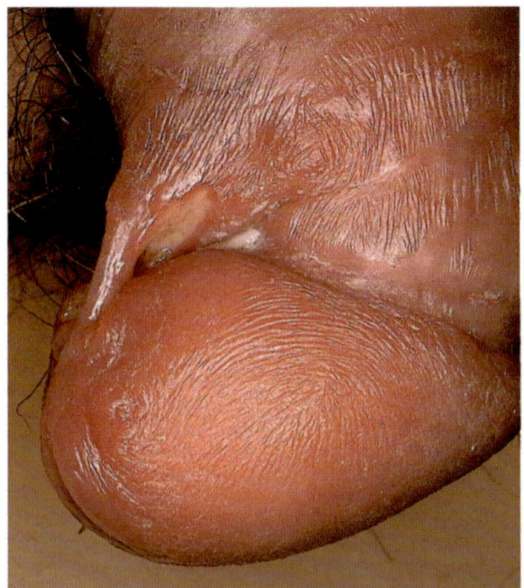

FIGURE 26-68. Very painful, small ulceration perforating the frenulum, a frequent site of chancroid.

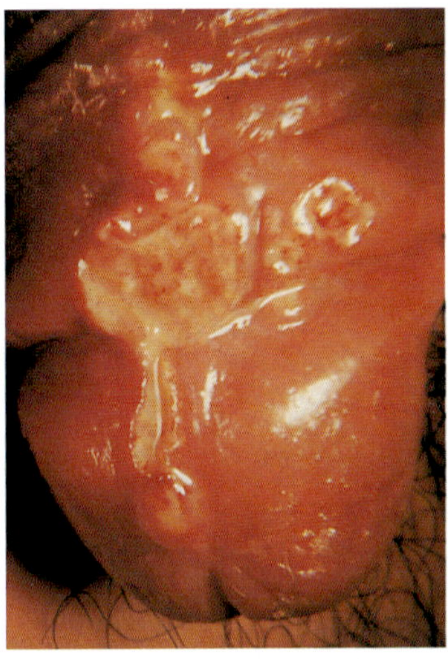

FIGURE 26-69. Characteristic, undermined, purulent ulcerations of frenulum, coronal sulcus, and prepuce in chancroid.

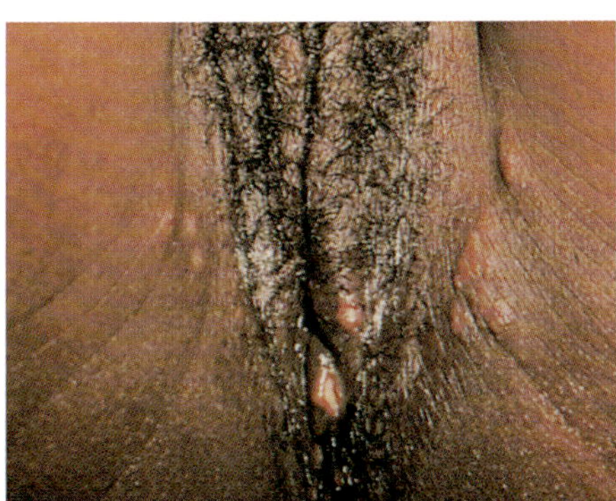

FIGURE 26-70. Painful chancroid lesions of labia. Herpes simplex infection can mimic or be coexistent with chancroid. (Courtesy of Dr. Antoinette Hood.)

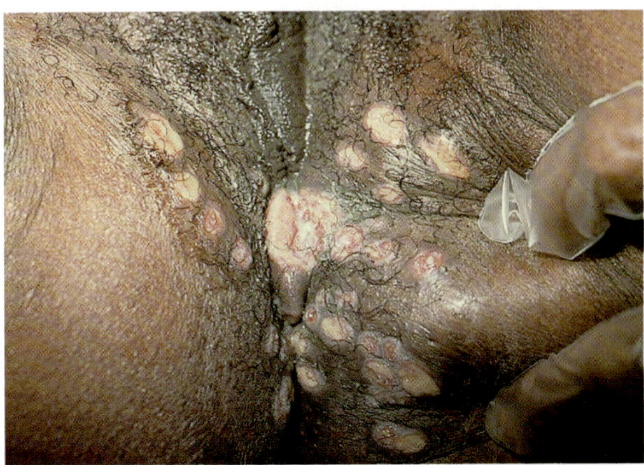

FIGURE 26-71. Multiple chancroidal ulcerations of the labia and perineum. Women tend to have more numerous lesions. (Courtesy of Dr. Antoinette Hood.)

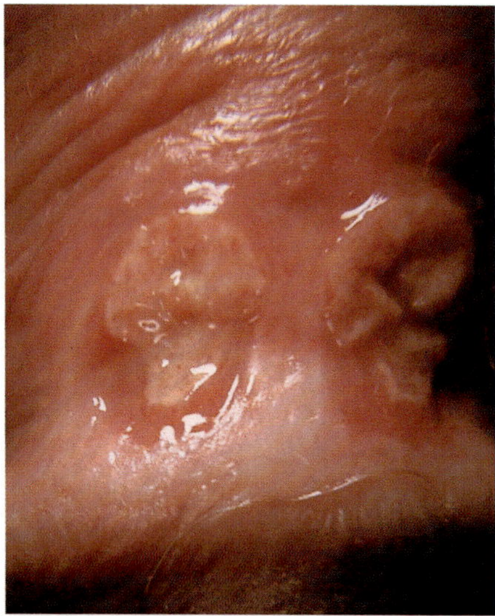

FIGURE 26-72. "Kissing ulcers" in chancroid. Autoinoculation frequently produces these typical lesions.

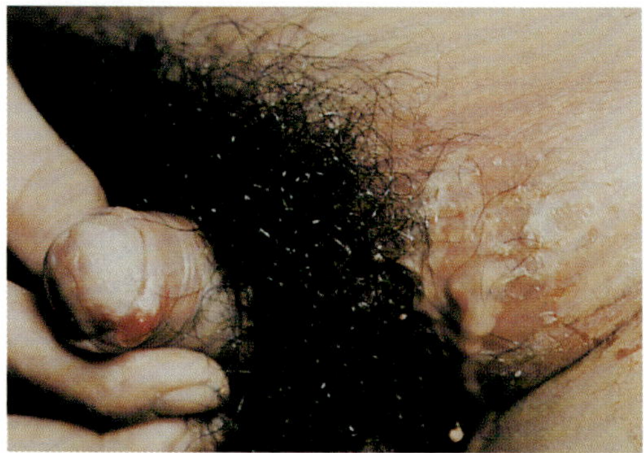

FIGURE 26-73. This patient's pain was greatly reduced following rupture of his chancroidal adenopathy. Lymphogranuloma venereum can mimic this picture (see Chapter 27).

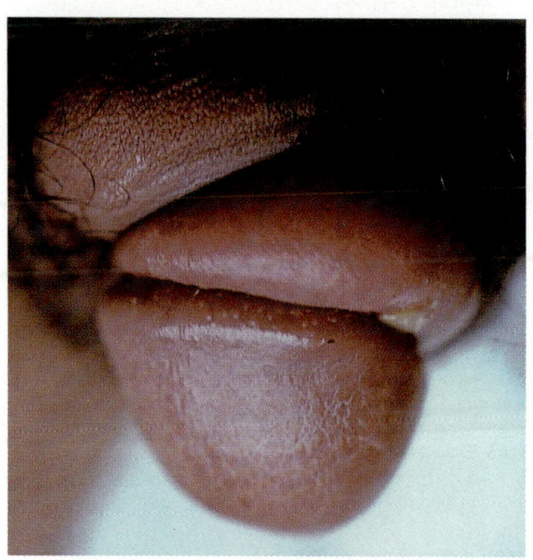

FIGURE 26-74. Paraphimosis as complication of chancroid.

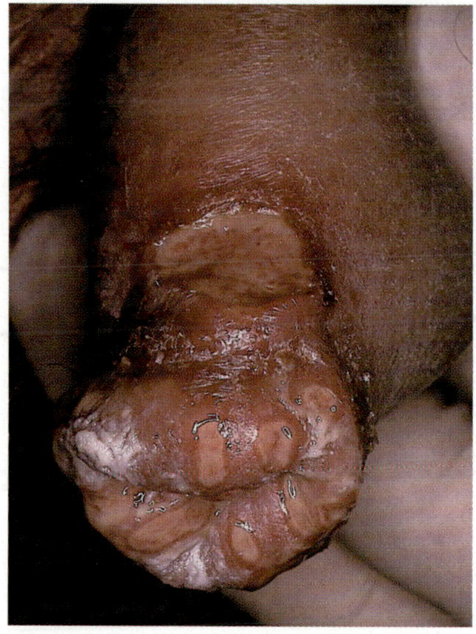

FIGURE 26-75. Phimosis in severe chancroid with multiple very painful lesions. Patient refused dorsal slit surgery but recovered with several weeks of antibiotic treatment and saline soaks.

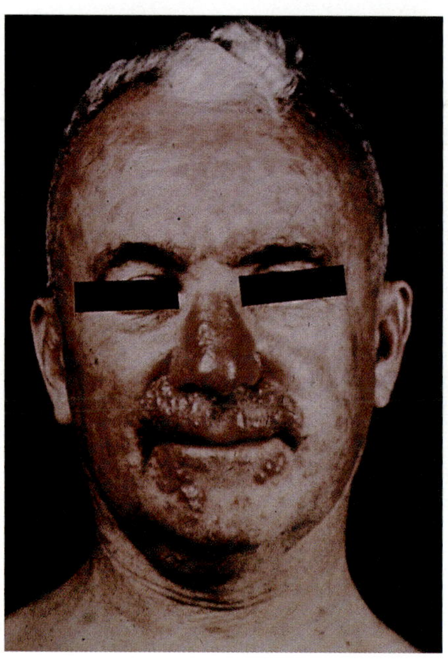

FIGURE 26-76. Glanders. Patient has primary nasal infection with multiple perinasal and perioral nodules. (Courtesy of Armed Forces Institute of Pathology.)

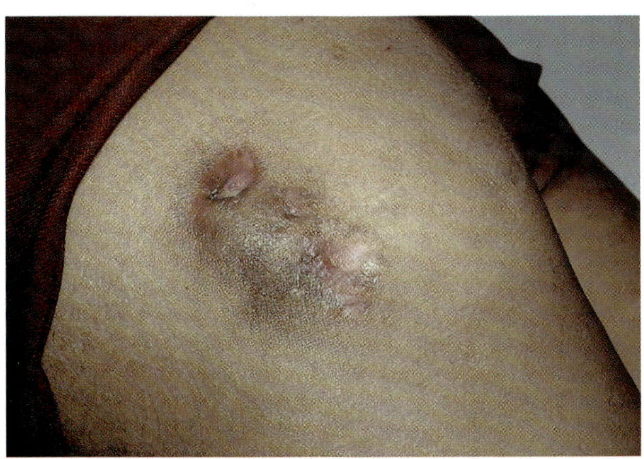

FIGURE 26-77. Melioidosis. The patient, a woman from Cambodia, had suffered from these abscesses and draining sinuses for more than 10 years. Surgical resection, after failure of long trials with antibiotics, cured her infection.

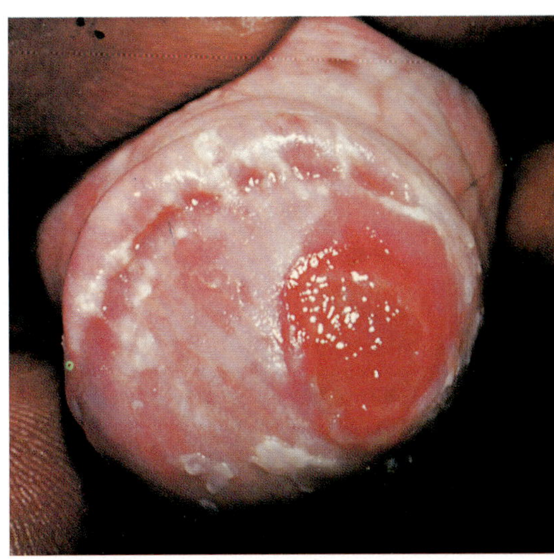

FIGURE 26-78. Granuloma inguinale showing typical friable beefy lesion. (Courtesy of Dr. William Henessy.)

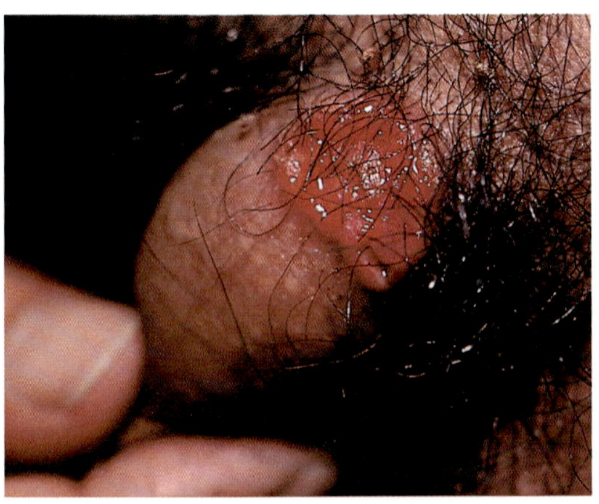

FIGURE 26-79. Granuloma inguinale with rolled borders mimicking carcinoma of the penis. (Courtesy of Dr. Steve Smith.)

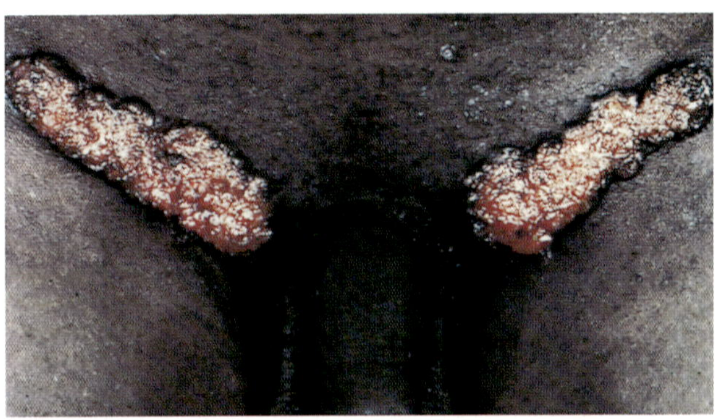

FIGURE 26-80. Granuloma inguinale of the groin untreated for many years. (Courtesy of the Communicable Disease Center, Atlanta, GA.)

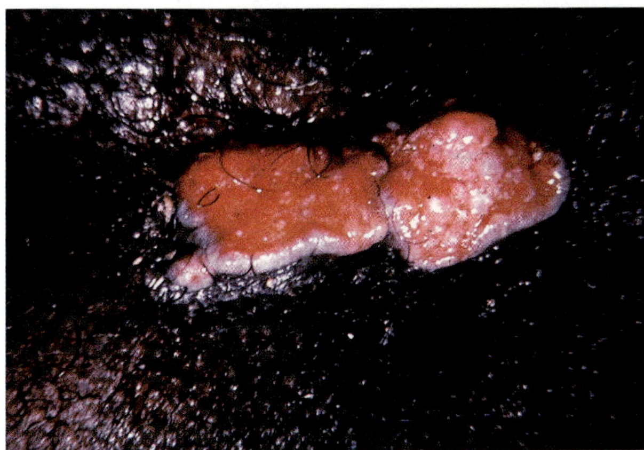

FIGURE 26-81. Granuloma inguinale of pubic area. Note typical rolled margin and beefy granulating base. (Courtesy of the CDC.)

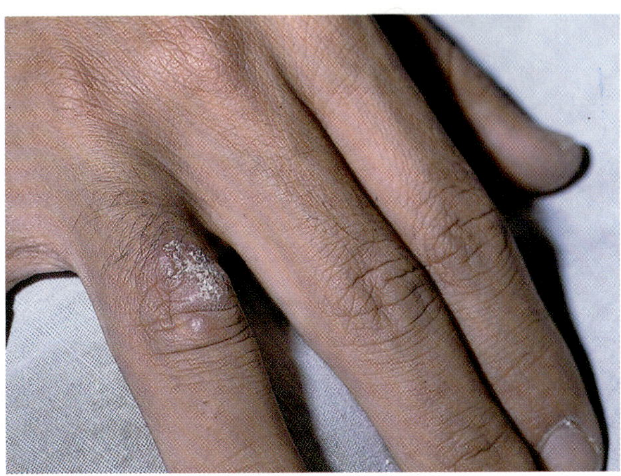

FIGURE 26-82. Tuberculosis verrucosa cutis showing an early nodule that could easily be mistaken for a traumatic or verrucous lesion.

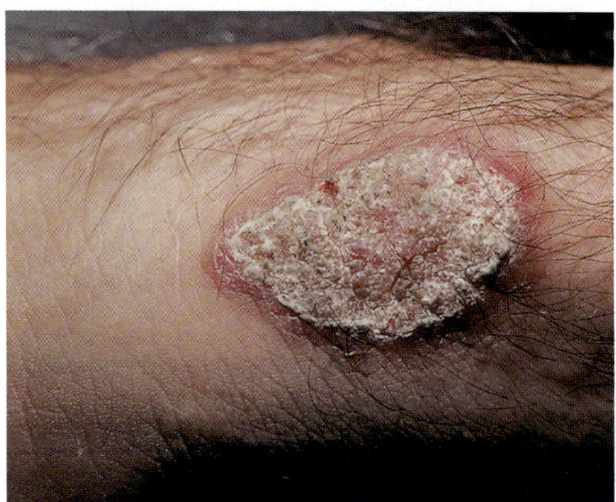

FIGURE 26-83. Tuberculosis verrucosa cutis of the wrist.

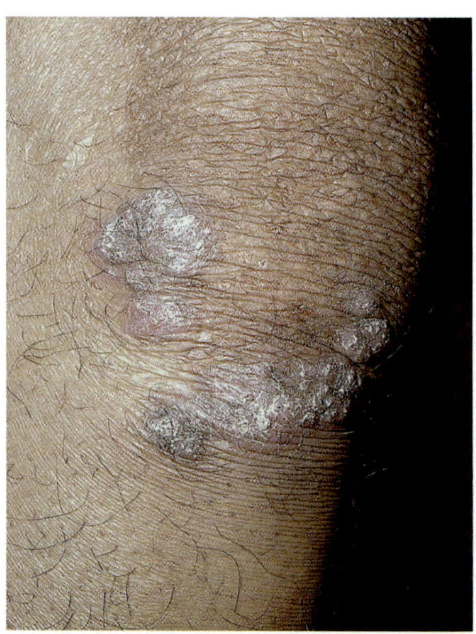

FIGURE 26-84. Tuberculosis verrucosa cutis of the knee, a common site.

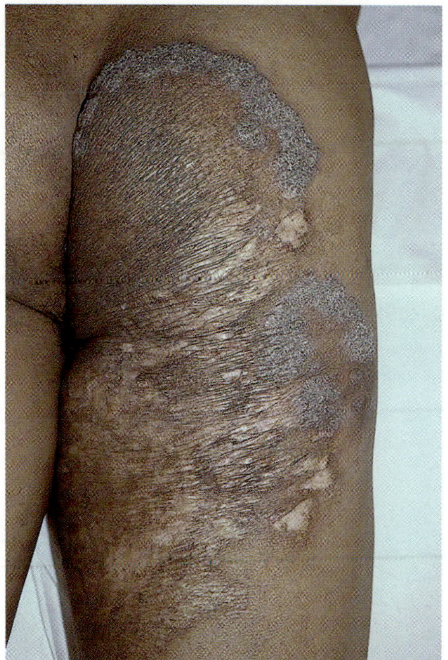

FIGURE 26-85. Tuberculosis verrucosa cutis. These lesions could be confused with tertiary syphilis, deep fungal infections or cutaneous lymphomas.

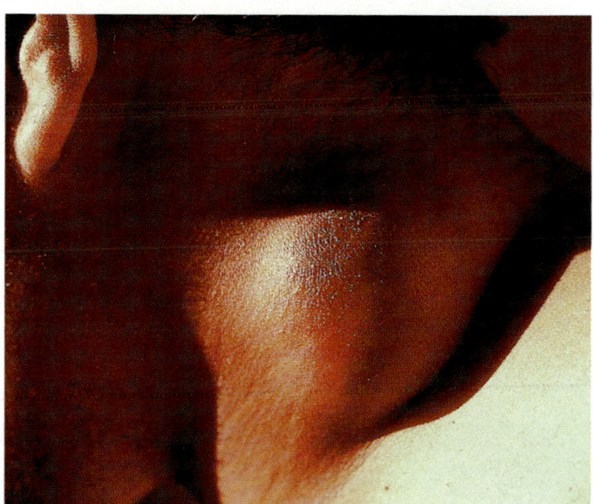

FIGURE 26-86. Tuberculosis lymphadenitis, a frequent site. This painful abscess was aspirated before it could spontaneously rupture.

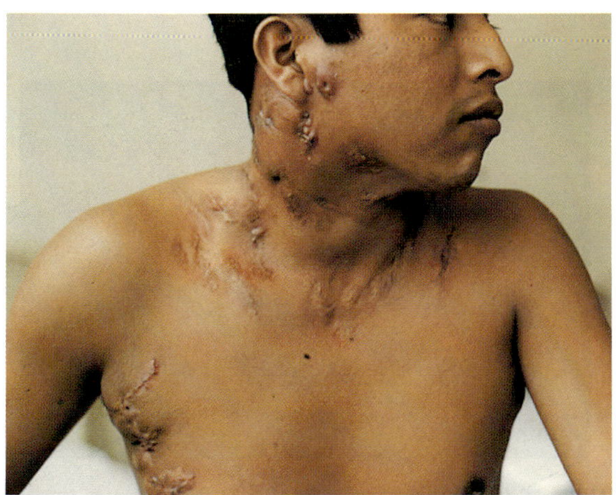

FIGURE 26-87. Scrofuloderma with drainage from the neck and right axillary nodes in an Indian from Costa Rica.

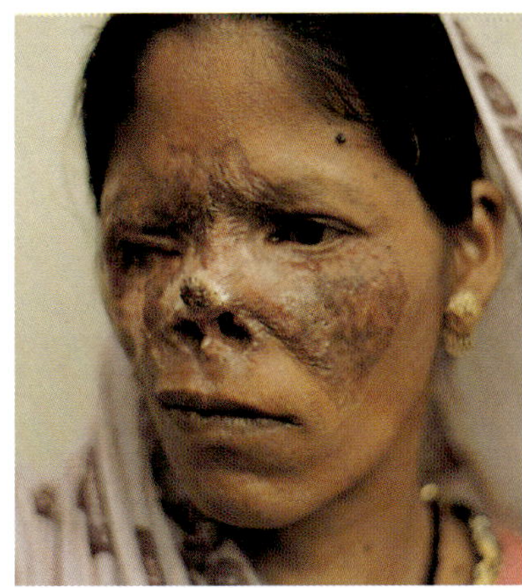

FIGURE 26-88. Lupus vulgaris with destruction of the nose. Note scarring of the lid with lagophthalmos on the right side. (Courtesy of Dr. David Lakes.)

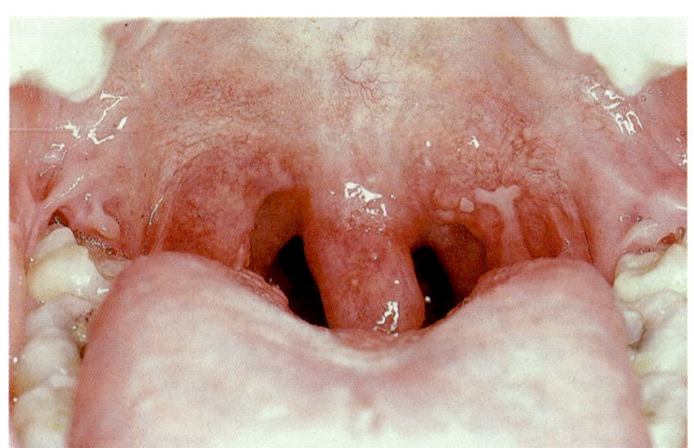

FIGURE 26-89. Tuberculosis of the pharynx in patient with fulminant pulmonary tuberculosis. Note erythema with small mucoid-appearing patch on right phauces.

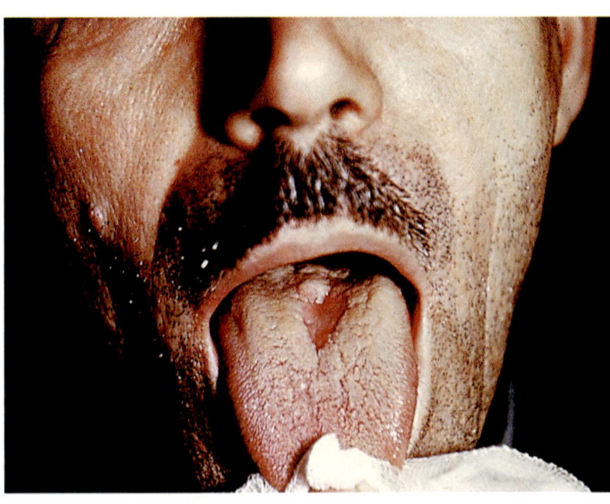

FIGURE 26-90. Tuberculosis of the tongue. The central location is typical. Carcinoma and tertiary syphilis can mimic this picture.

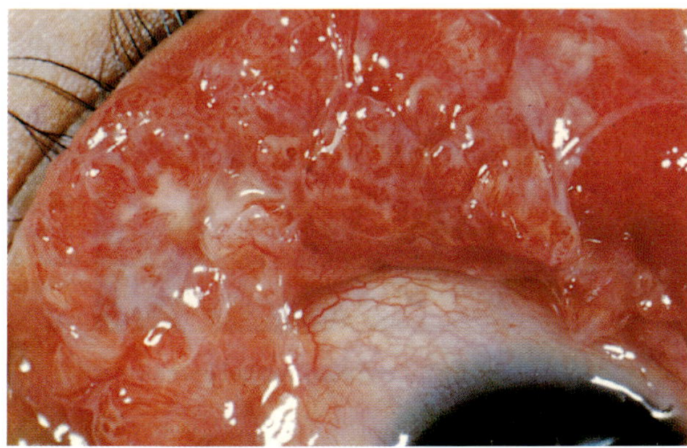

FIGURE 26-91. Conjunctival granulomas in tuberculosis. (Courtesy of Dr. Mario Valenton.)

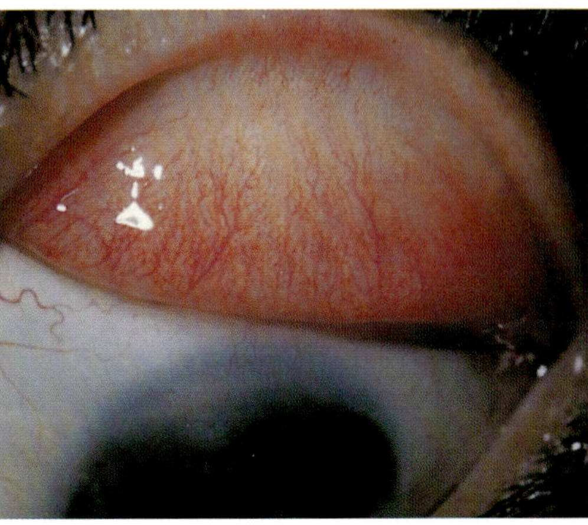

FIGURE 26-92. Characteristic, almost pathognomonic, corneal scar arising from tuberculous phlyctenular keratoconjunctivitis.

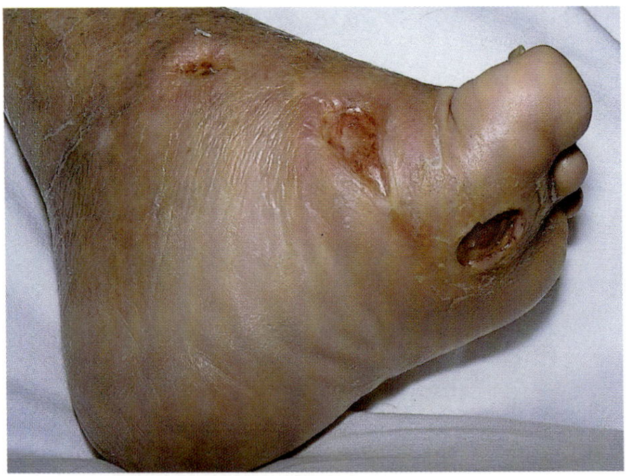

FIGURE 26-103. Multiple trophic ulcers of foot and sole with marked resorption of toes, making walking difficult in this patient with advanced leprosy seen in the tropical disease ward in London.

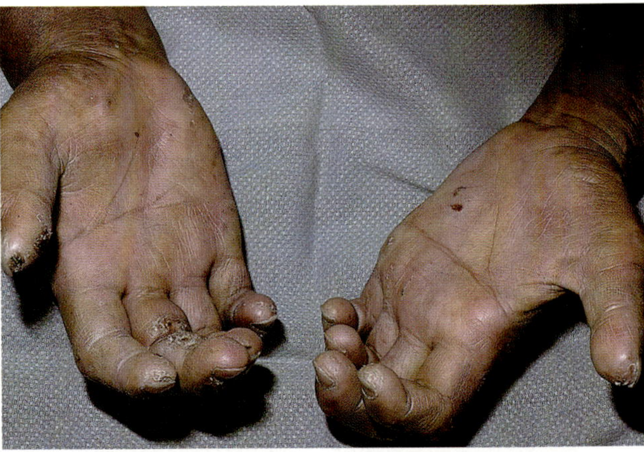

FIGURE 26-104. "Claw hand" resulting from destruction of ulnar and median nerves. The flexors are stronger than the extensors of the hand, eventually overpowering them, producing the "claw hand." Note flattening of thenar and hypothenar eminences due to muscle atrophy, and burn scars of fingers and thumb from sensory loss.

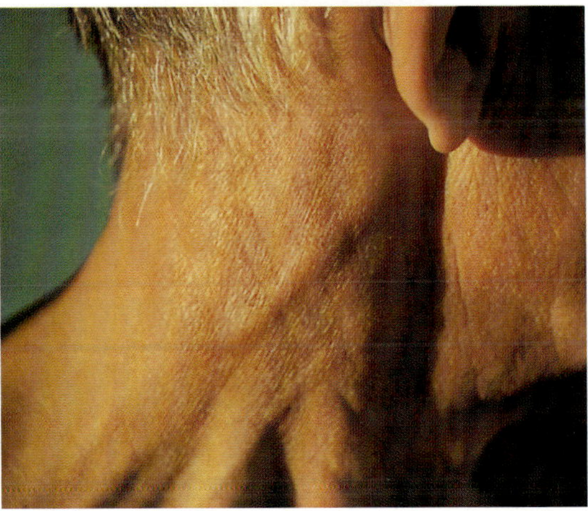

FIGURE 26-105. Enlarged and "ropy" nonpainful greater auricular nerve in patient who contracted leprosy while working in Africa for many years as a missionary.

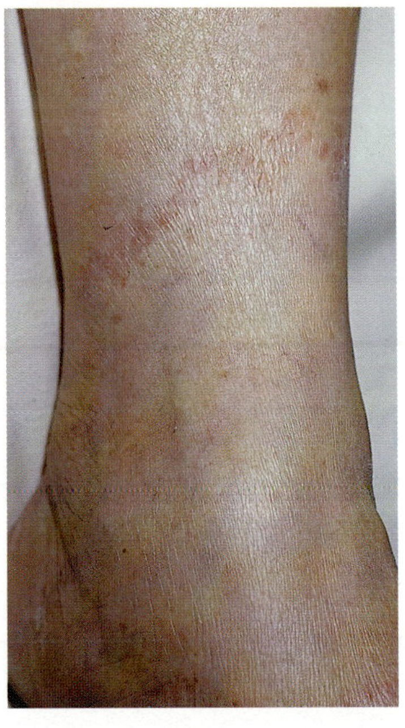

FIGURE 26-106. Tuberculoid leprosy. This faintly hypopigmented, sharply marginated patch showed slightly decreased perception to cold and light touch. It was the only lesion found in this 72-year-old Filipino lady, which is frequently the case in persons with good immunity to *Mycobacterium leprae*.

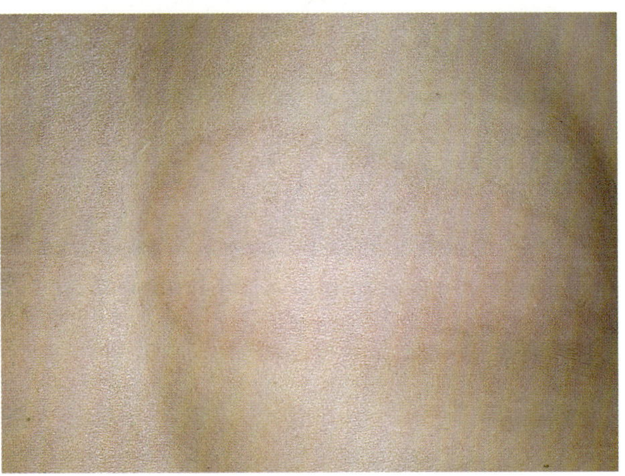

FIGURE 26-107. Tuberculoid leprosy. This young man, who had spent several years in American Samoa, was referred by his family doctor, whom he had seen for minimal burning pain of one hand and wrist (tuberculoid neuritis). His astute physician noted this slightly erythematous, asymptomatic plaque with faintly perceptible elevated border and sought consultation. The area was anesthetic to light touch with a wisp of cotton and the patient could not tell heat from cold.

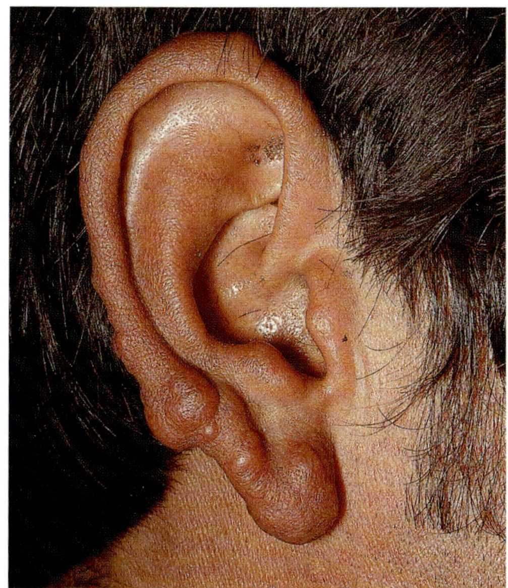

FIGURE 26-108. Lepromatous leprosy showing flesh-colored, moderately firm nodules of ear lobes. Note similarity to lupus pernio (sarcoidosis). The leprosy bacillus prefers cooler skin and mucosal sites, especially ear lobes, where the earliest nodules are often found, and the nasal and upper respiratory mucosa (see Fig. 26-111).

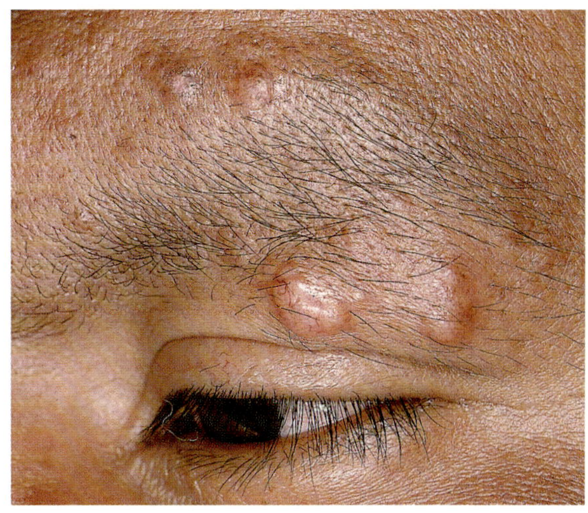

FIGURE 26-109. Nodules of eyelids and brows in lepromatous leprosy.

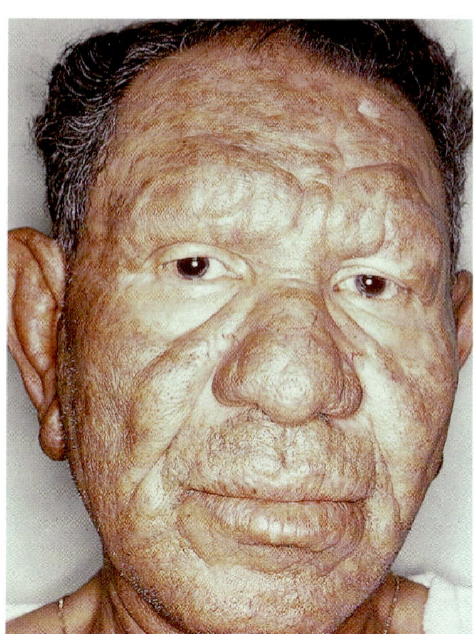

FIGURE 26-110. "Leonine facies" in advanced lepromatous leprosy. This patient, a tailor, had complained for several years of not being able to feel his needle and thread. His internist assured him that this was caused by his diabetes. In the United States, the diagnosis of leprosy is usually delayed 2 to 3 years after the onset of symptoms because it is not considered.

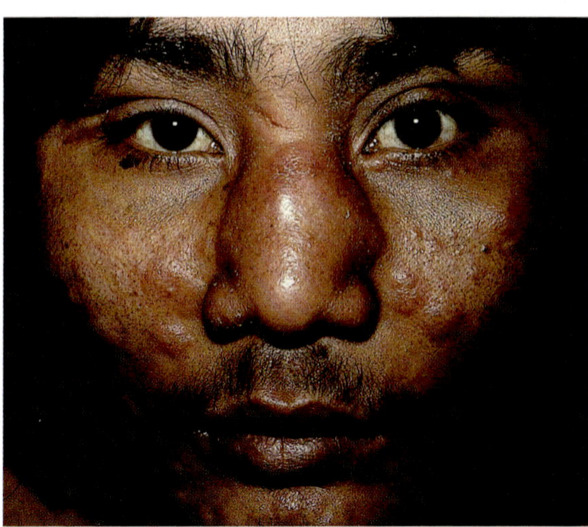

FIGURE 26-111. Nasal mucosal involvement in lepromatous leprosy. The patient had complained of nasal stuffiness, discharge, and epistaxis for several months before the suspicious nodules appeared on his face. These nasal symptoms, as well as hoarseness, are fairly common and early in lepromatous leprosy.

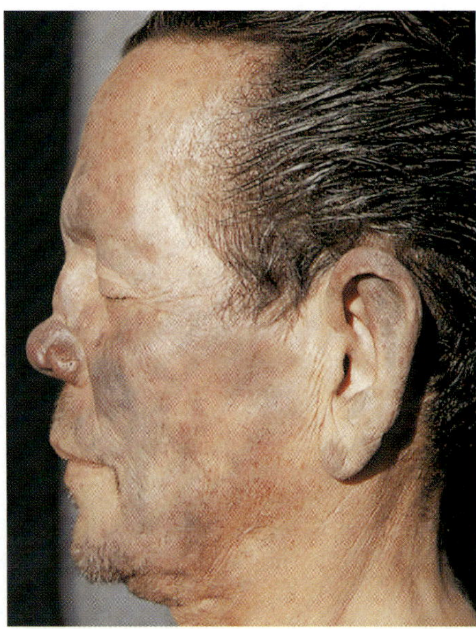

FIGURE 26-112. Collapse of nasal septum in patient whose lepromatous leprosy was not treated for many years. Note absence of brows and lashes and purplish patches resulting from treatment with clofazimine. The patient died a few years after this photo was taken from renal amyloidosis, a complication of leprosy now rarely seen.

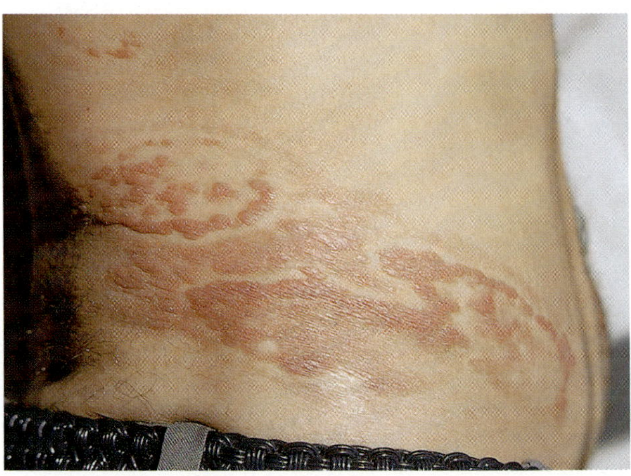

FIGURE 26-113. Borderline tuberculoid. Lesions are similar to those seen in tuberculoid leprosy but show less tendency to central clearing and may have satellite nodules. Note striking similarity to mycosis fungoides.

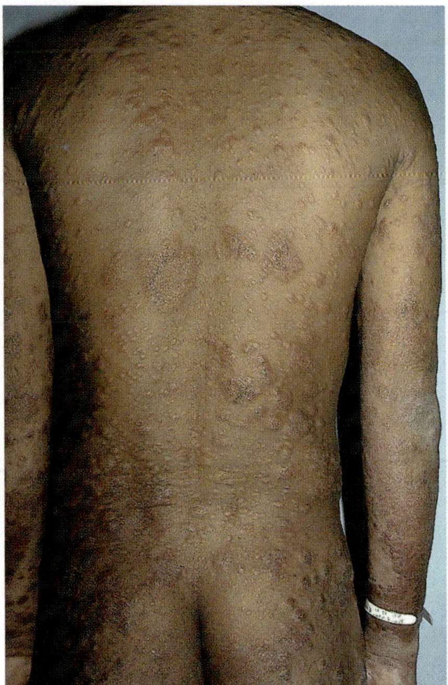

FIGURE 26-114. Borderline lepromatous leprosy. Lesions are numerous, symmetric and include annular plaques (some with central clearing suggesting partial immune response) as well as nodules.

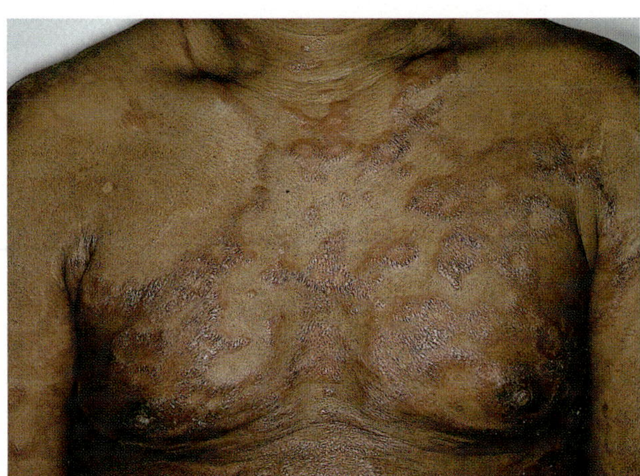

FIGURE 26-115. Lepra reaction (reversal) in patient with borderline tuberculoid leprosy. This Samoan patient developed fever, malaise and pain in previously enlarged ulnar nerva and swelling of old plaques as well as appearance of new skin lesions 6 weeks after beginning treatment of previously untreated leprosy.

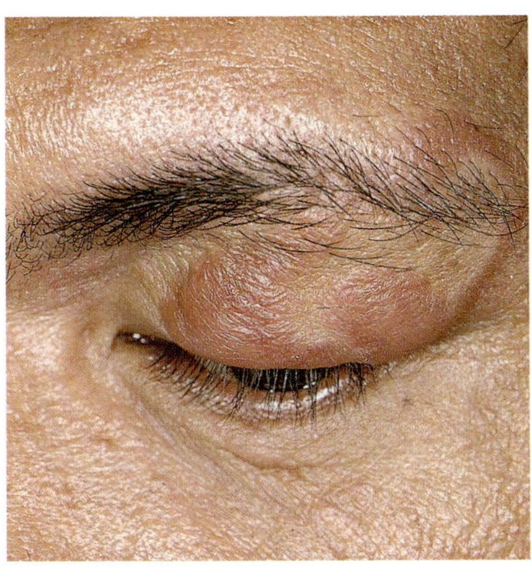

FIGURE 26-116. Lepra reaction with new lesions on eyelid. (Same patient as pictured in Fig. 26-115.)

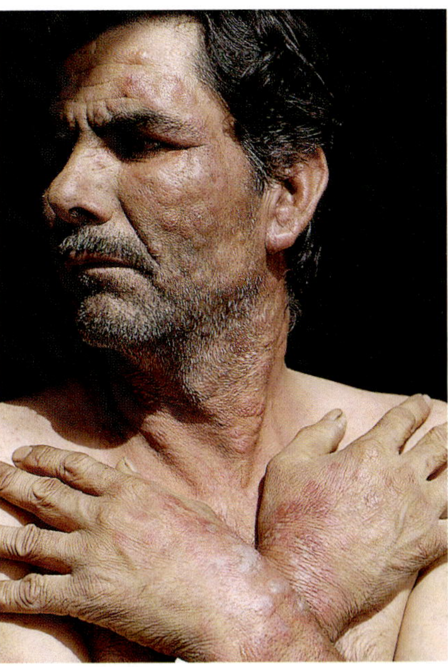

FIGURE 26-117. Erythema nodosum leprosum. The patient was acutely ill with fever, arthralgias, lymphadenopathy, and orchitis. Crops of painful erythematous nodules appeared on the face and upper extremities.

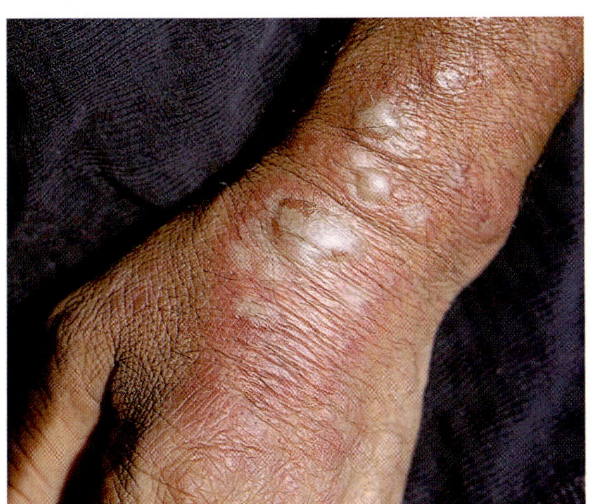

FIGURE 26-118. Erythema nodosum leprosum (ENL). Close-up of wrist and arm of patient pictured in Fig. 26-115. Note that these nodules have become bullous. ENL is somewhat of a misnomer since the nodules in erythema nodosum are usually confined to the lower extremities and do not become bullous or break down.

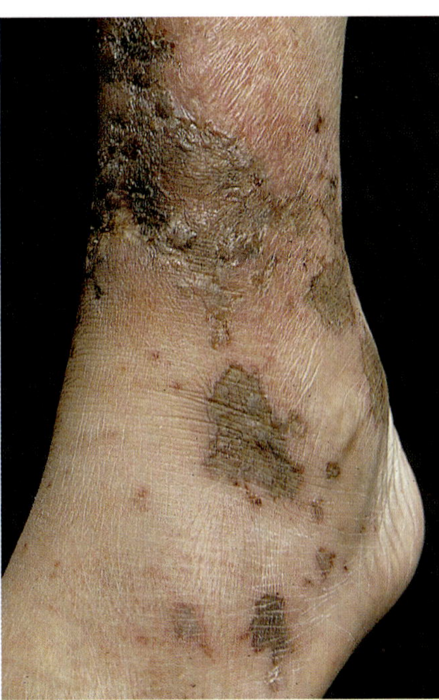

FIGURE 26-119. Erythema necroticans (Lucio phenomenon) in patient with diffuse lepromatous leprosy. Unlike erythema nodosum leprosum, which is usually precipitated by therapy of lepromatous leprosy, this is not.

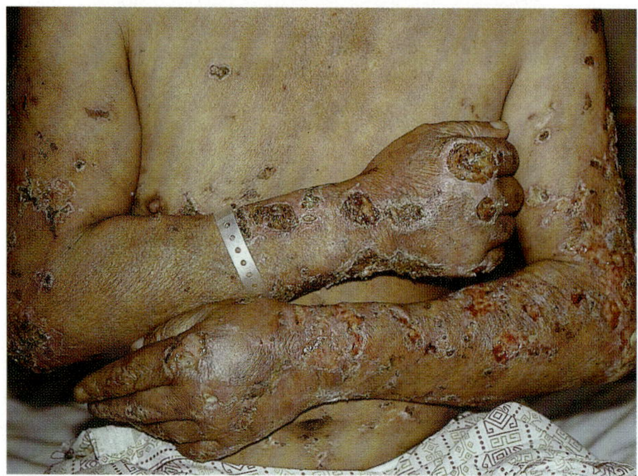

FIGURE 26-120. Lucio phenomenon in patient from western Mexico. His multiple painful sloughing, bullous and necrotic lesions became secondarily infected and required many months of treatment in the hospital.

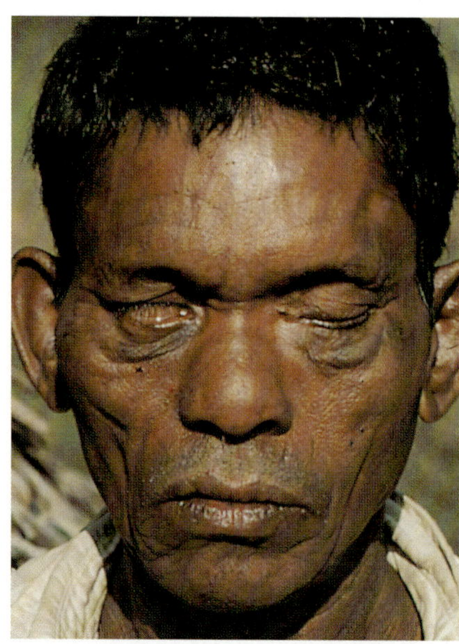

FIGURE 26-121. Lagophthalmos and thickening of the left supraorbital nerve as it passes under the skin of the forehead in this patient with tuberculoid leprosy.

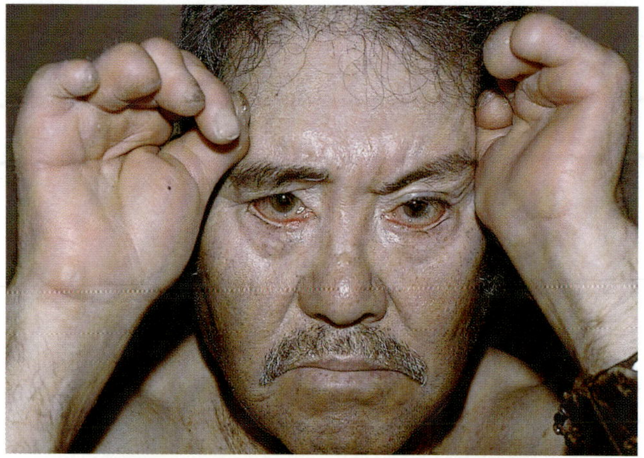

FIGURE 26-122. Tuberculoid leprosy with severe resorption of digits and contractures of hands and also ectropion.

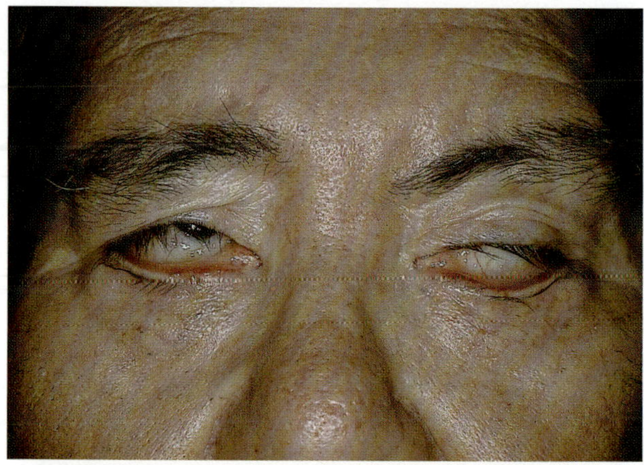

FIGURE 26-123. Lagophthalmos and ectropion. (Same patient as in Fig. 26-122.)

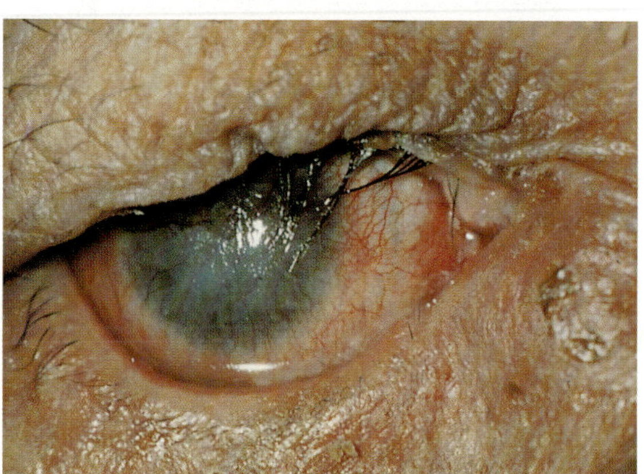

FIGURE 26-124. Entropion, trichiasis, lagophthalmos, and exposure keratitis in this patient with tuberculoid leprosy. Trichiasis, perilimbal injection, mucous strands in the tear film, and corneal neovascularization and scarring are apparent.

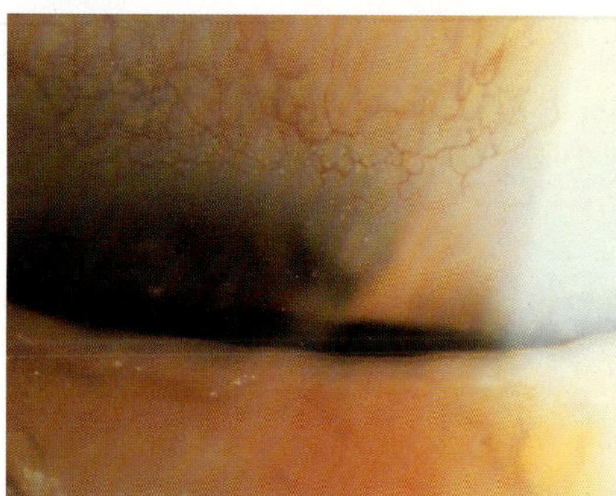

FIGURE 26-125. Early punctate keratitis caused by lepromatous leprosy. The minute, chalklike lesions can be seen on both the scleral and corneal sides of the limbus.

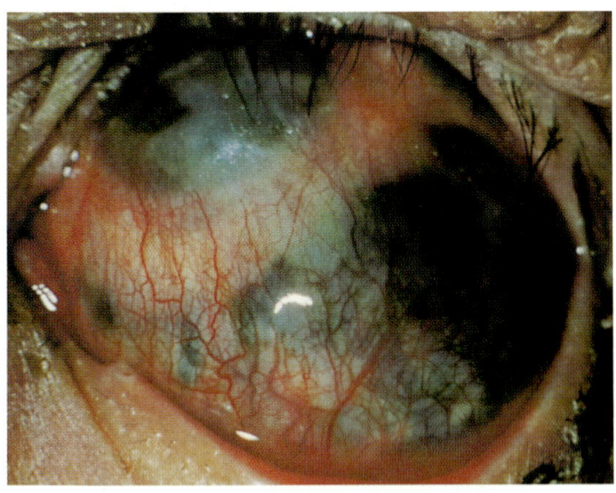

FIGURE 26-126. Severe scleritis with scleral thinning, staphyloma, and exposure keratitis in lepromatous leprosy.

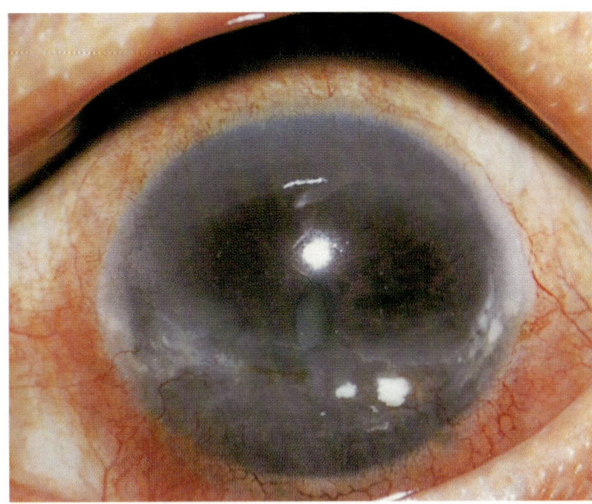

FIGURE 26-127. Iris pearls in Hansen disease. Moderate injection, inferior corneal scarring, and iris pearls are evident. The iris pearls appear as tiny white dots on the face of the iris to the left of the pupil.

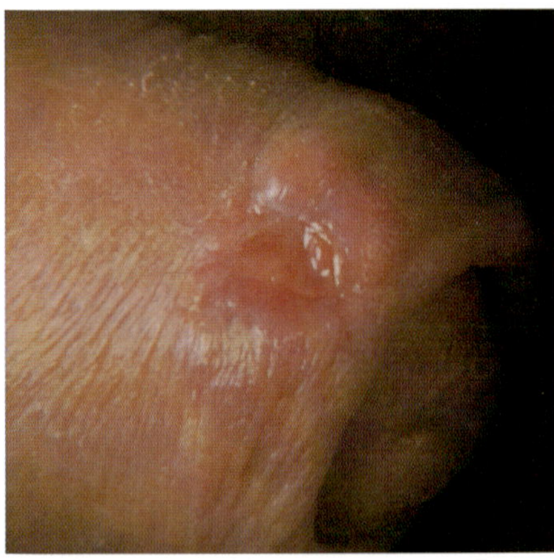

FIGURE 26-128. Penile syphilitic chancre. Note nonpurulent ulcer with moderately firm rolled margin. This classic presentation is now seen in less than half of primary syphilis patients.

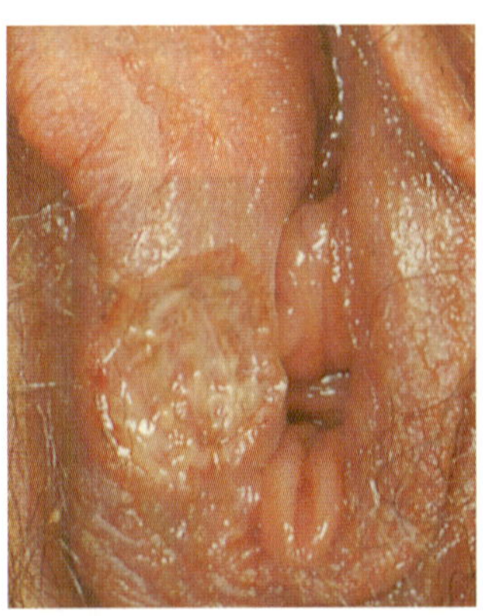

FIGURE 26-129. Syphilitic chancre in the female. The majority of chancres in women are overlooked, since they are usually asymptomatic and hidden.

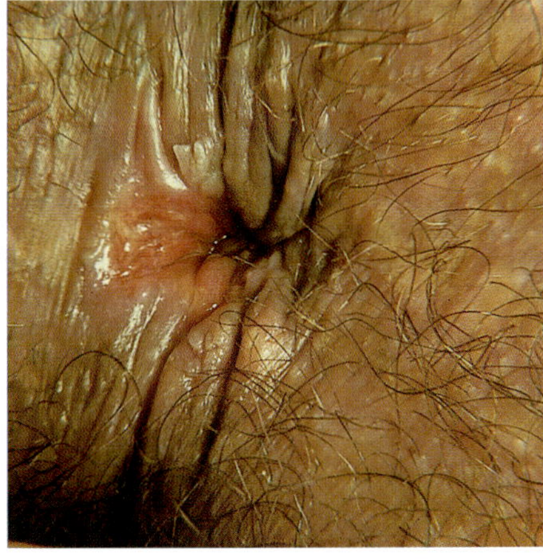

FIGURE 26-130. Anal chancre, a frequent site.

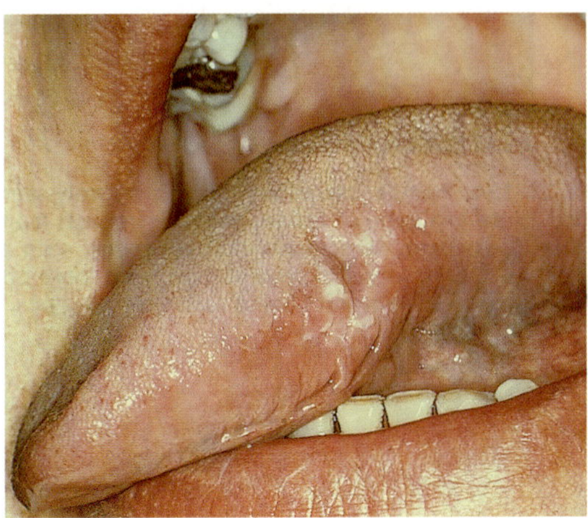

FIGURE 26-131. Chancre of the tongue. (Courtesy of Dr. Kuffer.)

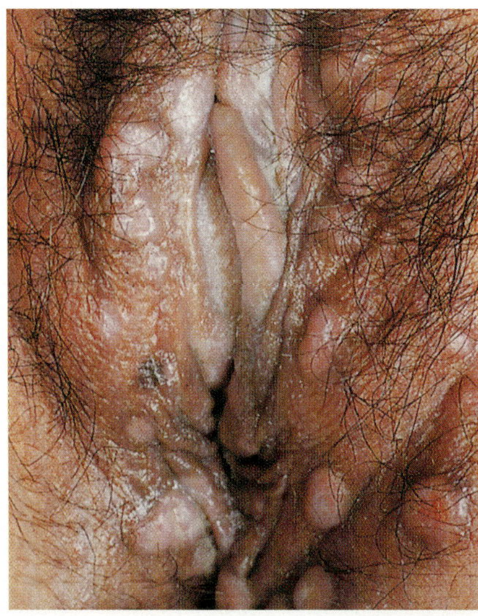

FIGURE 26-140. Condyloma lata of the labia in secondary syphilis. The flat, moist appearance of these lesions helps to differentiate them from warts. (Courtesy of Dr. John Reeves.)

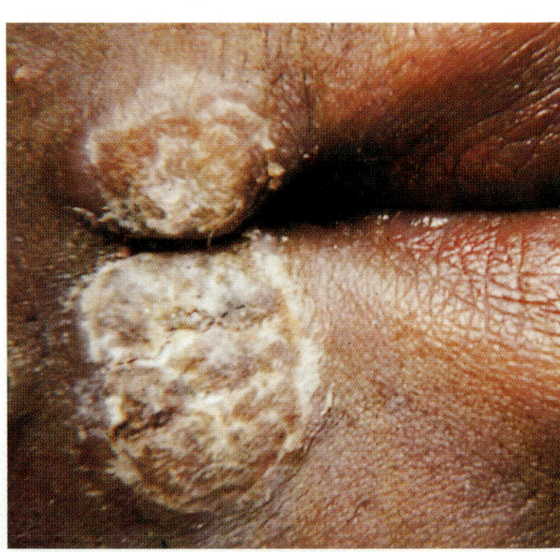

FIGURE 26-141. Split papule of the lip in secondary syphilis. Such a lesion is highly infectious.

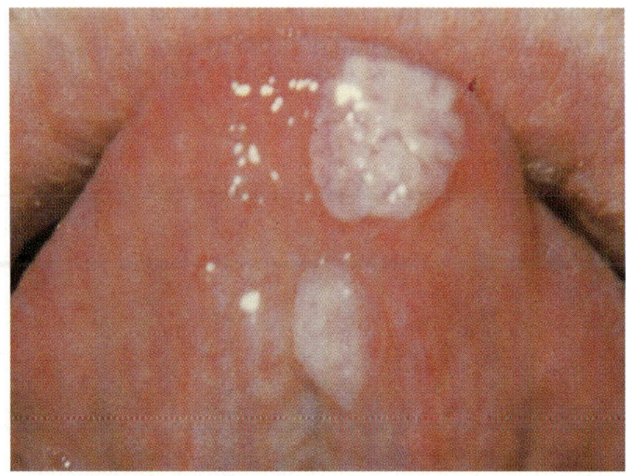

FIGURE 26-142. Mucous patches of the tongue in secondary syphilis. These lesions are teeming with spirochetes. (Courtesy of Dr. Richard Odom.)

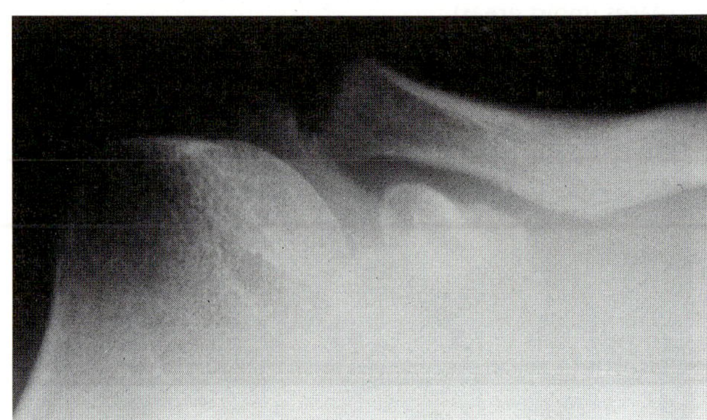

FIGURE 26-143. Syphilitic osteomyelitis of the lateral aspect of the clavicle. (Same patient as in Fig. 26-138.) The bone lesion healed completely several months after the patient was treated for his syphilis.

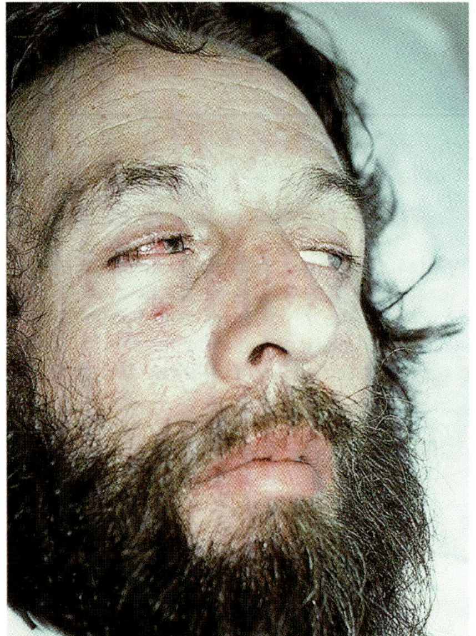

FIGURE 26-144. Early meningeal neurosyphilis in a patient with secondary syphilitic lesions of palms and soles pictured in Fig. 26-137. The patient experienced sudden onset of severe headache, confusion, loss of hearing, pain and visual loss in the right eye, and papilledema.

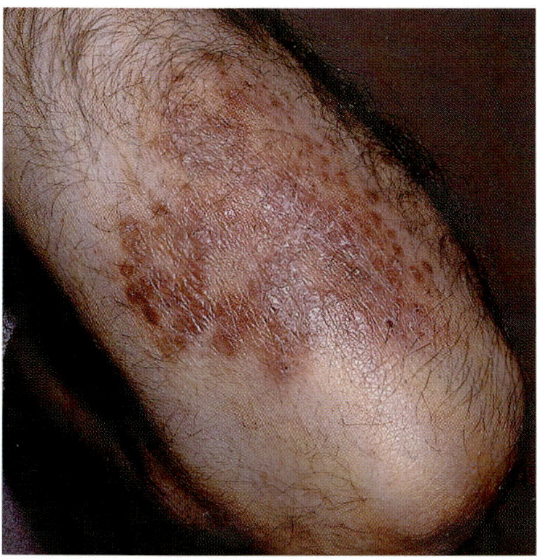

FIGURE 26-145. Tertiary cutaneous syphilis appearing as a coppery-red confluent nodules on the elbow. Note similarity to cutaneous tuberculosis.

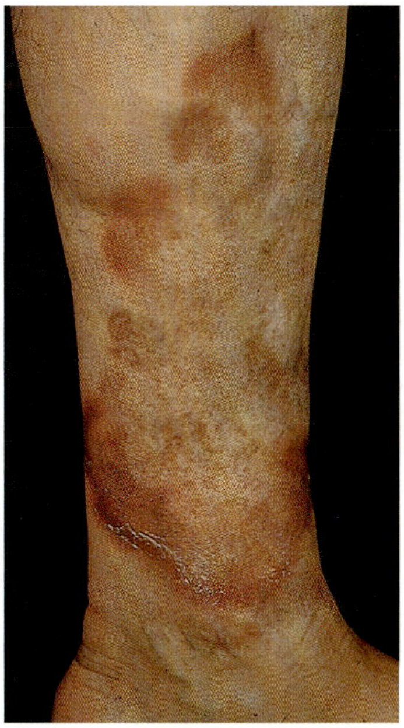

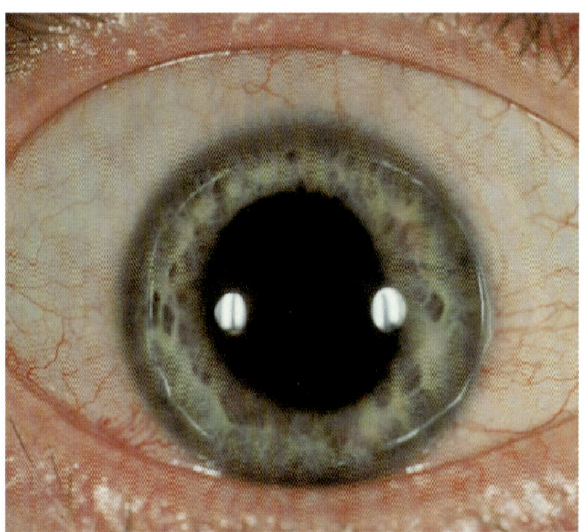

FIGURE 26-146. Tertiary cutaneous syphilis, nodular type, showing arcuate and annular lesions that tend to slowly extend peripherally while healing with scarring centrally. (Courtesy of the CDC.)

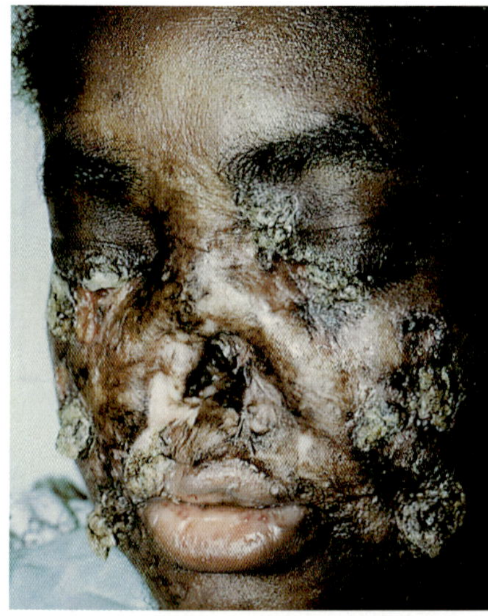

FIGURE 26-147. Severely destructive gummata in tertiary syphilis. (Courtesy of Dr. John Reeves.)

FIGURE 26-148. Roseola of the iris in secondary syphilis. The dilated vessels are evident near the pupillary margin at 2, 4, and 6 o'clock. (Courtesy of Dr. Lee Schwartz.)

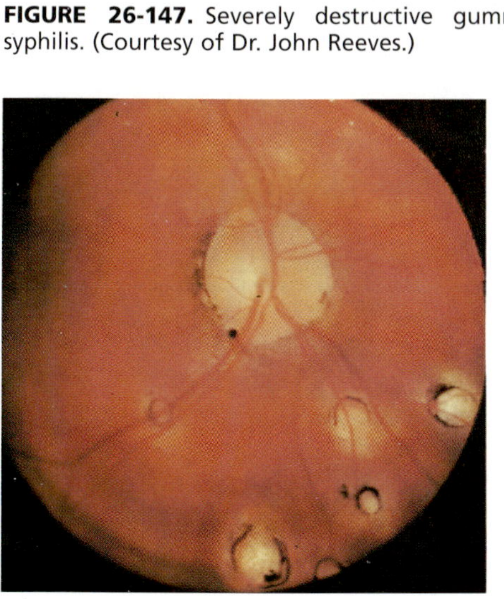

FIGURE 26-149. Disseminated syphilitic chorioretinitis. (Courtesy of Dr. Michael Hogan.)

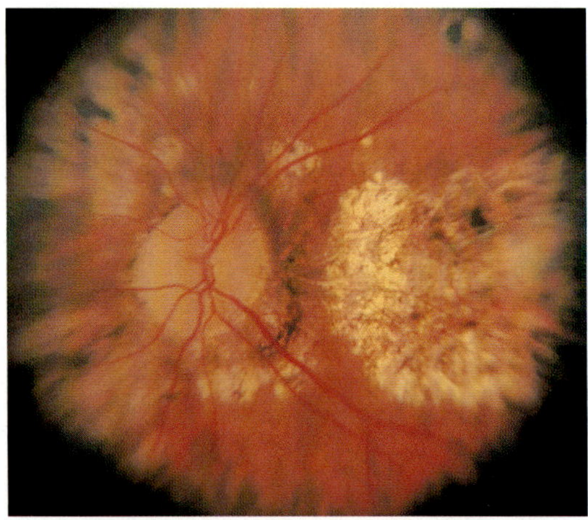

FIGURE 26-150. Chorioretinitis in syphilis. (Courtesy of Dr. Michael Hogan.)

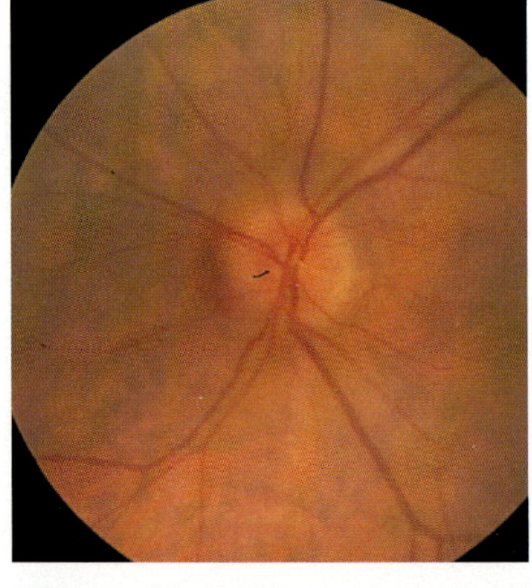

FIGURE 26-151. Papillitis in secondary syphilis.

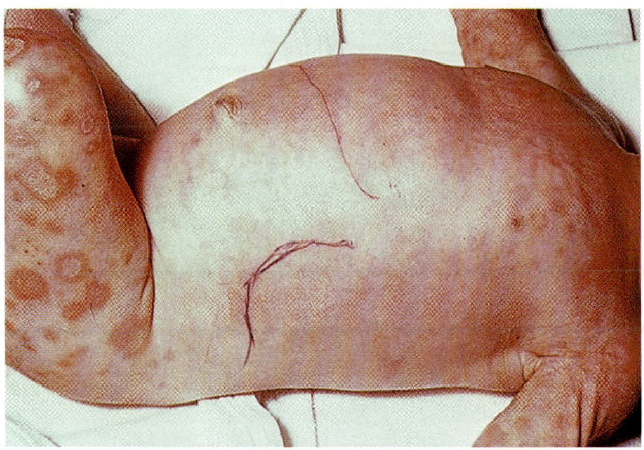

FIGURE 26-152. Skin lesions of early congenital syphilis. Note copper-colored annular scaly macules of legs. The infant exhibited hepatosplenomegaly, a common complication in early congenital lues. (Courtesy of the CDC.)

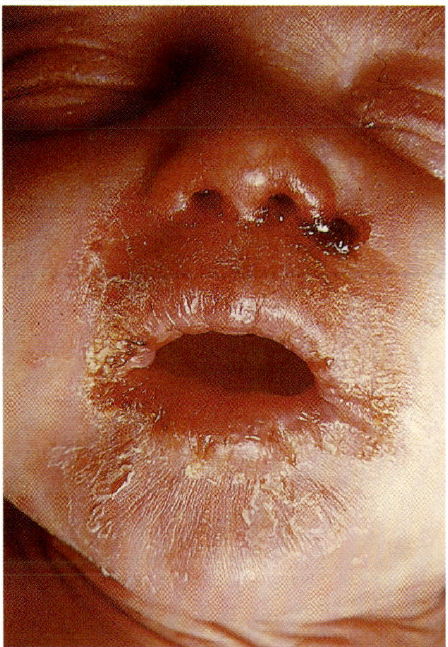

FIGURE 26-153. Early congenital syphilis showing perinasal and perioral condylomata lata and snuffles. (Courtesy of Dr. Alagil.)

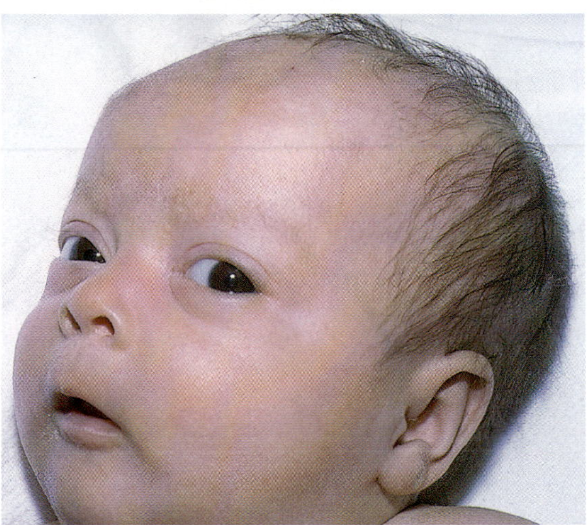

FIGURE 26-154. Congenital syphilis in 4-week-old infant with irritability, failure to thrive, and problems with nursing due to copious mucoid nasal discharge (snuffles). The mother had carefully wiped the infant's nose before allowing me to take this photo.

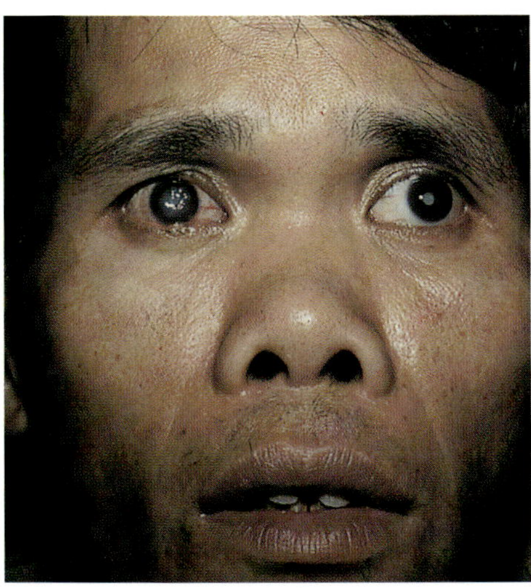

FIGURE 26-155. Saddle nose and corneal scarring in a patient with prenatal syphilis. A cataract is evident in the other eye.

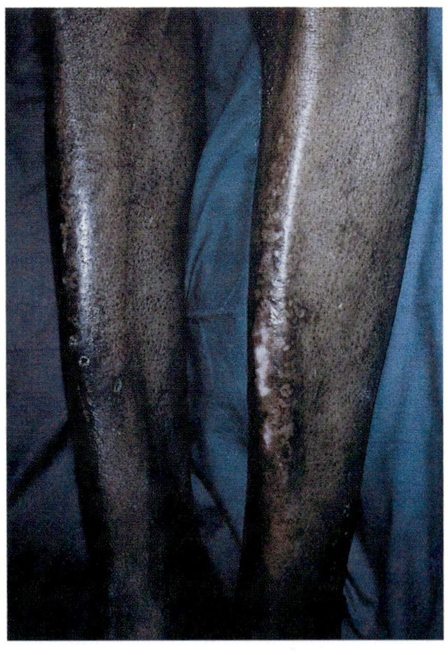

FIGURE 26-156. Saber shins in congenital syphilis. (Courtesy of the CDC.)

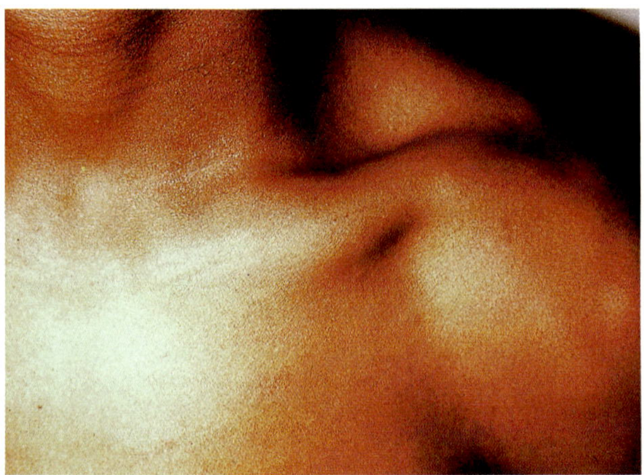

FIGURE 26-157. Higoumenaki sign in congenital syphilis. (Courtesy of the CDC.)

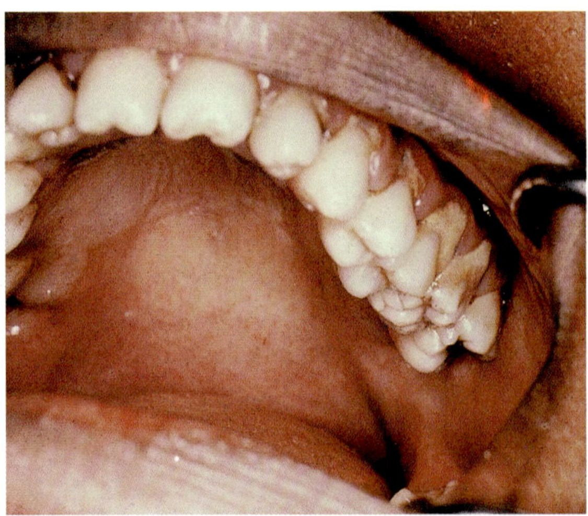

FIGURE 26-158. Hutchinson teeth and mulberry molars. (Courtesy of the CDC.)

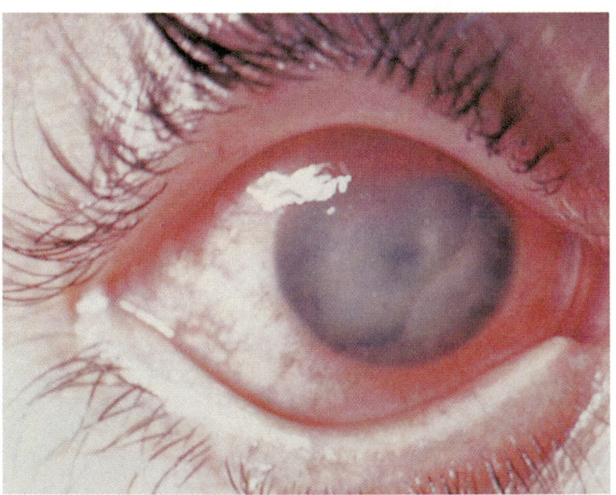

FIGURE 26-159. Epaulet in interstitial keratitis of syphilis.

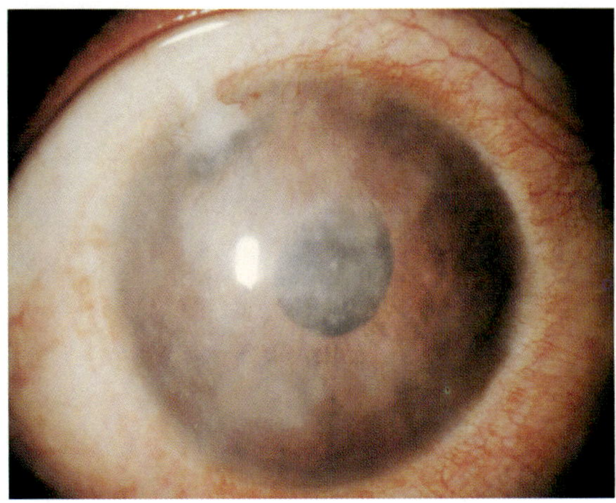

FIGURE 26-160. Quiet interstitial keratitis with corneal scarring.

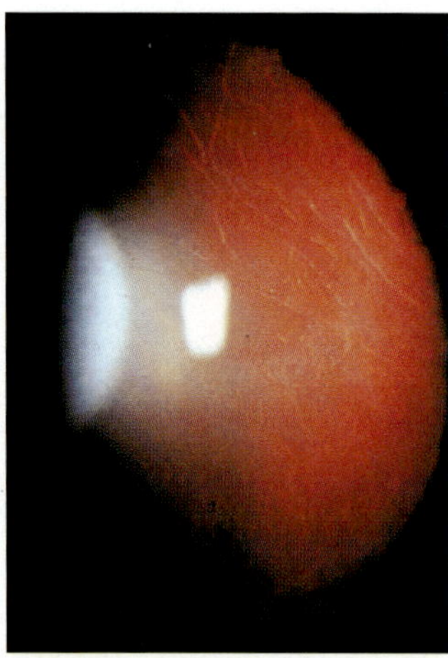

FIGURE 26-161. Deep ghost vessels. (Courtesy of Dr. John Belmont.)

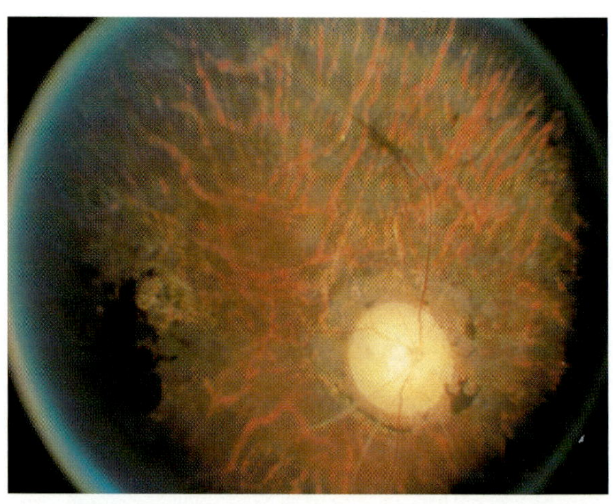

FIGURE 26-162. Optic nerve atrophy in syphilis. (Courtesy of Dr. Michael Hogan.)

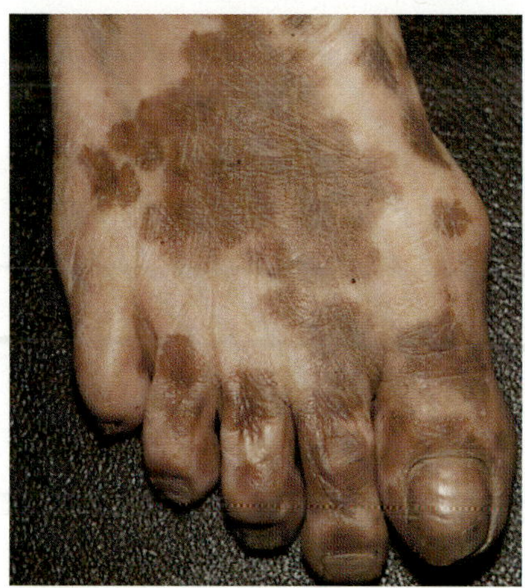

FIGURE 26-163. Hypopigmented skin lesions in pinta. (Courtesy of Dr. Paul Fasal.)

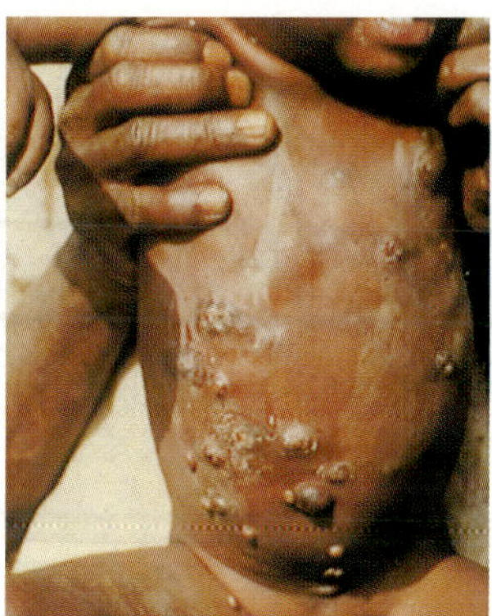

FIGURE 26-164. Skin lesions of secondary yaws in a young boy living in the central Ivory Coast in Africa. The photograph shows multiple warty papillomas over the trunk. (Courtesy of Dr. David Lakes.)

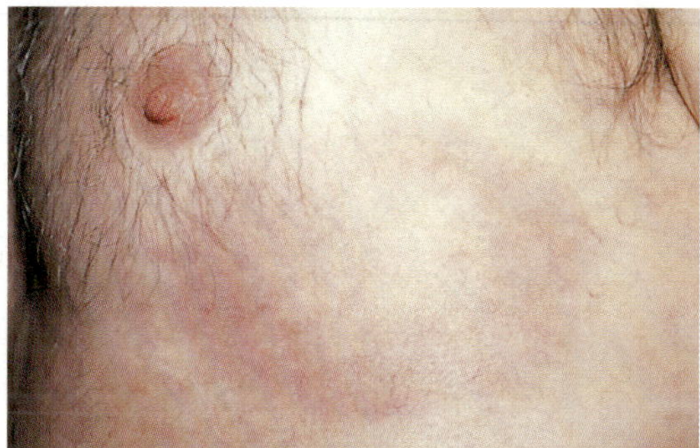

FIGURE 26-165. Erythema chronicum migrans in Lyme disease.

CHLAMYDIAL INFECTIONS

Both lymphogranuloma venereum and psittacosis have skin and ocular features.

LYMPHOGRANULOMA VENEREUM

Lymphogranuloma venereum (LGV) is a sexually transmitted disease caused by the *Chlamydia trachomatis* group of organisms, serotypes L1, L2, L3. Surface antigens allow separation from chlamydia, causing urethritis, cervicitis, trachoma, and inclusion conjunctivitis. The primary lesion, usually anogenital sites, appears several days to weeks after infectious contact. Beginning as a small, painless vesicle or erosion (Fig. 27-1), it is often overlooked and the patient does not seek medical help until several weeks later, when painful regional lymphadenopathy appears, usually accompanied by malaise and fever. The adenopathy is most often unilateral (Fig. 27-2), though bilateral inguinal and femoral nodes may be found (Fig. 27-3). The adenopathy is characteristically quite painful, with matted nodes and periadenitis producing dusky erythema of the overlying and surrounding skin (Fig. 27-3). Adenopathy above and below the inguinal ligament (Poupart ligament) results in the characteristic, though not diagnostic, "groove sign" (Fig. 27-4). Untreated buboes frequently rupture, resulting in draining sinuses (Fig. 27-5). In women, primary lesions of LGV are usually not noticed. Lymphatic drainage mostly leads to pararectal or iliac, rather than inguinal or femoral adenopathy (Fig. 27-6). Thus in women, the diagnosis of LGV is usually not considered until mucopurulent rectal discharge and rectal strictures appear, sometimes requiring colostomy (Fig. 27-7).

Primary rectal infections are more common in the homosexual population, leading to proctitis and strictures. Women may be asymptomatic and shed the organisms from the cervix. In late stages, LGV in women may result in elephantiasis, with ulcerations and scarring of the genitals (esthiomene) (Fig. 27-8). During primary and secondary stages of LGV, one may occasionally see erythema nodosum, erythema multiforme, and photosensitivity.

Ocular Features

A fleshy conjunctival lesion may occur at the superior limbus or as a granulomatous conjunctivitis (Fig. 27-9).

Dacryoadenitis occasionally develops in association with the lid edema and conjunctivitis, and punctal stenosis is often a late sequela of the chronic conjunctivitis. Conjunctivitis may occur by spreading from the genital tract to the eye by way of the fingers. It is manifested by a primary chancre (small nodule or ulcer); an infiltrative, follicular, or granulomatous conjunctivitis (Fig. 27-9); a purulent discharge; and striking bulbar chemosis with minimal or no pain. It usually subsides without sequelae; occasionally, it becomes chronic and persists for years and may lead to lymphatic obstruction and severe persistent lid swelling (elephantiasis). Regional lymphadenopathy develops 2 to 3 days following infection. The nodes are firm, often grossly visible, and occasionally suppurate, producing a draining fistula. The lids, especially the lower lid, become swollen and red with the conjunctivitis, and permanent lid edema may occur.

Corneal involvement includes an epithelial keratitis; small, discrete marginal infiltrates, which may coalesce; corneal ulcers and perforation; a dense pannus and opaque and heavily vascularized cornea with an associated anterior uveitis; and sectorial interstitial keratitis in all layers of the cornea, usually involving the upper corneal quadrants.

The episcleritis and scleritis usually occur near the limbus (Fig. 27-10). The episcleritis and scleritis usually develop from laboratory infections and occur near the limbus. They represent chronic granulomatous reactions and are associated with chronic nongranulomatous iridocyclitis.

Other findings include acute anterior uveitis with hypopyon, retinal hemorrhages, optic neuritis, and papilledema.

PSITTACOSIS

Psittacosis is acquired by contact with infected birds. Ocular infections generally occur from laboratory sources. Fever, chills, headache, backache, malaise, myalgia, epistaxis, sore throat, depression, disorientation, insomnia, dry cough, prostration, and gastrointestinal symptoms often occur during the prodromal period. The fever usually persists 10 to 21 days, then it gradually declines with treatment.

Patients often complain of a mild respiratory infection, and pneumonia, pericarditis, and myocarditis have been observed. Hepatosplenomegaly and icterus may also occur. Nervous system involvement includes polyneuritis, peripheral facial paralysis, unilateral radicular syndrome, paresis of the peripheral nerves, and meningismus.

Skin Features

In the more severe infections, rose spots or a morbilliform eruption are occasionally evident. Erythema nodosum and a few cases of erythema multiforme have been observed.

Ocular Features

A mild to severe follicular conjunctivitis accompanied by a mucopurulent discharge is uncommon. The conjunctivitis is subacute in onset and lasts 3 to 4 months without treatment. It is usually accompanied by a mild preauricular adenopathy.

Other ocular changes include the following:

1. A diffuse epithelial and subepithelial keratitis that accompanies the conjunctivitis.
2. An interstitial keratitis associated with uveitis and otologic and cardiovascular complications.
3. A nonspecific iritis.
4. Macular edema and focal subretinal retinitis.

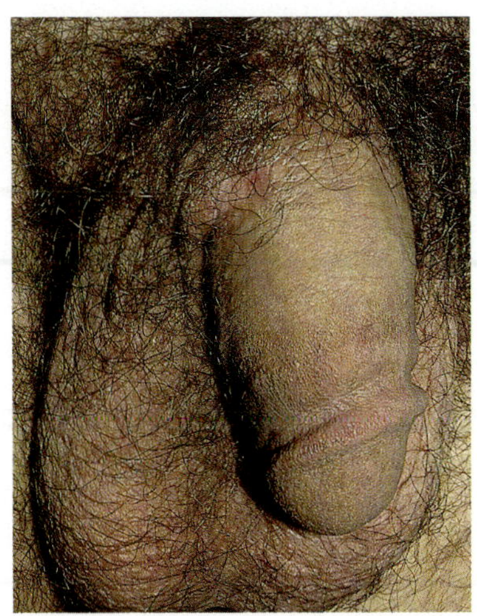

FIGURE 27-1. Lymphogranuloma venereum. Primary lesion is a small, asymptomatic erosion at base of penis. (Patient had used a condom during his extramarital sexual contact.) He later infected his wife (see Fig. 27-6).

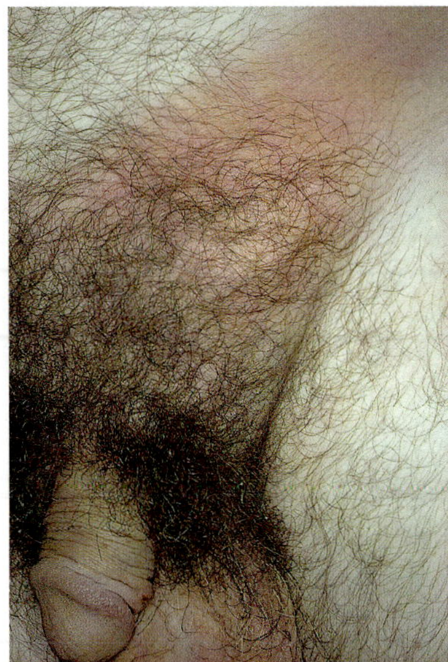

FIGURE 27-2. Lymphogranuloma venereum with resolving primary lesion on the distal shaft of the penis and very painful regional lymphadenopathy and periadenitis.

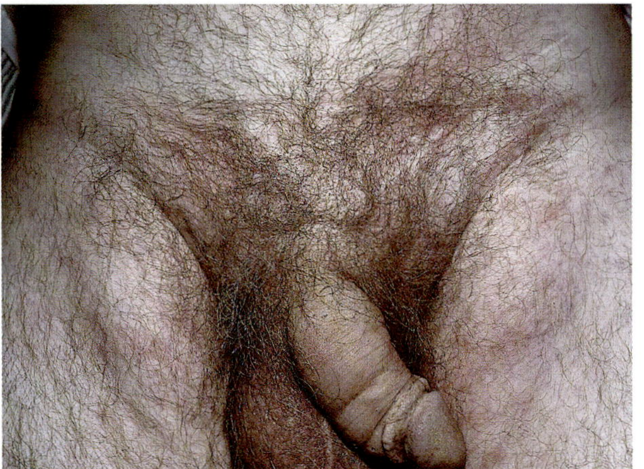

FIGURE 27-3. Lymphogranuloma venereum (LGV) with less commonly seen bilateral inguinal and femoral adenopathy. On palpation, one could feel the chain of matted nodes characteristic of LGV, as is the erythema of overlying skin.

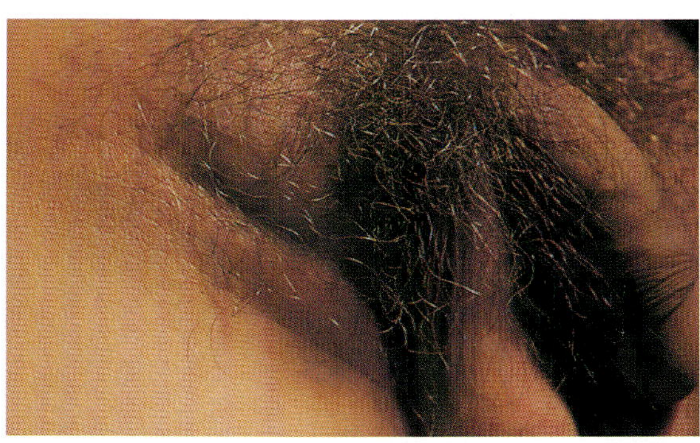

FIGURE 27-4. "Groove sign" characteristic in lymphogranuloma venereum, resulting from adenopathy above and below the inguinal (Poupart) ligament.

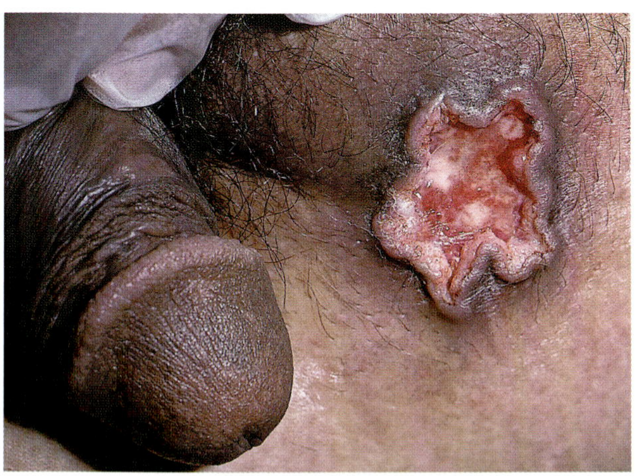

FIGURE 27-5. Buboes of lymphogranuloma venereum (LGV) often rupture. Ruptured bubo in LGV. Note the healed small primary lesion on the foreskin.

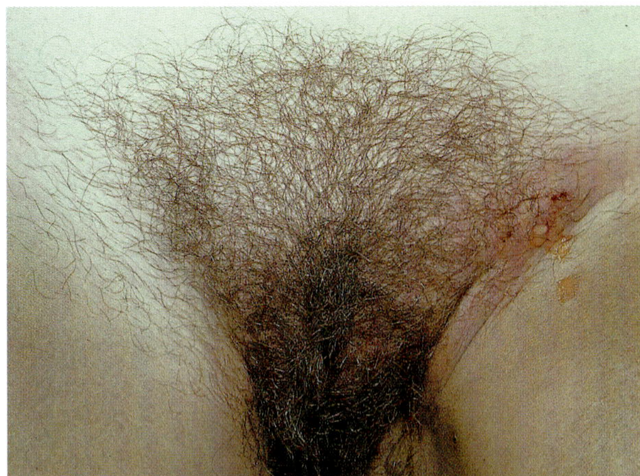

FIGURE 27-6. Ruptured lymphogranuloma venereum (LGV) bubo in wife of patient pictured in Fig. 27-1. Most adenopathy in women with LGV is pararectal, leading to rectal discharge and eventual stricture.

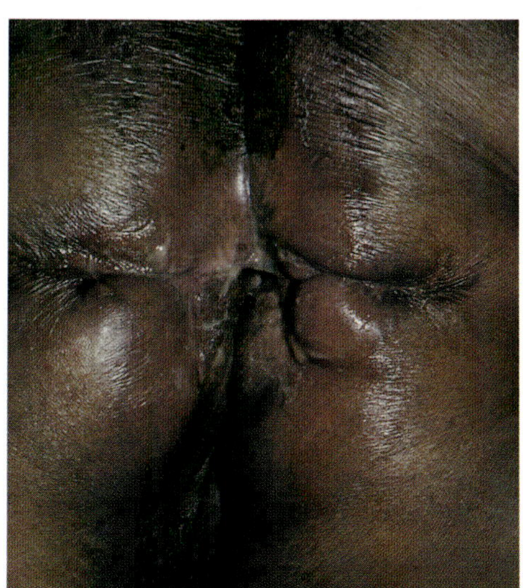

FIGURE 27-7. Rectal stricture as late complication of lymphogranuloma venereum in this elderly woman who required a colostomy.

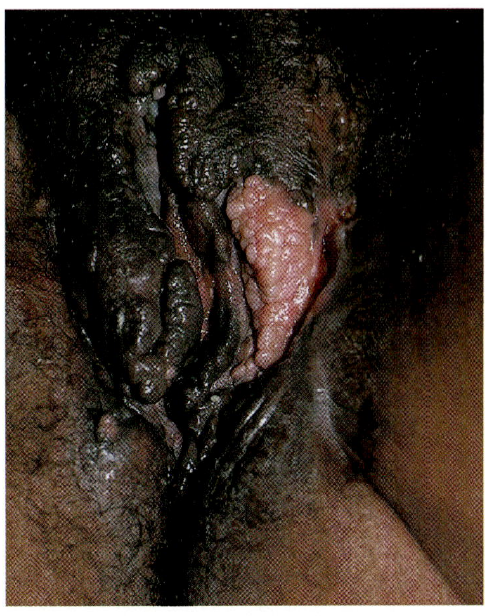

FIGURE 27-8. Esthiomene in lymphogranuloma venereum (edema, scarring, and ulcerations) of genitals in 70-year-old black lady who remembered being told as a teenager that she had "blue balls" (buboes). (Courtesy of Dr. Karl Beutner.)

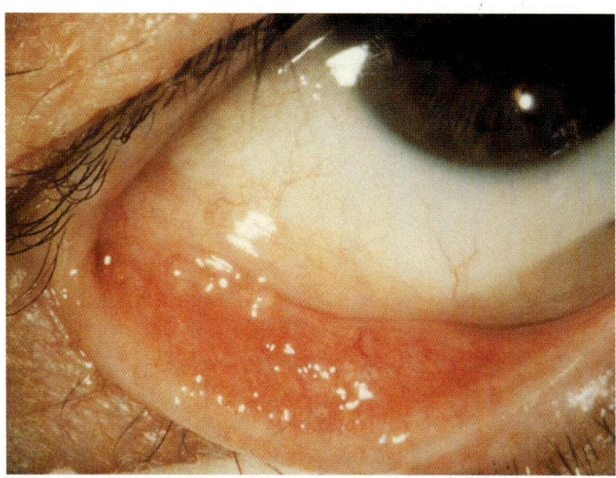

FIGURE 27-9. Granulomatous conjunctivitis of moderate intensity in a 28-year-old male with lymphogranuloma venereum. The patient had an enlarged preauricular lymph node. His granulomas were originally mistaken as follicles.

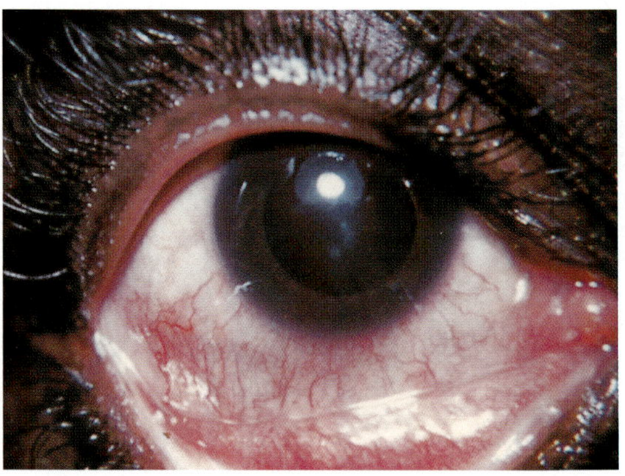

FIGURE 27-10. Sclerokeratitis in lymphogranuloma.

RICKETTSIAL INFECTIONS

Rickettsia often infect endothelial cells, causing vascular infarcts, extravascular fluid loss, and disseminated intravascular coagulation.

EPIDEMIC TYPHUS

Epidemic typhus occurs through the bite of the infected louse or inhalation of louse feces.

Infections are clinical, subclinical, or recurrent (Brill disease). Prodromal symptoms include intractable headache, chills, high fever, prostration, myalgia, delirium, and stupor. The infection and fever last 13 to 16 days before recovery occurs.

The findings include the following:

1. Signs of pulmonary consolidation.
2. Splenomegaly.
3. Renal insufficiency.
4. Meningeal symptoms (almost a constant feature). Stupor and coma often occur late in the illness.
5. A peripheral neuritis of the cutaneous twigs of the femoral and ulnar nerves during the acute stage of the disease.
6. Deafness from 8th cranial nerve involvement.
7. Gangrene of the digits, genitalia, or nose from vascular obstruction.

Skin Features

The face is usually flushed, and about 80% of patients develop a typical skin rash during the fourth to seventh day of illness. At first, the rash is macular but quickly becomes papular. It begins in the axilla, then it spreads to the trunk and extremities. The face, palms, and soles are rarely involved. In severely ill patients, it is often purpuric during the second week of infection and may be accompanied by hypotension.

Ocular Features

Photophobia is common.

Conjunctival hyperemia is a constant feature, and in a few cases there is a mild catarrhal conjunctivitis with mild discharge. In other patients, small, purple colored conjunctival spots and large subconjunctival hemorrhages may be observed at the time of the skin eruption. A few patients have reduced tearing.

Other changes include orbital edema during the acute stage; an anterior or diffuse posterior uveitis; retinal edema, hyperemia, venous thrombosis, hemorrhages and exudates, exudative retinal detachment, retinal pigment epithelial degeneration, Jensen chorioretinitis; and optic neuritis.

BRILL DISEASE

Brill disease represents the recurrent form of infection. It is usually milder and of shorter duration than the classic epidemic typhus. Often there is no rash.

MURINE TYPHUS

Murine typhus is transmitted by the rat flea. Its manifestations are similar but much milder than in epidemic typhus and usually persist 1 to 2 weeks.

ROCKY MOUNTAIN SPOTTED FEVER

Rocky Mountain spotted fever is transmitted by wood ticks, dog ticks, or other hard-shelled ticks. Headache, malaise, anorexia, nausea, and sore throat develop 3 to 10 days following the tick bite. Soon thereafter, chills, fever, myalgia, arthralgia, nausea and vomiting, abdominal pain, restlessness, insomnia, and irritability become manifest. The fever persists 2 to 3 weeks.

The systemic features include cough and pneumonitis, myocarditis, hepatosplenomegaly, uremia, and central nervous system symptoms of delirium, lethargy, stupor, coma, nervousness, irritability, insomnia, hyperreflexia, and deafness. Convulsions occasionally occur in children.

Skin Features

Three to 4 days after onset of infection, a red, macular rash begins at the ankles and wrists, then it spreads centripetally to the legs, arms, trunk, palms, and soles. The maculae increase in size and become petechial in character. There is usually facial flushing. The rash fades and desquamation occurs at about the same time that the fever disappears. In occasional instances, gangrene necessitating amputation has been observed.

Ocular Features

Lid edema and conjunctival congestion occur during the acute phase of the infection. A mild, subacute catarrhal conjunctivitis is a constant finding.

Fundus findings include striate and punctate hemorrhages, cotton-wool exudates, and venous distention during the acute infection. Papilledema occurs if there is central nervous system involvement.

TICK TYPHUS

The various tick typhus infections vary only in the severity of the constitutional symptoms and the extent of the skin eruptions. They are known variously as Boutonneuse fever (Mediterranean fever, Kenya tick typhus, and African and Indian tick typhus); Siberian tick typhus (occurring in Russia and Central Asia); Queensland tick typhus (occurring in Australia); and Flinders Island spotted fever (occurring in Bass Strait, Tasmania). They are characterized by a primary lesion that progresses to an eschar at the site of the tick bite. The lesion is associated with fever and influenza-like symptoms. Later, a generalized maculopapular eruption occurs that, in some instances, becomes purpuric.

Boutonneuse fever is sometimes associated with a severe granulomatous or ulcerative conjunctivitis and a grossly enlarged preauricular node. Uveal and retinal changes include exudative uveitis, retinal edema, central serous retinopathy, perivasculitis with venous and arteriolar occlusions, serous retinal detachment, and papillitis.

RICKETTSIALPOX

Rickettsialpox causes the sudden onset of chills, fever, headache, and disseminated aches and pains. The primary skin lesion develops at the site of the bite of the mite several days before, or at the same time as, the fever. It is a red papule that vesiculates, then it forms a black eschar. A widespread papular eruption develops 2 to 4 days later that quickly becomes vesicular, then crusts.

Photophobia is one of the early manifestations of infection. Frequently, the papular skin rash involves the eyelids and progresses to vesiculation and crusting. The crusts persist for about 10 days.

SCRUB TYPHUS

Scrub typhus is an acute febrile illness that is transmitted by the bite of a mite. At onset, it is characterized by constitutional symptoms of fever, severe headache, dizziness, malaise, and generalized aching and backache. The fever persists 2 to 3 weeks before subsiding with lysis. Splenomegaly is common, and during the third week of infection, a pneumonitis, myocardosis, and cardiac failure may occur.

The initial skin lesion develops at the site of the bite. It is characterized by a papule that progresses to vesiculation and crusting with a black eschar. A macular or maculopapular skin rash may occur but is rare. If the rash develops, it usually occurs on the trunk about the third day, then occasionally spreads to the face and extremities over the next 6 to 7 days, persisting for about 5 days. Discrete, tender, regional, or generalized lymphadenopathy is a constant finding.

Ocular Features

Pain, photophobia, irritation, and tearing often occur at onset of the disease. If the initial lesion occurs on the eyelid, there is severe swelling, edema, and sometimes ecchymosis.

Conjunctival injection occurs in about one-third of patients and accompanies the primary lesion. Occasionally, subconjunctival hemorrhages, considerable chemosis, and moderate conjunctival discharge occur during the acute phase of the illness.

Uveal involvement includes severe iridocyclitis. Neuroretinitis or other retinal changes, such as retinal vascular engorgement, edema, hemorrhages, and exudates, may occur during the tenth to seventeenth day. Vitreous opacities are associated with the retinal changes. Papilledema may be evident.

Q FEVER

Although Q fever has constitutional and ocular features, the skin is not involved. Q fever is a possible cause of bilateral optic neuritis and has been associated with choroidal neovascularization during its course as well.

29

VIRAL INFECTIONS

MOLLUSCUM CONTAGIOSUM

Molluscum contagiosum is caused by a pox virus. Infections are most often seen in children, sexually active adults, and immunocompromised patients.

The lesions present as single (Fig. 29-1) or multiple small, firm, flesh-colored or slightly erythematous, pearly papules with a characteristic central white umbilication. They may become irritated and inflamed, causing confusion with bacterial infections or skin tumors. Sexual transmission is common and may be a clue to other sexually transmitted diseases, for which the patient should be evaluated.

In patients with AIDS, *molluscum contagiosum* may be a fairly early cutaneous marker of immunosuppression. Lesions favor the cheeks (Fig. 29-2) and the eyelids (Fig. 29-3), and are often large, confluent, and atypical, causing confusion with basal cell carcinoma and occasionally cutaneous cryptococcosis or histoplasmosis.

Ocular Features

Conjunctival molluscum nodules present as a nonspecific growth with no associated conjunctivitis or keratitis. The lesion is usually macerated by tears. Molluscum nodules may involve the lid and lid margin (Fig. 29-4). The lid margin nodules are similar to other molluscum nodules and often cause photophobia, tearing, burning, chronic catarrhal or follicular conjunctivitis (Fig. 29-5), superior pannus, and keratitis simulating trachoma. The conjunctivitis involves both the upper and lower palpebral conjunctivae. The keratitis comprises fine, superficial, grouped epithelial erosions and subepithelial and intraepithelial infiltrates that stain only slightly with fluorescein. It is more pronounced superiorly but usually involves the entire cornea.

ORF (ECTHYMA CONTAGIOSUM; CONTAGIOUS PUSTULAR DERMATITIS)

Orf (ecthyma contagiosum; contagious pustular dermatitis) is caused by a parapox virus closely related to the causative agent of milker's nodules, which it can resemble.

Orf causes a pustular dermatitis in sheep and goats. Humans become infected by contact with skin lesions of infected animals or, since the virus is resistant to drying, contaminated objects such as hides and structures on a farm.

Skin Features

Skin lesions are usually solitary but may be multiple. Most often they are seen on the fingers, hands, or occasionally, face. The infection begins as an erythematous papule that develops a white halo, producing a target-like appearance. A hemorrhagic bulla then ensues, eventuating in a thick brownish-black eschar (Fig. 29-6). The lesion heals spontaneously without scarring usually in 6 to 8 weeks. Immunosuppressed patients may develop large, fungating lesions, appearing as pyogenic granulomas or malignant tumors. Erythema multiforme or toxic erythema infrequently occurs 10 to 14 days following onset of the infection.

Ocular Features

Preauricular and submandibular lymphadenopathy usually accompanies both lid and conjunctival lesions. Periocular lesions and lid lesions cause lid edema. The lid lesions usually occur at the medial or lateral canthus (Fig. 29-7) and are similar to other skin lesions causing minimal pain and inflammation. Rarely, lid lesions cause a follicular conjunctivitis.

ERYTHEMA INFECTIOSUM (FIFTH DISEASE)

Erythema infectiosum (fifth disease) is a common viral infection caused by the parvovirus B-19. It is most often seen in childhood and is usually manifested by a characteristic flushlike exanthem on the cheeks, producing a "slapped-check" appearance (Fig. 29-8), hence the common name *slapped cheek disease*. The exanthem may be preceded by prodromal symptoms such as fever, headache, sore throat, coryza, sore eyes, photophobia, abdominal pain, anorexia, joint pains, and pruritus. These symptoms, especially the arthritis, are more frequently found in and are more severe in adults.

A few days after the onset of the slapped cheek appearance, small, discrete erythematous macules and papules appear on the extremities and trunk and soon evolve into a reticulated or lacy pattern (Fig. 29-9) characteristic of this viral exanthem.

In adults, the disease may present with acute arthritis and arthropathy, most commonly of the hands, feet, and knees, often without a rash. Both the rash and the arthralgias are thought to be postinfectious, immune-mediated phenomena. In patients with chronic hemolytic anemia, infection with the B-19 virus can result in transient aplastic crisis. In immunocompromised patients, it can lead to prolonged anemia. Infection during pregnancy, and especially in the third trimester can result in fetal hydrops.

HERPES SIMPLEX INFECTIONS

Of the two antigenic types of herpes simplex virus (HSV), HSV-1 causes most ocular infections, gingivostomatitis, labial lesions, and eczema herpeticum (Kaposi varicelliform eruption). HSV-2 is more often the cause of genital and neonatal infections, and infections below the waist or on the fingers and hands. HSV-2 is usually transmitted sexually. Most HSV infections are localized to the skin and mucous membranes; occasionally, they disseminate.

The infections are primary, latent, or recurrent. The primary infection represents the initial infection, and serum antibodies are formed during this stage. The site of primary infection in infants over the age of 2 is usually the mouth. In the 5- to 14-year-old the primary infection usually occurs on the skin, eye, and occasionally the genitalia, and in the central nervous system. After the age of 14 it occurs most often on the genitalia.

In latent infections, the virus lies dormant in one or more sensory ganglia.

Recurrent infections usually develop at the site of the previous primary lesion. (A nonprimary first-episode infection represents a recurrent infection where HSV lesions occur at a new site.) Recurrent infections are often triggered by fever, sun exposure, trauma, emotional stress, onset of the menstrual period, and sudden extreme temperature changes.

Clinical Features—Primary Infection

The primary infection causes fever, toxicity, regional lymphadenitis or lymphadenopathy, local edema, pain, tenderness, and discomfort. The virus infects the skin, lips, eye, genital tract, upper respiratory tract, or mouth, or it may disseminate to the viscera or brain. Disseminated infection (Kaposi varicelliform eruption) occurs mainly in immunosuppressed and in atopic patients.

Mucous Membrane Features

HSV gingivostomatitis usually causes fever, pain, irritability, general malaise, myalgia, chills, and a sore throat, followed in 1 or 2 days by an oral vesiculo-bullous eruption. The vesicles quickly erode to form small gray-white plaques, which then break down to form an ulcer with elevated, inflamed margins, and a base covered by a yellowish pseudomembrane. They occur in the anterior or posterior oral cavity and on the tongue.

The gums are usually swollen and edematous. The vermilion border of the lips and the glabrous skin about the mouth are commonly affected (Fig. 29-10). There the vesicles usually pustulate, form crusts, and heal without scarring unless secondarily infected. Dysphagia, fetor oris, increased salivation, soreness of the mouth, and diarrhea may occur. The cervical lymph nodes are often tender.

Neonatal Infections

Transplacentally acquired infections are rare occuring primarily in mothers who acquired primary genital herpes during pregnancy. Infections in utero may result in scarring of the skin, microcephaly, encephalitis, intra cerebral calcifications, chorioretinitis, microphthalmos, and permanent neurologic sequelae or death.

A neonatal infection may cause only local lesions of the skin, oral mucosa, eyes, or central nervous system. The skin lesions often occur on the crown of the head in vertex presentations and the perianal area in breech presentations. Sometimes there is a generalized erythematous rash; at other times, there are recurrent clusters of vesicles. Recurrent clusters of vesicles are usually associated with severe disease. Petechial rashes may develop with or without evidence of disseminated intravascular coagulation.

Most disseminated neonatal infections develop when the mother has a primary HSV infection at the time of delivery. Skin and mucous membrane lesions are usually absent. The child usually appears normal at birth, then after 2 or 3 days becomes listless, stops eating, and develops a high fever. The lungs, liver, adrenal glands, gastrointestinal tract, and central nervous system may be involved. Prompt treatment is essential and may prevent death or serious disability.

Meningoencephalitis

HSV-1 is the major cause of meningoencephalitis in children and adults, causing death in about 50% of cases. It occurs in both primary and recurrent infections and is probably unrelated to the patient's humoral immune status. It is clinically indistinguishable from other forms of viral meningoencephalitis.

HSV-2 infections, except in the newborn, are usually benign but sometimes cause recurrent aseptic meningitis without encephalitis; occasionally they cause an ascending myelitis.

Genital Infections

The uterine cervix is the principal site of genital herpes in women. It is usually asymptomatic, and the cervix appears inflamed. Primary vulvar or vaginal infection (Fig. 29-11) usually causes fever, dysuria, leukorrhea, genital soreness, and inguinal lymphadenopathy. (Recurrent vulvar HSV is usually associated with dysuria only.) Vesicles develop at the site of infection and quickly break down to form erosions or ulcers that gradually heal. Occasionally, the primary lesions extend to the perineum, buttocks, and thighs.

Herpes genitalis in the male is manifested by vesicles or ulcers on the glans penis, prepuce, penile shaft, or infrequently, scrotum and adjacent perineum. It is usually associated with fever, dysuria, and tender regional lymphadenopathy.

Skin Features—Primary Infection

Primary HSV skin infections occur in any location and often cause fever, lymphangitis, regional lymphadenopathy, and edema. Usually, only a small area is infected, but sometimes many lesions appear at various sites at about the same time. The lesions are limited to the skin and mucous membranes, and viremia is uncommon in otherwise normal patients.

The lesions begin as small patches of erythema followed by thin-walled vesicles filled with clear fluid, which gradually pustulate, crust, and heal without scarring. (Several grouped vesicles may form a plaque on an erythematous base.)

Features—Disseminated Infections in the Child and Adult

Eczema herpeticum (Kaposi varicelliform eruption) usually occurs during the primary infection but may also occur in recurrent HSV infections. It usually occurs in patients with atopic eczema or other eczematoid diseases (e.g., Wiskott–Aldrich syndrome) and is occasionally associated with Darier disease, congenital ichthyosiform erythroderma, pemphigus, seborrheic dermatitis, impetigo, scabies, sycosis vulgaris, and diaper rash.

The skin lesions are accompanied by malaise, toxicity, and fluctuant or unremitting fever. The lesions begin as 1- to 2-mm round vesicles and are frequently mistaken for worsening of the atopic disease or development of pyoderma. Gradually, the vesicles umbilicate, enlarge peripherally, and pustulate or become hemorrhagic while crops of new lesions develop. Facial skin lesions are painful and accompanied by edema of the skin and subcutaneous tissue, which causes marked facial distortion. Confluent lesions occur in areas of severe eczematoid disease, whereas in pre-

viously normal skin, the lesions are few and are often scattered. A massive generalized lymphadenopathy may be found, and secondary infections are common. After 7 to 10 days the lesions crust and often heal with hypopigmentation and scarring. The virus sometimes disseminates to the visceral organs or central nervous system, where it causes symptoms referable to those sites.

Features—Generalized Herpetic Infections

Generalized herpetic infections occur in immunosuppressed patients (e.g., patients with severe burns, measles, kwashiorkor, Wiskott–Aldrich syndrome). They cause fever, headache, severe malaise, and generalized lymphadenopathy. The skin lesions are often atypical, and although initially vesicular, they may enlarge, coalesce, and ulcerate. Oral lesions are an almost constant feature. The infection usually affects the visceral organs, causing hepatosplenomegaly. Meningoencephalitis may occur, causing meningeal irritation and mental deterioration.

Features—Chronic Cutaneous Infections

Recurrent Infections

Prodromal symptoms are common in recurrent infection and include paresthesia, pain, burning, stinging, and itching. The symptoms are quickly followed by erythema and vesiculation at or near the initial infection site (Fig. 29-12). The vesicles pustulate, crust, and heal without scarring. Skin edema, regional lymphadenopathy, fever, and signs of toxicity do not develop.

Atypical Recurrent HSV Skin Infections

Atypical recurrent infections may cause regional lymphangitis and skin edema. Eczema herpeticum occasionally occurs, and HSV infections may serve as a trigger for erythema multiforme (Fig. 29-13). Characteristics of atypical skin lesions include extensive and deeply destructive very painful lesions (Fig. 29-14), persistent lesions, and lesions that have a dermatomal distribution, such as of the 5th cranial nerve, suggesting herpes zoster (zosteriform herpes simplex).

Herpes Labialis

Herpes labialis may affect the mucocutaneous border of the lip. There is often a 1- or 2-day prodromal period of hyperesthesia and burning followed by vesicles that persist 2 to 10 days. The recurrences may occur at the same or at an adjacent site at any time. Healing occurs without scarring.

Herpes Genitalis

Recurrent genital infections are often triggered by the trauma of sexual relations. Recurrent vulvar infections usu-

in a series of anomalies, including hypoplastic limbs, ocular and central nervous system disorders such as bulbar palsy and Horner's syndrome, and cutaneous scars. A mature cortical cataract, chorioretinitis with subsequent scarring, posterior synechiae, and microphthalmos may be found. Chickenpox is usually severe in the woman, with a significant risk of pneumonia as a complication. If varicella develops within 5 days before to 2 days after delivery, there is a significant risk that the baby will acquire neonatal varicella, which, without treatment, has significant mortality.

In immune-suppressed patients (e.g., persons with AIDS, bone marrow transplant recipients, patients on long-term corticosteroid treatment, or severely malnourished persons), varicella can result in necrotic skin lesions and life-threatening complications, such as pneumonia, hepatitis, or meningoencephalitis (Fig. 29-30).

Ocular Features

Varicella lid and lid margin lesions are not uncommon and are usually associated with edema (Figs. 29-29, 29-31, and 29-32). Trichiasis, entropion, necrosis, and lid gangrene are occasional sequelae.

Varicella often causes a mild catarrhal conjunctivitis with watery discharge. Follicles may also occur.

Individual pock lesions associated with a small subconjunctival hemorrhage and resembling conjunctival phlyctenules sometimes occur on the bulbar conjunctiva, semilunar fold, or limbus. They often ulcerate and are associated with a mucopurulent discharge.

Limbal pocks cause superficial marginal infiltration and stromal vascularization. They often resemble corneal phlyctenules and begin at, or shortly after, onset of the skin rash. They resolve rapidly, with little or no scarring.

The corneal sensation is markedly reduced or absent in varicella keratitis. Corneal findings include pseudodendrites; vesicular corneal epithelial lesions; superficial round, focal, peripheral corneal infiltrates; a disciform keratitis; interstitial keratitis; and a shallow, round corneal ulcer with underlying infiltrates.

Uveal tract involvement may occur before, during, or more commonly, after the skin eruption disappears. It includes a mild, nongranulomatous iritis or iridocyclitis, a severe recurrent and granulomatous iridocyclitis, a focal area of chorioretinitis, and neuroretinitis.

Retinal involvement includes diffuse retinitis, exudative retinitis, hemorrhagic retinopathy, and periphlebitis.

In rare instances, there is optic neuritis or papilledema.

Other ocular findings include secondary glaucoma, external and internal ophthalmoplegia, and phthisis bulbi.

Congenital Varicella Syndrome

Congenital malformations are uncommon but may occur when varicella is contracted during the first or second trimester of pregnancy. The child is usually born with a low birth weight and often has learning difficulties, bulbar palsy, and Horner syndrome. More than two-thirds of the children die during infancy.

Cicatricial skin lesions in a dermatomal distribution may be seen, and about 80% of infants have atrophic limbs.

A mature cortical cataract, chorioretinitis with subsequent scarring, posterior synechiae, and microphthalmos may be found.

Herpes Zoster (Shingles)

Herpes zoster (shingles) represents reactivation of the varicella-zoster virus. The incidence of zoster increases with advancing age from 2.5 per 1,000 in the 20- to 50-year-old group to 5 per 1,000 in those 51 to 79 years of age, and 10 per 1,000 in those beyond the age of 80. Immunosuppression dramatically increases the incidence of zoster.

Clinically, in most patients, predrome of intense pain in the involved dermatome precedes by a few days the cutaneous manifestations. The pain may be burning, sharp, lancinating, intermittent, or continuous with paresthesia and dysesthesia. Pruritus is sometimes present, especially in younger patients in whom pain may be minimal or absent. When the cranial nerves are affected, intense headache and sometimes meningeal symptoms may be evident.

Skin and Mucous Membrane Features

Herpes zoster classically appears in a unilateral dermatomal pattern within a spinal sensory or cranial nerve, with some overflow into the adjacent nerves. The dermatomes most frequently affected are the thoracic (55%); the cranial (20%), especially the trigeminal (Fig. 29-33); the lumbar (15%); and the sacral (5%). The eruption may begin as a single painful lesion often mistaken both by the patient and the physician as an insect or spider bite (Fig. 29-34). More often, grouped herpetiform vesicles on an erythematous base are seen (Fig. 29-35). In more severe cases, the vesicles may become confluent, pustular, and necrotic (Figs. 29-36 and 29-37). In immunocompromised patients, zoster is far more frequent and severe. About 20% of patients with Hodgkin disease develop zoster, usually late in the course of their disease. Lesions in these patients are severe and often show widespread varicella-like hemorrhagic eruptions (disseminated zoster) (Fig. 29-38). Zoster, usually severe, may be an early cutaneous sign of AIDS. It occurs 30 times more frequently in those with AIDS than in those with normal immunity.

Zoster is infrequent in young children (Fig. 29-39); when it occurs in day care or kindergarten, it often leads to many cases of chickenpox in unvaccinated playmates.

Zoster in pregnancy, unlike varicella, rarely poses problems for the fetus.

Ramsey Hunt Syndrome

The Ramsey Hunt syndrome is the result of herpes zoster involvement of the geniculate ganglion. The facial and auditory nerves on one side become inflamed, leading to motor and auditory signs and symptoms. Initially, there may be mild to severe tinnitus, decreased hearing, vertigo, and occasionally nausea, vomiting, and nystagmus. Zoster lesions may be found on the external ear (Fig. 29-40) or tympanic membrane, accompanied by ipsilateral facial paralysis (Fig. 29-41).

Less common sites of herpes zoster include the palm and arm (C7–C8) and sacral nerves resulting in unilateral anogenital lesions.

Central Nervous System Features

Central nervous system features include neck stiffness and a positive Kernig sign during the prodromal phase, 7th cranial nerve paralysis, parasympathetic and sympathetic nerve palsies, contralateral hemiplegia, mononeuritis affecting the lower motor neurons of either the cranial or spinal nerves, myelitis, meningoencephalitis, and hemiplegia.

Ocular Features

Nasociliary or lacrimal branch involvement of the trigeminal nerve usually leads to ocular involvement (Fig. 29-42.)

Ocular features include: lid edema, ptosis, lash loss, scarring, trichiasis, entropion, ectropion, and lid necrosis. The conjunctivitis is usually papillary, occasionally follicular, or, rarely, pseudomembranous or membranous. Petechial subconjunctival hemorrhages may occur.

Cornea

The corneal findings in herpes zoster include epithelial keratitis, pseudodendrites, corneal neovascularization; disciform keratitis, which may lead to scarring; absent corneal sensation; an immune ring, which surrounds the disciform lesion; round, 1- to 2-mm nummular opacities at various levels in the stroma; interstitial keratitis characterized by deep corneal vessels and prominent Descemet folds; and lipoidal, amyloid, or calcium deposition (Figs. 29-43 and 29-44). Mucous plaque keratitis is also a common finding in patients with chronic corneal inflammation secondary to varicella-zoster virus.

Herpes zoster may cause dacryoadenitis or canaliculitis that may lead to puncta or canalicular occlusion.

Sclera

Scleral and episcleral features of herpes zoster include diffuse or nodular episcleritis or scleritis (Fig. 29-45). The scleritis often develops several months after the skin eruption and may be associated with iridocyclitis. It is usually painful, and relapses are common; new nodules may occur with relapses, and scleral thinning becomes evident after healing occurs. Rarely, it leads to an intercalary staphyloma or perforation.

Uveal tract involvement includes mild or, rarely, severe nongranulomatous or granulomatous iridocyclitis; focal or sector-like areas of iris atrophy or heterochromia; a plastic form of iritis with pain, keratic precipitates, and a tendency to form synechiae; and focal chorioretinitis. Herpes zoster sine eruptium (without skin eruption) may present as profound iridoplegic granulomatous iridocyclitis with high intraocular pressure. Retinal involvement with herpes zoster may also occur without skin eruptions.

Retina

Herpes zoster may lead to vitreitis, retinal vasculitis, and vascular occlusion (Fig. 29-46). Other retinal findings include nonrhegmatogenous detachment, hemorrhages, periphlebitis, central retinal artery and vein occlusion, cotton-wool patches, necrotizing retinitis, and fulminant acute retinal necrosis. The latter is characterized by peripheral to midperipheral pale yellow exudates extending for 360 degrees, vitreous opacities, and anterior uveitis. The exudates often become confluent and lead to retinal detachment. Rarely, the exudates remain isolated.

Other Ocular Findings

Other ocular findings include retrobulbar involvement with proptosis and ophthalmoplegia, neuroophthalmic findings, cataracts, secondary glaucoma, and phthisis bulbi, although the latter is uncommon following herpes zoster ophthalmicus.

Neuroophthalmic findings include blindness from optic neuritis or retrobulbar neuritis; extraocular muscle paralysis from involvement of the 3rd, 4th, or 6th cranial nerves; ipsilateral 7th cranial nerve involvement; contralateral hemiplegia; pupillary abnormalities (Horner syndrome, Argyll Robertson pupil, Adie pupil, and paralytic mydriasis); and loss of accommodation.

Variola (Smallpox)

In 1967 the World Health Organization (WHO) began a campaign to eradicate smallpox. By 1980 the World Health Assembly declared the world free of smallpox. The last endemic case of smallpox occurred in Somalia in 1977, and by 1984 all countries had ceased vaccination of the general public.

With the recent growing threat of bioterrorism, smallpox has become a potentially dangerous agent because most of the world's population is not immune to this infection, no effective treatment is available, the attack rate is 25% to 40%, and the fatality rate is 30%.

There are four clinical types of smallpox: variola major (the severe form), modified (by previous vaccination), variola minor (alastrim), and hemorrhagic.

The incubation period averages 12 days, after which there is sudden onset of fever and malaise, followed in 2 to 4 days by the appearance of the exanthem. The rash typically favors the face and extremities more than the trunk

(Figs. 29-47 and 29-48). The lesions evolve from erythematous macules to papules, vesicles, and pustules, which become umbilicated and crusted (Figs. 29-49 and 29-50). Smallpox lesions are all at the same stage, whereas in chickenpox multiple crops produce lesions at varying stages. Also, in smallpox, lesions favor the extremities, especially the palms (Fig. 29-51) and soles (Fig. 29-52).

Complications of smallpox include secondary bacterial infections of skin lesions, pneumonia, encephalitis, osteitis, joint effusions, and frequent corneal destruction resulting in blindness (Fig. 29-53).

Ocular Features

An active case of smallpox has not been seen in the world in more than 20 years. Hence these descriptions are limited to historical information. The potential for variola as an agent of bioterrorism raises the possibility for additional outbreaks of this disease; hence the clinical findings are included.

Ocular involvement follows the exanthem by about 4 or 5 days. This may present as a simple, self-limited conjunctivitis. Hemorrhagic or even purulent conjunctivitis with bacterial superinfection may occur. Phlyctena-like lesions may present on the bulbar or tarsal conjunctiva and follow shortly thereafter with subsequent necrosis. These lesions are painful, with a marked reaction and discharge. Corneal involvement may occur with a poxlike lesion, as mentioned earlier with frank keratitis. The superficial ulceration may develop necrosis and eventual scarring. Interstitial and disciform keratitis have also been reported. If the cornea is not involved, the prognosis is generally good, but corneal involvement may lead to blindness. Dense corneal leucomata and even phthisis have been seen following corneal involvement. In the nineteenth century, smallpox was believed to be the cause of 25% of the total blindness in some countries.

Vaccinia

Vaccinia virus used for smallpox vaccination can cause serious local (Fig. 29-54) as well as disseminated reactions in patients with impaired immunity and occasionally in immunocompetent persons (Fig. 29-55). Eczema vaccinatum represents vaccinia virus infection superimposed on previous eczematous skin lesions in atopic individuals (Fig. 29-56). Lesions can resemble those seen in smallpox (Fig. 29-57) and may be accompanied by fever, prostration, encephalitis and result in ocular paralysis, postvaccinial retinitis, and, rarely, death. Vaccinial roseola is a transient, generalized, morbilliform exanthem that occasionally appears 2 weeks after vaccination.

Vaccinia necrosum is rare, occurring mostly in infants less than 6 months old who are immunocompromised (Fig. 29-58).

Ocular Features

Vaccinia infection of the eyelid, conjunctiva, or cornea following immunization for smallpox has recently been seen following the vaccinations of the military, first responders and health care personnel. Ocular infections can occur because of contamination after contact with the vaccination vesicle of another person, or inadvertent self-inoculation. Clinically, these infections can resemble other microbial agents, such as herpes simplex, varicella zoster, or even molluscum contagiosum. Inoculation of the eyelid may produce a remarkable acute blepharoconjunctivitis with vesicles that progress to pustules. This may have the appearance of an orbital cellulitis. Conjunctival involvement may be nonspecific conjunctivitis or may produce an ulcerative indurated lesion. Corneal involvement may be mild or lead to more serious problems, such as stromal keratitis with keratouveitis. Disciform or necrotizing stromal keratitis even with eventual perforation has been reported. Immunocompetent individuals have a self-limited and benign course with a good prognosis. Immunoincompetent individuals such as those with HIV or even with atopic dermatitis may have a risk of more severe and prolonged disease.

CYTOMEGALOVIRUS INFECTIONS

Cytomegalovirus (CMV) infections in newborn infants and other immunosuppressed patients (especially those with AIDS) cause colitis, meningitis, hepatitis, and sight-threatening retinitis; not infrequently, infected fetuses are stillborn or grossly abnormal. The viral infection persists for life, and periodic viral shedding may occur during periods of stress (e.g., pregnancy) or other causes of immunosuppression.

Infants are infected *in utero*, during the birth process, or from exposure to the virus in infected breast milk. Oral secretions and urine are important sources of infection in toddlers. Sexual transmission, blood transfusions, and organ donors are important sources in older patients.

Clinical Features

Most infected infants are asymptomatic; others are premature or have growth retardation, microcephaly, periventricular calcification, encephalitis, hydrocephalus, decreased hearing, or hepatosplenomegaly.

In the acute acquired infection, symptomatic CMV may cause an infectious mononucleosis-like syndrome with fever, malaise, muscle and joint pains, generalized lymphadenopathy, and hepatomegaly. In other patients, it may cause severe progressive opportunistic pneumonia; it sometimes causes immunosuppression itself, which allows other infections such as *Pneumocystis carinii* to occur.

Skin Features

Infected newborn infants may exhibit jaundice, thrombo-cytopenic purpura, or purple or red papules or nodules ("blueberry muffin" lesions). The latter are caused by development of erythropoietic tissue in the dermis.

The skin eruption in the infectious mononucleosis-like syndrome affects the legs and is follicular, maculopapular, rubelliform, or urticarial. Sometimes the rash is triggered by ampicillin.

CMV vasculitis causes a widespread papular, purpuric, or vesiculobullous eruption or indurated pigmented nodules or plaques. Sharply demarcated ulcers may develop around the genitalia, perineum, buttocks, and thighs.

Ocular Features

Ocular disease is more common in newborn infants with severe cerebral involvement and may cause microphthalmia. Diffuse corneal opacities, keratomalacia, and perforating corneal ulcers with hypopyon occasionally develop in moribund infants. The eye may be involved without systemic signs.

CMV conjunctivitis is usually an acute bilateral membranous conjunctivitis with severe lid edema or, occasionally, mild follicular conjunctivitis. AIDS patients may develop keratoconjunctivitis sicca as a result of CMV dacryoadenitis.

About 25% of CMV-infected infants develop focal retinochoroiditis of the posterior pole or peripheral retina and a hazy vitreous. The lesions appear white and heal with a gliotic scar and retinal pigment epithelial disturbances suggestive of secondary retinitis pigmentosa. Infrequently, they lead to total retinal necrosis.

Adult CMV retinal infection may cause bilateral visual loss (Fig. 29-59). Perivasculitis and exudative retinitis (white fluffy areas of retinal necrosis) develop along the vascular arcades and resemble a brush fire because of cell-to-cell viral spread. Within months obliteration of the retinal architecture occurs and retinal pigment epithelium mottling and atrophic scars form. Other findings include venous and arterial occlusions, retinal aneurysms, retinal detachment, hazy vitreous, and hyaloid precipitates.

Infectious Mononucleosis

Infectious mononucleosis is caused by the Epstein–Barr virus. It is transmitted through saliva and occasionally through blood transfusions. In Western countries it is more common in patients between the ages of 15 and 25.

Clinical Features

Initially, the patient develops exudative pharyngitis with inflammation, edema, and a gray-white exudate of the tonsillar region. Petechiae often develop at the junction of the hard and soft palate (Fig. 29-60) after the first week of illness.

The anterior and posterior cervical lymph nodes are tender and discretely enlarged. Hepatomegaly and splenomegaly may occur. Chest pain, dyspnea, cough, tachycardia, arrhythmias, and hepatitis sometimes occur. Central nervous system involvement may cause headache, stiff neck, photophobia, neuralgia, acute cerebellar ataxia, and Guillain–Barré syndrome.

Skin Features

Infectious mononucleosis causes a morbilliform (maculopapular or petechial) or a scarlatiniform rash of the trunk, upper arms, and occasionally, face, forearms, thighs, and legs, especially following the use of ampicillin (Fig. 29-61). Urticaria and thrombocytopenic purpura are uncommon.

Ocular Features

Hoglund sign, which is bilateral supraorbital and lid edema, develops early. Burning and photophobia sometimes occur and are caused by conjunctivitis or uveitis.

Conjunctival injection is occasionally the presenting sign of infection and may be associated with conjunctival chemosis and subconjunctival hemorrhages. An infiltrative, follicular, pseudomembranous, membranous, or granulomatous conjunctivitis, which is often unilateral, may occur. It is self limited and clears spontaneously but may be associated with a large preauricular node.

The conjunctivitis may cause lid edema and a large preauricular lymph node (Fig. 29-62).

Keratitis is uncommon. It begins as a sectorial epithelial keratitis and eventually involves the stroma. It causes neovascularization, multiple epithelial microdendrites, a disciform keratitis, or a nummular keratitis. The nummular lesions are located in the peripheral superficial stroma and appear as discrete, sharply demarcated, pleomorphic, or ring-shaped granular opacities with normal intervening stroma or as blotchy, soft, pleomorphic multifocal infiltrates.

Other ocular findings include the following:

1. Nodular episcleritis, diffuse scleritis, and icterus.
2. Acute dacryoadenitis; acute dacryocystitis.
3. Mild or acute bilateral iridocyclitis.
4. Retinal edema, preretinal hemorrhages, and venous thrombosis.
5. Nystagmus, hippus, conjugate gaze paralysis, isolated 3rd nerve palsies, ptosis, facial diplegia and monoplegia, scotomata and hemianopia, papillitis, optic neuritis, and papilledema.

Verrucae

Verrucae are common warty elevations that occur anywhere on the skin and mucous membranes. They are uncommon in infants, become frequent from ages 12 to 16, then they gradually become less frequent. They often spontaneously resolve, but recurrences are frequent.

Skin Features

Verrucae usually cause no symptoms and are classified by their size, shape, and location.

Verruca vulgaris is a painless, firm papule with a rough, horny surface. It is usually 0.5 cm or less in diameter but may be large because of confluence. Most occur on the hands (Fig. 29-63), fingers, and knees in children but may be found anywhere on the skin, including the genitalia (Fig. 29-64) and periungually (Fig. 29-65). They usually resolve spontaneously within 2 years.

Plantar warts (Fig. 29-66) begin as small, shining papules and quickly develop a rough, keratotic surface surrounded by a smooth, keratinous ring. They are sometimes painful and are usually flat but may have finger-like projections.

Plane (flat) warts are smooth, flat, occasionally slightly elevated, skin-colored or grayish-yellow growths that usually involve the forehead (Fig. 29-67), back of the hands, or shins. They often occur in linear patterns as a result of inoculating the virus following minor injury or scratches.

Filiform or digitate warts are common on the face (Fig. 29-68). When they occur on the bearded area in men or axilla or legs in women, shaving must be temporarily avoided to prevent spreading the lesions while undergoing treatment.

Condyloma acuminata usually occur on moist surfaces, such as the angle of the lips (Fig. 29-69) and the anogenital region (Fig. 29-70). They may be asymptomatic or sometimes cause bleeding, discharge, and discomfort. They appear as pink, fleshy, lobulated, or pedunculated masses. They usually resolve spontaneously after many years, but recurrences occur in about one-fourth of cases. They may undergo malignant changes, especially in immunocompromised individuals.

Butchers' warts often occur on the hands of meat, poultry, and fish handlers, and are usually larger than other warts.

Verrucae sometimes involve the mucous membranes (Fig. 29-71). Laryngeal papillomatosis, presenting as recurrent hoarseness, may occur in children born to mothers with genital condylomata. Carcinoma develops in 10% to 15% of these patients and may be fatal.

Epidermodysplasia Verruciformis

Epidermodysplasia verruciformis (EV) is a rare, inherited disorder characterized by extensive verrucae that begin in childhood and continue throughout the patient's life. Squamous cell carcinoma may develop in one-third to two-thirds of these persons, especially when the warts are on sun-exposed sites. Clinically, the lesions are flatter than the typical warts and may become confluent (Fig. 29-72).

Ocular Features

Lid verrucae are often multiple. They may be flat, digitate (Fig. 29-73), or filiform in type and occur between the eyelashes or on the skin of the eyelid proper. Filiform warts usually involve the face and neck, and often occur in clusters. Condyloma acuminata are uncommon on the lid. The lesions are similar to those of the skin.

Lid margin verruca may produce a chronic, low-grade, papillary conjunctivitis with minimal or no discharge. Occasionally, they cause a fine, grouped punctate epithelial keratitis that is sometimes associated with the conjunctivitis.

The keratitis is usually located in the sector nearest the lid lesion and causes irritation, pain, and photophobia. In severe, long-standing cases, a superficial wedge-shaped pattern of neovascularization may also develop.

Conjunctival verrucae (Figs. 29-74 and 29-75) are usually located on the bulbar conjunctiva near the lower fornix. They are pedunculated; have delicate, frondlike processes; or are pedunculated with a cauliflower-like appearance. The lesions may cause a foreign body sensation.

Measles (Rubeola)

Rubeola is highly infectious. In the setting of a refugee camp, it is a major cause of morbidity and mortality. Infection occurs through aerosolized droplets reaching the conjunctiva or mucous membrane of the upper respiratory tract.

Clinical Features

Measles is manifested by malaise, fever, cough, coryza, periorbital edema, conjunctivitis, and photophobia. The fever is usually moderate to marked; the cough may be severe but is generally nonproductive; the malaise and fever usually subside as the rash develops.

Pathognomonic Koplik spots develop on the conjunctiva and buccal mucosa within 2 to 3 days of onset of symptoms. They appear as bluish, white specks on an erythematous base.

Measles encephalopathy, acute retinitis, pneumonia, myocarditis, keratitis, and death commonly occur in immunosuppressed (especially malnourished) patients.

Skin Features

Typically, the macular rash of measles begins at the hairline, then over the next 2 to 3 days spreads to the face, trunk, and extremities (Fig. 29-76). It often becomes confluent on the face and areas above the shoulders. After 4 to 6 days, the rash subsides, disappearing first from the head. Desquamation may or may not occur.

Ocular Features

Photophobia and lid edema are common. The rash often involves the lids, and the lesions may coalesce.

An acute catarrhal conjunctivitis with hyperemia and mucoid discharge is quite common. Koplik spots occur on the conjunctiva and resemble specks of sand surrounded by a red areola. Hirschberg's sign (Koplik's spots on the caruncle and semilunar fold) may also occur.

Most patients develop a superficial, fine, epithelial keratitis consisting of fine gray or white epithelial dots grouped into larger lesions (Fig. 29-77). The keratitis clears spontaneously, leaving no permanent visual loss. In immunosuppressed patients, especially in patients with hypovitaminosis A with or without kwashiorkor, the epithelial keratitis is usually severe and may progress to keratomalacia, perforation, and blindness.

Other ocular findings include keratoconjunctivitis sicca, chorioretinitis, central retinal vein occlusion, isolated extraocular muscle paralysis, and optic nerve involvement.

German Measles (Rubella)

Postnatal Rubella Infection

Rubella is an acute, mild, moderately contagious viral infection. There is no geographic or racial preponderance of the disease, although a mild rash may be missed in darker-pigmented skin.

Rubella infection of a pregnant woman may cause a severe generalized and persistent fetal infection with severe sequelae. Abnormalities occur by the fourth year of life in about 85% of fetuses infected before the fourth week of gestation. Infants infected during the ninth to twelfth week of gestation have defects about 50% of the time. Infection during the thirteenth to the twentieth week causes defects in about 16% of infants. Occasionally, defects occur in infants infected as late as the seventh lunar month of pregnancy.

Clinical Features—Postnatal Infection

Characteristically, there are small, shotty, and occasionally, tender postoccipital, postauricular, and cervical lymphadenopathy during the incubation period. Sometimes mild, generalized lymphadenopathy and splenomegaly occur.

Mild malaise, low-grade fever, headache, anorexia, conjunctivitis, and mild respiratory symptoms usually develop before the skin rash in older children and adults. About one-fourth of adults develop polyarthritis. The prodromal symptoms, except for fever, disappear at the onset of the rash. The fever usually persists until the exanthema fades.

Skin Features

The eruption is characterized by a discrete, fine, pink, macular, papular, scarlatiniform, and rarely, petechial or acne-form rash, or a transient erythematous flush that begins on the face and neck, then spreads (usually within a day) to the trunk and extremities. Occasionally, the rash is biphasic and accompanied by pruritus. It persists for about a day in each involved area, evolving and disappearing by the third or, occasionally, fourth or fifth day. It fades in the order in which it develops. On the second day, the rash on the trunk may be almost confluent. In severe infections the rash fades with a fine, branny desquamation.

Forchheimer spots develop before or at the time of the skin rash in about 20% of patients. They are confined to the soft palate and appear as small erythematous macules or petechiae but are not distinctive for rubella.

Ocular Features

A mild acute catarrhal conjunctivitis or occasionally a follicular conjunctivitis may develop 2 to 3 days before the skin eruption. It is usually self-limited and lasts for only a few days. Often the conjunctivitis is associated with a fine, grouped epithelial keratitis.

The ocular manifestations associated with postnatal rubella meningoencephalitis include irregular pupils, oculomotor palsies of supranuclear or nuclear origin, and papilledema.

Congenital Rubella Syndrome

Clinical Features

The rubella virus infects virtually any fetal organ during the first 4 months of pregnancy. It causes absorption of conceptual products, abortion, stillbirth, intrauterine and extrauterine growth retardation, and severe multiple birth defects. The triad of congenital heart defects, deafness, and cataracts are usually evident at birth.

The hearing loss may be sensorineural, arising from damage to the organ of Corti, or peripheral, arising from otitis media. It varies from mild to severe, is permanent, is frequently progressive, and may be bilateral.

Congenital heart disease is the leading cause of death in congenital rubella. The defects usually involve the pulmonary arterial system and the aorta. Myocarditis may also occur in these infants.

Musculoskeletal abnormalities usually arise from chronic disturbance of the blood supply, from specific cellular dysfunction, or from immunologic deficiencies. Micrognathia, metaphyseal rarefaction of the long bones, a high-arched palate, talipes equinovarus, depressed sternum, pes cavus, elfin facies, clinodactyly, brachydactyly, syndactyly, myositis, and dental abnormalities may be observed.

Central nervous system abnormalities include microcephaly, calcification of the brain, bulging fontanels, anencephaly, encephalocele, meningomyelocele, spastic quadriparesis, active encephalitis or extensive meningoencephalitis, chronic progressive panencephalitis, and psychomotor abnormalities.

Gastrointestinal abnormalities include cleft palate, esophageal atresia, tracheoesophageal fistula, indirect inguinal hernia, giant cell and cholangiolitic hepatitis, and diarrhea.

The genitourinary abnormalities include cryptorchidism; hypospadias; interstitial nephritis; polycystic kidney; bilobed kidney with reduplication of the ureter, hydroureter, and hydronephrosis; renal artery stenosis and hypertension; and unilateral agenesis of the kidney.

Other clinical features include acute, subacute, or chronic interstitial pneumonia that may be progressive.

Immunologic dyscrasias, although rare, may occur but are usually masked by maternal immunoglobulins in the early months of life. Both depressed humoral and cellular immunity may also occur.

Skin Features

A maculopapular rash ("blueberry muffin" lesions) is usually present at birth or occurs within 2 days. It may involve the face, scalp, back of the neck, and trunk, and persists for several weeks before fading. The lesions represent foci of dermal erythropoiesis. Other skin changes include abnormal dermatoglyphics, cutis marmorata (a reticular blue vascular pattern), skin dimples over the bony prominences (especially the patellae), seborrhea, and hyperpigmentation of the forehead, cheeks, and umbilical area.

Ocular Features

More than 50% of infants with congenital rubella have ocular stigmata. The most common are microphthalmia (>40%) and cataracts (>40%) (Fig. 29-78). The congenital cataracts are usually evident at birth and may be nuclear or cortical in type; the Y-sutures are often distinctly visible. The abnormalities are usually bilateral. Microphthalmos and cataracts often occur together.

In many instances, moderate papillary conjunctivitis is present and is associated with corneal involvement at birth. Corneal clouding is sometimes present at birth and is usually more dense centrally; it gradually clears after a few weeks.

Fundus changes are common and are frequently progressive (Fig. 29-79). The fundus has a mottled appearance with black spots of varying magnitude. The pigment is aggregated into small, round, irregular, or in some instances, filiform masses of black or leaden-gray color and is most pronounced in the macular region. In the periphery, the lesions are more diffuse and less pronounced. The pigmented lesions are rarely larger than the diameter of the retinal vessels, which appear normal. The retinal changes usually do not affect vision, but subretinal neovascularization and hemorrhage or a disciform scar with significant loss of central vision has been reported. A coloboma of the retina has also been observed.

Other ocular findings include the following:

1. Dacryoadenitis and nasolacrimal duct obstruction.
2. Iris hypoplasia, incomplete iris coloboma, a small pupil that is hard to dilate, and nongranulomatous iritis.
3. Bilateral glaucoma.
4. Searching nystagmus, convergent alternating strabismus, and optic atrophy.

Yellow Fever

Yellow fever is a mosquito-borne viral infection that predominantly involves the liver. The principal skin and eye manifestations are jaundice and icterus.

Dengue Fever

Dengue fever is transmitted by the bite of the Aedes mosquito. It is often called breakbone fever because of the severe aching that occurs.

Clinical Features

The clinical features include the following:

1. Symptoms of chilliness, high fever, severe frontal headache, backache, and aching of the extremities. The fever has a saddle-back character.
2. Prostration, depression, and occasionally, meningeal irritation.
3. Nausea and vomiting in children, pharyngitis, and gastrointestinal hemorrhages in Southeast Asian patients.
4. Palsies of the 7th cranial nerve (Bell palsy), long thoracic nerve, peroneal nerve, and ulnar nerve; palatal paralysis; and sciatic neuritis.

Skin Features

Flushing or blotching of the skin often develops during the initial period of fever. During remission or during the recurrent period of fever, a scarlatiniform, morbilliform, maculopapular, or petechial eruption occurs that begins on the dorsum of the hands and feet, then spreads to the arms, legs, trunk, and neck. It rarely involves the face. The rash fades after a few hours or days and is occasionally followed by desquamation.

Children who develop a second dengue infection from a different serotype of virus may develop hemorrhagic diathesis manifested by petechiae, followed after 2 to 7 days by decreased body temperature, shock, and sometimes death.

Ocular Features

During the acute episode, photophobia and tearing are prominent and may be persistent; the eyes feel sore to touch, and retrobulbar pain occurs, which is especially severe on movement of the eyes.

Lid edema and bulbar conjunctival redness, most marked near the fornices, develop during the acute stages of the illness.

The febrile episodes are sometimes associated with a punctate epithelial keratitis, disciform keratitis, or marginal corneal ulcer.

Mild iritis, manifested by anterior chamber cells and flare with very little tendency to cause posterior synechiae, occasionally occurs during the first or third week of illness.

Other findings include retinal vascular engorgement, retinal hemorrhages and vitreous hemorrhages, dacryoadenitis, and weakness of accommodation.

Lassa Fever

Lassa fever occurs in West Africa, where the rat is the natural host, although human-to-human transmission may occur.

The infection begins with fever, malaise, headache, a nonproductive cough, and in some patients, joint and lumbar pain. The patient develops a sore throat, followed by high fever and prostration by the fifth day of illness; diarrhea frequently occurs within the first week. Unilateral or bilateral deafness occurs in about one-fourth of the patients and may be permanent.

Respiratory complications sometimes occur within the first week of the illness; bleeding, although uncommon, portends a poor prognosis. Confusion, coma, and convulsions may develop early in the infection.

A petechial rash sometimes occurs, and conjunctivitis is common.

HIV, HIV-1 AND HIV-2

Infection with HIV-1 (the most common cause of AIDS in the United States) or HIV-2 (the most common cause of AIDS in West Africa) produces a spectrum of disease that progresses at a variable rate (from a few months to 17 years) from latency to AIDS. At this writing, an estimated 40 million persons worldwide are infected with HIV and 16,000 people become infected with this virus every day.

HIV is primarily transmitted through blood and semen, with the major routes of infection being sexual, contaminated blood (intravenous drug use and transfusion), and mother to fetus. Cofactors for sexual transmission include sexually transmitted diseases that cause genital ulcers (herpes simplex, syphilis, and chancroid).

With the introduction of multiple new drugs, including protease inhibitors combined with nucleoside and nonnucleoside reverse transcriptase inhibitors [highly reactive antiretroviral therapy (HAART)], there has been a significant reduction in HIV-associated morbidity and mortality. Though HAART can profoundly suppress viral replication and allow increase in CD-4 positive lymphocytes, it has not been able to eliminate the virus completely.

Patients with persistent generalized lymphadenopathy, depleted T-helper lymphocytes, and HIV infection were considered to have AIDS-related complex, at one time called ARC.

Clinical Features

The infection has four phases:

Phase I (acute infection) is variable in severity. About 50% of patients are asymptomatic. Others develop the acute retroviral syndrome characterized by fever, lymphadenopathy, malaise, headache, sore throat, arthralgia, rash, abdominal pain, and diarrhea. It usually lasts up to 2 weeks, and seroconversion may occur as early as 4 to 6 weeks, but may take as long as 1 year.

Phase II develops between 2 months to more than 7 years following infection. It is usually asymptomatic, although 10% to 20% may develop neurologic symptoms.

Phase III is associated with a persistent generalized lymphadenopathy of two or more extragenital sites without other manifestations. The lymph nodes are rubbery, mobile, and sporadically tender.

Phase IV represents symptomatic AIDS and is subdivided into:

Phase IV A: patients with AIDS-related constitutional disease previously called ARC; Patients with Phase IV A often present with fever, weight loss, chronic diarrhea, oral candidosis (Fig. 29-80), and lymphadenopathy. At this point in their infection, they have not developed AIDS-defining infections or neoplasms.

Phase IV B: patients with AIDS who have neurologic disease (HIV encephalopathy). (HIV encephalopathy defines AIDS.)

Phase IV C: patients with secondary infectious diseases.

Phase IV C1: patients with secondary infectious diseases defining AIDS, such as disseminated *Mycobacterium avium* complex or *M. kansasii* extrapulmonary cryptococcosis, *Pneumocystis carinii* pneumonia, cerebral toxoplasmosis over 1 month of age, or retinal CMV, among others, should be suspected of having AIDS, and diagnostic studies should be carried out with the patient's consent.

Phase IV C2: patients with other infectious diseases.

Phase IV D: patients with malignancies that occur secondary to AIDS.

Phase IV E: patients in whom other conditions develop.

HIV Infection in Infants

HIV infection in infants causes failure to thrive, developmental delay from encephalopathy, chronic parotid swelling, hepatosplenomegaly, and major bacterial infections.

Pulmonary Disease

Prior to the advent of HAART, *Pneumocystis carinii* pneumonia was a major cause of death in AIDS patients. Other pulmonary infections, which sometimes occur, include cytomegalovirus, *Mycobacterium avium* complex, and *Mycobacterium tuberculosis*.

Neurologic Disease

HIV probably infects the central nervous system in all cases of AIDS and causes clinical neurologic signs in up to 40% of patients. Subacute encephalitis (AIDS dementia) may occur and is manifested by motor and behavioral disorders and cognitive dysfunction. Opportunistic neurologic infections, such as cerebral toxoplasmosis, cryptococcal meningitis, herpes zoster of the central nervous system, and neurosyphilis, are more common in AIDS.

Other System Disease

Diarrhea and, occasionally, malabsorption may be caused by direct HIV infection, infection by the CMV virus, *Salmonella* spp., *Shigella* spp., *Campylobacter* spp., and mycobacteria, as well as *Cryptosporidium, Isospora belli,* and *Giardia lamblia* protozoa.

Renal disease is caused by AIDS-associated nephropathy, ischemic injury, or drugs.

A seronegative oligo- or polyarthritis of unknown etiology may also occur.

Skin Features

The acute infection, during which the patient is highly contagious (Phase I), causes an asymptomatic fine morbilliform eruption of the face, neck, and trunk that evolves over 1 to 3 days. The extremities are only mildly involved, if at all. Occasionally, the patient develops urticaria. Perleche, palatal, and esophageal ulcers and candidiasis may also be seen.

Skin manifestations arising during the other phases of AIDS are the result of immunosuppression. They include Kaposi sarcoma (Chapter 20), other neoplasms, severe skin infections, skin infections caused by unusual pathogens, and other skin lesions. For example, immunosuppressed patients may develop a chronic cutaneous HSV infection in which the skin lesions increase in size, often become confluent, then form an ulcer with a sharp, erythematous border, covered by a purulent exudate or pseudomembrane (Fig. 29-14). Visceral dissemination is common in these instances.

The neoplasms include lymphomas that may present as skin nodules, malignant melanomas, basal cell carcinomas, intraoral squamous epithelioma (especially of the tongue), cervical intraepithelial neoplasia, and intraepithelial carcinoma in association with anogenital verruca.

Other Skin Diseases

Diseases that are sometimes modified by the presence of AIDS or in which AIDS is a definite risk factor include seborrhea (Fig. 29-81), papulonecrotic folliculitis, ecthyma (Fig. 29-82), eosinophilic folliculitis (Fig. 29-83), xeroderma, acquired ichthyosis, atopic disease, psoriasis, drug eruptions, and drug reactions (e.g., fever, thrombocytopenia, etc.), and generalized or extensive local granuloma annulare. Significant generalized pruritus is a troublesome problem, as is photosensitivity.

Bacterial Infections

The bacterial skin infections and skin manifestations of bacterial infections that are increased in frequency or appear to be more severe in AIDS patients include *Mycobacterium marinum, M. avium* complex, secondary syphilis, tertiary benign syphilis, neurosyphilis, bacillary (epithelioid) angiomatosis, and severe mixed bacterial gingivitis.

Viral Skin Infections

Viral skin infections, which are often more severe and persistent in AIDS patients, include herpes zoster, herpes simplex, cytomegalovirus, Epstein–Barr virus (Fig. 29-84), molluscum contagiosum (Fig. 29-3), and verruca (Fig. 29-85).

Fungal Infections

Fungal infections that are often more extensive and severe in AIDS patients than in others include *Cryptococcus neoformans* (a specific indicator disease of AIDS), *Pityriasis versicolor,* dermatophyte infections (Fig. 29-86), candidosis (Fig. 29-80), and *Histoplasma capsulatum*.

Demodicidosis (a parasitic infection) is also more common and modified in its presentation in AIDS patients.

Ocular Features

Kaposi sarcoma, the second most common AIDS-associated opportunistic disease, may involve the lid. It presents as a purple subcutaneous nodule or plaque and occasionally ulcerates (Chapter 20). Massive swelling of the lid, entropion, and trichiasis are sometimes caused by the tumor.

Conjunctiva

About 10% of AIDS patients develop conjunctival Kaposi sarcoma (Chapter 20). At first, it resembles a subconjunctival hemorrhage of the fornix; later, it gains bulk and appears more like a tumor.

Other conjunctival findings include conjunctival vascular changes (the vessels appear curved, comma-shaped, globular, or aneurysmal), transient conjunctivitis, mild follicular conjunctivitis caused by CMV infection, bilateral pseudomembranous conjunctivitis, and eratoconjunctivitis sicca.

Other Ocular Findings

Other ocular findings include the following:

1. Orbital pseudotumors in the region of the lacrimal fossa.
2. Chronic iridocyclitis with anterior vitreitis and nongranulomatous choroidal inflammation subjacent to CMV-involved retina.
3. Cotton-wool spots, which develop spontaneously and resolve after 4 to 6 weeks; retinal hemorrhages and microaneurysms; retinal periphlebitis; CMV retinopathy (the most serious opportunistic infection in this group); opportunistic retinal necrosis (usually caused by CMV infection and manifested by occlusion of retinal vessels or nonperfusion of large areas of retina; and acute retinal necrosis.
4. Papilledema, papillitis, optic atrophy, retrobulbar neuritis, visual field defects, cortical blindness, visual allesthesia, oculomotor nerve palsies, and vertical diplopia.

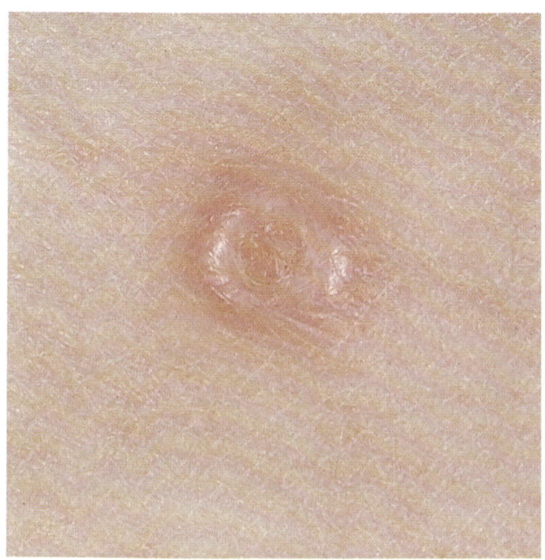

FIGURE 29-1. Solitary molluscum contagiosum showing small, pearly papule with characteristic central light-colored umbilication.

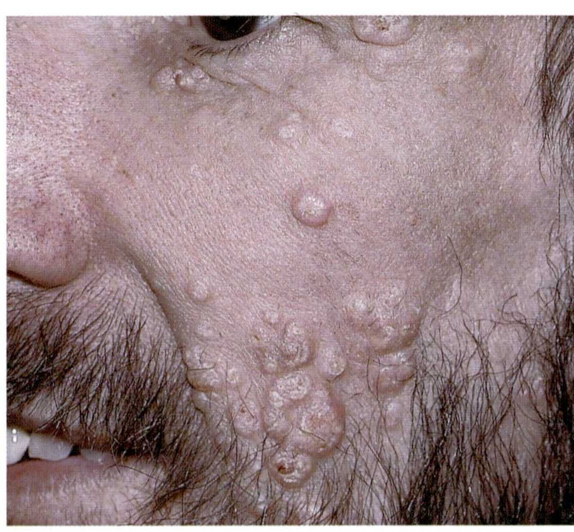

FIGURE 29-2. Atypical giant molluscum lesions in a patient with AIDS. These viral lesions are often an early cutaneous clue of significantly reduced immunity.

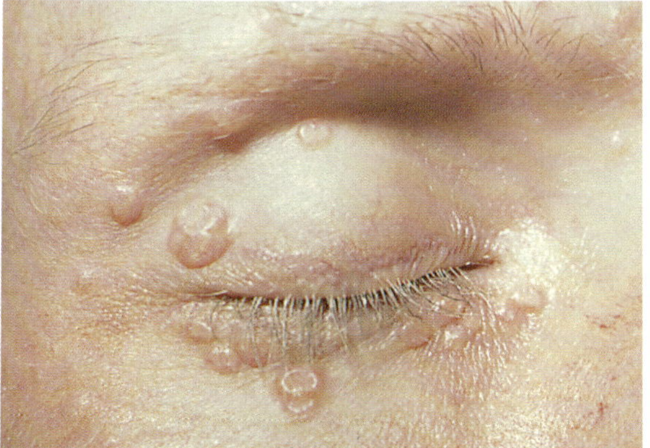

FIGURE 29-3. Molluscum contagiosum of eyelids in a patient with AIDS. Note similarity to basal cell carcinoma.

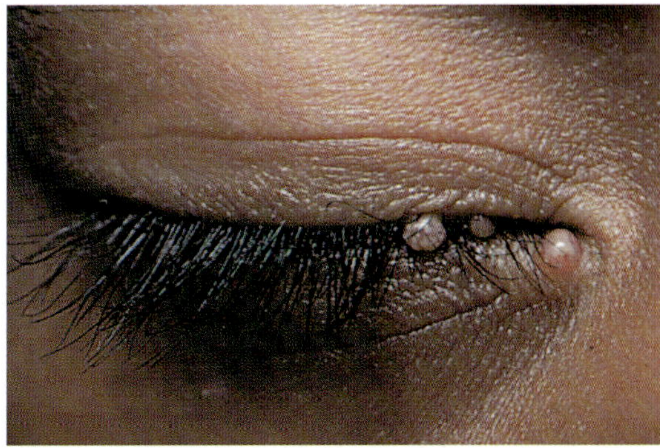

FIGURE 29-4. Molluscum contagiosum of the lid margin.

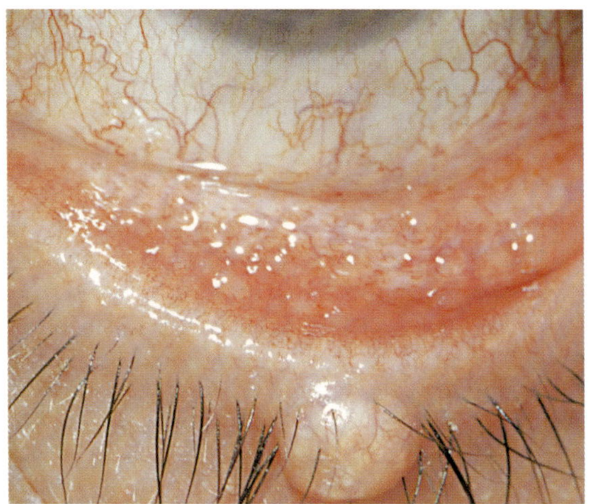

FIGURE 29-5. Follicular conjunctivitis associated with molluscum nodule of the lid margin.

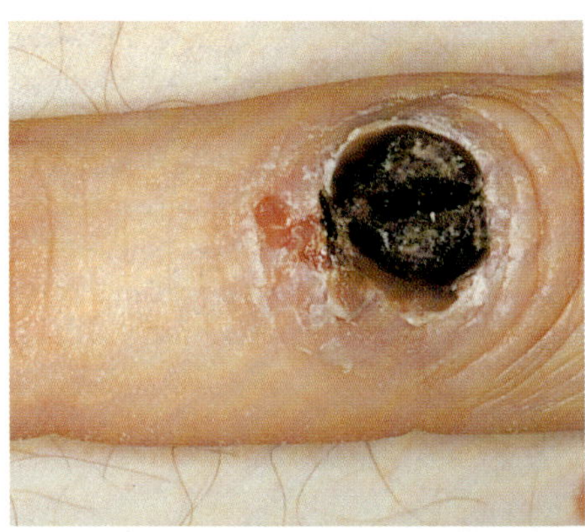

FIGURE 29-6. Skin lesion of the finger in orf. (Courtesy of Dr. John Reeves.)

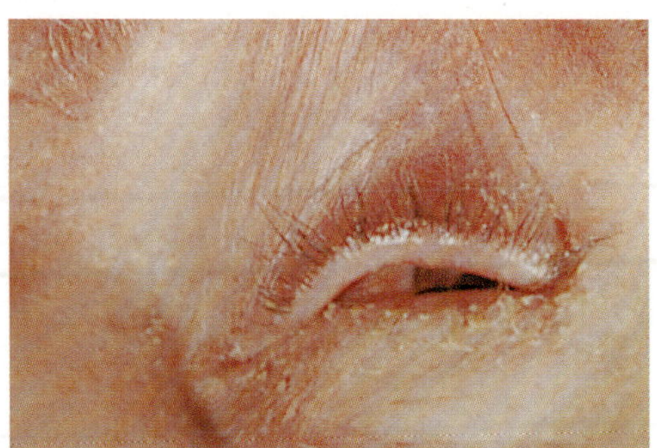

FIGURE 29-7. Orf skin lesion just below and lateral to the lid. This 43-year-old sheepherder developed pustules on the face, lid margin, neck, forearm, and hand.

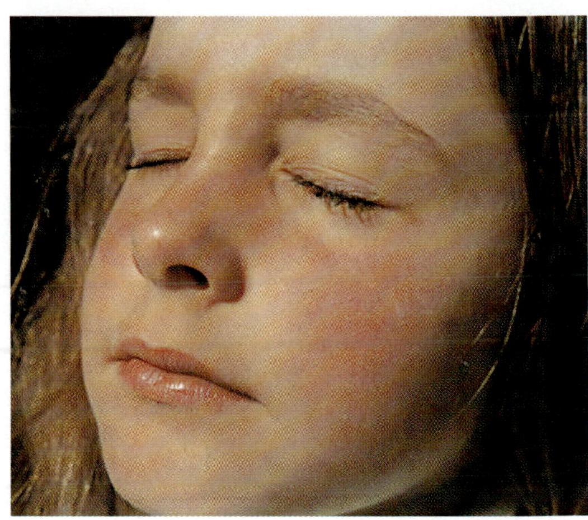

FIGURE 29-8. Erythema infectiosum (fifth disease) showing the characteristic "slapped cheek" for which this infection is often named.

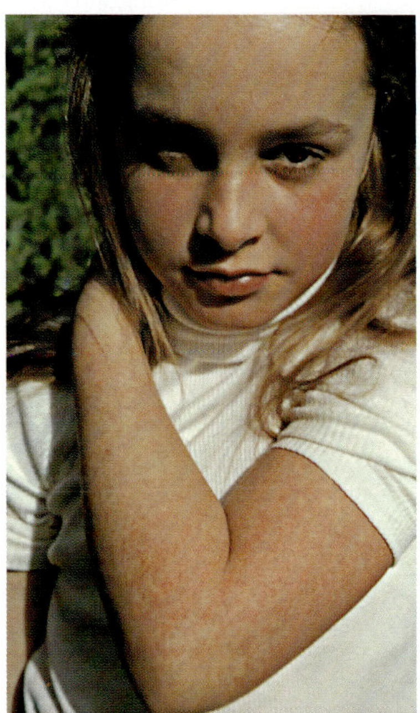

FIGURE 29-9. Fifth disease showing fading "slapped cheeks" and the characteristic lacy reticulated exanthem of the arms (same patient as pictured in Fig. 29-8).

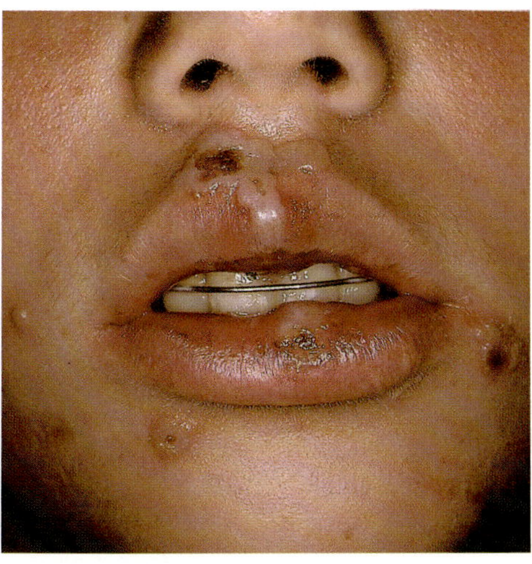

FIGURE 29-10. Primary herpes gingivostomatitis with perioral, labial, and intraoral vesiculopustular and bullous lesions accompanied by a severely sore throat, tender cervical adenopathy, fever, and malaise in this 15-year-old girl.

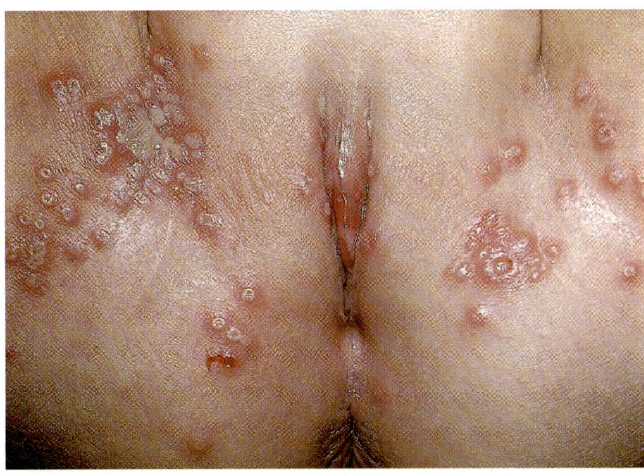

FIGURE 29-11. Primary anogenital herpes in an infant girl. Sexual abuse was suspected, though an uncle said he had only "kissed the baby on her bottom."

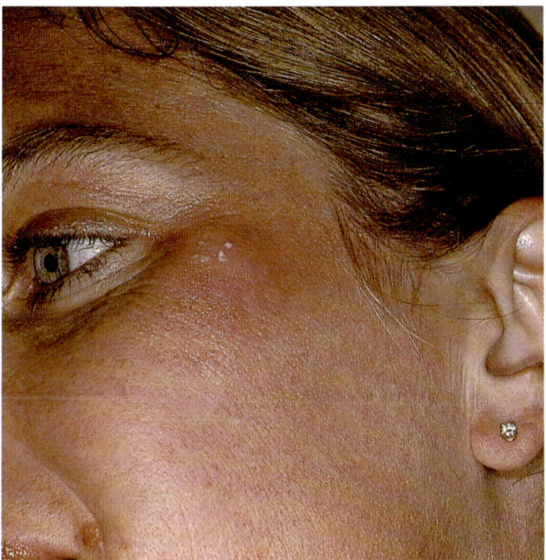

FIGURE 29-12. Recurrent herpes of cheek treated as impetigo. To reduce chance of autoinoculation of eye, patient was placed on suppressive long-term antiherpes treatment.

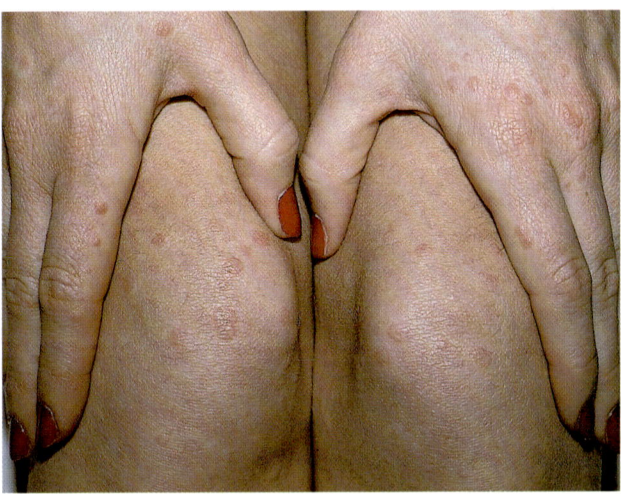

FIGURE 29-13. Recurrent erythema multiforme occurring several days to weeks after each episode of herpes simplex. Both problems were eliminated by chronic suppressive oral antiviral therapy.

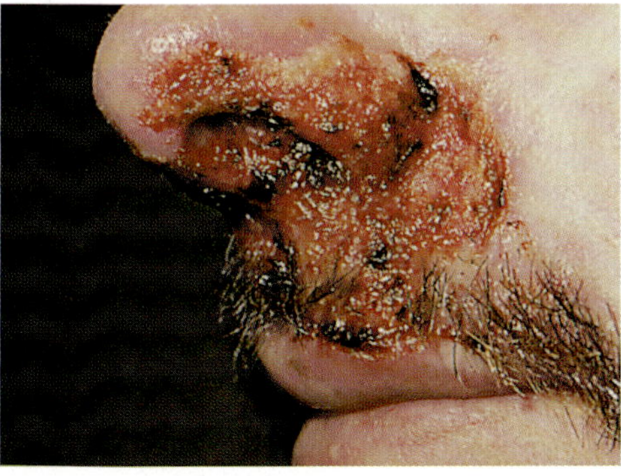

FIGURE 29-14. Chronic destructive herpetic lesions in a patient with AIDS.

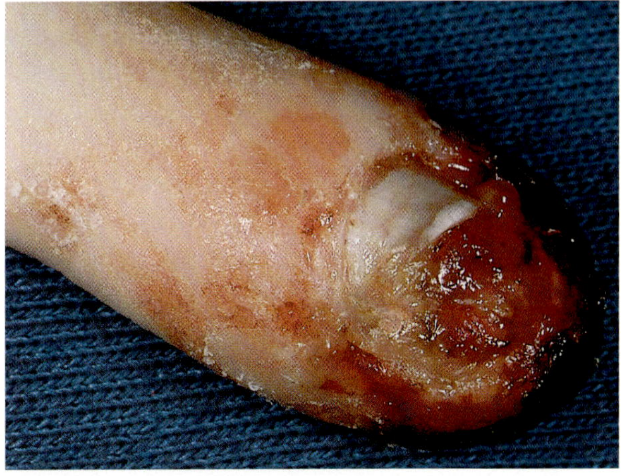

FIGURE 29-15. Herpetic whitlow. This very painful and destructive lesion had plagued this patient for many months. Intravenous antiviral therapy and aggressive management of his AIDS infection resolved the problem.

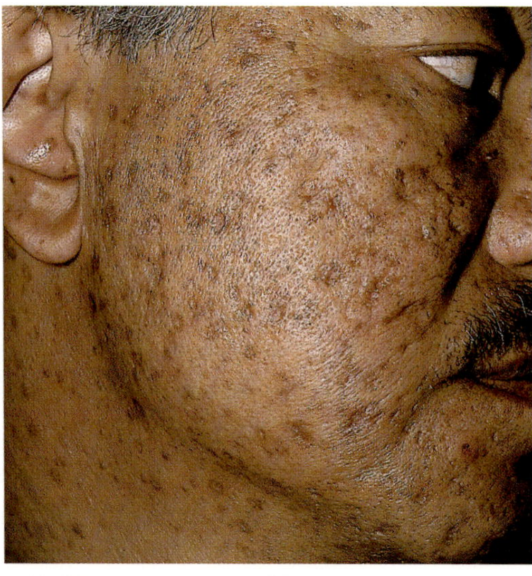

FIGURE 29-28. A severe case of chickenpox as an adult left this middle-aged man with multiple pox scars, causing him significant distress and depression. Early aggressive treatment of his infection might have prevented this.

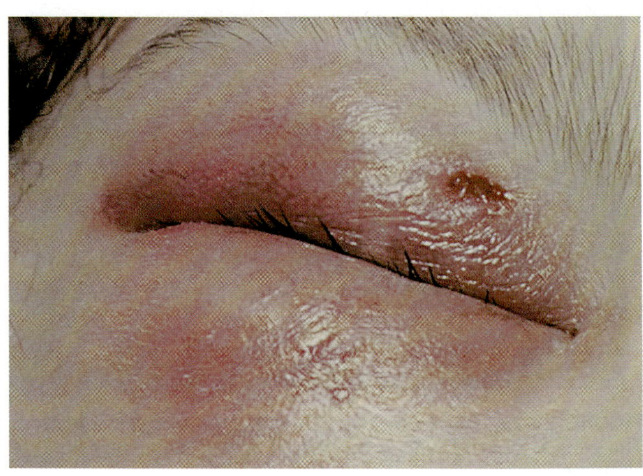

FIGURE 29-29. Varicella of the eyelid. (Courtesy of Dr. Phillips Thygeson.)

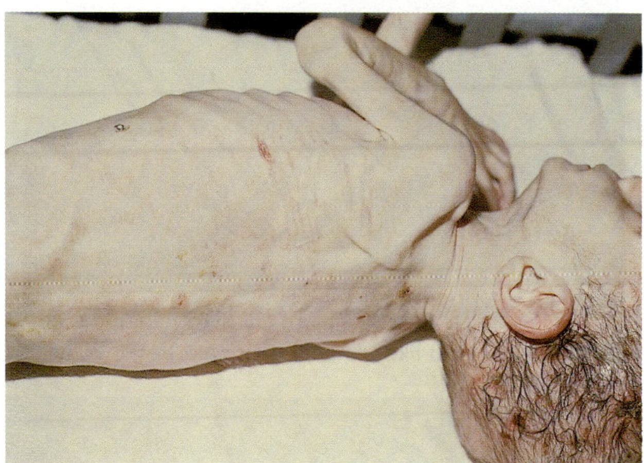

FIGURE 29-30. Meningoencephalitis (note marked opisthotonos) as complication of chickenpox in this extremely malnourished infant seen in Central America. The patient died the day after this photo was taken.

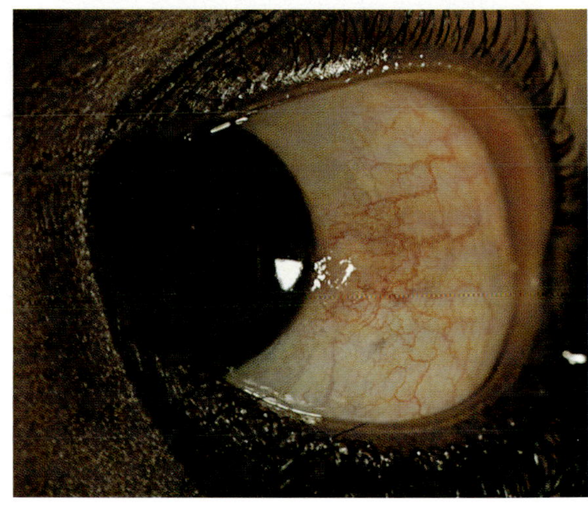

FIGURE 29-31. Pock lesion at the limbus.

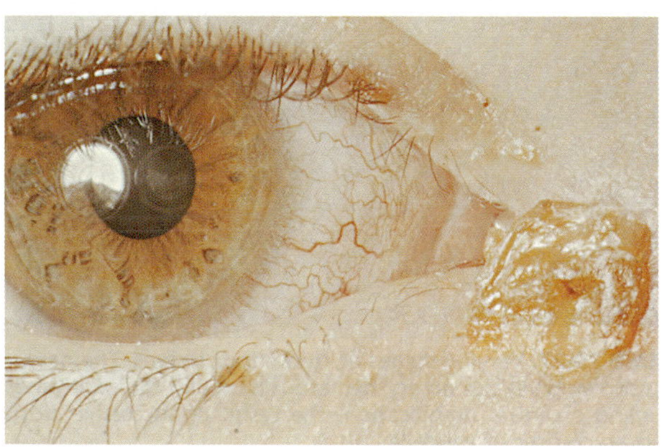

FIGURE 29-32. Pock lesion on the medial canthus associated with mild corneal scarring.

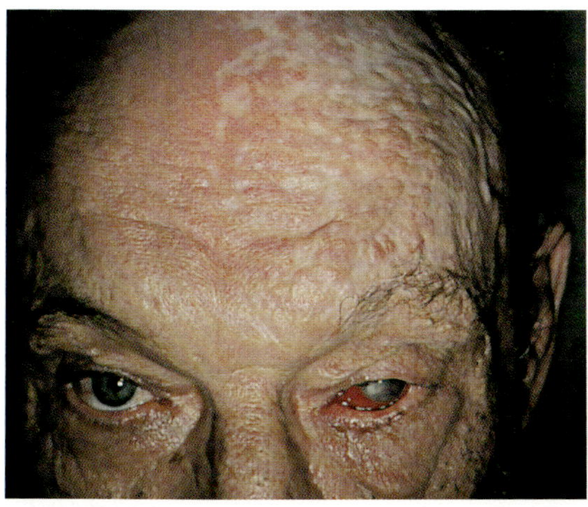

FIGURE 29-33. Severe scarring of the skin in ophthalmic zoster associated with corneal ulceration and eventual loss of the left eye. The patient experienced chronic pain and dysesthesia of the affected skin.

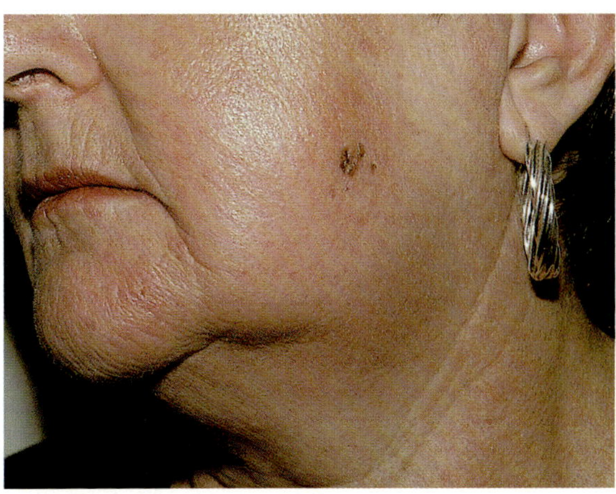

FIGURE 29-34. Initial solitary painful vesiculocrusting lesion of zoster (maxillary branch of trigeminal nerve) misdiagnosed as insect bite with secondary impetigo.

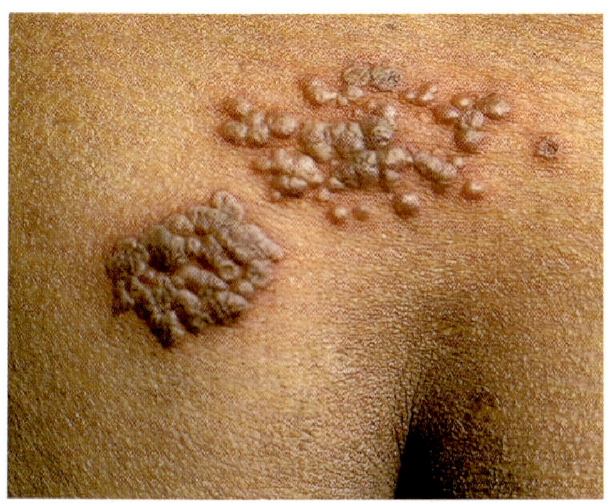

FIGURE 29-35. Grouped (herpetiform) vesicles on an erythematous base in sacral herpes zoster.

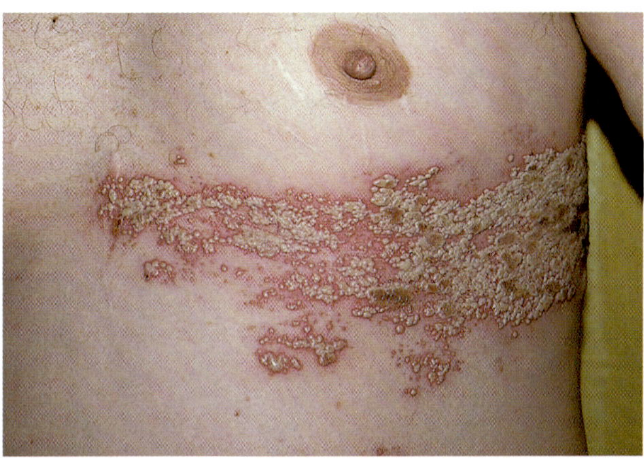

FIGURE 29-36. Thoracic zoster with confluent vesiculopustular and necrotic lesions. This young man was partially immunocompromised because of chronic corticosteroid treatment for his atopic eczema.

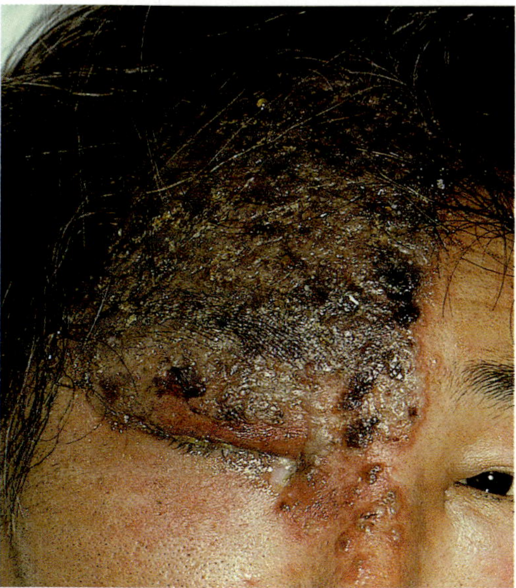

FIGURE 29-37. Severe zoster ophthalmicus.

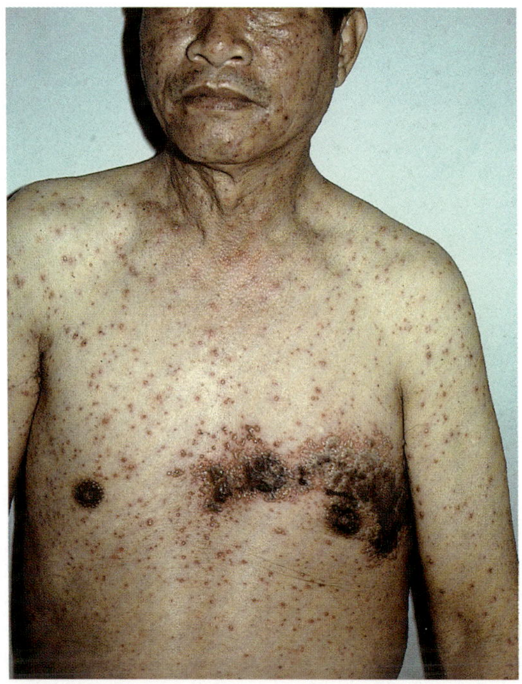

FIGURE 29-38. Disseminated zoster (Herpes zoster generalisatus) with hemorrhagic varicelliform lesions.

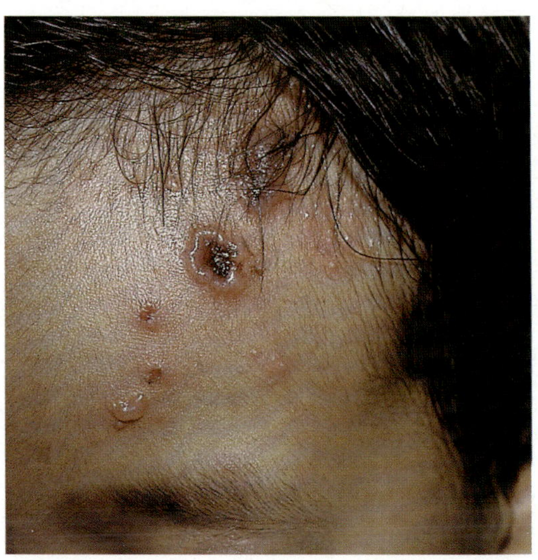

FIGURE 29-39. Zoster in a child. This often leads to chickenpox in his playmates who have not been vaccinated.

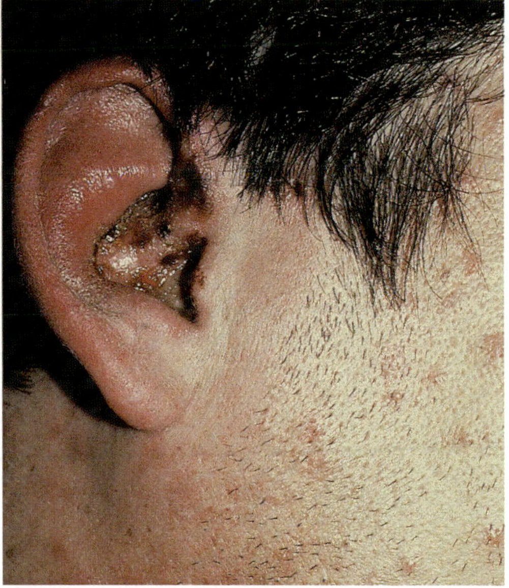

FIGURE 29-40. Hemorrhagic vesicles of external ear in a patient with Ramsey Hunt syndrome. He had experienced tinnitus and marked pain in the ear as well as ipsilateral facial weakness.

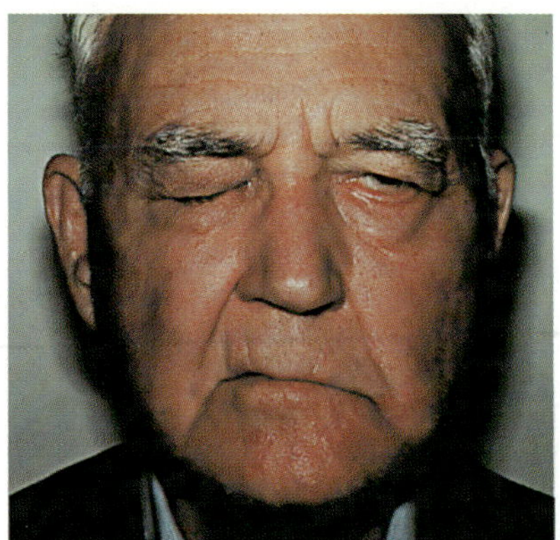

FIGURE 29-41. Facial palsy arising in the Ramsey Hunt syndrome.

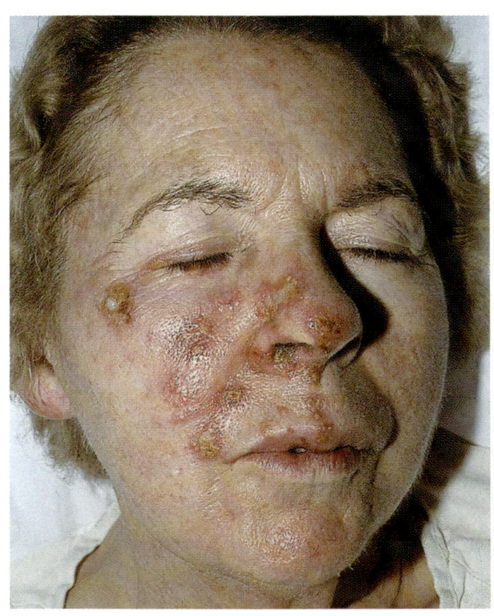

FIGURE 29-42. Zoster V1 and V2. Note lesions on tip of nose (nasociliary branch of trigeminal nerve), indicating eye involvement. This lady continued to have pain and dysesthesia of her eye and cheek for the remainder of her life.

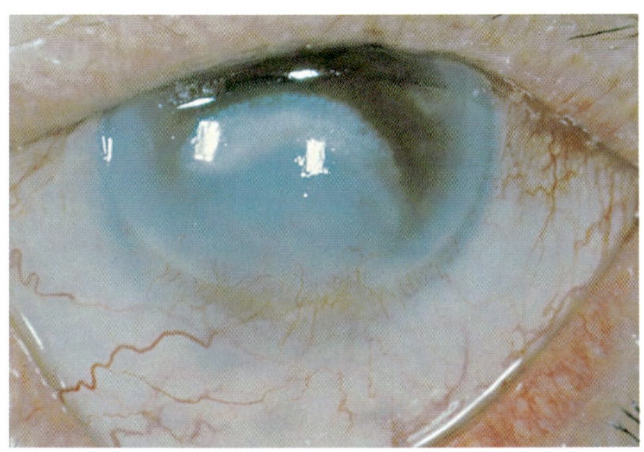

FIGURE 29-43. Sclerokeratitis in herpes zoster. A corneal opacity and superficial and deep corneal vessels are evident.

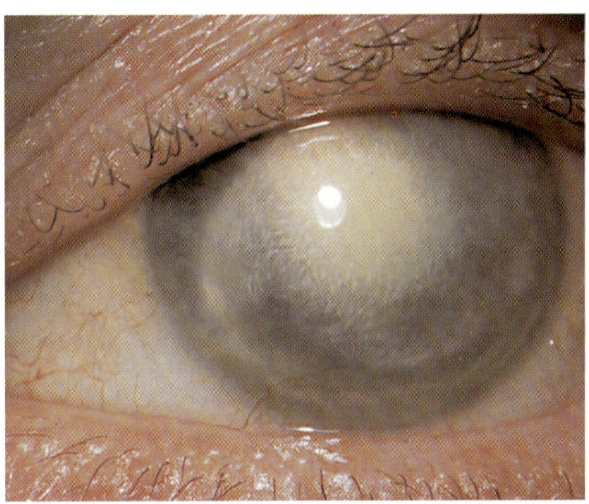

FIGURE 29-44. Lipoidal deposits in the cornea following herpes zoster keratitis. This 57-year-old man developed severe lipoidal deposition in the cornea following herpes zoster ophthalmicus. There is very little neovascularization.

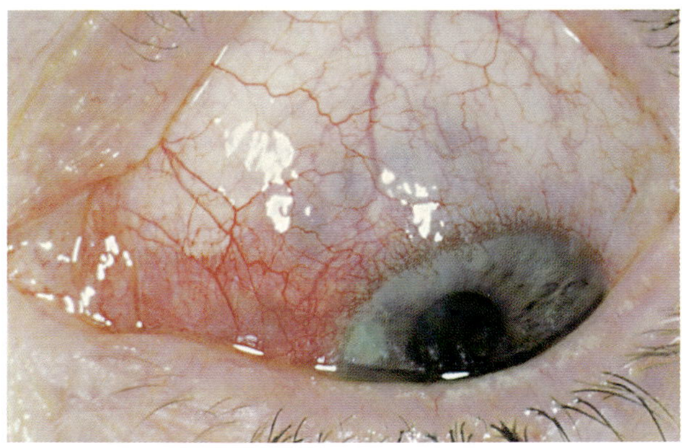

FIGURE 29-45. Scleral thinning together with an active diffuse scleritis are evident in this patient.

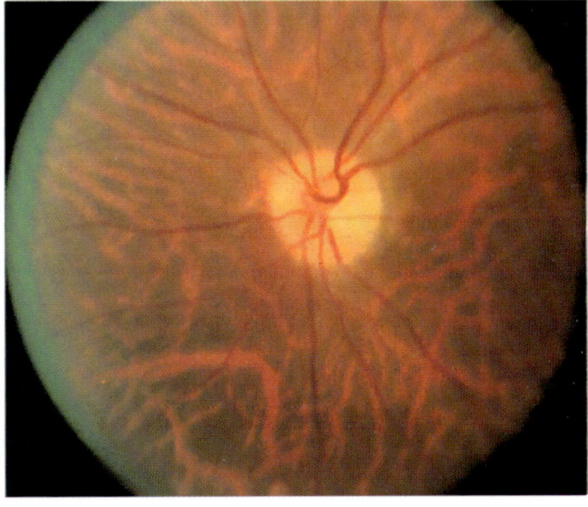

FIGURE 29-46. Central retinal artery occlusion in herpes zoster ophthalmicus. (Courtesy of Dr. John Belmont.)

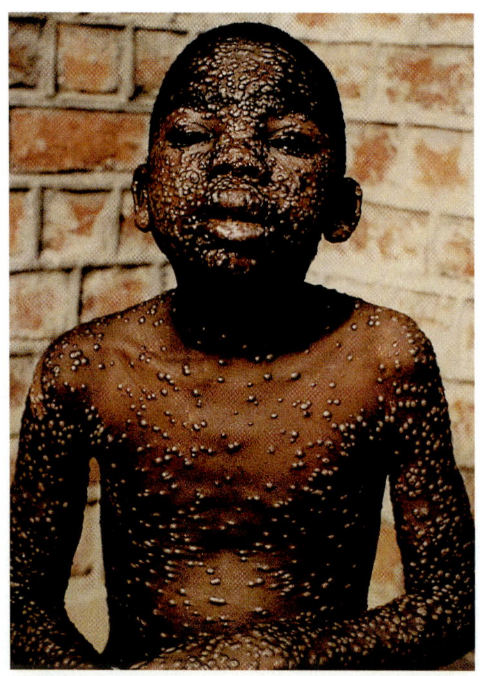

FIGURE 29-47. Smallpox. Note papulopustules all at same stage. Also note multiple lesions of face. (Courtesy of the World Health Organization.)

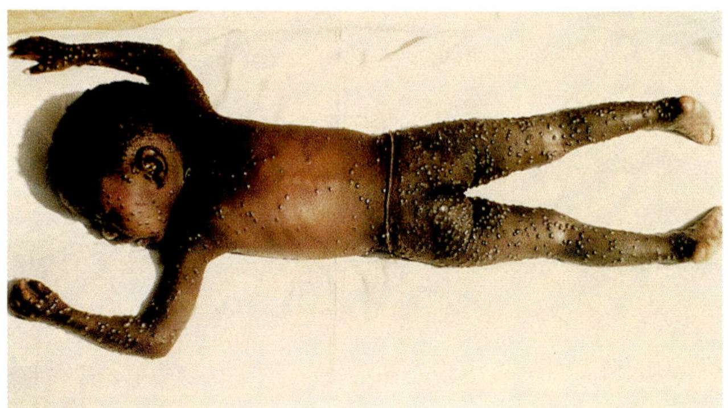

FIGURE 29-48. Smallpox showing central centrifugal pattern with more lesions on face and extremities than on trunk. (Courtesy of the CDC.)

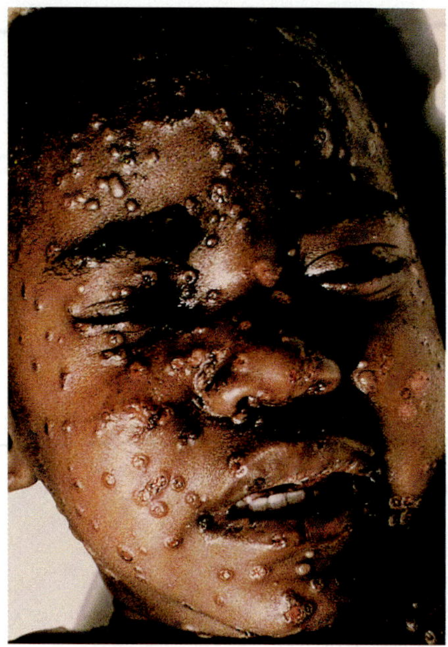

FIGURE 29-49. Smallpox showing classic umbilicated papulopustules of face. (Courtesy of the CDC.)

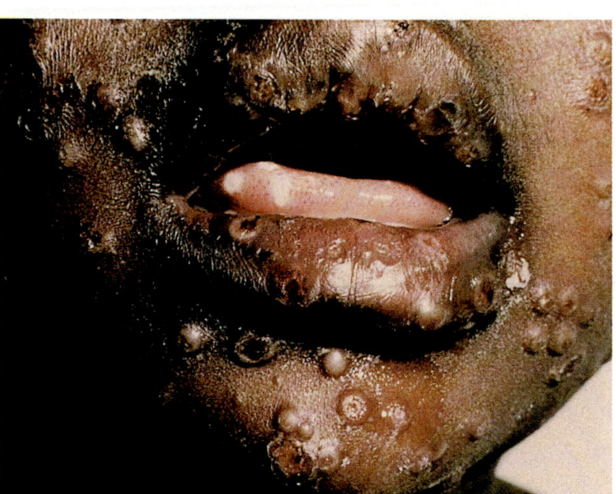

FIGURE 29-50. Close-up of Fig. 29-49 showing smallpox lesions of lips. (Courtesy of the CDC.)

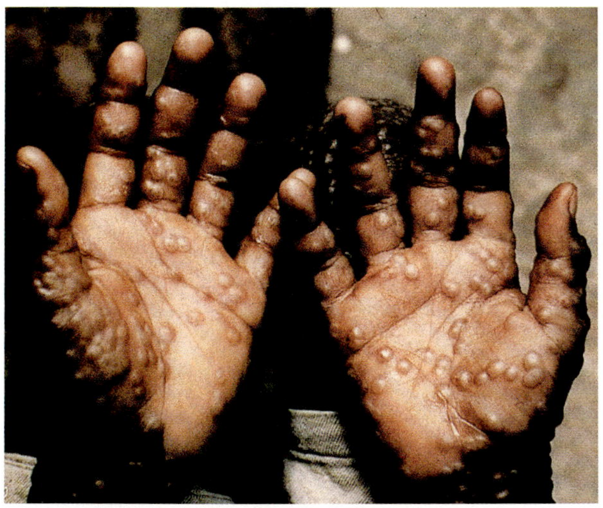

FIGURE 29-51. Multiple vesiculopapules of palms in child with smallpox. (Courtesy of the CDC.)

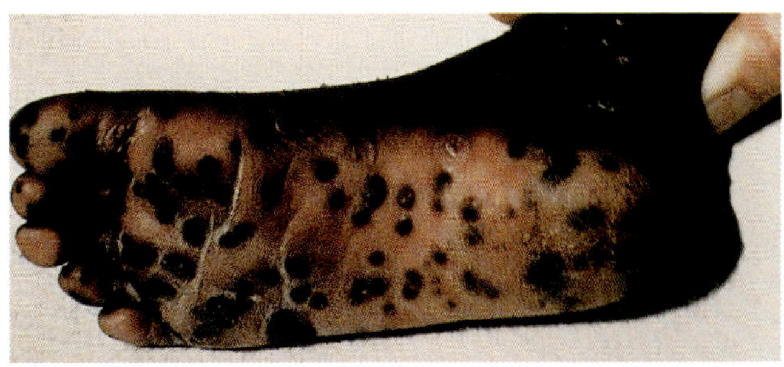

FIGURE 29-52. Hemorrhagic necrotic smallpox lesions of soles. (Courtesy of the CDC.)

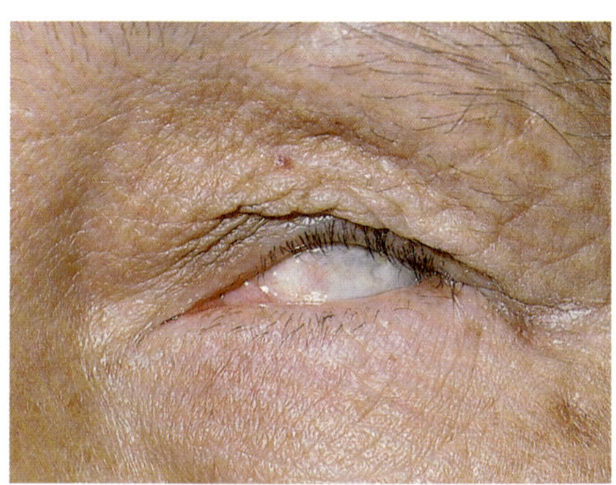

FIGURE 29-53. Corneal scarring from smallpox resulting in blindness.

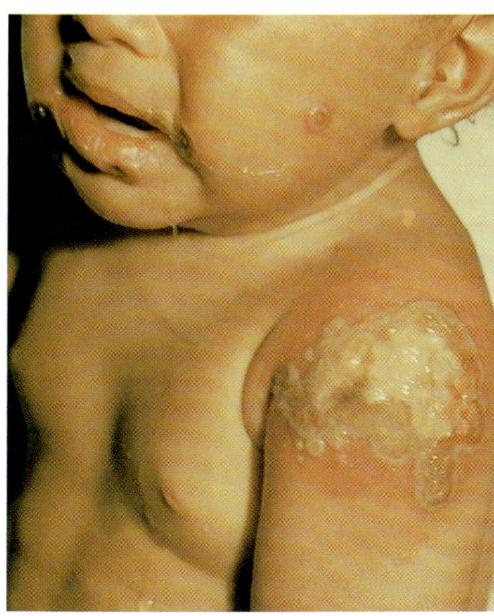

FIGURE 29-54. Vaccinia showing severe local reaction with confluent pustules, edema, and erythema. (Courtesy of Dr. Paul Fasal.)

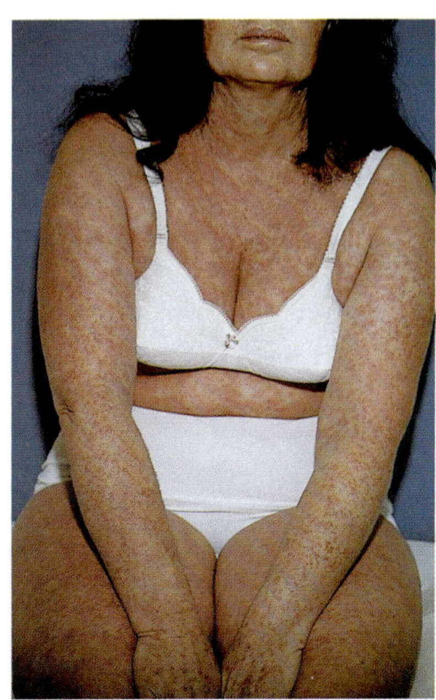

FIGURE 29-55. Erythema multiforme 10 days after smallpox revaccination in this immunocompetent female. Her widespread morbilliform eruption was accompanied by fever, malaise, pruritus, and cervical adenopathy. She fully recovered in 2 weeks.

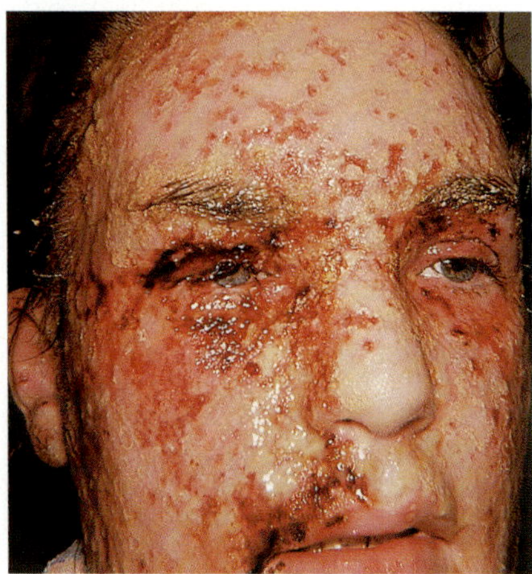

FIGURE 29-56. Eczema vaccinatum (Kaposi varicelliform eruption) in a man with a history of atopic eczema. Note significant eye involvement which can result in ocular paralysis and postvaccinial retinitis.

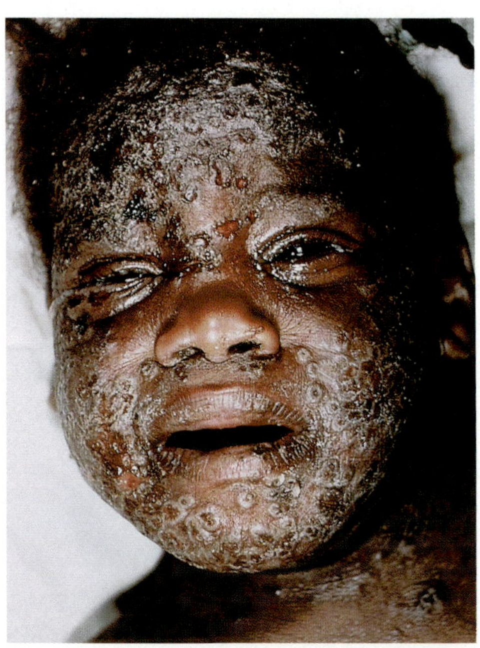

FIGURE 29-57. Eczema vaccinatum following primary smallpox vaccination in this young child with eczema. Note close resemblance to smallpox. (Courtesy of CDC.)

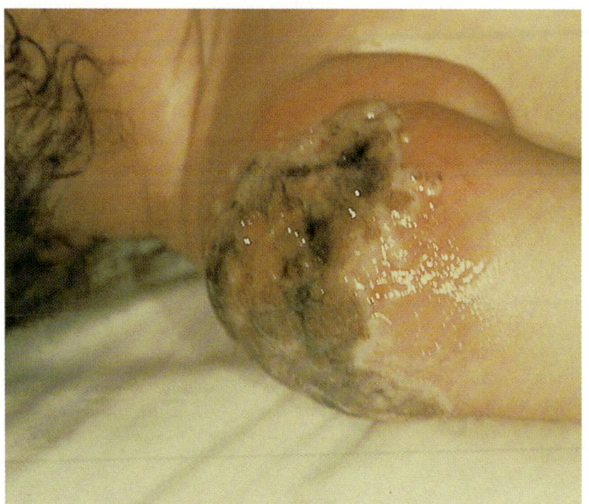

FIGURE 29-58. Vaccinia necrosum. Necrotizing cellulitis in immunocompromised infant. (Courtesy of Dr. Paul Fasal.)

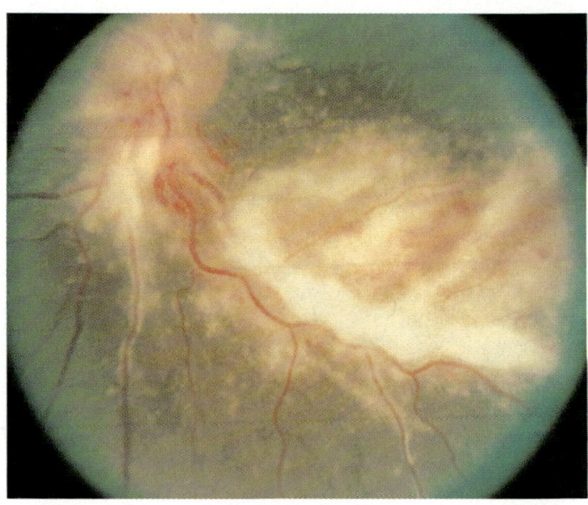

FIGURE 29-59. Cytomegaloviral retinitis. (Courtesy of Dr. John Belmont.)

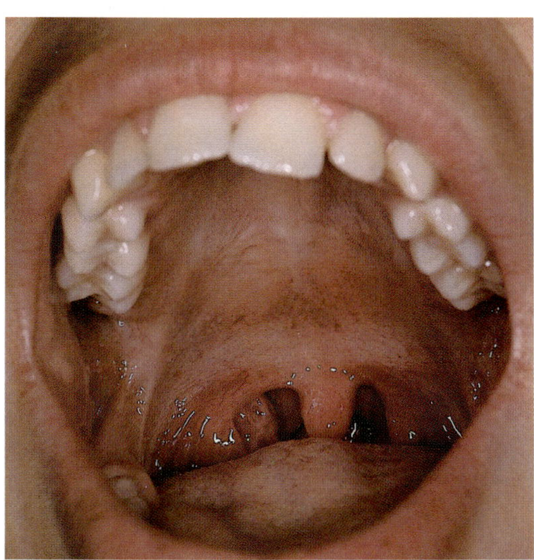

FIGURE 29-60. Petechiae at junction of hard and soft palate in a patient with infectious mononucleosis.

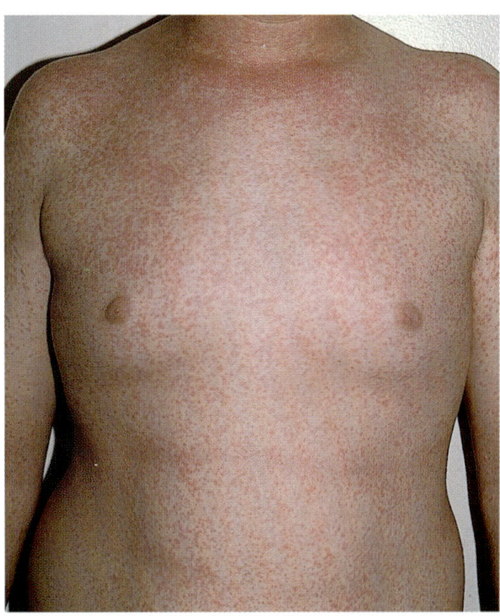

FIGURE 29-61. Morbilliform rash after 5 days of ampicillin in a teenaged boy with infectious mononucleosis.

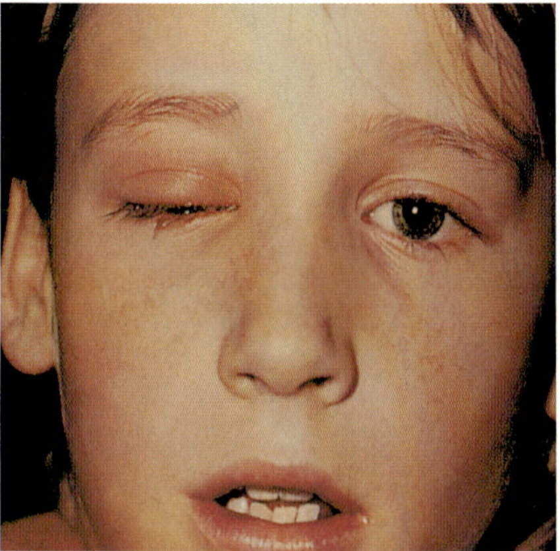

FIGURE 29-62. Erythema and edema of the lid and enlarged lymph node in infectious mononucleosis.

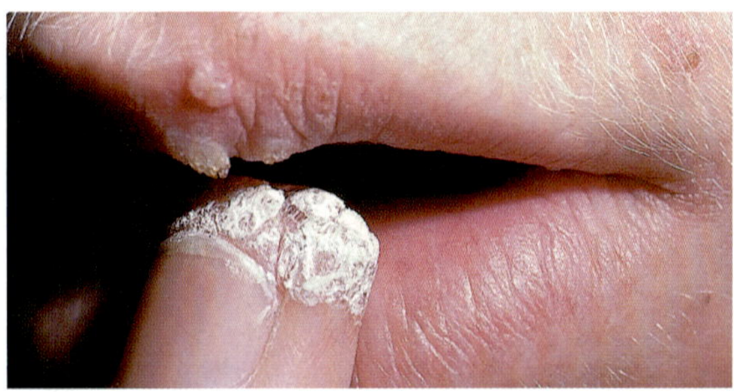

FIGURE 29-63. Wart on finger transferred to lip by the child chewing on the wart.

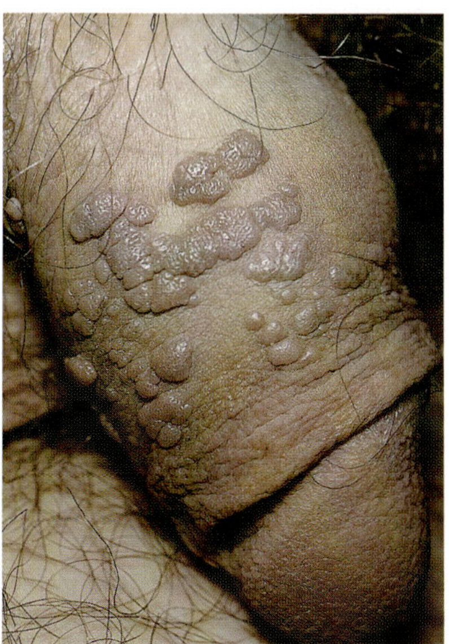

FIGURE 29-64. Multiple penile warts. The somewhat flattened and slightly brown appearance can indicate bowenoid papulosis. A biopsy did not reveal that diagnosis in this patient.

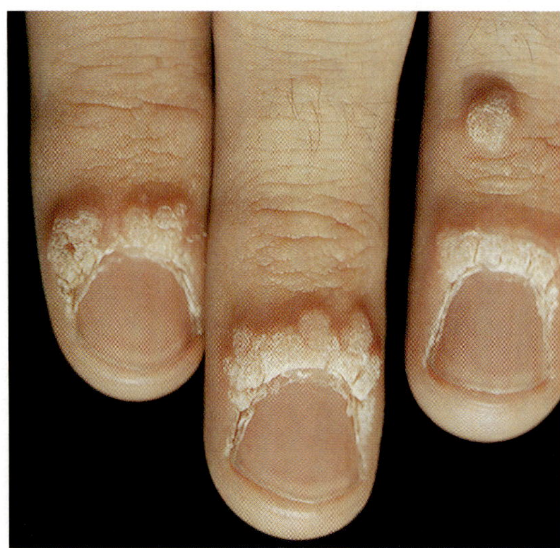

FIGURE 29-65. Multiple periungual warts. These are often refractory to treatment, which must be done cautiously to avoid permanent damage to the nail matrix.

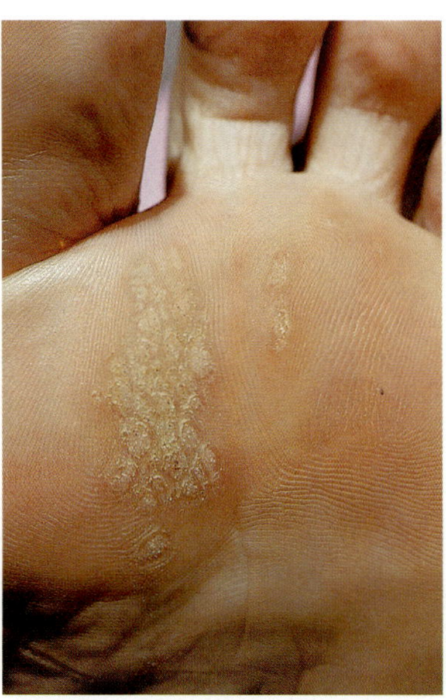

FIGURE 29-66. Confluent plantar warts producing mosaic pattern. This site must be carefully treated to avoid producing a permanent painful scar.

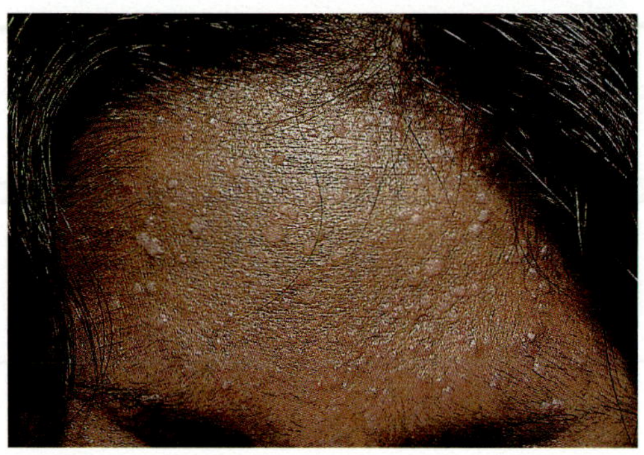

FIGURE 29-67. Flat warts (verruca plana) of forehead. This type of wart responds readily to conservative treatment, which also avoids producing scars.

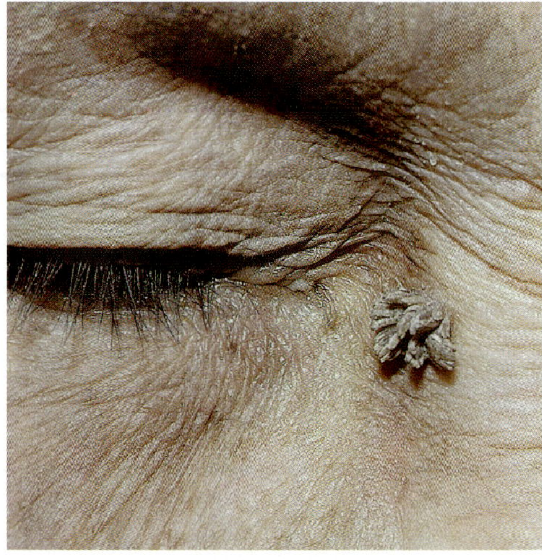

FIGURE 29-68. Digitate warts on face, a common site.

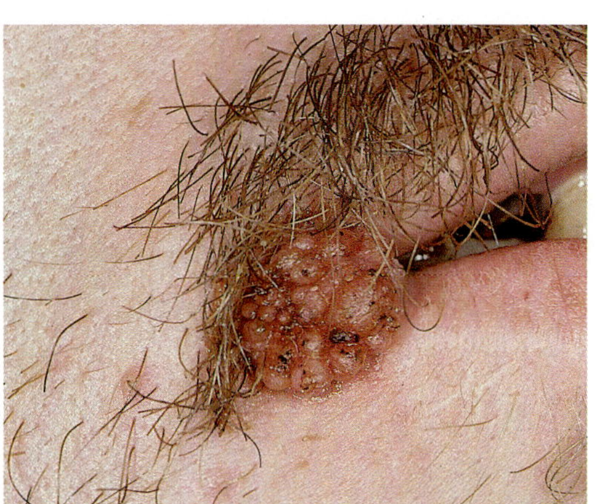

FIGURE 29-69. Condyloma acuminata at angle of mouth. Lesions were resistant to treatment in this man who had AIDS.

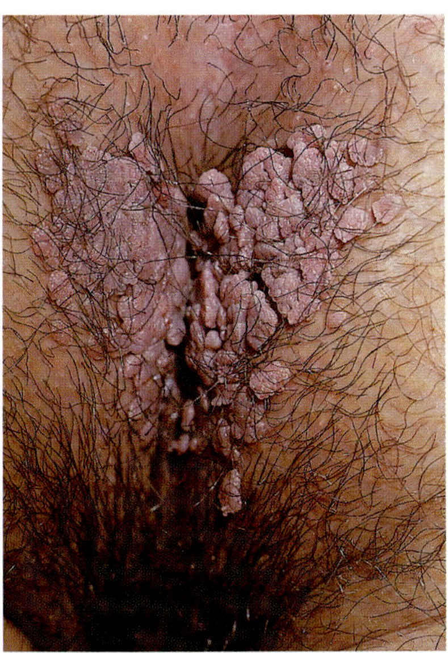

FIGURE 29-70. Anal warts (condyloma acuminata). Lesions at this site have a significant incidence of malignant transformation in patients who are immunocompromised.

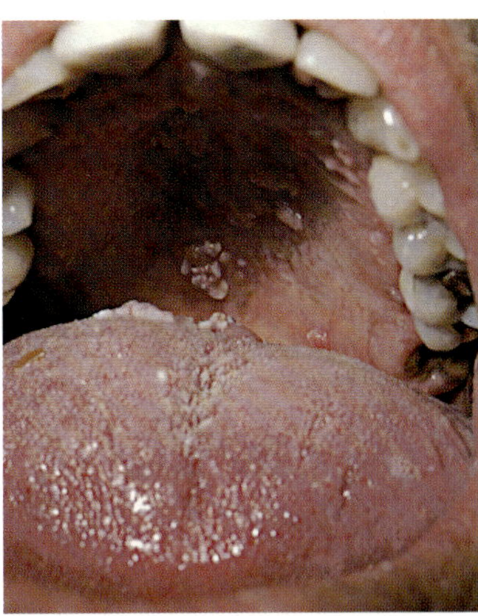

FIGURE 29-71. Warts on palate and tongue in patient with HIV.

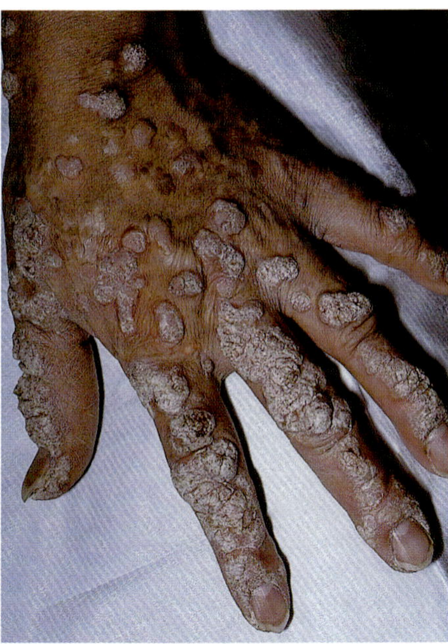

FIGURE 29-72. Epidermodysplasia verruciformis with multiple verrucae of dorsum of hands. This young man, who, unfortunately, was lost to follow-up, has a high probability of developing squamous cell carcinomas at this sun-exposed site.

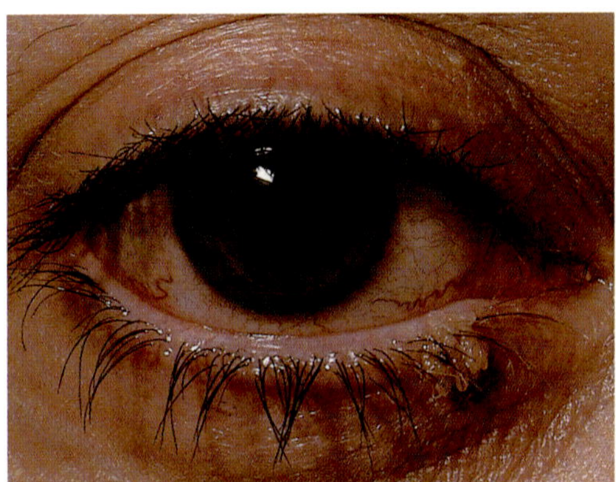

FIGURE 29-73. Digitate wart on eyelid.

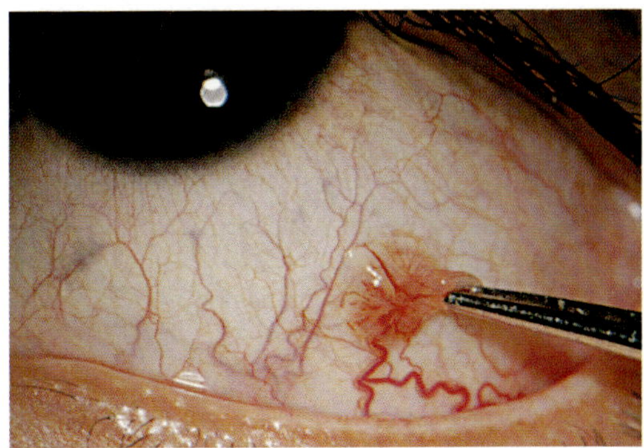

FIGURE 29-74. Verruca of the conjunctiva.

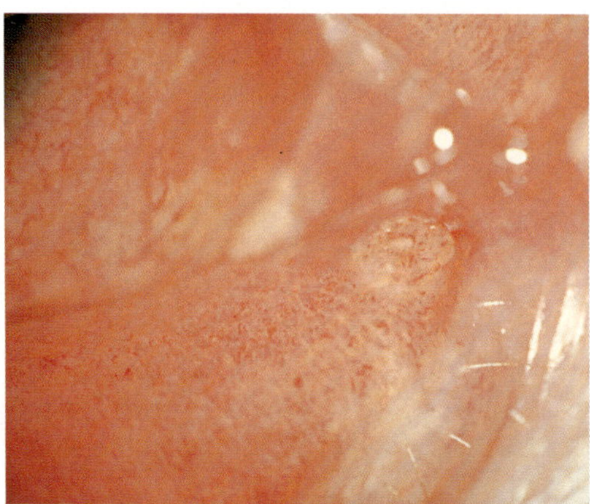

FIGURE 29-75. Verruca of the lacrimal punctum. The lesion is evident in the orifice of the punctum or becomes evident with pressure upon the canaliculus. Verruca of the lacrimal punctum may cause bloody tears and epiphora.

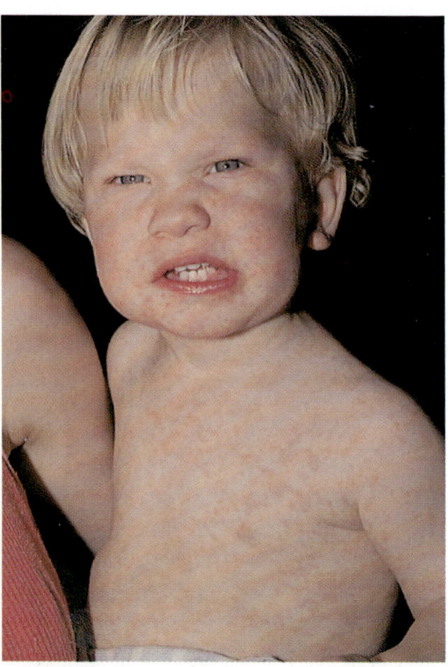

FIGURE 29-76. Skin rash in measles. Note periorbital edema and photophobia.

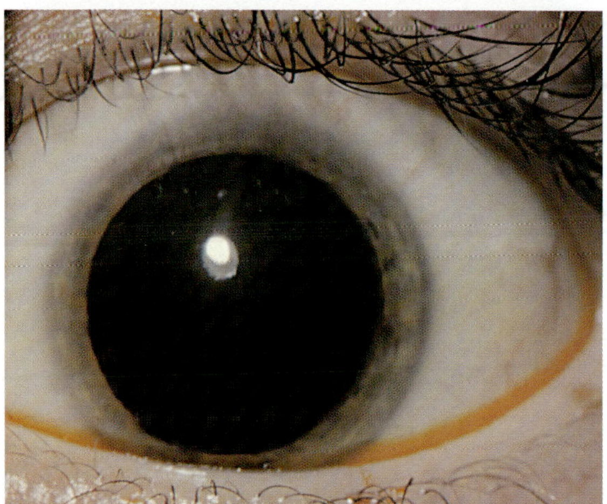

FIGURE 29-77. Measles keratitis. The epithelial keratitis is most evident near the light reflex in this photograph.

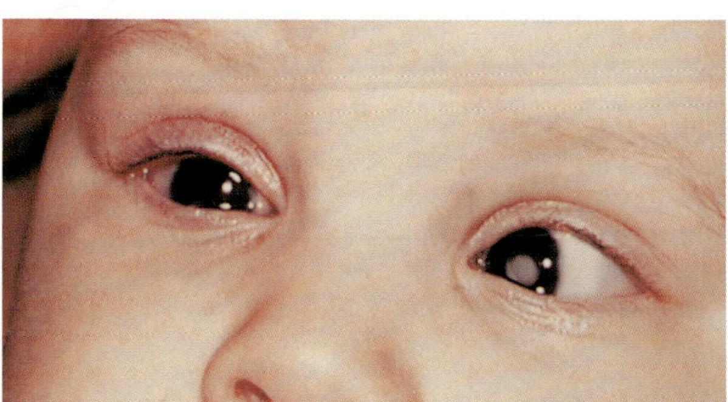

FIGURE 29-78. Esotropia and cataract of left eye and conjunctivitis and corneal opacity of right eye in congenital rubella syndrome. The cataract is readily visible on the left eye, and there is moderate esotropia. The conjunctivitis is readily visible on the right eye.

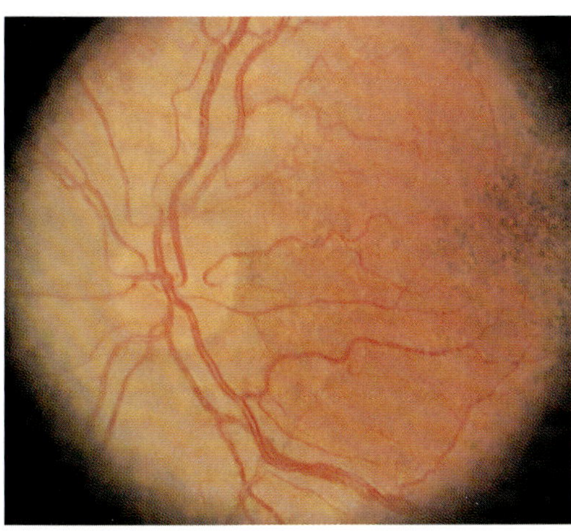

FIGURE 29-79. Rubella retinopathy. (Courtesy of Dr. John Belmont.)

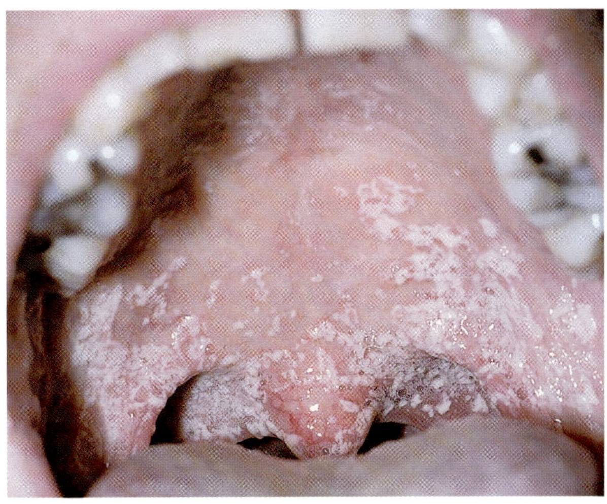

FIGURE 29-80. Extensive lesions of oral candidiasis in patient with HIV infection.

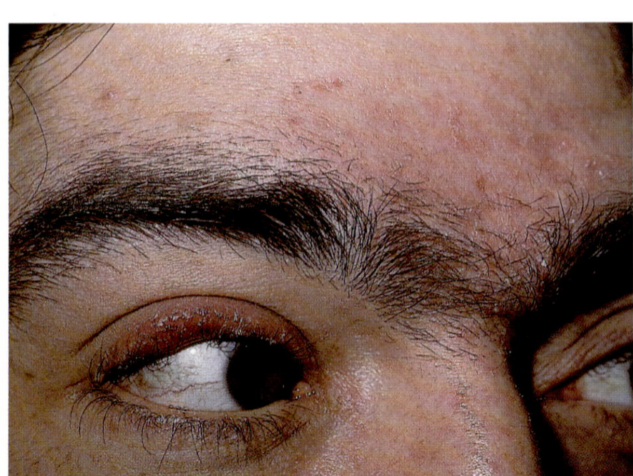

FIGURE 29-81. Seborrheic dermatitis and blepharitis in a patient with AIDS. This is a common early cutaneous clue.

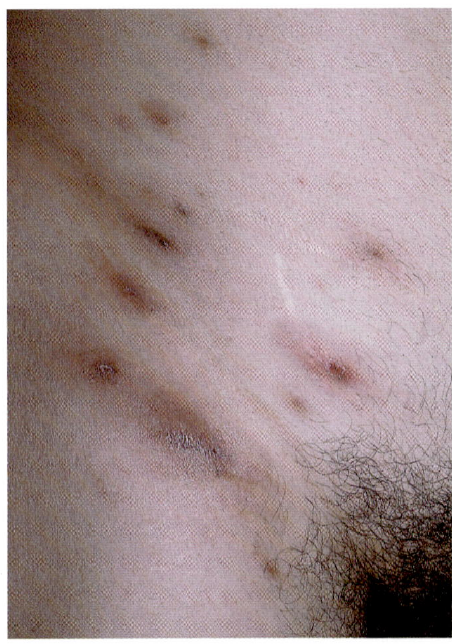

FIGURE 29-82. Ecthyma following recurrent staph folliculitis suggested HIV infection, as was the case in this patient.

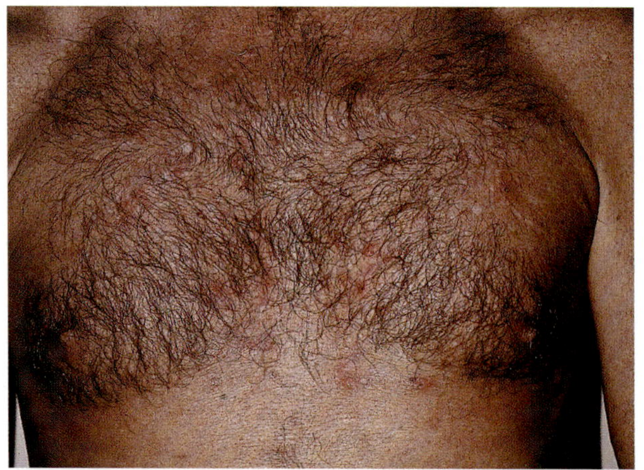

FIGURE 29-83. Eosinophilic folliculitis, this common pruritic follicular eruption, appears when the CD-4 lymphocyte count drops to about 200. The follicular papules are classically above the nipple line, as is seen in this patient.

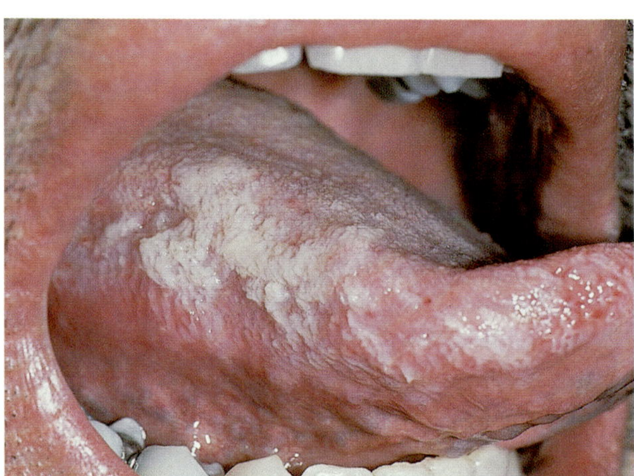

FIGURE 29-84. Oral hairy leukoplakia caused by the Epstein–Barr virus in a patient with AIDS. This is commonly seen before the onset of AIDS. It may also be found in organ transplant recipients on immunosuppressive therapy.

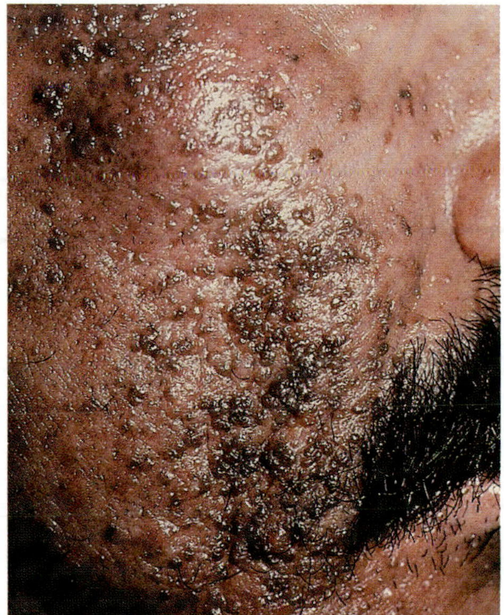

FIGURE 29-85. Extensive recalcitrant warts in a patient with AIDS.

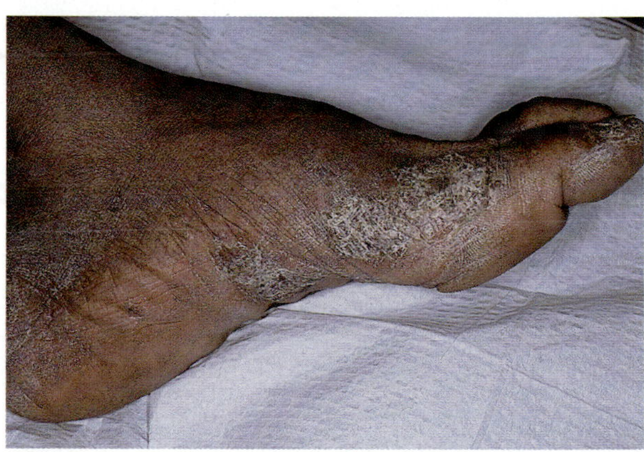

FIGURE 29-86. Severe recalcitrant tinea pedis in this man with AIDS.

30

FUNGAL INFECTIONS

SUPERFICIAL (CUTANEOUS) MYCOSES (DERMATOPHYTOSIS)

Fungi that cause primarily only superficial skin infections are called *dermatophytes.* Sources of infection include other humans (anthropophilic), animals (zoophilic), and soil (geophilic). Anthropophilic infections are sometimes epidemic and associated with only mild inflammation; zoophilic and geophilic infections are usually endemic and inflammatory in character. Susceptibility to infection with dermatophytes is determined by genetic factors as well as the immunologic status of the host.

Tinea Versicolor (Pityriasis Versicolor)

Tinea versicolor (TV) (pityriasis versicolor) is caused by the yeast phase of *Pityrosporum orbiculare* known as *Malassezia furfur.* It is a common superficial skin infection that thrives on moist, oily skin, hence its prevalence in the tropics. The lesions appear as fine, scaling, discrete, and confluent guttate macules, which, in pale skin, assume a fawn or slightly pink color and which may be slightly itchy and which in darker skin are hypopigmented (Figs. 30-1 and 30-2). Most lesions are seen on the trunk and arms, though in infants and especially immunocompromised people the infection may be widespread, extending to the face (Fig. 30-3), brows, and lids. Sites involved by this yeast infection tend not to tan well, thus remaining as relatively light spots and patches in summer, whereas in winter on skin without a tan they appear darker than the rest of the skin. The name *tinea versicolor* (variable colors) stems from this variable appearance. When there are extensive large patches of TV, it is sometimes difficult to determine which areas are involved versus which areas represent normal skin. It is then helpful to gently scrape the skin with a blade, which will reveal somewhat greasy scaling of the involved sites. Also, if the lesions have a convex border, the involved areas are usually inside the arc. Examination under a Wood's light gives a pale-yellow fluorescence. The organism is easily demonstrated under the microscope especially when the Schwartz-Lamkin stain (Fig. 30-4) is added to the specimen. *M. furfur* colonizes not only the superficial epidermis but also follicular areas, including the scalp, which is frequently the source of reinfections if only the skin is treated.

Tinea Corporis

Tinea corporis involves the trunk and extremities. Variable pruritus is common.

Individual lesions begin as red macules that extend centrifugally and superficially while healing centrally, giving a ring appearance with sharp margins (Fig. 30-5). Several lesions may coalesce to produce polycyclic patches with raised, erythematous, scaly margins.

The degree of inflammation varies according to the amount of inoculum, the organism's pathogenicity, the extent of follicular invasion, and the patient's immune status (Fig. 30-6). Sometimes, the lesion resembles a pyoderma. Occasionally, the central area does not heal; in other instances, the central area may become pigmented. Regional lymphadenopathy may occur.

Immunosuppressed patients with specific defects may develop extensive, persistent, dermal, and subcutaneous involvement manifested by nodules, abscesses, and draining sinuses.

Tinea Capitis

Tinea capitis (scalp ringworm) represents a dermatophytic scalp infection with invasion of the hair shaft. It is most often seen in children and at times in adults in whom it may be asymptomatic, providing an often overlooked source of reinfection in the family. Occasionally, it involves the eyebrow or lashes. The infection may be ectothrix, endothrix, or favic in type. Zoophilic organisms usually cause more severe inflammatory reactions, such as a kerion.

Ectothrix hair invasion is characterized by spore growth over the surface of the hair shaft. It causes often subtle scaly patches of partial alopecia, which contain many dull-gray, broken-off hairs. Occasionally, it causes a kerion, which begins as a small furuncle and progresses to form multiple follicular abscesses, discharge of pus, sinus formation, and loss of hair in the involved areas, while the surrounding hair is matted and crusted (Fig. 30-7). Untreated, a kerion persists for months and often results in scarring and permanent madarosis. Lid involvement causes lid edema and a purulent blepharitis.

In endothrix hair invasion, the arthrospores invade the hair shaft, resulting in the hair being easily broken off close to the scalp, causing classical black-dot ringworm (Fig. 30-8). (The black dots represent swollen hair shafts, which are broken off at the surface of the skin.) The black dots are seen in patches of noninflammatory areas of alopecia; infrequently, there is a low-grade folliculitis and, rarely, a kerion. Usually, multiple, scaling, angular-shaped patches of alopecia are evident.

The infected hair in favus (tinea favosa) often grows to normal length. The infection begins as a small red pimple surrounding a hair follicle. The scalp surface appears scaly and is quickly covered by a characteristic sulfur-yellow, shield-shaped, or cup-shaped crust called a scutula. Satellite lesions develop around the lesion, and each scutula is pierced by a hair shaft. The crusts eventually become confluent, forming a large yellow mass. Favus often causes scarring, atrophy, and permanent madarosis.

Tinea Barbae

Tinea barbae represents ringworm of the coarse facial hairs. It is characterized by a pustular folliculitis of the beard or moustache regions (Fig. 30-9), although sometimes it involves the lashes or eyebrows. Red, inflammatory pustules develop and discharge pus, and the area crusts. The involved hair is easily removed. Occasionally, the lesions are dry, circular, reddish, scaling areas containing lusterless stumps of hair.

Tinea Faciei

Tinea faciei encompasses dermatophyte infections of the face, excluding tinea barbae. The diagnosis is frequently initially mistaken as other entities because many times lesions lack the typical presentation of ringworm (Fig. 30-10). Among entities that tinea faciei may mimic are atopic eczema (Fig. 30-11), seborrheic dermatitis, photodermatitis and impetigo (Fig. 30-12). Failure to respond to treatment for these various other entities finally leads to the correct diagnosis, which is usually easily confirmed by finding hyphae on a potassium hydroxide (KOH) prep or culturing for the dermatophyte.

Tinea Cruris (Jock Itch)

Tinea cruris (jock itch) is a common dermatophytosis of the groin. It is seen most frequently in men, especially in warm, humid conditions. Erythematous scaling or vesicular patches with an advancing, well-defined border at times extending from the groin to the medial thighs and pubic area may be seen (Fig. 30-13). Itching is variable. Differential diagnosis includes psoriasis, in which one finds other areas of psoriasis as well; yeast intertrigo, in which lesions are usually more deeply erythematous, have small satellite scaling pustules, and often extend to the scrotum and penis,

which happens rarely, if ever, with tinea (Fig. 30-14); and erythrasma, which presents with more delicate, dry, brownish patches that usually do not itch and that, on Wood's light examination, show striking coral fluorescence (Figs. 30-15 and 30-16).

Tinea Manus (Tinea Palmaris)

Most tinea infections of the hands are confined to one palm, a phenomenon that has thus far not been satisfactorily been explained. Generally, the patient presents with slight scaling and dryness of one palm, which does not bother the patient except for the appearance (Fig. 30-17). Occasionally, one may see bilateral tinea palmaris and more inflammatory, pruritic, and fissuring lesions.

Tinea Pedis (Athlete's Foot)

Tinea pedis (athlete's foot) is the most common superficial fungal infection in man. The most frequent sites are the toe webs, especially the third one with the presenting complaint of itching. Scaling and maceration are usually evident, and secondary infection can lead to cellulitis (Fig. 30-18). Condylomata lata in secondary syphilis is occasionally misdiagnosed as athlete's foot both by the patient and occasionally by the physician (Fig. 30-19).

Another common presentation of tinea pedis is dry, slightly scaly erythema of the sole, which may extend to the edges of the foot, producing the so-called moccasin type of athlete's foot. When caused by *Tricophyton rubrum,* it is usually asymptomatic, but when the fungus is *Tricophyton mentagrophytes,* intense itching and painful vesicopustules and, at times, secondary bacterial infection can ensue (Fig. 30-20).

Onychomycosis

Tinea unguium, or onychomycosis of nails, frequently accompany tinea of other sites such as tinea palmaris or tinea pedis. Most onychomycotic fingernails are caused by true dermatophytes, whereas those of the toenails may also be due to nondermatophyte molds. There are several different types of onychomycosis. Most are distal subungual with slow destruction of the nail beginning at the distal edge (Fig. 30-21). Proximal white onychomycosis is less common and may be a cutaneous marker of AIDS.

Ocular Features of Ringworm Infections

Dermatophyte lid infections are similar to skin infections (Fig. 30-12). Individual lesions begin as red spots that extend centrifugally and superficially while healing centrally, giving a ringlike appearance with sharp margins. Several lesions may coalesce to produce a polycyclic, erythematous eruption.

Lid infections may cause a chronic papillary conjunctivitis with mild discharge or, occasionally, a severe conjunctivitis and keratitis. Favus has been reported to cause a painful, ulcerative conjunctivitis covered by a crust, fine petechiae, and superficial punctate keratitis.

Chronic dacryocystitis is extremely uncommon but has been described.

SUBCUTANEOUS FUNGAL INFECTIONS

Maduromycosis (Mycetoma)

Maduromycosis comprises any mycetoma caused by true fungi. It occurs from direct inoculation into traumatized skin. The lesions are relatively painless. Skin papules or nodules develop at the site of inoculation and are followed over many months by subcutaneous nodules that break down to form abscesses and chronically draining sinuses. Sometimes, they involve deep muscle and even bone (Fig. 30-22). The entire area becomes indurated and discolored, and skin ulcers may develop because of secondary infection. Elephantiasis of the limbs may occur from lymphatic scarring.

Maduromycosis may cause a lump of the lid or sometimes distinct nodules in the orbit. The latter leads to proptosis and orbital fistulas.

Sporotrichosis

Sporotrichosis is a chronic fungal infection, characterized by skin or subcutaneous nodules and a regional lymphangitis. There are five clinical forms, namely:

1. Lymphocutaneous (most common and often painful).
2. Fixed cutaneous (limited to the site of inoculation).
3. Mucocutaneous (rare except in disseminated disease).
4. Disseminated and extracutaneous. Dissemination usually occurs in association with systemic glucocorticoid use.
5. Pulmonary (arising from spore inhalation).

Lymphocutaneous Sporotrichosis

At first a small, hard, freely movable, nontender subcutaneous nodule develops at the site of inoculation and is quickly followed by regional lymphadenitis. The nodule becomes fixed to the overlying skin, turns red, violaceous, or black and ulcerates, discharging a thin, seropurulent discharge (Fig. 30-23). The ulcer eventually heals, but further nodules and buboes develop along the involved lymphatics, which then soften and ulcerate. Healing occurs by secondary intention and scarring, while the draining lymphatic channels are indurated and cordlike.

Fixed Cutaneous Sporotrichosis

Fixed cutaneous sporotrichosis usually involves the neck or trunk and presents as an ulcerative, verrucous, acneform,

infiltrated, or erythematous plaque, or as a scaly macular or papular rash. The skin lesions are localized to the site of inoculation, and the local lymphatics are not involved. The lesions occasionally heal spontaneously or heal only to break down again.

Mucocutaneous Sporotrichosis

The morphology is quite similar for the skin and mucous membrane lesions. Erythematous, ulcerative, or suppurative lesions develop in the mucous membranes of the mouth, pharynx, or nose and gradually become granulomatous. They typically scar and heal, causing little or no deformity. Regional lymphadenitis usually occurs.

Extracutaneous and Disseminated Sporotrichosis

Fever, anorexia, weight loss, and joint stiffness are common. Disseminated sporotrichosis is typified by scattered multiple, hard, subcutaneous nodules. Lesions of the bones of the hand, wrist, feet, ankle, forearm, leg, thigh, and ribs may occur, and usually occur from spread of skin infection. They may lead to pathologic fractures. Joint involvement is characterized by pain, swelling, effusion, and progressive limitation of movement.

Visceral involvement is quite rare in disseminated sporotrichosis and usually occurs in the presence of sarcoid, diabetes mellitus, AIDS, or long-term use of glucocorticoids or alcohol.

Meningitis is very rare and causes dizziness, headache, confusion, and weight loss.

Pulmonary Sporotrichosis

Most pulmonary sporotrichosis cases represent primary lung infection. There are two forms: (a) acute pneumonitis, or bronchitis, which later involves the apex of the lung; and (b) one that involves the tracheobronchial lymph nodes while sparing the lung parenchyma. Nodular masses, thin-walled cavities, fibrosis, and pleural effusions occur, and the infection may be fatal.

Ocular Features

Ocular adnexal infection is usually primary and arises from inoculation, whereas involvement of the globe arises from direct trauma, contiguous extension, or hematogenous dissemination.

Lid involvement is in the form of lymphocutaneous sporotrichosis or fixed cutaneous sporotrichosis (see earlier).

Conjunctival sporotrichosis begins as yellow, soft, conjunctival or limbal nodules that ulcerate and form granulomas. They cause purulent discharge and regional lymphadenitis. Occasionally, the infection causes conjunctival scarring or spreads to the sclera, causing perforation.

Other ocular findings include stromal keratitis, canaliculitis with ulceration of the wall of the canaliculus, purulent dacryocystitis, scleral infection (see earlier), orbital abscess or granuloma, uveitis, iris abscess, necrotizing retinitis, endophthalmitis, and panophthalmitis.

SYSTEMIC FUNGAL INFECTIONS

North American Blastomycosis

The initial infection in blastomycosis occurs in the respiratory tract; cutaneous, osseous, and other lesions occur from metastasis. The lid skin usually becomes involved by extension of facial lesions.

Clinical Features

Except for primary inoculation cutaneous blastomycosis, the infection begins in the lung. Metastatic spread leads to rapidly evolving multiple organ system involvement, chronic skin disease that waxes and wanes, or bone lesions that are usually associated with the skin disease. Primary inoculation cutaneous infection is self-limited and generally involves only the area of inoculation.

Primary Pulmonary Blastomycosis

Primary pulmonary blastomycosis causes a mild, progressive pulmonary infection associated with a dry cough, hoarseness, dyspnea, low-grade fever, and occasionally, pleuritic pain. Arthralgias and myalgia occasionally occur. This disease usually resolves spontaneously with a small fibrotic scar.

Infrequently, blastomycosis causes acute lobar pneumonia, acute bronchopneumonia, or chronic pulmonary infection with fever, dyspnea, weight loss, night sweats, productive cough, and increased weakness.

Inoculation (Primary Cutaneous) Blastomycosis

Inoculation (primary cutaneous) blastomycosis occurs in the laboratory, in the autopsy room, or at the mortuary. It is manifested as a mild, indurated skin ulcer with regional lymphangitis and lymphadenopathy and heals spontaneously, without dissemination.

Chronic Skin Infection

About 80% of patients have single or multiple skin lesions that begin as subcutaneous nodules or papulopustular lesions on exposed areas (e.g., face, hand, wrist, and leg) and that eventually ulcerate. The granulomatous ulcers (Fig. 30-24) have a reddish or purplish base and an overlying thick crust. The ulcer base contains black dots representing degen-

erating papillary vessels; the edges are sharp and sloping, and microabscesses are common in the periphery. Healing occurs from the center outward, leaving a thin, atrophic scar and deformity. Regional lymphadenopathy is common.

Other skin manifestations include erythema nodosum, which occasionally develops during pulmonary infection.

Osseous Blastomycosis

Single bony lesions occur from chronic, low-grade infection; multiple bony lesions from generalized systemic disease. The lesions present as a monarticular septic arthritis or an osteolytic lesion.

Systemic Blastomycosis

Systemic blastomycosis involves multiple organ systems, and the disease course is often rapid and downhill. Liver, spleen, and gastrointestinal involvement are rare. Adrenal involvement may cause Addison disease.

Central Nervous System Blastomycosis

Central nervous system blastomycosis causes confusion, aphasia, convulsions, coma, paraplegia, and hemiparesis.

Ocular Features

An ulcerative, pseudomembranous, or granulomatous conjunctivitis with seropurulent discharge is very uncommon (Fig. 30-24). Dry areas that suggest Bitot spots or small granulomata may occur on the bulbar conjunctiva. Rarely, a superficial yellowish tumor develops at the medial canthus.

Small limbal granulomata occasionally develop, then spread circumferentially around the cornea. Central corneal ulcers with hypopyon are sometimes associated with lid infection. Lesions of the lid skin are similar to other skin lesions. Small abscesses may occur around the base of the lashes. Scarring is common.

Other ocular features include dacryocystitis from infection of the skin of the face and lid; orbital cellulitis and abscess formation in systemic blastomycosis; iritis, iridocyclitis, and multifocal choroiditis with resultant scarring; iris nodules with an intense anterior chamber reaction and hypopyon; ciliary body involvement with destruction of the ciliary processes; and endophthalmitis or panophthalmitis arising from generalized or pulmonary disease.

Coccidioidomycosis

Pulmonary coccidioidomycosis is usually subclinical and self-limited. Occasionally, it presents as an acute, self-limited respiratory tract infection. A very small number develop chronic disseminated disease with visceral, skin, bone (Fig. 30-25), meningeal, and, rarely, ocular involvement. Risk factors include race (dark-skinned individuals), pregnancy, males, individuals working in dusty areas, glucocorticoid use, malignancy, and AIDS.

Immune Hypersensitivity Reactions

About 25% to 30% of patients develop an immune hypersensitivity reaction (a generalized, erythematous macular or papular rash, erythema nodosum, erythema multiforme, episcleritis, scleritis, or phlyctenular keratoconjunctivitis). Erythema nodosum develops about 1 to 2 weeks after onset of symptoms and usually involves the anterior tibia. The nodules are dusky, erythematous, and tender or painful. They vary from several millimeters to several centimeters in diameter and are firm, elastic, and deeply imbedded in the skin.

Erythema multiforme (EM) is characterized by erythematous macules that, over a period of 24 to 48 hours, develop an erythematous ring while the center assumes a dusky, edematous appearance, producing the classic "iris" or "target" lesion of EM. They may become vesicular and, in the more severe forms, progress to hemorrhagic necrotic lesions, especially at mucosal sites such as the lips, eyes, and anogenital areas. Cutaneous lesions most frequently occur over the dorsa of forearms, hands, and feet, as well as palms, elbows, knees, and soles. Mucosal involvement primarily of the mouth occurs in about 25% of patients, with up to 50% mucosal lesions in erythema multiforme bullosum (Stevens–Johnson syndrome). Arthralgias and arthritis with pain and joint stiffness (often called desert rheumatism) may also occur, usually lasting from several days to 2 weeks.

Primary Cutaneous Coccidioidomycosis

Primary cutaneous coccidioidomycosis is very rare. The chancriform lesion is painless, nodular, and ulcerated in its center. It is associated with regional adenitis.

Ocular Features—Primary Coccidioidomycosis

The ocular features include small, generalized, erythematous macules or papules; and skin lesions similar to those seen in the disseminated form of the disease.

Conjunctival involvement includes self-limited, acute or chronic follicular conjunctivitis with minimal discharge and phlyctenules of the conjunctiva, limbus, or cornea (Chapter 26).

Other features include simple or nodular episcleritis, nodular scleritis, and endophthalmitis.

Clinical Features, Secondary Coccidioidomycosis

Less than 10% of patients with symptomatic coccidioidomycosis develop residual pulmonary disease with chronic cavitation or with the appearance of a tumor (coc-

cidioidoma). The cavitation is usually single, is thin-walled, and causes very few symptoms.

Infrequently, the pulmonary infection is progressive, and extrapulmonary extension may occur.

Secondary dissemination usually occurs from overwhelming exposure to the organism, especially if other risk factors are present (see earlier). Dissemination may lead to acute or chronic meningitis, cutaneous and subcutaneous abscesses, or multiple organ infection. This usually occurs within several weeks of the primary infection and often rapidly progresses to death.

Chronic Cutaneous Coccidioidomycosis

Chronic skin infections with coccidioidomycosis occur primarily in native Americans and Afro-Americans as well as patients of Mexican and Filipino extraction. The lesions may appear on the trunk, face (especially nasolabial folds), scalp, neck, and extremities. They are noninflammatory and gradually enlarge to form verrucous granulomas. Some lesions remain small and resolve to form atrophic scars; others develop into indolent draining skin lesions, especially over joints. Ulcerated skin lesions arise from infection of the underlying tissues.

Lid (Fig. 30-26), brow, and canthal granulomas similar to other facial lesions occur as part of the chronic cutaneous disease. They represent individual lesions or part of extensive facial involvement and are usually found in dark-skinned patients. Occasionally, a semifluctuating mass develops that drains pus.

Mucous membrane involvement may also occur in coccidioidomycosis (Fig. 30-27).

Ocular Features—Chronic Ocular Coccidioidomycosis
Conjunctiva
Conjunctival coccidioidal granulomas (Figs. 30-28 and 30-29) usually occur on the palpebral conjunctiva. They often resemble a chronic chalazion and are associated with a grossly enlarged preauricular node. The granulomas may be multiple and, especially in younger patients, are often associated with follicular conjunctivitis.

Conjunctival phlyctenules occasionally develop and resemble the phlyctenules seen in the primary disease but are not recurrent.

Uvea
Granulomatous iridocyclitis or panuveitis that is indistinguishable from sarcoid may be seen and will include granulomatous keratic precipitates in Arlt triangle, anterior and posterior synechiae, cataracts, vitreitis, papillitis, and vasculitis.

Choroidal involvement is often in the form of multifocal areas of choroiditis, which, upon healing, leave punched-out chorioretinal scars.

Other ocular findings include pannus and crescentic-shaped, superficial epithelial keratitis; necrotizing scleral granuloma associated with severe granulomatous iritis; chronic granulomatous iridocyclitis; iris nodules; juxtapapillary focal chorioretinitis; multifocal areas of choroiditis (Fig. 30-30); retinal scars; retinal infiltrates; hemorrhages; sheathing of retinal vessels; telangiectatic capillary changes; macular edema; proliferative retinitis; serous retinal detachment; endophthalmitis; orbital granuloma; and papilledema.

Cryptococcosis

Primary cryptococcosis almost always occurs in the lung. Cutaneous involvement is usually a component of disseminated infection but in exceptional cases is a localized process. It is an important complication in immunosuppressed patients, especially those with AIDS, where the infection may progress to systemic and even fulminant disease.

Clinical Manifestations

The major clinical forms of disease are pulmonary, central nervous system, cutaneous, mucocutaneous, osseous, and visceral. Chronic infection is very uncommon but occasionally occurs in normal patients. It is manifested by cutaneous, systemic, or meningitic manifestations and usually responds readily to treatment.

Primary lung infections are usually subclinical and the lesions are found only on x-ray. In severe infections, the patient may have a high fever and unilateral, bilateral, or miliary pulmonary involvement.

Central nervous system involvement causes headache, dizziness, vertigo, and fever. Signs of meningitis and pyramidal tract involvement may also be present. A single localized granuloma causes manifestations of a space-occupying lesion.

Chronic bone infections cause swelling and pain, usually in areas of bony prominences, cranial bones, and vertebrae. Joint involvement occurs by direct extension of infection.

Disseminated cryptococcal infections involve any organ system, especially the heart, prostate, testis, and eye.

Skin Features

Cryptococcal skin lesions present as papules, nodules, infiltrative plaques, pustules, ulcers, chancres, or subcutaneous abscesses and usually occur around the nose or mouth. The ulcers often have a punched-out appearance with a rolled edge, gelatinous to the touch. Approximately 50% of patients with HIV will develop lesions resembling molluscum contagiosum, often with a central hemorrhagic crust.

Primary cutaneous cryptococcal lesions are very rare and have a chancriform appearance with regional lymphadenopathy.

Mucocutaneous lesions (Fig. 30-31) are nodular, are granulomatous, or present as a superficial or deep ulcer.

Ocular Features

Lid infections in immunosuppressed patients are usually fulminant but may be prolonged. Occasionally, the skin of the lid, brow, or forehead is involved in disseminated cryptococcosis. The lesions are similar to the skin lesions (see earlier). Other ocular findings include the following:

1. Extensive and deep corneal infiltration, resulting in minimal scarring.
2. Chronic dacryocystitis.
3. Orbital cellulitis.
4. Severe anterior uveitis with secondary glaucoma.
5. Bilateral chorioretinitis with extensive retinal detachment and single or multiple focal lesions.
6. Retinal lesion with overlying vitreitis.
7. Endogenous endophthalmitis leading to panophthalmitis.
8. Papilledema and optic atrophy.

Histoplasmosis

Histoplasmosis usually involves the lungs. It is usually chronic and progressive but is rarely fatal.

Clinical Manifestations

Most patients experience asymptomatic infection. Some develop acute or chronic pulmonary symptoms, and only a few develop acute or chronic disseminated disease.

Acute pulmonary infections are characterized by fever, cough, congestion, and sometimes pleurisy. Chronic pulmonary histoplasmosis has many characteristics of tuberculosis and occurs primarily in adults.

Acute disseminated histoplasmosis usually occurs in AIDS patients, causing fever, loss of appetite, manifestations of pulmonary infection (e.g., consolidation), and hepatosplenomegaly. It often leads to skin and mucous membrane changes.

Chronic disseminated disease develops months or years following the acute infection. The patient may present with a chronic oral (Fig. 30-32) and/or laryngeal ulcer and often has Addison disease from adrenal gland involvement.

Skin Features

Primary cutaneous histoplasmosis is uncommon but arises from skin inoculation. The lesion presents as a nodule or ulcer associated with regional lymphadenopathy. AIDS patients develop multiple, small skin nodules.

Sometimes erythema multiforme or erythema nodosum develops a few weeks after onset of the acute pulmonary infection.

Ocular Features

The "presumed ocular histoplasmosis syndrome" (Fig. 30-33) is characterized by multifocal choroiditis without overlying retinal or vitreous reaction. The focal areas eventually evolve into atrophic scars with a characteristic central or eccentric fleck of pigment. Subretinal neovascularization may lead to loss of central vision from serous detachment and progressive scar formation. Peripapillary scars may also occur.

Histoplasmosis may also cause an infectious granulomatous uveitis and retinitis.

African Histoplasmosis

Patients in sub-Saharan Africa occasionally develop characteristic cutaneous lesions, associated with lymphadenopathy, and bone and other visceral involvement. The lung is usually spared.

Skin nodules, papules, or ulcers develop at the site of infection. Sometimes the lesions resemble molluscum contagiosum nodules. The regional lymph nodes are markedly enlarged and frequently soften from liquefaction.

Infrequently, patients have developed a swelling over the upper eyelid. Other findings have included a suppurative dacryoadenitis and orbital or orbital bone involvement.

Rhinosporidium Infection

Rhinosporidiosis is a chronic granulomatous, mucocutaneous disease typified by papillomas, wartlike lesions, or large, highly vascularized and friable polyps. It usually infects the nasal mucous membranes but may involve the lid margin, conjunctiva (especially the inner canthal region), sclera, lacrimal system, ears, mouth, pharynx, larynx, vagina, penis, anus, and skin. The disease is endemic in Sri Lanka and India, and is also seen in Argentina, Brazil, Mexico, and Cuba. Occasional cases have been reported in Italy, England, and southern areas of the United States.

Clinical Manifestations

The infection is usually confined to the local area of infection, sparing the lymph nodes and deep tissue. Rarely, it infects the lung, liver, spleen, other viscera, striated muscle, brain, or bone.

Nasal infection begins with symptoms of coryza and a foreign-body sensation, followed by mild to intense pruritus, obstruction of nasal breathing, blood-tinged nasal discharge, and occasionally, epistaxis. The most common sites of nasal infection are the septum, inferior turbinate, and floor of the nose. At first, there is a pink or red, sessile growth composed of granulation tissue that later becomes pedunculated and polypoid in appearance. The lesion is friable and often lobulated, giving the appearance of a cauliflower. As the growth becomes vascularized, it becomes deep red in color, and hemorrhages occur in its substance. If viewed closely, numerous white spherules may be seen studding its surface.

Tumors of the superior part of the nose may spread to the nasopharynx, producing nasal obstruction and difficulty in swallowing. Their appearance is similar to other nasal lesions. Pharyngeal lesions are usually associated with nasal involvement and cause dyspnea and dysphagia. Rhinosporidiosis may also involve the hard palate, uvula, epiglottis, and larynx.

Anal, vaginal, and penile lesions resemble rectal or meatal polyps, hemorrhoids, or condyloma. External ear lesions resemble aural polyps.

Skin Lesions

Most skin lesions are associated with infection of the contiguous mucous membranes. Solitary skin lesions have been found on the scalp and abdomen, and multiple skin lesions without mucous membrane involvement have also been reported. They are relatively asymptomatic unless repeatedly traumatized or secondarily infected, at which time they cause pain and discomfort.

The lesion begins as a papule that develops into a verrucous, friable, occasionally pedunculated lesion. Ulceration and secondary bacterial infection are common. Subcutaneous lesions arise from hematogenous dissemination, feel firm or hard, and may or may not involve the overlying skin.

Ocular Manifestations

Lid margin (Fig. 30-34) and conjunctival lesions appear as small, red, freely movable, papillomatous, pedunculated growths that may become verrucous. They are frequently flattened between the eyelid and globe. Yellow and white dots representing the sporangia may be evident in the tumor mass.

About two-thirds of ocular infections involve the conjunctiva (usually the tarsal conjunctiva and less frequently the limbus, caruncle, or canthus). The lesions are often small or flat, pedunculated, freely movable, pink or red in color, and granular in appearance. Sometimes they resemble a ruptured chalazion.

The scleral lesions are similar to the conjunctival lesions.

Rhinosporidiosis may also infect the canaliculi, lacrimal sac, and orbit.

Paracoccidioidomycosis (South American Blastomycosis)

Paracoccidioidomycosis usually involves males in their second to fifth decade.

Clinical Manifestations

The disease infects the skin, mucous membranes, lymph nodes, and internal organs, and is only slowly progressive. Pulmonary infection is the most common and causes a mild productive cough. Hepatosplenomegaly, ulcers of the upper gastrointestinal tract, destruction of the adrenal glands, and central nervous system involvement may occur. The lymph nodes draining ulcerative areas such as the nasopharynx and pharynx enlarge, suppurate, and drain, forming chronic draining sinuses. They are sometimes enlarged early in the disease and are often painful. In some instances, suppuration and drainage of the involved lymph node through the skin are the earliest manifestation of the infection.

Skin Features

Skin lesions preferentially occur around the mouth and may arise by extension of the oral and pharyngeal mucosal infection. They are characterized by a necrotic central crater and a hard hyperkeratotic border.

Nasal and oropharyngeal ulceration is usually the first manifestation of paracoccidioidomycosis. Lesions may be seen at the mucocutaneous border, or satellite lesions may occur from autoinoculation. The oral ulcers are painful and often present as a "mulberry-like" erosion because of their granulomatous character. Progressive ulceration may cause extensive destruction of the larynx, epiglottis, uvula, and tongue. Gum lesions cause loss of the teeth. Mucous membrane lesions also occur in the anus.

The lid lesions usually involve the lower lid and are similar to other skin lesions.

OPPORTUNISTIC FUNGI

Candidosis (Moniliasis)

Candidosis encompasses a diverse group of clinical infections. Cutaneous lesions, thrush, onychia, and paronychia are common in the very old or very young, the very ill or debilitated (e.g., diabetics, patients with leukemia, AIDS), and those with chronic mucocutaneous candidiasis. Systemic candidosis often occurs in immunosuppressed patients and in those receiving broad-spectrum antibiotics or intravenous injections.

Most infections remain localized to the site of origin, and systemic invasion is unusual.

Clinical Manifestations

Superficial Infections

Small numbers of *Candida* are often found on the mucosal surfaces of apparently normal patients. Moderate to severe local infection usually occurs from excessive numbers of organisms. Invasion and dissemination may occur in immunocompromised patients or those in whom the nor-

mal defense mechanisms of the body are bypassed (e.g., intravenous injections). Oropharyngeal infections occur in patients with AIDS (Fig. 30-35), those who are immunosuppressed from other causes, diabetics, and those on long-term antibiotic therapy.

Thrush usually occurs in the first few weeks of life, in neutropenic patients, or in those with AIDS. It is characterized by a sharply defined, creamy-white membranous plaque that, when removed, leaves a moist, reddish, macerated base, often, with small bleeding areas. Areas of involvement include the buccal mucosa, tongue, gums, palate, and occasionally, pharynx or palate.

Acute atrophic candidosis causes pain. The tongue appears smooth and may have localized erosions. Cheilitis also occurs.

Candidal leukoplakia resembles other forms of leukoplakia. The lesions are firm, irregular, persistent white patches of the buccal mucosa, tongue, and other areas of the mouth. A small rim of erythema usually surrounds the leukoplakic patch.

Chronic atrophic candidosis is usually found in patients who wear dentures. It is usually located on the upper gums and palate and is characterized by a variable bright red or dusky erythema at the margin of the denture area, edema, shiny and atrophic-appearing epithelium, and angular cheilitis.

Candida is a common cause of angular stomatitis or perlèche with cracking and fissuring at the angles of the mouth.

Esophageal infection causes severe retrosternal pain and dysphagia (Fig. 30-35).

Vaginal infection may spread to the perianal skin or groins. *Candida balanitis* may also involve the scrotum (Fig. 30-36).

Skin Features

Candidal skin infection may be primary or may occur in chronic mucocutaneous candidiasis.

Primary skin infections usually occur around the nails and in the intertriginous areas. Candidal intertrigo is common in obese patients and is an important cutaneous marker for diabetes. Frequent sites include inframammary, inguinal, and axillary areas. Congenital candidosis is present at birth or develops within a few hours of birth. The lesions begin as diffuse, pinkish maculopapules that quickly become vesicular and then pustular or bullous in character. Occasionally, it affects the entire skin surface, including the palms and soles. Healing occurs with desquamation.

Candidosis of the diaper area (Fig. 30-37) is manifested by erythema or, in some instances, subcorneal pustules, satellite lesions, and a fringed border. Lesions of the hand probably arise from oral candidosis in a thumb sucker.

Skin lesions associated with systemic candidosis usually begin as erythematous macules, which become papular or nodular and have a pale center. Sometimes ecthyma gangrenosum–like lesions occur, and frequently the hair follicles of the coarse, hair-bearing areas are invaded.

Infection around the nails presents as an acute (Fig. 30-38) or chronic paronychia with marked tenderness, sometimes with pain, swelling, redness, and occasionally, scaling. It begins with erythema and moist exudation in the skinfold with a discharge of small amounts of creamy white pus. Secondary mixed infection with bacteria soon change the color to yellow (*Staphylococcus*) or green (*Pseudomonas*). The paronychial tissue is boggy and painful to pressure. The lateral borders of the nail slowly erode with gradual thickening and brownish discoloration of the proximal and lateral nail plate. Candidal paronychia occurs most often in persons whose hands are frequently moist, such as bartenders, dishwashers, food handlers, and young mothers with twins.

Chronic Mucocutaneous Candidiasis

Chronic mucocutaneous candidiasis (CMC) usually begins in childhood. It is autosomal recessive or dominant. Diffuse CMC is autosomal dominant and represents the most severe form. Patients often develop bronchiectasis and other systemic infections, such as miliary tuberculosis and cryptococcosis. Many die in childhood.

The candidiasis endocrinopathy syndrome [chronic mucocutaneous candidiasis, hypothyroidism, adrenal cortical failure (Addison disease), and keratoconjunctivitis] or type I autoimmune polyglandular syndrome usually develops in early childhood. Other findings include alopecia, vitiligo, gonadal failure, chronic active hepatitis, autoimmune thyroid disease, and insulin-dependent diabetes mellitus.

Chronic mucocutaneous candidiasis occurs in four clinical forms, namely:

1. Chronic oral candidal leukoplakia (as described earlier) sometimes associated with chronic hypertrophic changes.
2. Chronic localized mucocutaneous candidiasis.
3. Chronic localized mucocutaneous candidiasis associated with candidal granulomas of the face (Fig. 30-39) paronychial areas.
4. Chronic localized mucocutaneous candidosis beginning in the first decade. Chronic localized mucocutaneous candidosis that begins in the first decade usually involves the oral mucosa, then extends to involve the skin (Fig. 30-40.) It may also involve the larynx, esophagus, and vagina.

Deep (Systemic) Infections

Systemic infection arises from intestinal tract invasion; from use of contaminated needles, solutions, or intravenous catheters; or from cardiovascular surgery. Multiple organ systems are usually involved.

Candidal septicemia causes chills; high-spiking fever; prostration; hypotension; erythematous, maculopapular rash of the trunk and extremities; muscle tenderness; and oral and esophageal involvement. Pulmonary infiltrates may be evident on x-ray, and retinal lesions develop 1 to 6 weeks later.

Candidal endocarditis is clinically similar to bacterial endocarditis, with the exception that the major emboli often occlude medium-sized arteries of the brain, spleen, kidneys, and extremities. Petechiae and splenomegaly are common.

Pulmonary involvement as a primary nonhematogenous infection is very rare. Asymptomatic urethritis and cystitis sometimes occur, and candidal pyelonephritis causes fever, nausea, vomiting, flank pain, and, in some instances, dysuria. The kidneys are usually involved from hematogenous dissemination.

Candida only rarely infects the bones and joints. The manifestations suggest osteomyelitis. Hematogenous dissemination occasionally leads to central nervous system involvement.

Ocular Features

Candidal blepharitis is usually associated with use of broad-spectrum antibiotics (Figs. 30-41 to 30-43). It resembles staphylococcal blepharitis, causing discharge, erythema, thickening of the lid margin, ulcers, collarettes, canities, and broken, shortened, and absent lashes. Exceptionally, there are vesicles that later pustulate. The presence of small granulomas near the lash follicles serves as a useful clue of a candidal infection. Rarely, candidal blepharitis resembles ringworm (see ringworm). The id reaction sometimes occurs in the skin of the eyelid. It is pruritic, eczematoid, or vesicular in character.

Candidal conjunctivitis produces a picture similar to thrush or a follicular or ulcerative conjunctivitis, with the latter leading to scarring.

Other ocular features include corneal ulcers similar to other fungal ulcers, a chronic epithelial keratitis, superficial corneal vascularization and infiltrates reminiscent of phlyctenulosis, canaliculitis, orbital abscess, severe iritis, iridocyclitis with edema of the retina and optic nerve, chronic uveitis, and papillitis or papilledema.

Aspergillosis

Aspergillosis represents a spectrum of diseases, including toxicity from ingestion of contaminated food, allergic reactions, colonization in debilitated tissue and preformed cavities without actual invasion, invasive infections of lungs and various organs, and dissemination. Less common forms of human infection include mycetomas, otomycosis, corneal ulcers, endophthalmitis, and nasoorbital infection. The host–parasite reaction helps to determine the type of disease produced. Pulmonary disease is the most common.

Clinical Manifestations

Invasive Aspergillosis

Invasive pulmonary aspergillosis is uncommon and usually occurs in patients with lymphoma, leukemias, or lung conditions, as noted previously. It causes manifestations of a pneumonitis with fever, cough, respiratory distress, and leukocytosis. As the infection becomes chronic, recurrent hemoptysis is common.

Disseminated Aspergillosis

Disseminated aspergillosis is probably related to antibiotics, glucocorticoids, or immunosuppressives. The patient is acutely ill and has fever, arthralgia, and skin eruptions. Areas of dissemination include the lungs, central nervous system, kidney, and bone.

Nasal-Orbital Aspergillosis

Granulomas occur in the nasal cavity, paranasal sinuses, orbit, brain, eye, or cavernous sinus. They slowly enlarge and frequently simulate neoplastic lesions. Abscesses cause severe pain, lid and conjunctival edema, marked proptosis, and concomitant sinusitis (see "Ocular Manifestations" later).

Cutaneous Aspergillosis

The skin becomes infected by inoculation, during dissemination, or by colonization of third degree burns (Fig. 30-44). Inoculation leads to erythematous or violaceous edematous skin nodules or plaques. They usually ulcerate and develop a black eschar. The skin lesions from dissemination begin as small, red, discrete papules that pustulate.

Ocular Manifestations

Ocular findings include the following:

1. Severe lid edema associated with *Aspergillus* orbital abscess.
2. A localized lid aspergilloma from direct inoculation that presents as a chronic ulcerative, granulomatous papilloma.
3. Chronic granulomatous lid lesions in disseminated aspergillosis.
4. Conjunctival chemosis with orbital abscesses.
5. *Aspergillus* conjunctivitis associated with canaliculitis.
6. *Aspergillus* corneal ulcer.
7. A paracentral corneal infiltrate that quickly ulcerates and vascularizes, producing a fascicular keratitis.
8. Granulomatous dacryoadenitis that results from nasoorbital aspergillosis. A canaliculitis.
9. Progressive scleritis.
10. A slowly progressive orbital granuloma or abscess in the nasoorbital form of infection.
11. Optic atrophy in orbital aspergillosis.
12. Multifocal choroiditis with yellow-white choroidal lesions and clouding of the overlying vitreous.
13. Retinal vasculitis.
14. Endophthalmitis.

Mucormycosis

Mucormycosis, zygomycosis, or phycomycosis is the most common fungal orbital infection and often causes death. It occurs in poorly controlled diabetic patients in ketoacidosis, cirrhotics, and patients on treatment for leukemia, lymphoma, or terminal carcinomatosis, especially if chemotherapy or glucocorticoid therapy is being given. Other associated conditions include malnutrition, thermal burns, severe gastroenteritis, and renal failure.

Clinical Manifestations

Mucormycosis usually causes an acute orbital apex syndrome, cerebral infarction, and contralateral hemiplegia. Other findings include coma, nuchal rigidity, and involvement of the 8th through 12th cranial nerves. Prodromal symptoms include headache, lethargy, facial pain, lid swelling, periorbital numbness, tearing, blurred vision, rhinorrhea, nasal stuffiness, sinusitis, pharyngitis, and epistaxis. The patient is often semicomatose or comatose.

Skin Features

Cutaneous mucormycosis arises from extension of nasal mucormycosis or develops in association with burn infections and is usually limited to cellulitis. Localized subcutaneous granulomatous infections by *Absidia* spp. may occur with no evidence of underlying disease.

Facial Features

Facial anhidrosis and pain are common. The hard and soft palates are markedly swollen; the septum and turbinates may become necrotic; the cheek may be hypesthetic. A black nasal turbinate is very suggestive of rhinomucormycosis, and a copious purulosanguineous exudate drains from the nose. Necrosis of the nasal mucosa and perforation of the nasal septum occur.

Ocular Features

Orbital mucormycosis is usually acute and frequently fulminating (Fig. 30-45). It is characterized by:

1. Severe lid edema, ptosis, proptosis, and limited extraocular movements.
2. Ecchymosis, gangrene, and necrosis of the periocular tissue.
3. Involvement of the 7th cranial nerve with inability to close the lids.
4. Conjunctival hyperemia, chemosis, necrosis, subconjunctival hemorrhages, and purulent discharge.
5. Decreased corneal sensation, corneal edema, and ulceration.
6. Scleral infection.

Thrombosis of the orbital vessels causes ischemic necrosis and rapid development of a unilateral orbital apex syndrome with involvement of 2nd, 3rd, 4th, 5th, and 6th cranial nerves. Other manifestations of intraorbital involvement include cavernous sinus thrombosis, thrombosis of the ophthalmic artery or its branches, involvement of the orbital bones, and infection of the extraocular muscles.

Iridocyclitis and anterior chamber exudates are common. The organism frequently invades the eye, and central retinal arterial thrombosis and retinal infarction have been observed. Optic neuritis and ischemic infarction of the optic nerve are frequent complications.

Cephalosporium Spp.

Cephalosporium infections are uncommon. The organism occasionally produces maduromycosis (see earlier).

Cephalosporium has been found to cause blepharitis, conjunctivitis, canaliculitis, purulent dacryocystitis, and corneal ulcers.

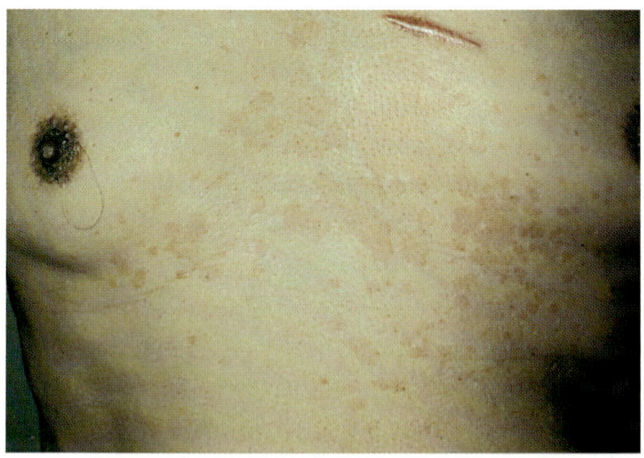

FIGURE 30-1. Tinea versicolor in a light-skinned patient without a tan. Lesions appear as pale pink discrete and confluent macules.

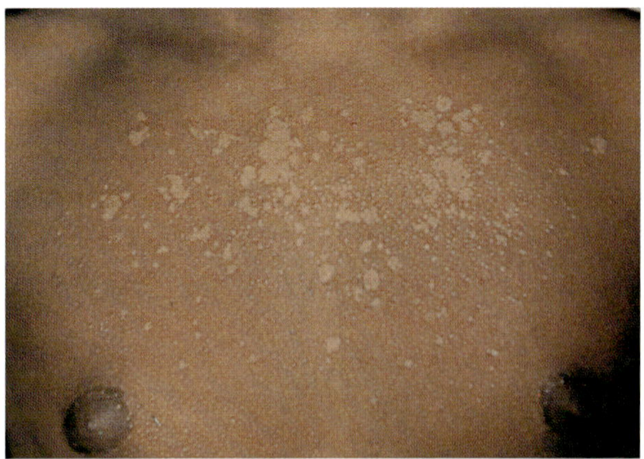

FIGURE 30-2. Hypopigmented scaly macules of tinea versicolor in dark skin.

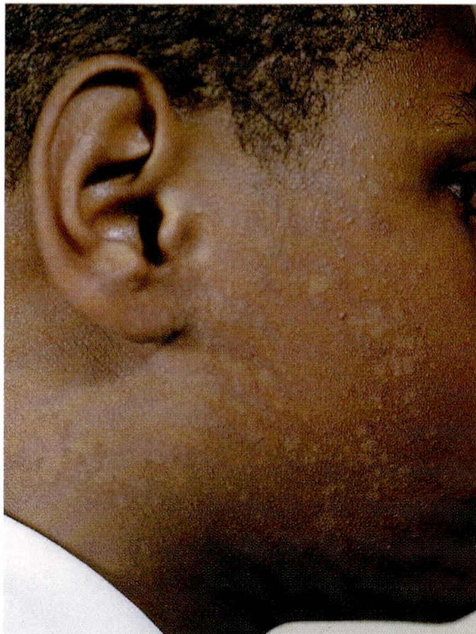

FIGURE 30-3. Tinea versicolor of the face with lesions extending to brow. The scalp is often colonized by the fungus and can be the source of recurrent infections with tinea versicolor if not treated as well as the skin.

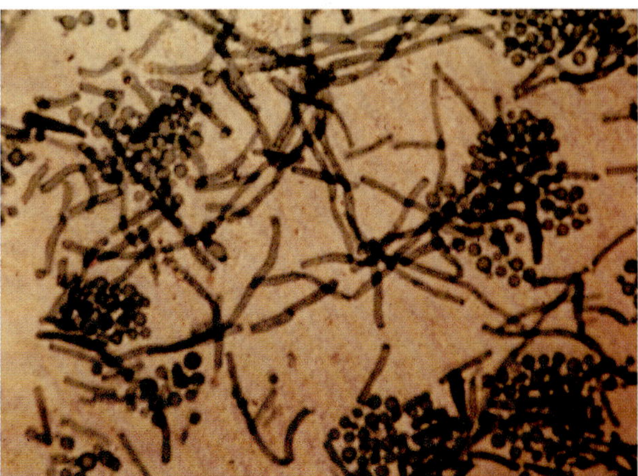

FIGURE 30-4. Short, thick fungal hyphae and clusters of spores giving the "meatballs and spaghetti" appearance of *Malassezia furfur* on a skin scraping stained with Schwartz–Lamkin.

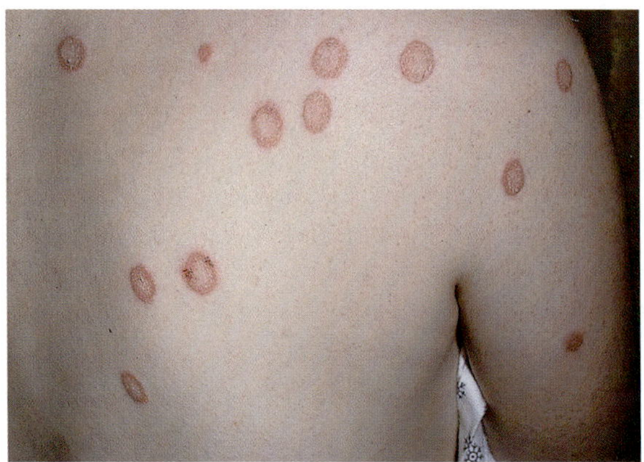

FIGURE 30-5. Tinea corporis with typical annular lesions ("ringworm") in young girl who slept with her newly acquired kittens, a common source of this infection. Note the inflammatory reaction, which is more often seen when the source of the tinea is zoophilic.

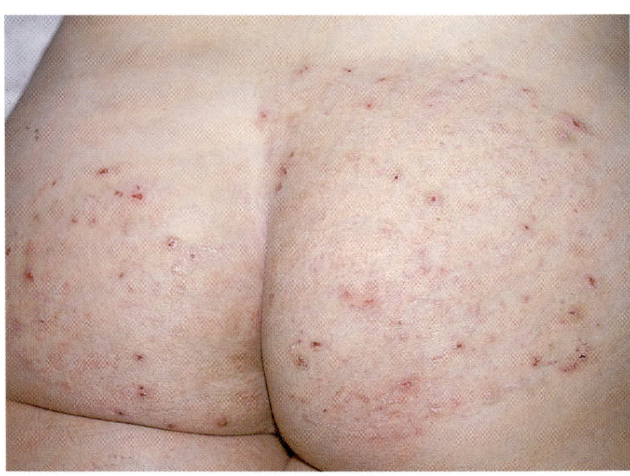

FIGURE 30-6. Tinea corporis treated as eczema with topical steroids for 2 years by her physician. Note the sharp annular margin, which should alert the examiner to the correct diagnosis of tinea.

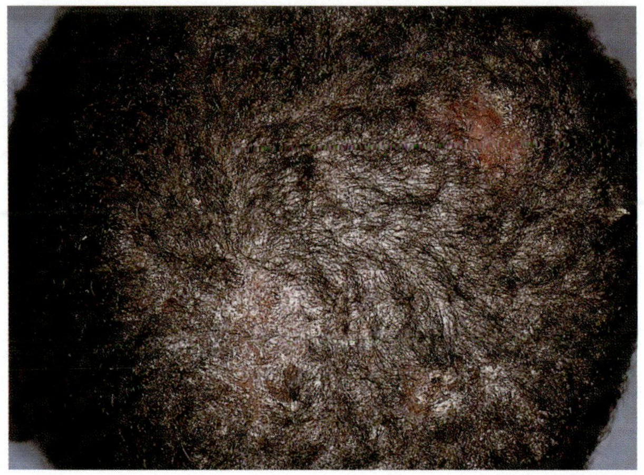

FIGURE 30-7. Kerion. Painful, multiple oozing and crusting accompanied by scaling and hair loss had plagued this 6-year-old boy from Eritrea for more than half a year.

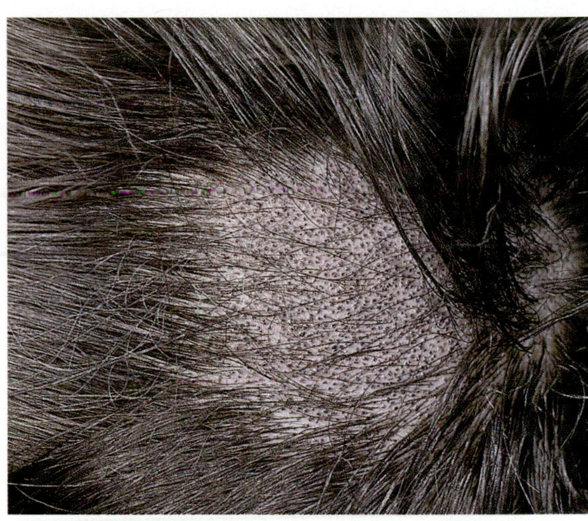

FIGURE 30-8. "Black dot" ringworm. The area of alopecia is studded with black dots from infected hairs broken off at the surface of the scalp. Most of these infections seen in the United States are caused by *Trichophyton tonsurans*.

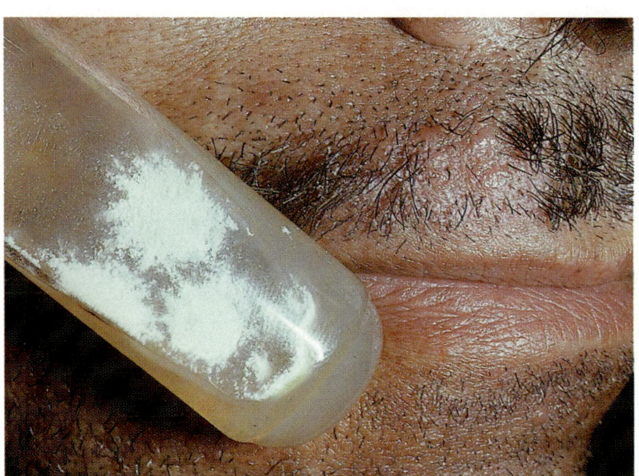

FIGURE 30-9. Tinea barbae showing improvement after 2 weeks of topical antifungal therapy. Note culture showing *Trichophyton mentagrophytes,* granular type.

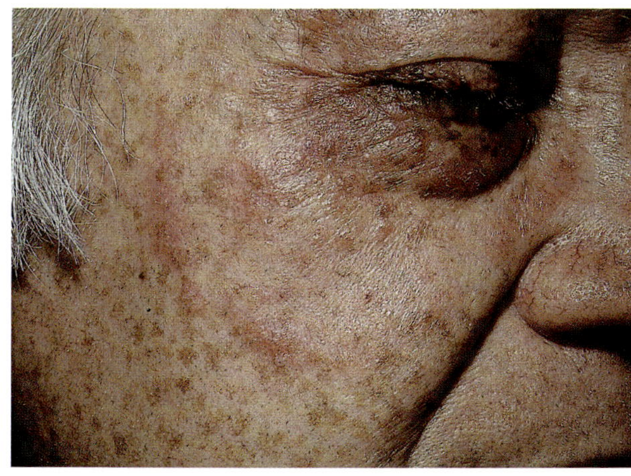

FIGURE 30-10. Tinea faciei. Note arcuate inferior margin bordering these scattered erythematous papules extending onto the eyelid.

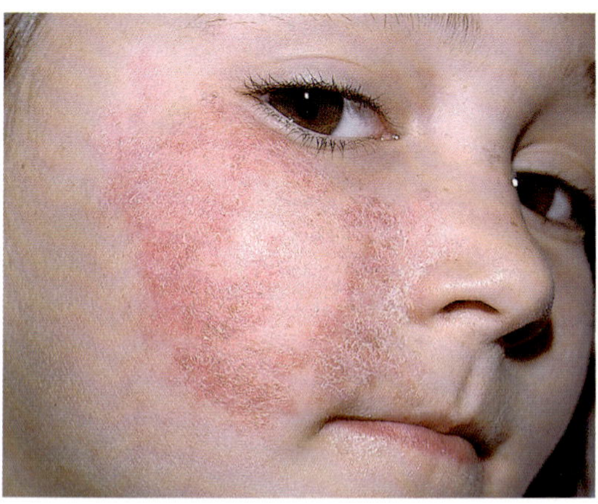

FIGURE 30-11. Tinea faciei originally misdiagnosed as an inflamed eczema by the patient's dermatologist. Failure to respond to treatment with mild topical steroids and additional history of exposure to a pet gave the correct diagnosis.

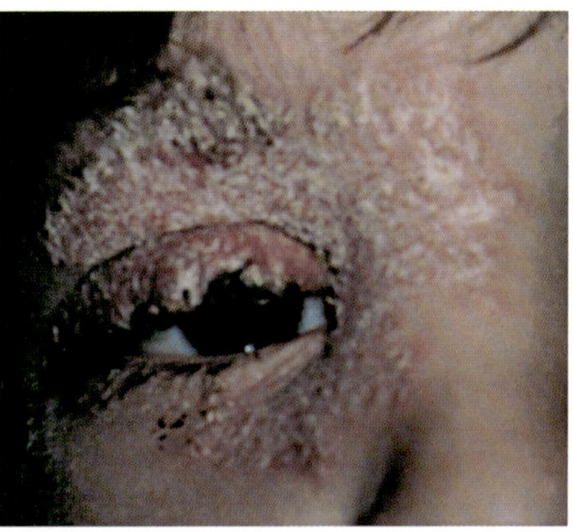

FIGURE 30-12. Tinea faciei extending to the eyelid. The marked inflammatory reaction is characteristic of dermatophyte infections transmitted by animals (zoophilic), in the case of this 3-year-old boy, from his pet rabbit.

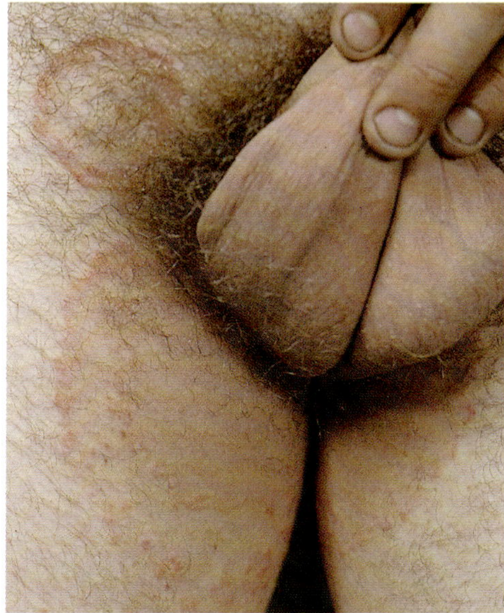

FIGURE 30-13. Tinea cruris showing classic annular and bordered lesions. Note absence of extension to scrotum, which is rarely affected by tinea but often by yeast infection (see Fig. 30-14).

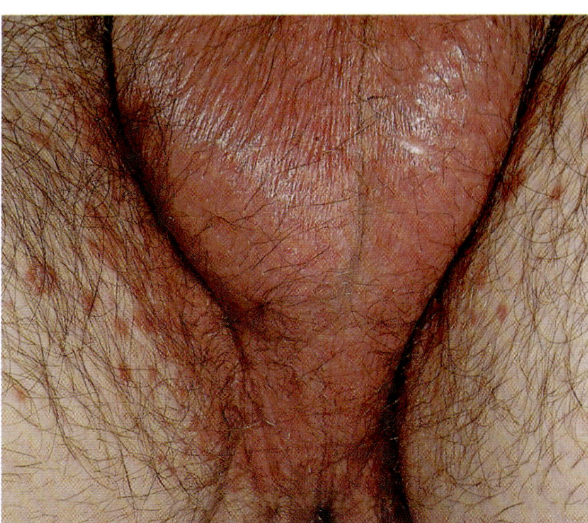

FIGURE 30-14. Candidal (yeast) intertrigo. Note deeper erythema than in tinea cruris (Fig. 30-13) as well as presence of small satellite scaling papulopustular lesions. Psoriasis may closely resemble this picture.

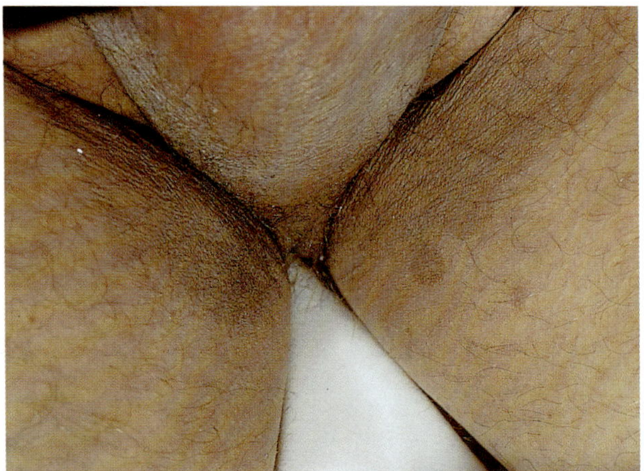

FIGURE 30-15. Erythrasma showing characteristic pale brown delicate scaling patches.

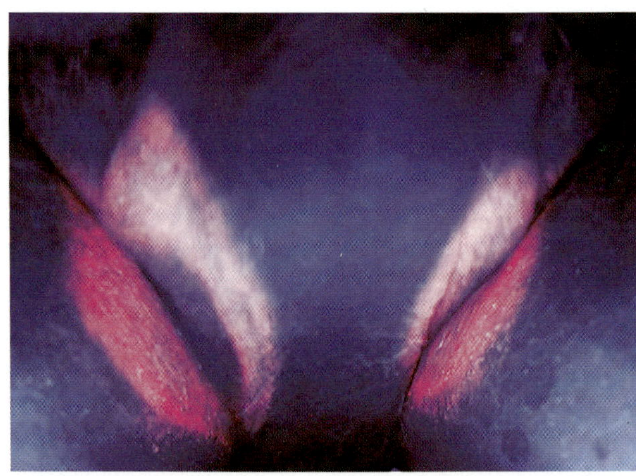

FIGURE 30-16. Erythrasma of genitocrural creases showing striking coral red fluorescence on Wood's light examination. The fluorescence is due to the presence of porphyrins, which, when washed off, do not fluoresce.

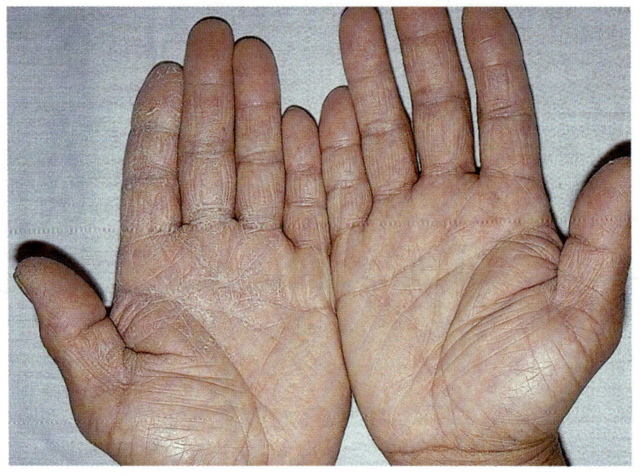

FIGURE 30-17. Tinea palmaris (*T. manum*) manifest by mild scaling of one palm. Typically, only one palm and both soles are affected ("one-palm, two-foot disease").

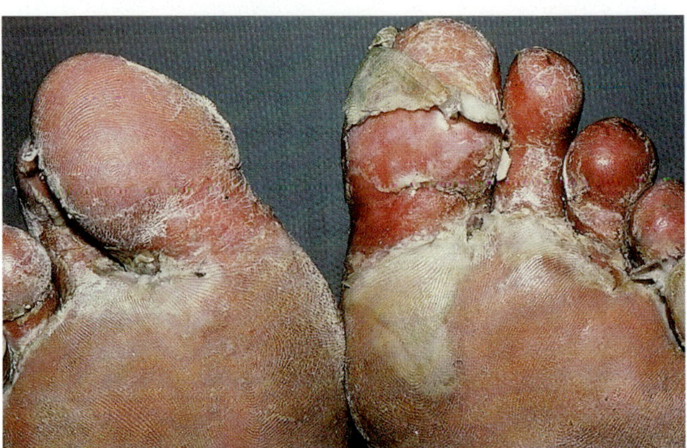

FIGURE 30-18. Tinea pedis with secondary bacterial infection resulting from overtreatment with Clorox soaks.

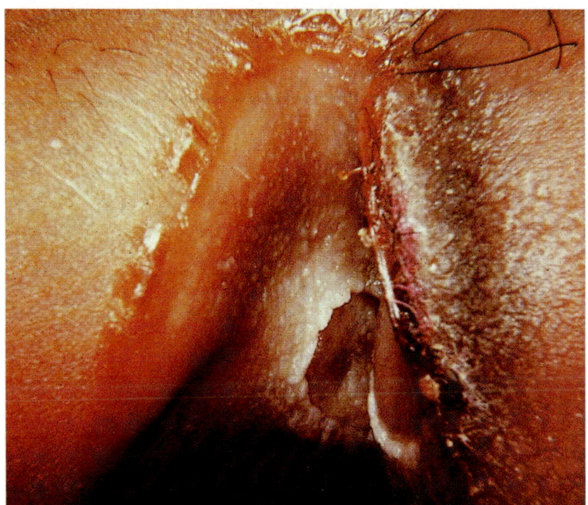

FIGURE 30-19. *Condylomata lata* (secondary syphilis) of toe web treated as athlete's foot with Gentian violet by the patient.

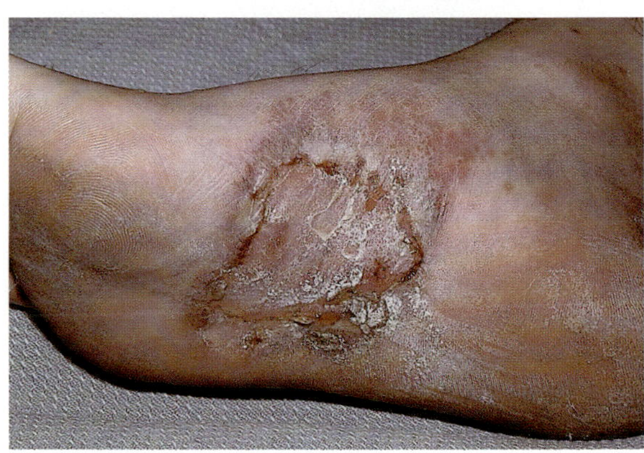

FIGURE 30-20. Tinea pedis, vesiculobullous type, with secondary cellulitis. Most of these types of tinea pedis are caused by *Trichophyton mentagrophytes*.

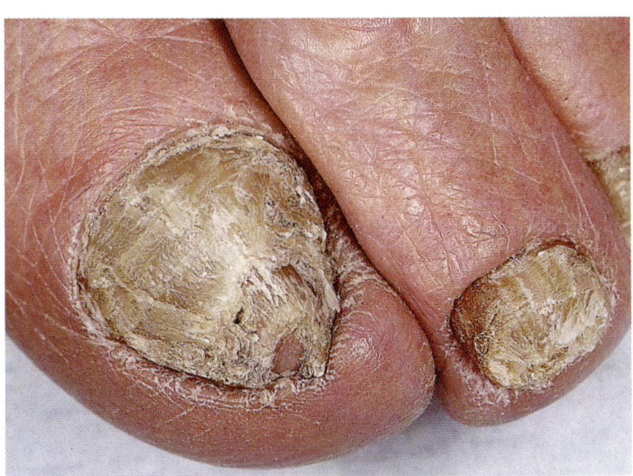

FIGURE 30-21. Onychomycosis of toenails. Newer oral therapies, though expensive, have changed the outlook for this common annoying and, at times, painful condition.

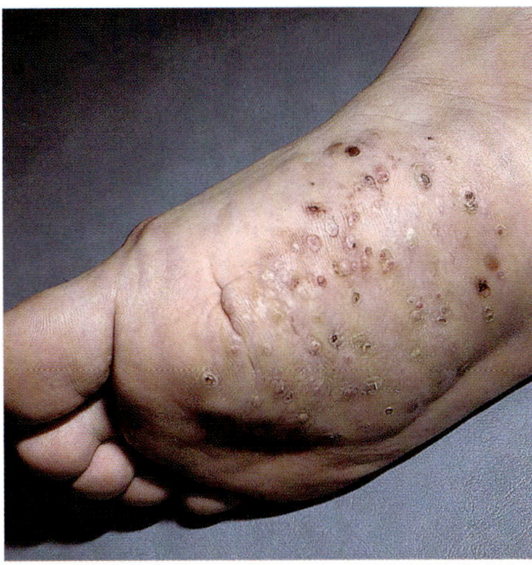

FIGURE 30-22. Nocardial mycetoma in a 35-year-old athlete who used to run barefoot in his native Mexico. He had been plagued by this slowly enlarging, painful boggy mass with multiple small draining sinuses for several years. His nocardial infection was complicated by osteomyelitis of the foot which fortunately responded to appropriate intravenous antifungal therapy.

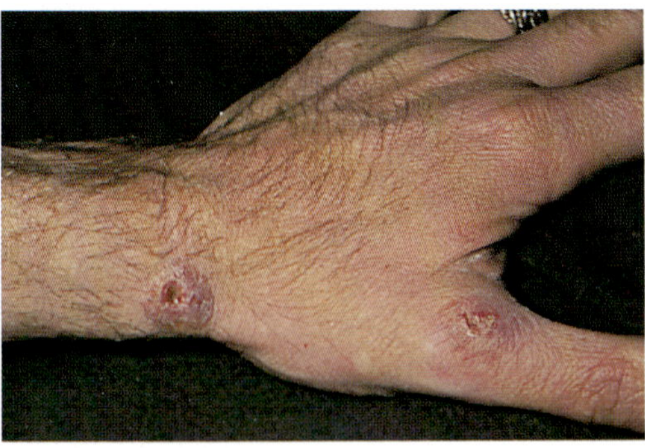

FIGURE 30-23. Sporotrichosis showing typical lymphocutaneous pattern of lesions in this 34-year-old gardener. Common sources of infection include rose thorns and sphagnum moss in this occupation as well as injury from wood splinters especially in African gold mines.

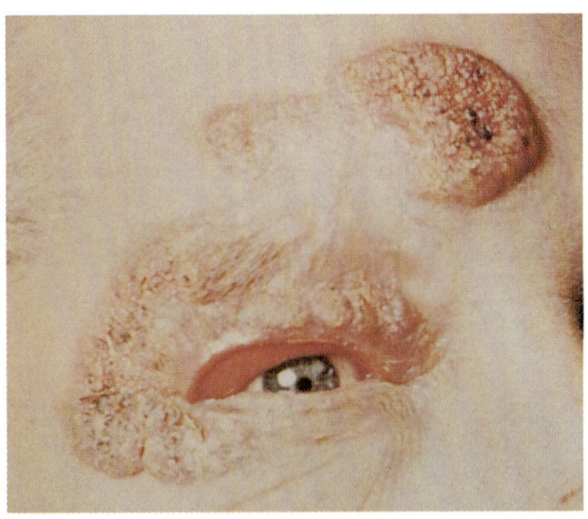

FIGURE 30-24. Blastomycosis of face and eyelid. (Courtesy of Dr. Alson E. Braley.)

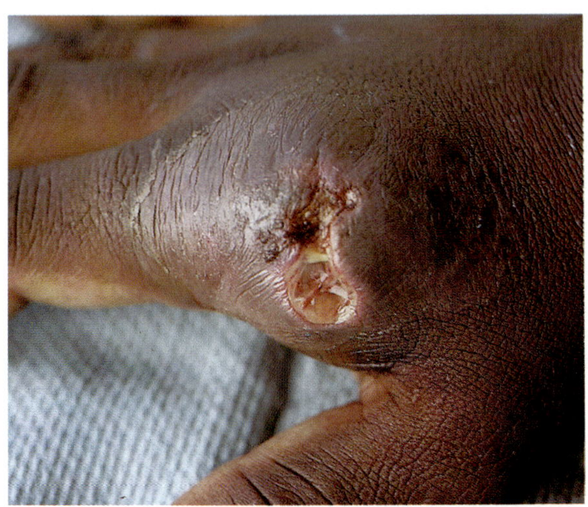

FIGURE 30-25. Coccidioidomycosis producing deep, painful abscess and local bone invasion. Infection developed following injury to hand. (Courtesy of Dr. Jane Rosensweig.)

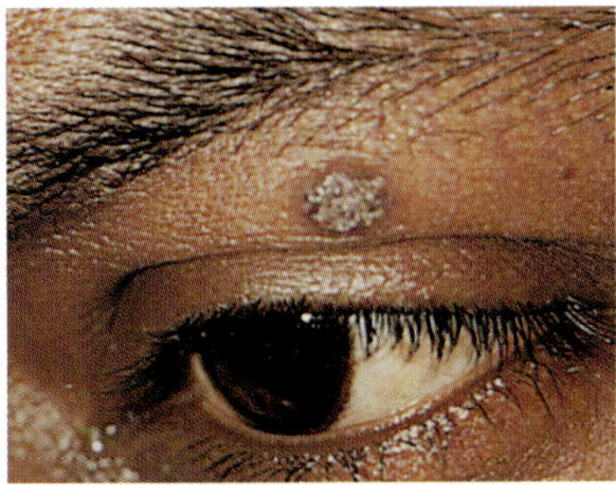

FIGURE 30-26. Cutaneous coccidioidomycosis lesion of eyelid.

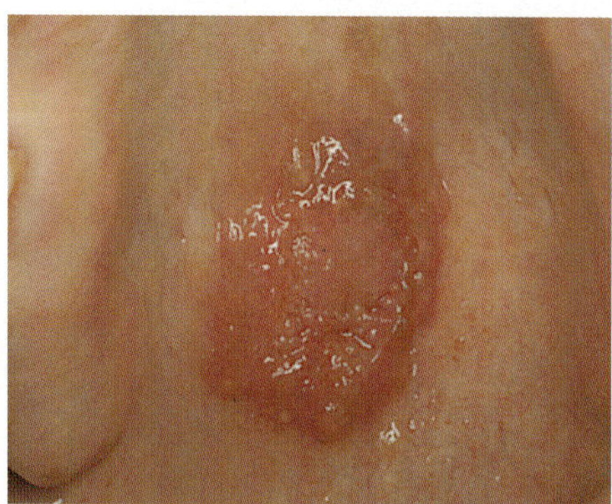

FIGURE 30-27. Coccidioidomycosis of palate.

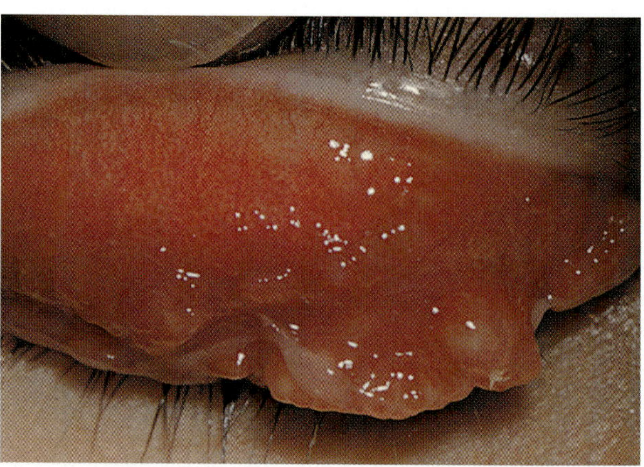

FIGURE 30-28. Conjunctival granulomas in coccidioidomycosis. (Courtesy of Dr. Philips Thygeson.)

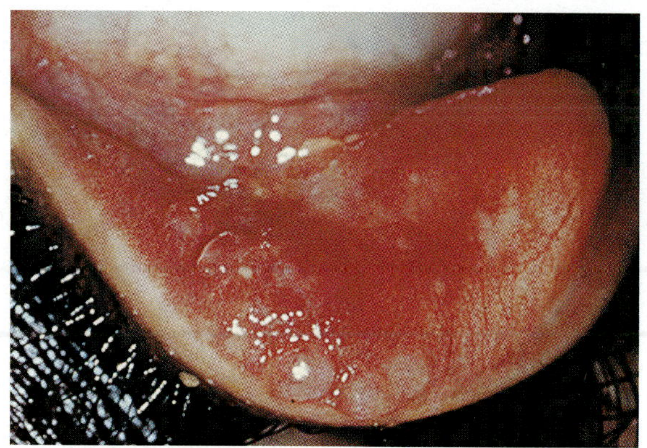

FIGURE 30-29. Conjunctival granulomas in coccidioidomycosis. (Courtesy of Dr. Philips Thygeson.)

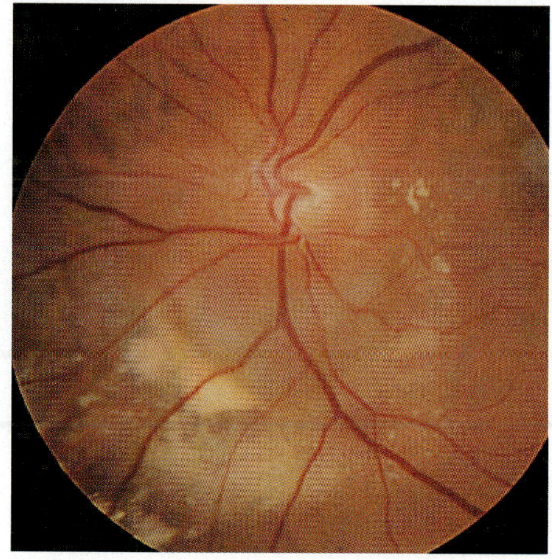

FIGURE 30-30. Choroidal involvement in chronic coccidioidomycosis. Note choroidal scarring just temporal to the nerve head and below the macular region. (Courtesy of Dr. John Belmont.)

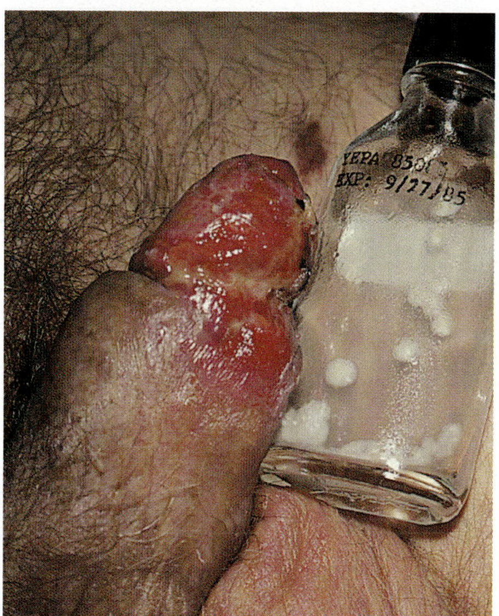

FIGURE 30-31. Painful erosive purulent lesions of mucocutaneous cryptococcosis in a patient with AIDS. Note the Kaposi sarcoma lesion on the thigh and culture showing mucoid white growth of cryptococcus.

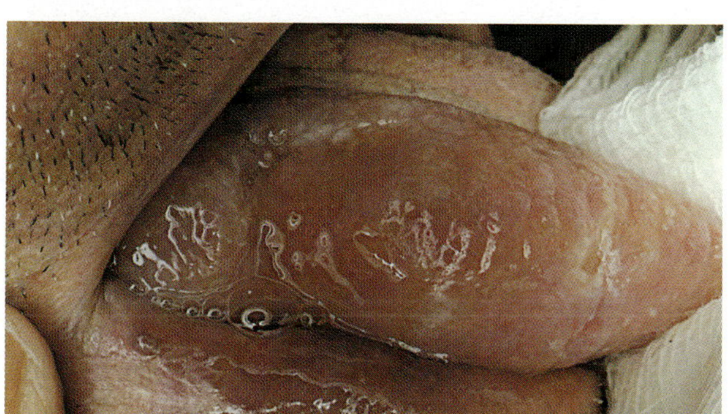

FIGURE 30-32. Histoplasmosis of the tongue. About 20% of patients with disseminated disease will develop ulcerations and granulomas of oropharynx.

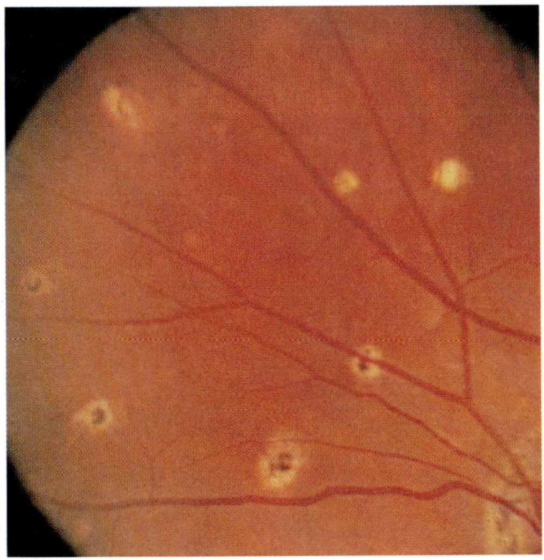

FIGURE 30-33. "Presumed ocular histoplasmosis syndrome." Multiple focal atrophic scars with a central pigment fleck and peripheral scarring are evident. (Courtesy of Dr. John Belmont.)

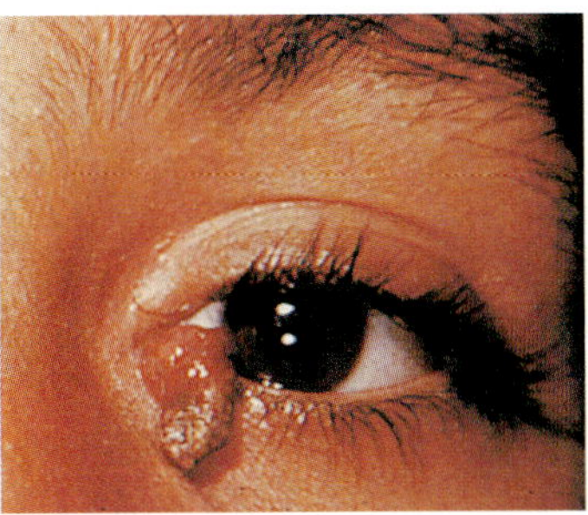

FIGURE 30-34. Rhinosporidiosis of the conjunctiva. Small ocular lesions usually cause no symptoms other than complaints of a growth in the eye. Large lesions occasionally cause tearing, discharge, photophobia, ectropion, and conjunctival injection.

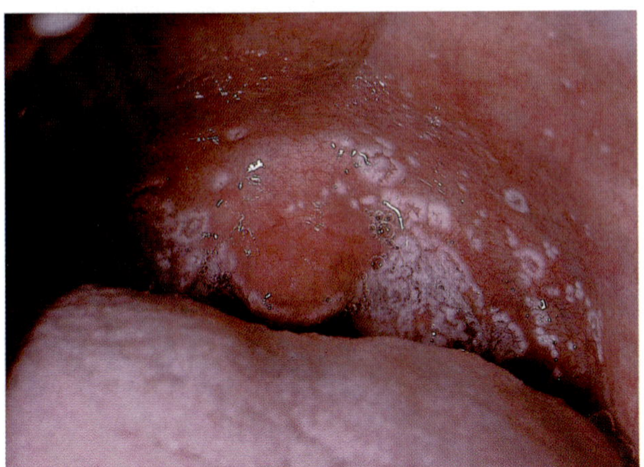

FIGURE 30-35. Oropharyngeal candidiasis in a patient with AIDS. He also experienced retrosternal pain and dysphagia due to esophageal candidiasis, a common problem in severely immunocompromised patients.

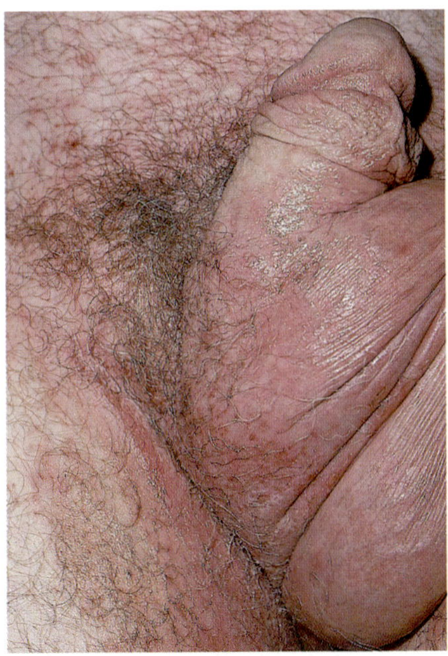

FIGURE 30-36. Candidal intertrigo with extension to scrotum and penis in a patient with AIDS. Therapy required systemic as well as topical agents.

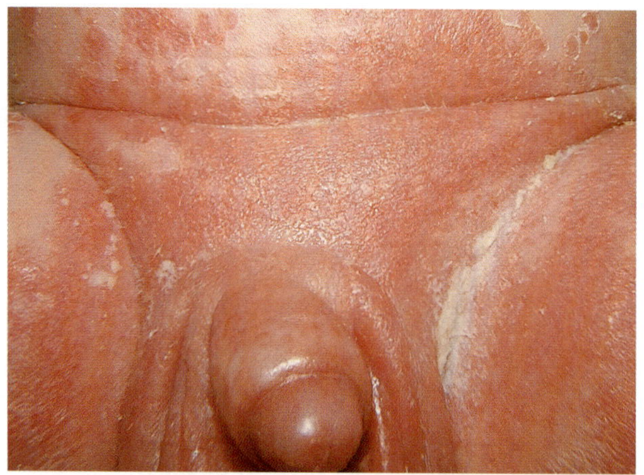

FIGURE 30-37. Candidal diaper dermatitis. Note involvement of inguinal folds, which are usually spared in contact dermatitis.

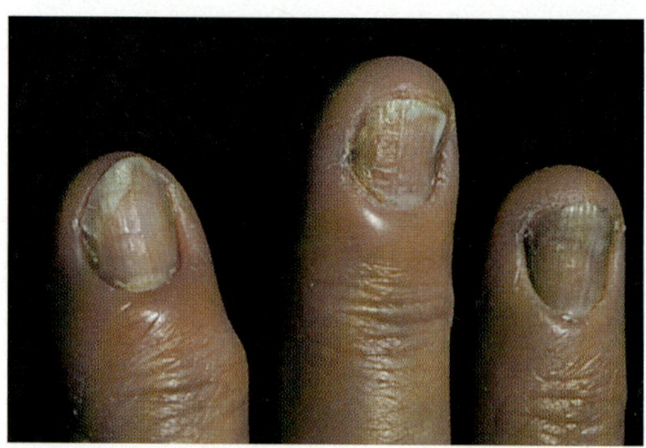

FIGURE 30-38. Acute candidal paronychia in a patient with diabetes.

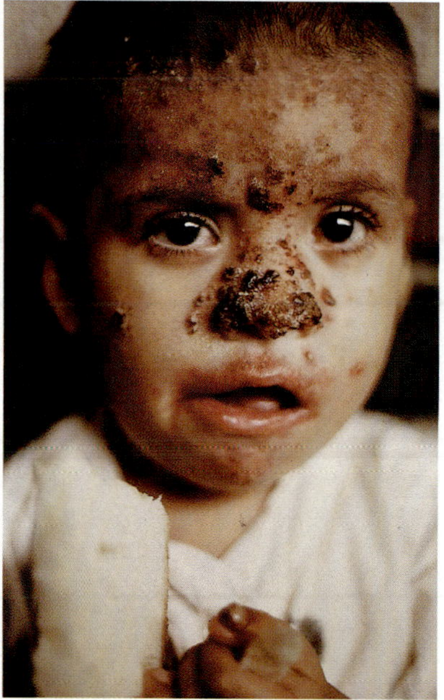

FIGURE 30-39. Severe mucocutaneous candidiasis with candidal granulomas. Note thickened thumbnail.

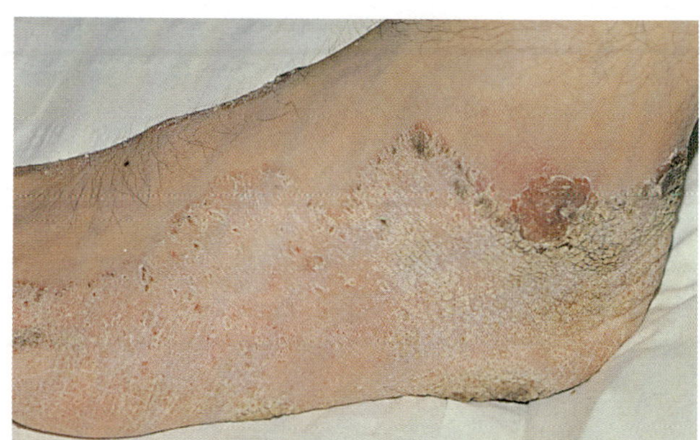

FIGURE 30-40. Candidal granulomas of skin in a patient with mucocutaneous candidiasis.

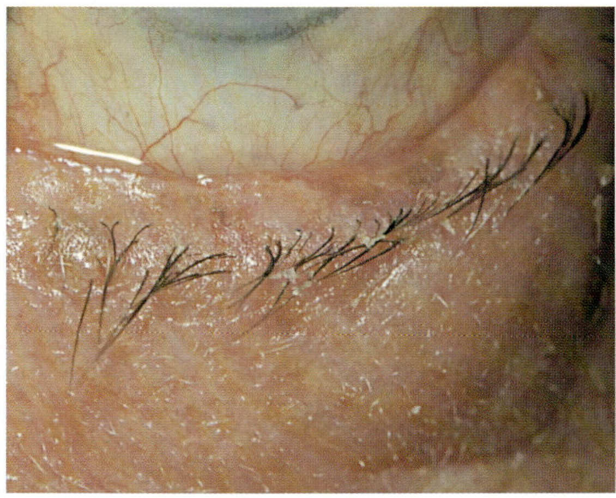

FIGURE 30-41. Candida blepharitis with granulomas.

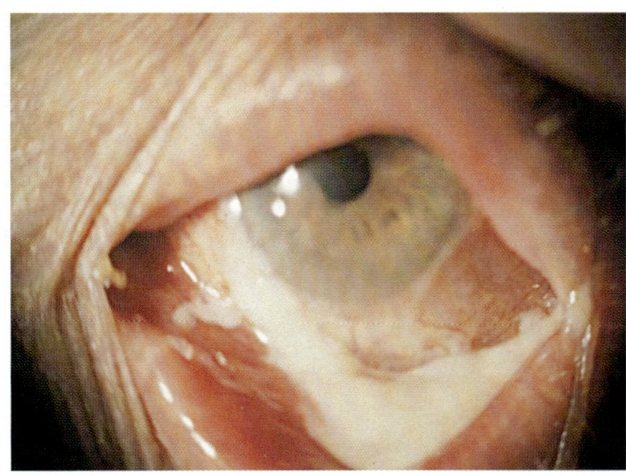

FIGURE 30-42. Conjunctival candidal infection.

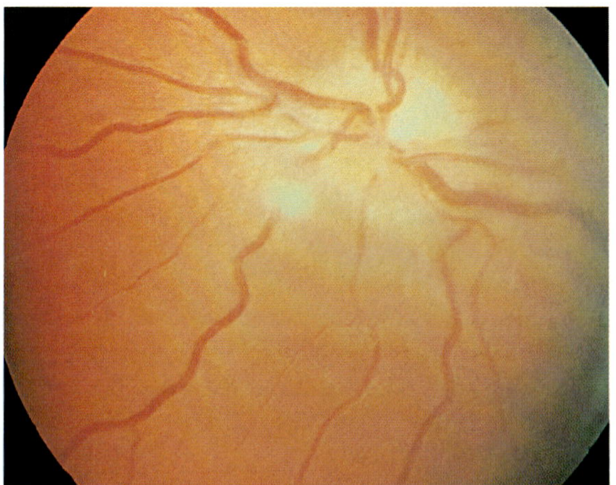

FIGURE 30-43. Candida metastatic endophthalmitis. Moderate vitreous haze and several round, small, white "puff ball" exudates in the retinal area are visible.

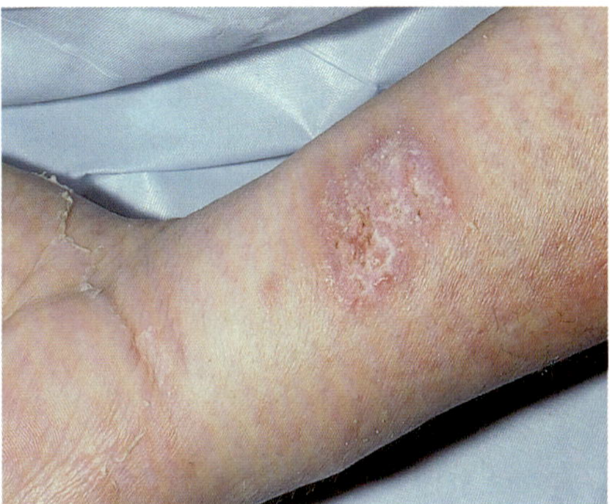

FIGURE 30-44. Cutaneous aspergillosis in a burn patient who had been on multiple antibiotics.

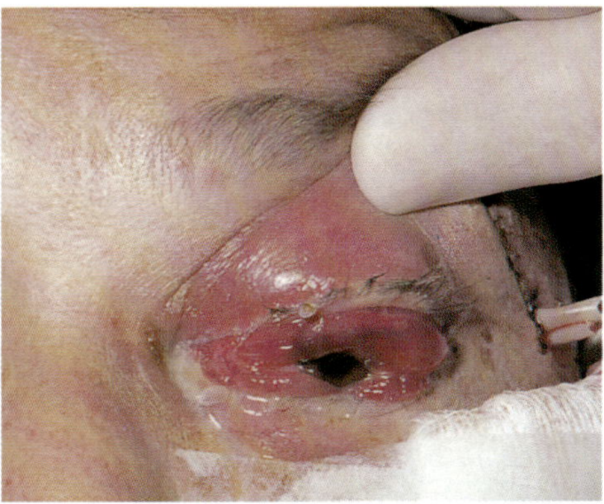

FIGURE 30-45. Mucormycosis infection of the eye. The patient, who was in renal failure, presented with rapidly progressive pain in one eye, accompanied by headache, confusion, reduced vision and proptosis. Emergency enucleation failed to save his life and he died 4 days later from renal complications.

31

PARASITIC INFECTIONS

A parasitic infection is one in which the parasite must invade a host to obtain its essential metabolic requirements. Sometimes the parasite invades several hosts before reaching sexual maturity, and in such instances the host in which sexual maturity occurs is considered to be the definitive host. An intermediate host is one in which the parasite undergoes larval development or an asexual stage of its life cycle. The exception occurs when the life cycle includes both arthropods and humans, and in such cases humans are considered to be the definitive host, whereas the arthropod is considered the vector or intermediate host.

PROTOZOAL INFECTIONS

Leishmaniasis

Visceral, cutaneous, and mucocutaneous leishmaniasis are caused by different *Leishmania* species, and skin lesions occur in each form. All leishmanial infections except for Indian kala-azar (transmitted from human to human) are transmitted through the bite of the sandfly.

Visceral Leishmaniasis (Kala-Azar)

Visceral leishmaniasis (Kala-Azar) occurs in Asia, East Africa, the Mediterranean basin, the Middle East, and Central and South America. The epidemiologic features vary from region to region. Mammals—especially humans and, less often, dogs, foxes, and wild rodents—serve as the reservoir of infection.

Clinical Manifestations

The initial inoculation site is usually inapparent. Infection causes chills, fever (often peaking twice daily), weakness, epistaxis, cough, and diarrhea, followed by progressive emaciation.

Massive splenomegaly and, occasionally, hepatomegaly are prominent findings. Inguinal and femoral lymphadenopathy and, sometimes, generalized lymphadenopathy occur. Occasionally, the manifestations are limited to mouth, oropharyngeal, or skin ulcerations. Death is usually caused by intercurrent infections.

Skin Features

In the Sudan, a nodular lesion resembling an epithelioma develops at the inoculation site. Prominent hyperpigmentation (hence the name *kala-azar,* which means "black fever") of the hands, feet, abdomen, and forehead occurs in light-skinned patients. In dark-skinned patients the hyperpigmentation may go unnoticed, although verrucous lesions or skin ulcers may be seen. Jaundice sometimes occurs.

Post-kala-azar dermatitis may develop 1 to 10 years following apparent cure. The lesions include multiple hypopigmented macules or nodules and erythematous patches in previous areas of skin involvement.

Ocular Features

The lid skin is sometimes involved with the facial skin in visceral leishmaniasis. The lesions may be hyperpigmented, depigmented, verrucous, or ulcerated. In some instances, the lesions resemble xanthomata, although the lid tissues are substantially thickened.

Cutaneous and Mucocutaneous Leishmaniasis

Cutaneous and mucocutaneous leishmaniasis causes self-healing ulcers (Oriental sore), chronic mutilating ulcers (espundia), and disseminated nonulcerating cutaneous lesions (disseminated cutaneous leishmaniasis).

Old World Cutaneous Leishmaniasis (Oriental Sore)

Old World cutaneous leishmaniasis caused by *L. major* occurs in North Africa, the Middle East, Pakistan, India, and Central Asia. *L. tropica* is found in the Mediterranean basin, the Middle East, and Centra Asia. *L. aethiopica* is found in Ethiopia and Kenya. *L. infantum* occurs on the northern Mediterranean littoral west of Greece and in North Africa.

The initial lesion occurs at the inoculation site, usually the face, neck, hand, arm, or leg.

Four forms of Old World cutaneous leishmaniasis are self-limited and heal spontaneously, whereas two are chronic.

The self-limited forms are the following:

1. Cutaneous leishmaniasis caused by *L. major.* It is a rural disease characterized by acute onset and single or multiple wet, rapidly ulcerating sores with considerable tissue reaction. The ulcer is usually crusted and has a raised red margin that sometimes reaches a diameter of up to 6 cm (Fig. 31-1). Secondary lymphatic nodules may develop around the initial lesion. Healing occurs with scarring.
2. Cutaneous leishmaniasis caused by *L. tropica.* It is a chronic urban disease characterized by a single sore, which may or may not ulcerate. The tissue reaction is mild; there are many parasites, and the healing period is more than a year. The skin lesion begins as a small, brownish nodule that enlarges in a 6-month period to form a plaque several centimeters in diameter. The plaque ulcerates, is covered by an adherent crust, and heals by scarring in 8 to 12 months. Sometimes multiple secondary nodules occur. The organism is transmitted from human to human.
3. Cutaneous leishmaniasis caused by *L. aethiopica* occurs as a single lesion on the central part of the face. Satellite lesions develop and coalesce to form a large, spreading nodule, which usually ulcerates and crusts before healing with scarring.
4. Cutaneous leishmaniasis caused by *L. infantum* causes visceral leishmaniasis in infants, whereas in adults it causes a mild, slowly developing but self-limited skin ulcer with minimal associated inflammation. Infrequently, it causes solitary mucosal lesions.

The two chronic forms are:

1. Chronic leishmaniasis (leishmaniasis recidivans), found in Iraq and Anatolia. It resembles lupus vulgaris (Fig. 31-2) with apple-jelly nodules and begins near or in a leishmanial scar and is characterized by brown-red or brown-yellow papules, which coalesce to form a plaque and sometimes ulcerate (Fig. 31-3).
2. Diffuse cutaneous leishmaniasis caused by *L. aethiopica* is characterized by the following:
   a. An initial lesion at the inoculation site that spreads locally while the organism disseminates to cause other skin lesions.
   b. Nodular lesions.
   c. The presence of many parasites and Leishman-Donovan bodies—macrophages full of amastigotes—in the lesions.
   d. The infection is confined to the skin.
   e. All tests for specific cell-mediated immunity (including the Leishman skin test) are negative.
   f. Frequent relapses even though gradual improvement seems to occur with specific therapy.

Ocular Features (Old World Cutaneous Leishmaniasis)

The typical oriental sore may occur on the upper or lower lid (see earlier).

Clinical Manifestations (American Cutaneous Leishmaniasis)

American cutaneous leishmaniasis is endemic in Central and South America. It occurs in rural areas and especially in individuals who work in the forest. In Mexico and Guatemala, the infection is caused by *L. mexicana* subspecies; in Peru and Argentina, by *L. peruviana;* and in other areas of South and Central America, by *L. braziliensis* subspecies.

The major cutaneous lesions are the following:

1. The chiclero ulcer, caused by *L. mexicana,* is a single, nonmetastasizing, self-limited lesion. It occurs on exposed body areas, most often on the ear and the face. The lesion of the ear is ulcerative and destructive (Fig. 31-4) and often persists for many years. In other areas, the lesions are small and heal spontaneously after about 6 months; they often behave like those described for *L. major* or *L. tropica.*
2. A diffuse cutaneous leishmaniasis similar to its counterpart in the Old World (see earlier) caused by *L. amazonensis.*
3. Deep ulcers with a raised edge caused by *L. braziliensis* and subspecies, *L. peruviana, L. guyanensis* results in multiple, fleshy, and protuberant lesions on the extremities. Secondary nodular lesions develop along the draining lymphatics.

Ocular Features (American Cutaneous Leishmaniasis)

A chiclero lid ulcer is similar to chiclero ulcers on other facial areas (see earlier). Sometimes the lids are involved by the widespread destructive process of espundia; chronic lower lid edema occurs with the oronasal lesions of espundia.

Keratitis from exposure and secondary infection also occurs.

Clinical Manifestations (American Mucocutaneous Leishmaniasis)

Disseminated cutaneous leishmaniasis occurs in the Amazon region of Brazil and Venezuela and in Ethiopia and the Sudan. It begins as a single nodule but spreads to all body areas, especially the nose (Fig. 31-5). The lesions are papular, nodular, and verrucose; frequently, the pinna of the ear becomes infiltrated. The lesions do not ulcerate, and nasal septal destruction does not occur. The infection is not self-limited; treatment is unsatisfactory.

About 40% of patients with cutaneous lesions caused by *L. braziliensis* develop mucocutaneous lesions (espundia) (Fig. 31-6) after 1 to 10 years. Mucocutaneous lesions also develop, but in a less significant number, following infection with *L. b. panamensis* and *L. b. guyanensis.* Some patients have no history of previous skin lesions.

L. tropica causes primary mucocutaneous leishmaniasis of the vermilion border of the lip or the mucosal border of the nose. There is considerable swelling of the lips or nose, but less destruction is caused than by *L. brasiliensis*. The ulcerative skin lesion seems to heal spontaneously but later metastasizes to other skin and mucous membrane areas (especially the nose). About one-third of patients have involvement of a second mucous membrane site (pharynx, palate, larynx, and upper lip). The lesion causes severe destruction of the nasal cartilage and other nasopharyngeal tissues. Mucosal and cutaneous lesions occasionally occur concurrently. Regional lymphangitis and lymphadenopathy are common. Death eventually supervenes from secondary infection.

Clinical Manifestations (Disseminated Cutaneous Leishmaniasis)

The lesions of the skin of the lid are similar to those found in other areas of the body (Fig. 31-7).

African Trypanosomiasis (Sleeping Sickness)

Sleeping sickness is caused by *Trypanosoma brucei rhodesiense* and *T. brucei gambiense*. The two organisms are morphologically indistinguishable and are transmitted by the bite of the tsetse fly.

Rhodesian sleeping sickness occurs in the savanna regions east of the Rift Valley. Game animals serve as the principal reservoir; humans are infected only sporadically.

Gambian sleeping sickness occurs primarily in West and Central Africa and is especially important in Zaire. Humans serve as the principal reservoir of the organism.

Clinical Manifestations

The trypanosomal chancre develops at the site of the bite of an infected tsetse fly. It is pruritic or painful for several days or weeks and is dusky red, indurated, raised, and tender, measuring 2 to 5 cm or more. It is surrounded by an area of edema, and sometimes a fluid-filled blister develops on its surface. Regional lymphadenopathy usually occurs. The chancre fades after several weeks.

The bloodstream and reticuloendothelial system are invaded after a few weeks in the Rhodesian form of infection, whereas in the Gambian form invasion occurs only after several months. Invasion causes irregular fever, transient erythematous, or urticarial circinate or annular rashes on the trunk and scattered areas of nonpitting edema of the hands, feet, and face. Sometimes the rash is hemorrhagic. Hepatosplenomegaly usually occurs and may be accompanied by a mild jaundice. Lymphadenopathy, especially of the posterior cervical chain (Winterbottom sign), is common in the Gambian infection; in the Rhodesian infection the lymph nodes are often not enlarged.

A persistent tachycardia is characteristic, especially in the Rhodesian variety. Myalgias, arthralgias, delayed sensation to pain, and deep hyperesthesia also occur.

Early central nervous system symptoms include persistent headache, personality changes, inability to concentrate, and a feeling of oppression. As the disease progresses, apathy, somnolence, mania, disturbed speech and gait, and anorexia occur. Pruritus and excoriation of the skin occur from scratching. Finally, emaciation and coma supervene, and death occurs from secondary infection or malnutrition.

Ocular Features

The ocular findings include the following:

1. Tense urticarial lid swelling in the early stages of infection that involves only the lateral portion of the lower lid. It recurs at intermittent intervals.
2. Bilateral diffuse interstitial keratitis of all layers of the cornea.
3. Iridocyclitis coinciding with hematogenous dissemination.
4. Small hemorrhages on the surface of the iris and hyphemas.
5. Papilledema that may lead to optic atrophy from meningeal and central nervous system infection.

American Trypanosomiasis (Chagas Disease)

Chagas disease occurs in the Americas and is transmitted by the reduviid bug, also known as the "kissing" or assassin bug (Fig. 31-8).

Humans are usually infected at night when the vector defecates while taking a blood meal; the trypomastigotes contained in the feces penetrate broken skin or the mucous membranes of the conjunctiva when the unsuspecting patient rubs the skin.

Clinical Manifestations

Chagas disease frequently involves young children and may cause acute meningoencephalitis or myocarditis and death (Fig. 31-9).

The initial bite is usually not noticed. The chagoma that occurs 5 days later is usually the first manifestation of infection. It is characterized by an erythematous, desquamating, slightly indurated macule measuring up to 4 cm.

Romana Sign

Romana sign is almost pathognomonic of an acute infection in endemic areas and is characterized by unilateral lid edema and, often, conjunctivitis and dacryoadenitis (Figs. 31-10 and 31-11). Regional lymphadenitis or lymphadenopathy accompanies Romana sign.

A remittent or constant fever occurs, lasting 10 to 14 days. Other manifestations include the following:

1. Malaise, irritability, anorexia, and watery diarrhea.
2. Palpitations, arrhythmias, tachycardia with gallop rhythm, cardiac enlargement, cardiac failure, and generalized nonpitting edema.
3. Psychological changes, focal neurologic symptoms, and convulsions.
4. Tender hepatosplenomegaly.
5. Generalized nontender lymphadenopathy in children and young adults.

Chronic Chagas infection which is seen in 10% to 30% of patients years to decades after the acute manifestations causes cardiomyopathy, myocarditis, arrhythmias, cardiac failure, megaloesophagus, and megacolon. Asymptomatic patients may transmit the parasites by blood transfusions.

The ocular manifestations are limited to Romano sign.

MULTICELLULAR PARASITES

Helminths

Helminths are divided into roundworms (Nematoda) and flatworms (Platyhelminths). The latter contain the Trematoda (flukes), and Cestoda (tapeworms).

Nematoda

The nematode life cycle involves insects, crustaceans, or another vertebrate as the intermediate host.

Trichinosis

Trichinosis involves the muscles, heart, brain, and eye. It is acquired by eating inadequately cooked, tainted meat, especially pork.

There are three phases:

1. The intestinal phase, which begins when larvae are liberated in the intestine. It is associated with vomiting, diarrhea, and weakness.
2. The dissemination phase begins about the seventh day and is characterized by fever, sweating, urticaria, muscle pain, weakness, lid and facial edema, chemosis, leukocytosis, and eosinophilia. Subconjunctival, retinal, and nail splinter hemorrhages often occur. The fever may persist for several weeks.
3. The convalescence phase begins about the fifth to eighth week, during which time ocular and neurologic symptoms become prominent.

Focal central nervous system involvement often develops and is manifested by headache, stiff neck, mental confusion, delirium, psychosis, hemiplegia, aphasia, paraplegia, and paralysis of the cranial and peripheral nerves. Death or residual neurologic defects are common. Nonspecific central nervous system findings include headache, stiff neck, apathy, mental confusion, and diminished or absent deep tendon reflexes.

Skin Features

A transient erythematous, maculopapular rash of the extremities commonly occurs along with splinter hemorrhages of the nail beds between the sixth and twenty-second day of infection.

Ocular Features

The ocular symptoms include photophobia, pain on ocular rotation, blurred vision, strabismus, proptosis, and visual hallucinations.

The ocular findings include the following:

1. Pronounced bilateral lid edema, which often extends onto the cheeks and into the temples.
2. Lemon-yellow conjunctival chemosis that is usually localized over the insertion of the lateral and medial rectus muscles and persists for about a week. Diffuse conjunctival hemorrhages and subconjunctival petechiae also may be seen.
3. A unilateral or bilateral nonpurulent tenonitis or myositis of any extraocular muscle with mild proptosis and apparent immobility of the eyes from the pain that occurs with ocular motility.
4. Uveitis with small retinal hemorrhages and exudates.
5. Other ocular findings include paresis of the 6th cranial nerve, pupillary dilatation and sluggish reaction to light, decreased accommodation, diplopia, dyschromatopsia, decreased visual acuity, scotomas, visual field defects, secondary glaucoma, nerve head hyperemia, optic neuritis, and papilledema.

Ascariasis

Ascariasis occurs in areas of poor sanitation and hygiene and where human feces are used for fertilizer.

Clinical Manifestations

Humans become infected by ingesting food or water contaminated with the ascariasis eggs. The larvae hatch in the intestine; pass to the portal circulation, heart, and lungs; then migrate through the alveolar walls to reach the pharynx, where they are then swallowed to reach the small intestine.

Larval migration through the lungs causes a productive cough, often with blood-tinged sputum, low-grade fever, wheezing, rales, dyspnea, substernal pain, and signs of local consolidation.

Large numbers of intestinal parasites (Fig. 31-12) may cause vague pre- and postprandial pain and colic.

During their migration or because of reverse peristalsis, the larvae occasionally reach other body sites (e.g., kidney, spinal cord, eye), causing symptoms localized to those sites.

Central nervous system invasion probably does not occur, and the symptoms of meningitis, convulsions, choreiform movements, delirium, and paralysis of the lower extremities are caused by toxins released from the parasites.

Skin Features

Urticaria and angioedema often occur during migration of larvae through the lung.

Ocular Manifestations

Ocular involvement occurs from aberrant larval migration. The ocular findings include the following:

1. Unilateral or bilateral lid edema and urticaria, which may be recurrent.
2. Severe conjunctivitis caused by juices from the worm being squirted into the eye during cutting of meat.
3. Migration of the worm into the conjunctiva from the canaliculus.
4. Subconjunctival or intraocular ascarid resembling a white, undulating thread.
5. Occlusion of the nasolacrimal duct by the adult worm that causes dacryocystitis.
6. Orbital pseudotumor caused by toxins.
7. Acute, severe, iridocyclitis caused by toxins.
8. Acute iridocyclitis, elevated pressure, lens subluxation, retinal edema, macular changes, chorioretinitis, and papilledema caused by intraocular ascarids.
9. Retinal edema, periphlebitis, and macular changes caused by subretinal worms. Sometimes the worms cause minimal reaction and move freely during the period of observation.
10. Recurrent vitreous hemorrhages caused by worms in the vitreous.
11. Secondary glaucoma with visual field defects.

Filariasis (*Wuchereria* Spp., *Brugia* Spp., and *Dirofilaria* Spp.)

Wuchereria bancrofti occurs in the tropics and subtropics of both hemispheres. Humans are the only vertebrate host. *Brugia malayi* is found in South India, Sri Lanka, Southeast Asia, China, and South Korea. *B. timori* is found in some of the Indonesian islands. *Dirofilaria tenuis* is harbored by raccoons and is found in the southeastern and eastern United States. *D. repens* is found in the subcutaneous tissues of dogs, cats, and foxes in Africa, Europe, and Asia. *D. immitis,* the heart worm of dogs, is prevalent in many areas of the United States.

Clinical Manifestations

The organisms are transmitted by mosquitoes and often cause minimal or no manifestations.

Symptomatic early infections cause swelling, tenderness, and erythema of the arms, legs, or scrotum, along with periodic, irregular episodes of fever, sometimes associated with lymphadenitis, enlarged lymph nodes, orchitis, and epididymitis. The lymph nodes occasionally suppurate. Periodic inflammation may occur for months before signs of late infection develop.

Late filarial infection is manifested by the adult worm blocking the superficial and deep lymphatic channels, which causes a hydrocele, scrotal lymphedema (Fig. 31-13), lymphatic varices, lower leg edema (Fig. 31-14), and elephantiasis of the leg, breast, arm, or lids. The swelling is soft and pits easily at onset; later, it feels hard. The affected part becomes grossly enlarged from edema, skin hypertrophy, and proliferation of subcutaneous connective tissue.

Small, migratory subcutaneous nodules of the arm, leg, scrotum, and breast comprise the late manifestations of *Dirofilaria* species infection. The nodules become inflamed and are occasionally painful when the parasites die.

Ocular Manifestations

Lymphatic blockage by *W. bancrofti,* causes intense and enormous lid swelling; *B. malayi* and *B. timori* cause less intense lid swelling. *D. tenuis* and *D. immitis* cause lid edema by direct periocular tissue infection, and subcutaneous cysts containing *D. repens* and *D. tenuis* may be found in the lid.

Other ocular findings include the following:

1. Toxic, severe conjunctival suffusion during febrile episodes caused by *W. bancrofti.*
2. Small subconjunctival granulomas containing *D. repens* or *D. tenuis.*
3. Corneal edema caused by the organism in the anterior chamber.
4. Sclera nodules caused by *Dirofilaria.*
5. Chronic granulomatous orbital reaction simulating an orbital tumor caused by *W. bancrofti.* The reaction develops slowly and simulates an intraorbital tumor with only mild signs of inflammation and pain.
6. Lid edema, signs of orbital inflammation, tenonitis, or orbital pseudotumor caused by dirofilarial organisms.
7. Anterior chamber filaria appear as specks of dust; the adult worms, as threads 2 to 3 cm long. The organisms move rapidly in the aqueous.
8. Intense intraocular reaction, keratitis, vitreous opacities, and secondary glaucoma caused by living intraocular filaria.
9. Intense pain caused by ciliary body involvement.
10. Retinal hemorrhages from vitreous parasites.
11. Unilateral retinal pigment epithelial disturbances simulating retinitis pigmentosa from intraocular *Dirofilaria.*

Onchocerciasis

Onchocerciasis is caused by *Onchocerca volvulusa,* which is transmitted by the bite of a small black fly, genus *Simulium.* The fly breeds along fast-flowing streams and rivers, especially along the Victoria Nile, where onchocerciasis is known as "river blindness" because it so frequently leads to that complication. Worldwide, onchocerciasis is the second leading cause of infectious blindness. It occurs in tropical Africa, Yemen, Saudi Arabia, southern Mexico, Guatemala, northern Brazil, Venezuela, Ecuador, and Colombia. In humans, the larvae migrate to subcutaneous or deeper tissue and mature. The microfilaria (Fig. 31-15) measure 200 to 300 μm and live up to 30 months. The adult male measures 20 to 45 mm; the female measures 23 to 70 mm (Figs. 31-16 and 31-17) and lives up to 15 years.

Skin Features

The skin becomes thick, inelastic, and coarse in texture, and lies in thick folds.

Early in the infection and persisting throughout most of the infection, a mild, intermittent or constant, intense itching occurs. The first sign of infection is often an infiltrated appearance of the skin of the shoulders or around the pelvis associated with obliteration of skin marking. Later, papules or pustules (called craw craw or gale filarienne) may develop. They are associated with severe itch and represent intraepithelial abscesses that contain microfilariae. They exude clear fluid or pus. Focal edema (peau d'orange) or diffuse edema occurs as a reaction to the microfilariae. The infection evolves months or even years later into a chronic papular dermatitis with excoriated papules, flat-topped scars, and early lichenification, especially over the shoulders and buttocks.

Late in the infection, lichenified confluent papules and nodules develop on the leg, and spotty hyper- or hypopigmentation (leopard skin) develops on the lower trunk, buttocks, thighs, shins, and scrotum. The skin becomes atrophic, inelastic, wrinkled; appears shiny and dry (Fig. 31-18); and is associated with fibrosis of the dermal appendages and supporting tissue of the epidermis, including the areolar connective tissue. The extreme form of atrophy is often called "lizard skin" by the local population.

Onchocercomas

Palpable subcutaneous, asymptomatic, rubbery nodules (onchocercomas) contain the adult worms (Fig. 31-16). They occur on the head and above the pelvic girdle in Central America (Figs. 31-19 and 31-20), around the pelvis in Africa, and below the pelvic girdle in Yemen. Some nodules are deeply seated and not palpable. The nodules are well defined, 0.1 to 1.0 cm, nontender, firm, round or elongated; commonly, they are fewer than six in number. They are usually freely movable but may be fixed to fascia, periosteum, or skin.

Lymph Nodes

The superficial lymph nodes that drain the area of onchocercal dermatitis are often enlarged. The nodes, although bound together, feel discrete and are nontender.

Ocular Features

Ocular findings develop 15 months to 5 years after skin involvement.

The infection causes photophobia, redness, entopic vision (due to microfilaria), and visual disturbances.

Corneal and, occasionally, conjunctival involvement causes severe blepharospasm and needle-like pains (Figs. 31-21 and 31-22). Sclerosing keratitis begins in the peripheral cornea (about 1 mm from the limbus). The anterior stroma becomes hazy in the 2 to 4 o'clock and in the 8 to 10 o'clock areas. It is soon followed by superficial vascularization and migration of conjunctival pigment onto the corneal epithelium.

Other ocular findings include the following:

1. Lid and orbital edema with proptosis early in the infection; lid edema and skin pigmentation in the late stages. Permanent lid swelling may occur from lipomata formation.
2. Lid nodules may be found in Central American patients.
3. Chronic conjunctivitis manifested by lid edema, mild injection, chemosis, limbal swelling, and limbal pigmentation.
4. Lesions similar to conjunctival phlyctenulosis or small tumors.
5. Fine, peripheral epithelial keratitis located in the interpalpebral area. Corneal microfilaria seen on retroillumination at all depths of the peripheral cornea and even attached to Descemet membrane.
6. Nummular lesions located immediately beneath the epithelial keratitis and Bowman layer. The lesions have the appearance of white snowflakes in the anterior stroma and gray midstromal lesions. In severe cases, the nummular opacities coalesce to form a denser opacity.
7. Sclerosing keratitis. In advanced cases, deep stromal vessels accompanied by superficial and deep infiltration develop in the inferior cornea and gradually encroach on the visual axis. Eventually, the entire cornea is involved and calcific plaques may be seen.
8. An iritis accompanies the sclerosing keratitis. Microfilaria flitting about the anterior chamber.
9. A low-grade iridocyclitis with fine, white keratic precipitates, mild flare, and occasional cells. Severe iritis in severe infections.
10. Inferior distortion of the pupil with patches of iris atrophy, anterior and posterior synechiae, entropion uvea, and pupillary seclusion and occlusion.
11. Peripheral, asymmetric chorioretinal lesions.
12. Retinal changes include edema, retinal pigment atrophy, subretinal fibrosis, pigment disturbance of the choroid (appearing as fine, yellowish dots), retinal vasculitis (especially in the region of the central retinal artery), attenuation of retinal arteries, retinal hemorrhages, cotton-wool spots, and small, white retinal opacities.
13. Microfilaria are occasionally seen in the retrolental space and vitreous.
14. Cataracts and secondary glaucoma.
15. Papilledema, cupping, and optic atrophy.

Loiasis

Loiasis occurs in the damp forest areas of West and Central Africa. It is caused by the African eye worm and is manifested by transient painful swellings. The filaria are transmitted to humans by the bite of bloodsucking flies (deer, horse, and mangrove flies) and mature into adult worms over a 1- to 4-year period. The adult worms may live longer than 17 years.

Low-grade fever, malaise, myalgia, paresthesias, pleurisy, and glomerulonephritis are occasionally seen. Invasion of the central nervous system may lead to meningoencephalitis, encephalitis, coma, and death.

Skin Features

The adult worm is encountered from time to time in its aimless wandering throughout the body. Sites where it is commonly seen include the fingers, trunk, scalp, penis, and eyelid; sometimes it is found under mucous membranes. It usually causes itching or a creeping or pricking sensation during its wandering.

The adult worm occasionally causes Calabar swellings about the orbit, hands, and forehands. The swelling is probably an anaphylactic reaction and lasts 1 to 2 days. It develops rapidly and is firm, nonpitting, and tender or slightly painful.

Dead and dying organisms cause suppuration, granulomas, fibrosis, and sometimes generalized urticaria or angioedema, erythema, and pruritus.

Ocular Feature

The parasite favors facial regions, particularly regions about the eye (Fig. 31-23). Ocular involvement usually causes severe lid irritation and severe edema, which disappears quickly once the organism leaves the area. Often the organism is seen wriggling under the loose skin.

The adult worm may wander under the conjunctiva, where it causes itching, burning, and sometimes pain. The conjunctiva is red and edematous, and the organism may be seen wriggling under the conjunctiva. Occasionally, the organism encysts in the orbit.

Deep retinal hemorrhages and cotton-wool spots may be associated with the meningoencephalitis. Superficial retinal hemorrhages and yellow exudates have been observed with microfilaria in the retinal and choroidal blood vessels.

Gnathostomiasis

Gnathostomiasis is caused by *Gnathostoma* species. The infection occurs only in eastern and southern Asia. Humans become infected by eating the flesh of the intermediate host (fish, frogs, or snakes), by drinking water contaminated with the cyclops, or by the larvae gaining access through abraded skin. Since humans are facultative hosts, the larvae continue to migrate throughout the body.

Clinical Manifestations

Gnathostomiasis causes large, intermittent migratory subcutaneous swellings or abscesses. The lesions are usually firm and pruritic or, occasionally, painful. They occur anywhere on the body surface (usually on the upper part of the body) and may either migrate constantly or remain stationary for about 4 weeks. The worm is occasionally visible under the skin.

Central nervous system invasion causes encephalitis, paralysis, and subarachnoid hemorrhage. Pharyngeal and pulmonary invasion causes pharyngeal edema, pneumothorax, dyspnea, paroxysmal coughing, and hemoptysis. Cervical invasion causes leukorrhea.

Ocular Features

Invasion of the lid or a contiguous area causes severe lid edema and may simulate orbital cellulitis. In some instances, a lid abrasion serves as the portal of entry of the organism because of the tradition in Southeast Asia of patients using frog flesh as a poultice for ocular injuries.

Intraocular invasion usually causes corneal edema and severe iridocyclitis with iris nodules. Hypopyon, multiple retinal hemorrhages, and vitreous opacities may also occur.

Dracontiasis

The guinea worm infects only humans. It is found in rural farming communities, especially around communal drinking or washing areas and at wells in India; in West, East, and Central Africa; in the Arabian Peninsula, and the in western Pacific.

Infection occurs from drinking water containing the infected water flea (intermediate host) found in wells and ponds. The larvae mature and mate in the subcutaneous tissue. The female, which may measure about 1 m long, migrates to the skin surface of the lower extremity, provoking a blister that ruptures upon contact with water. Thousands of larvae are discharged from the ulcerated area over a period of 2 to 3 weeks whenever it comes in contact with water. The female worm is then extruded or retracts and reemerges. Other worms may die and induce a severe reaction.

Skin Features

About 24 hours before appearance of the worm at the skin surface, an allergic reaction occurs, characterized by generalized urticaria, pruritus, fever, dyspnea, nausea, vomiting, and diarrhea.

Local redness, burning, intense pruritus, and tenderness followed by a blister developing at the site of the head of the worm. The surrounding tissue is red, indurated, and tender. Part of the female worm then surfaces, forming an ulcer. Healing occurs after 4 to 6 weeks. The worm is occasionally visible as a palpable, cordlike structure deep to the skin. Infrequently, the adult worm migrates into a joint, such as the knee, where it causes an intraarticular infection.

Ocular Features

The urticaria is usually associated with intense lid edema. Infrequently, the worm migrates to the subcutaneous tissues of the lid, forming a nodule or subcutaneous abscess, which is sometimes intensely painful.

Conjunctival hyperemia occurs during the generalized urticaria. The worm occasionally invades the caruncle or orbit, producing periorbital swelling and proptosis.

Toxocariasis

Toxocariasis is caused by the roundworms of dogs, cats, and wild carnivores. Humans are incidental hosts who acquire the infection by ingestion of embryonate eggs. The second-stage larvae that develop are unable to continue the cycle and are distributed to all parts of the body, where they lodge in terminal vessels and invade the local tissue, including the brain, retina, conjunctiva, and cornea, inducing eosinophilic granulomas.

Many toxocariasis manifestations (i.e., visceral larva migrans) are also caused by other roundworms (e.g., *Ascaris suum*—the pig roundworm; *Capillaria hepatica*—the rat liver parasite; *Dirofilaria immitis*—the dog heartworm; and *Belascaris procyonis*—the raccoon round worm). Infections occur worldwide. Toxocariasis is very common in the United States, with most visceral larva migrans cases being found in the southeastern and south central areas.

Clinical Manifestations

Most human infections are asymptomatic or go unrecognized, whereas a few are associated with fever, cough, wheezing, pallor, malaise, irritability, weight loss, and hepatomegaly. Sometimes the patient develops splenomegaly, lymphadenopathy, vomiting, abdominal pain, papular skin rash, muscle pain, or myocarditis. The acute phase is self-limited, persisting 2 to 3 weeks. Central nervous system manifestations occur in 15% to 20% of cases and include ataxia, seizures, coma, encephalitis, Guillain-Barré syndrome, and hemiparesis.

Skin Features

A papular skin eruption of the legs often develops during the acute phase of the infection; occasionally, there is a generalized pruritic and urticarial or papular eruption (Fig. 31-24).

A migrating panniculitis may also occur, manifested by tender, subcutaneous nodules that persist for 1 to 2 weeks.

Ocular Features

Lid nodules represent an allergic reaction to migrating and degenerating nematodes. Conjunctival findings include injection and allergic nodules similar to those seen in the eyelids. Acute visceral larva migrans is occasionally associated with nummular keratitis.

Uveal and retinal findings (Fig. 31-25) in toxocariasis include the following:

1. Iris nodules (occasional).
2. Uniocular intermediate uveitis (common), characterized by anterior vitreous exudates; a large, gray mass at the ciliary body and ora or an elevated, dense, white inflammatory mass in the peripheral retina associated with central projecting retinal folds; and vitreous bands that extend to the nerve head.
3. Retinal granuloma.
4. Leukocoria appearing as a white retrolental mass with overlying blood vessels, retinal detachment, pseudoretinitis pigmentosa, and macular edema.
5. Diffuse painless endophthalmitis.
6. Diffuse unilateral subacute neuroretinitis with early loss of central vision, papillitis, vitreous inflammation, recurrent crops of evanescent gray-white lesions in the outer retina and pigment epithelium, progressive loss of the visual field, optic atrophy, narrowing of the retinal vessels, diffuse and focal atrophy pigment, and abnormalities in the electroretinogram.
7. Occasional live larva in the vitreous that causes severe inflammation when it dies.
8. Optic neuritis and papilledema from a granuloma of the optic nerve, cataracts, and strabismus.

Platyhelminths

The Platyhelminths, or flat worms, contain the classes Trematoda (flukes that are leaflike) and Cestoda (tapeworms that are ribbon-like).

Trematoda

The trematodes are nonsegmented flat worms that live in veins, the gut, bile duct, or lung of the definitive host.

Schistosomiasis (Bilharziasis)

Intestinal schistosomiasis (bilharziasis) is caused by *Schistosoma haematobium;* urinary schistosomiasis, by *S. mansoni;* and intestinal schistosomiasis, by *S. japonicum.* Other schistosomal species may secondarily infect humans and cause cutaneous manifestations, but their role in ocular disease is unclear.

S. haematobium is found in Egypt, Africa, the Middle East, India, south Portugal, and Cyprus. *S. mansoni* is found in Africa, South America, the West Indies, and the Arabian Peninsula. *S. japonicum* is common in the Philippines, China, the Far East, and occasionally, Japan. Humans become infected by cercaria (fork-tailed larvae) that invade the skin or mucous membranes, where they eventually migrate to the mesenteric venules (*S. mansoni* and *japonicum*), or venules of the bladder, prostate, and uterus (*S. haematobium*). Although most of the eggs produced by the adult organism are expelled, some lodge in the intestinal or bladder wall, producing inflammation, ulceration, granulomas, polyps, and fibrosis. Others lodge in veins around the rectum and colon or invade vesical and rectal veins to reach the surrounding tissue, where they incite a granulomatous reaction.

Clinical Manifestations

There are three separate phases of infection.

The initial phase persists up to 5 days and is characterized by an itchy, erythematous, and occasionally, petechial rash (swimmer's itch) at the site of skin penetration by the cercaria.

The second phase occurs 4 to 5 weeks later as the organisms migrate through the liver. This phase lasts 2 to 8 weeks, is allergic in origin, and consists of fever, malaise, headache, urticaria (especially severe in *S. japonicum* infection), pulmonary symptoms (especially a dry cough), and transitory hepatomegaly and splenomegaly.

The final phase begins 6 months to several years later. The manifestations and severity of the disease depend on the number of ova deposited, the type of infection, and the organ principally involved (intestinal symptoms from *S. mansoni* and *japonicum* and urinary symptoms from *S. haematobium*). During the final phase of the disease, paragenital granulomas; fistulous tracts in the perineum, groin, and buttocks; and cerebral and ocular involvement may occur.

The intestinal infection causes diarrhea, dysentery, and abdominal pain; later, anorexia, weight loss, polypoid intestinal lesions, signs of portal hypertension, and hepatic cirrhosis appear. Death occurs from secondary infection.

Genitourinary tract infection causes frequency, pain, and terminal hematuria. Death occurs from uremia or bladder carcinoma.

The central nervous system is infrequently affected; when it is affected, it is usually by *S. japonicum*. Acute manifestations usually include pyramidal tract signs, fever, headache, aphasia, nuchal rigidity, cranial nerve involvement, extrapyramidal signs, seizures, papilledema, paresthesias, and field defects. Late manifestations occur after 2 months and simulate a space-occupying lesion, with disorientation, aphasia, apathy, memory loss, personality changes, comas, clonic spasms, hemiplegia, field defects, paresthesias, and Jacksonian-type seizures. Photophobia and stiff neck may also occur. Ocular signs of cerebral involvement include the following: nystagmus, unilateral mydriasis, bilateral miosis with slow response to light, paralysis of accommodation, convergence, and 3rd, 4th, and 6th cranial nerve involvement.

The spinal cord is involved more frequently in *S. japonicum* infection and includes transverse myelitis.

Skin Features

In addition to the skin manifestations that sometimes occur in the early and late stages of the disease (see earlier), deposition of ova in the skin causes skin manifestations at distant sites, such as the trunk (especially the area around the umbilicus—the principal site), where firm, flesh-colored, oval papules develop, which then coalesce to form slightly elevated plaques with irregular, mamillated contours. The surface gradually becomes darker, scales, and sometimes ulcerates. Occasionally, the plaques become hypopigmented.

Ocular Features

Ocular disease is usually caused by *S. haematobium* and, rarely, by *S. japonicum*. The findings include the following:

1. Lid edema and urticaria, representing angioneurotic edema during the first phase of infection or in association with orbital involvement.
2. A localized granuloma caused by ova or adult forms of *S. haematobium*.
3. A chronic blepharitis from *S. mansoni*.
4. Conjunctival chemosis and inflammation during the initial phase of the infection, representing an allergic reaction or orbital involvement. It is usually mild and transient in type.
5. Small conjunctival granulomas near the caruncle, which cause few or no symptoms and appear as soft, smooth, pinkish-yellow polypoid masses from *S. haematobium* eggs in the conjunctival vessels.
6. Conjunctival scarring and subconjunctival hemorrhage in *S. mansoni* infections.
7. Fine corneal nebulae and interstitial keratitis in *S. mansoni* infections.
8. Localized granuloma or hyperplasia of the lacrimal gland from *S. haematobium* ova.
9. Lid edema, conjunctival chemosis, and proptosis, simulating an orbital pseudotumor from orbital *S. haematobium* infection. Either the adult parasite lodges in the orbital vein, causing symptoms of vascular occlusion, or an orbital granuloma develops in response to ova or to the adult form of *S. haematobium*.
10. Parasitic invasion of the anterior chamber.
11. Cataract from invasion of the lens by *S. mansoni*.
12. Central retinal artery embolism and recurrent intraocular hemorrhage from adult parasites lodging in retinal vessels.
13. Iritis, uveitis, chorioretinitis, and chorioretinal artery occlusion from deposition of *S. japonicum* ova in the uveal tract.
14. A healed chorioretinitis in *S. mansoni* infections.
15. Invasion of the vitreous cavity by adult organisms.
16. An optic neuritis from deposition of ova in optic nerve tissue.
17. Papilledema from cerebral involvement or invasion of the nerve head and retina by *S. mansoni*.

Paragonimiasis

Paragonimiasis is caused by various lung flukes. The disease occurs in the Far East, West Pacific, India, Africa, and Central and South America. Humans become infected by eating inadequately cooked crab or crayfish. The metacercaria that are released in the intestine penetrate the intestinal wall, pass through the diaphragm to the lung, and encyst and mature into adult worms.

Clinical Manifestations
Encysted adult worms in the lung cause fever, sweating, and chronic productive cough of brown-stained sputum.

Skin Features
Skin lesions are caused by ectopic localization of the fluke. Large, mobile subcutaneous lesions develop and often progress to cold abscesses. Larger lesions are often painful and may rupture spontaneously.

Ocular Features
Ectopic localization of the fluke in the conjunctiva may cause large granulomata.

Cestoda

The cestodes are flat, ribbon-like worms (tapeworms) composed of a variable number of segments (proglottids), an anterior segment (scolex) that comprises the head, and a narrow neck. Hooks or suckers are located on the head and serve to attach the worm to the intestinal mucosa.

Larval Cestodiasis

Echinococcus granulosus causes cystic hydatid disease; *E. multilocularis* causes alveolar hydatid disease; *Taenia solium* produces cysticercosis; *Multiceps* (Taenia) multiceps causes coenurosis; and *Spirometra* species cause sparganosis. The larvae of each of these organisms have a bladder-like form and possess one or more protoscolices. With the exception of *T. solium,* humans are nonessential hosts. In sparganosis, humans become infected by ingestion of first- or second-stage larvae of *Spirometra* species, from invertebrate or vertebrate intermediate hosts, respectively; or by contact with raw flesh of amphibians or reptiles infected with the spargana. Infection by the other cestodes occurs through ingestion of tapeworm eggs that are passed in the feces of infected, definitive hosts.

Because of differences in parasitic localization and host–parasite compatibility, the diseases have a broad range of manifestations.

Cystic Hydatid Disease

Cystic hydatid disease comprises infection with *Echinococcus granulosus* and *E. multilocularis.* The former is a small tapeworm parasitic for dogs, wolves, and occasionally cats. Its larva is known as the hydatid, which in humans, develops into a hydatid tumor or cyst of the liver, lungs, kidneys, or other organs, including the eye and orbit. The cyst is single and develops around the embryo.

E. multilocularis is parasitic for the red fox, arctic fox, mice, voles, and lemmings. The cyst in humans usually metastasizes to the liver, but occasionally, it metastasizes to all parts of the body, including the eye and orbit. Infection occurs through intimate contact with dogs, though ingestion of contaminated water or infected uncooked food, or through the intermediary of arthropods, such as flies.

Following ingestion, the cestoid eggs hatch in the small intestine where the embryos penetrate the wall to reach the portal circulation. The embryos are carried to the liver and other sites, where they produce cysts that slowly enlarge, eventually producing symptoms by virtue of their size or through spontaneous or traumatic rupture. Release of cyst fluid causes variable allergic reactions that may be severe.

Clinical Manifestations
The clinical manifestations vary according to the site, size, and condition of the cyst. Between 20% and 40% of primary human infections have multiple cysts or multiple organ involvement. The pastoral strain, in which dogs and other canids are the definitive host, involves the liver (>65%), the lungs (25%), and less commonly, the spleen, kidneys, heart, bone, and central nervous system. The northern sylvatic strain, in which wolves are the definitive host, preferentially involves the lungs, and the infection is less complicated and more benign.

Hepatic cysts cause right epigastric pain, nausea, vomiting, and liver enlargement. The liver and lung are often involved together.

Pulmonary cysts become symptomatic when ruptured, causing chest pain, cough, dyspnea, and hemoptysis. Cerebral cysts cause focal epilepsy and signs of increased intracranial pressure. Renal cysts cause hematuria and/or pain that extends into the loin. Hydatid bone cysts are usually asymptomatic but often lead to pathologic fractures.

Skin Features
Leakage of fluid from a cyst often causes generalized urticaria. A painless, sometimes fluctuant swelling may occur in muscle and subcutaneous tissue from cyst formation.

Ocular Features
Orbital involvement occurs in about 1% of cases. The manifestations begin insidiously and develop over a period of months; rarely, the onset is sudden. Findings include pain, unilateral proptosis, and a palpable orbital mass that is more common in the upper quadrants. The cyst usually protrudes under the skin of the eyelid or, occasionally, through the palpebral fissure as a tense elastic swelling. Eventually, the cyst may occupy most of the orbit, causing complete luxation of the globe.

Cerebral cysts may lead to papilledema and optic atrophy.

Cysticercosis

Cysticercosis is endemic in Mexico, Central and South America, Africa, Pakistan, India, and Asia. It represents an infection by the larval form of *Taenia solium,* with humans, instead of the pig, becoming the intermediate host. The eggs are ingested by humans and hatch in the intestine. The embryos are distributed to all parts of the body, especially to the skeletal muscle and brain and, rarely, to the eye, skin, or heart (Fig. 31-26). There the embryo is transformed into the larval stage (cysticercus).

Clinical Manifestations

Cysticercosis has a proclivity for involving the brain, eyes, subcutaneous tissue, and muscle, but it also involves the lungs, heart, liver, and peritoneum. Several sites may be involved simultaneously. Exceptionally, both eyes are involved at the same time.

Pain, muscle aches, and fever may occur, and the manifestations are determined by the location, number of cysticerci, and host's inflammatory response. The infection may therefore be relatively asymptomatic or very severe.

Manifestations of cerebral involvement include the following:

1. Progressive intracranial hypertension, with intermittent headaches, vomiting, and papilledema.
2. Convulsions, especially of the Jacksonian type.
3. Mental disturbances, such as amnesia, disorientation, confusion, and progressive deterioration.
4. Meningoencephalitis.
5. Less common findings include localized anesthesia and involvement of the 1st, 2nd, 3rd, 5th, 7th, 8th, 9th, 11th, or 12th cranial nerves.

Skin Features

Nodules often develop in the subcutaneous tissue and muscles. They are firm, round, rubbery, and painless; usually measure 1 to 2 cm; and often persist unchanged for many years.

Ocular Features

The ocular features of cysticercus (Fig. 31-27) include the following:

1. A localized, slowly growing subcutaneous cyst causing very few symptoms.
2. A localized, painless swelling or fleshy growth of the conjunctiva or, occasionally, a conjunctival abscess.
3. Enlargement of the lacrimal gland and manifestations of a chronic dacryoadenitis.
4. Severe orbital inflammation with pain, lid edema, ptosis, conjunctival chemosis, limitation of ocular movements, diplopia, and displacement of the globe.
5. Purulent tenonitis.

6. Intraocular cysticerci, which frequently move from one location to another. Early in the disease process, there is only mild inflammation; later, inflammation becomes intense.
   a. Anterior chamber cysticerci floating freely or attached to the corneal endothelium, iris, or anterior lens capsule.
   b. Cysticerci in the subretinal space near the posterior pole with signs of uveitis, chorioretinal scarring, and rhegmatogenous or exudative retinal detachment.
   c. Attachment to the optic nerve head.
7. Papilledema and optic atrophy from hydrocephalus.

Sparganosis

Sparganosis represents an infection by the second-stage larvae of the genus *Spirometra.* It is more common in Southeast Asia. Most cases in the United States occur in the Southeast.

Humans become infected by drinking water that contains the infected copepod, or by using frog flesh as a poultice for eye injuries.

Clinical Manifestations

There are two forms of infection: nonproliferating and proliferating. The proliferating form has an additional variant form.

The nonproliferating form is most common and causes tender, often migratory, subcutaneous, slow-growing nodules. Occasionally, it involves the lung, pulmonary artery, jejunum, colon, peritoneal cavity, epididymis, urethra, intracranial structures, and spinal cord. The nodules are associated with fever, chills, erythema, and edema, and sometimes cause local elephantiasis by obstruction of the lymphatics.

The proliferating form of sparganosis is characterized by extensive proliferation in the subcutaneous tissues, muscles, bone, viscera, and brain. Usually, there are multiple, painful, erythematous, subcutaneous nodules, and many of the nodules suppurate.

A second, variant form of proliferating sparganosis also occurs, which is associated with asymptomatic or pruritic skin papules and nodules. Occasionally, both forms of proliferating sparganosis occur together. Emaciation, weakness, prostration, and death eventuate.

Ocular Manifestations

Ocular involvement in the nonproliferating form of sparganosis causes irritation, pain, decreased vision, and blindness. The lid is swollen and painful. Subconjunctival hemorrhages, painful conjunctival swellings, chemosis, and proptosis may occur, suggesting an orbital cellulitis.

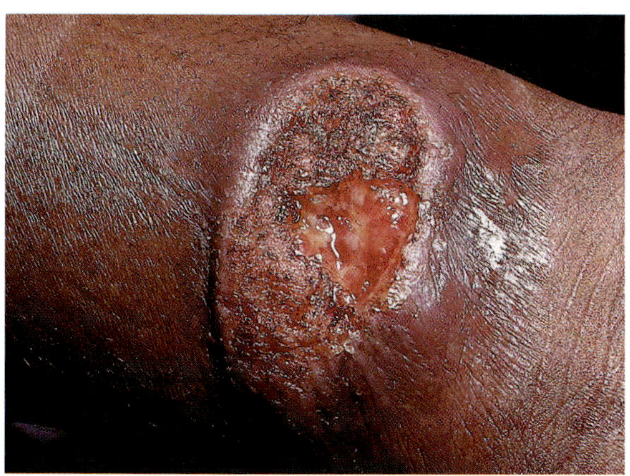

FIGURE 31-1. Cutaneous leishmaniasis showing large ulcer on wrist with typical indurated, raised margin. Infection acquired by an American soldier during Operation Desert Storm.

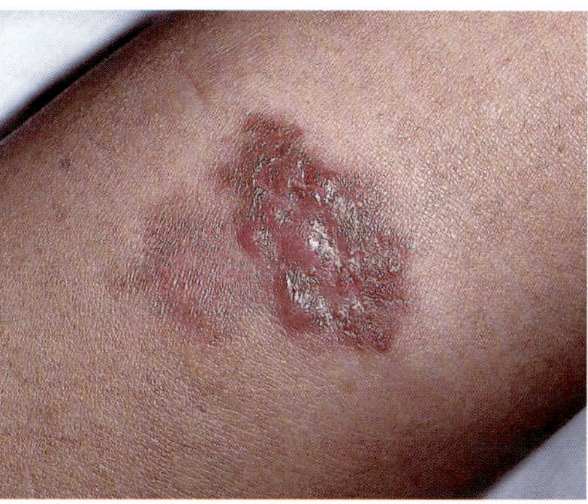

FIGURE 31-2. Chronic cutaneous leishmaniasis with grouped nodules resembling early lupus vulgaris and tertiary syphilis.

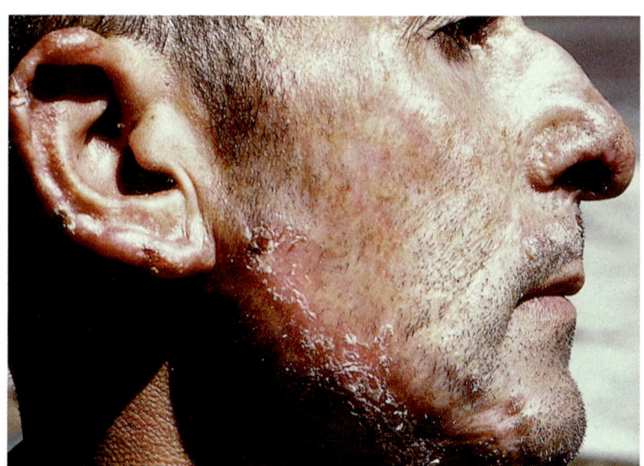

FIGURE 31-3. Chronic cutaneous leishmaniasis in a patient from Iran. Scarring of nose, ear, and mandible closely resemble lupus vulgaris.

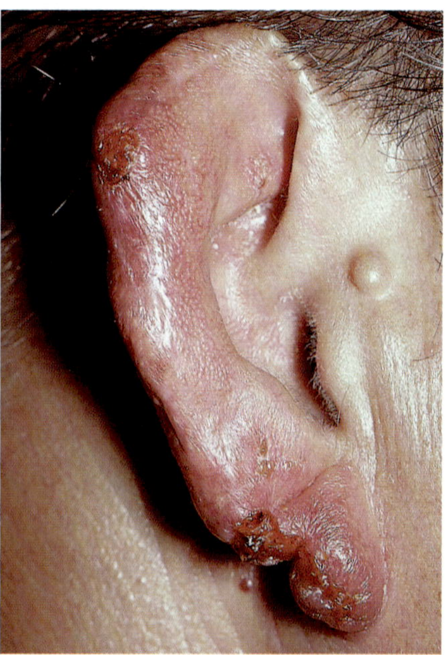

FIGURE 31-4. Chiclero ulcer, so called because these leishmanial infections are often found in workers who tap rubber trees to obtain chiclet for the manufacturer of chewing gum. Note resemblance to lupus vulgaris (tuberculosis) and lepromatous leprosy.

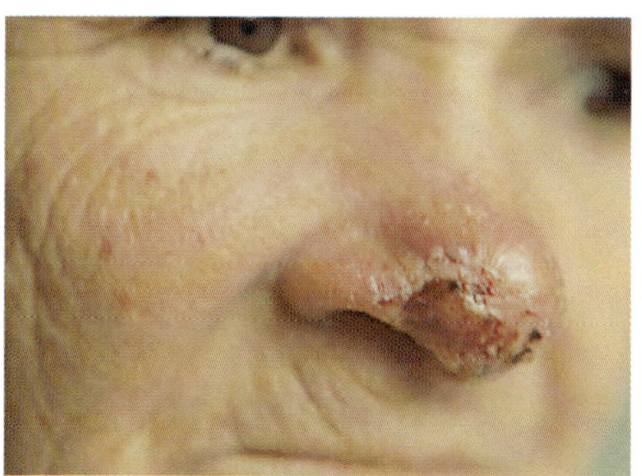

FIGURE 31-5. Mucocutaneous leishmaniasis in a Colombian patient. She had noticed these lesions only two months earlier. Untreated, this can progress to severe nasal destruction (see Fig. 31-6).

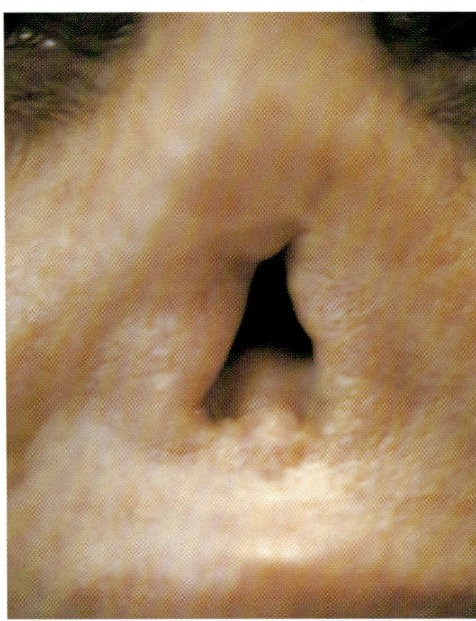

FIGURE 31-6. Espundia, late stage. Destruction of the septum has caused collapse of the nasal bridge and tip of the nose. Syphilis, tuberculosis, and leprosy share the predilection for this site with leishmaniasis.

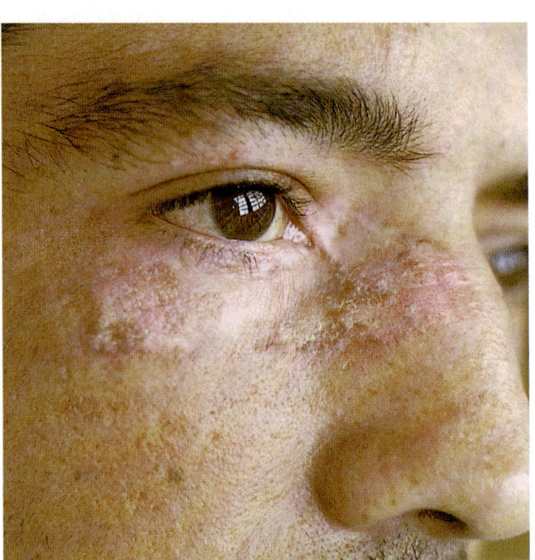

FIGURE 31-7. Mucocutaneous leishmaniasis of cheek, nose, and eyelid in a patient seen in Central America.

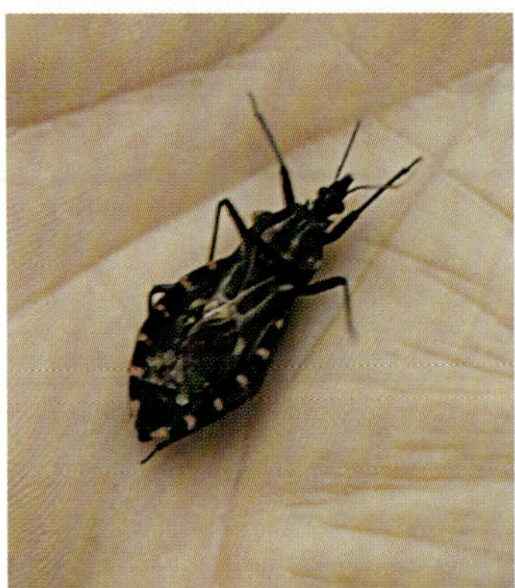

FIGURE 31-8. Reduviid bug transmits the pathogen causing American trypanosomiasis (Chagas disease) through its infected feces. It is also known as the "kissing" or assassin bug because it bites its sleeping victims at night.

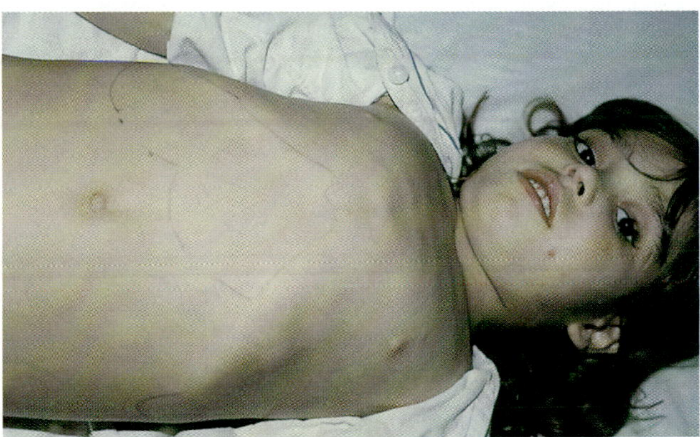

FIGURE 31-9. Acute Chagas disease in a young girl with a 4-month history of fever, malaise, and cough. She presented with cardiomegaly, hepatosplenomegaly, and resolving Romana sign.

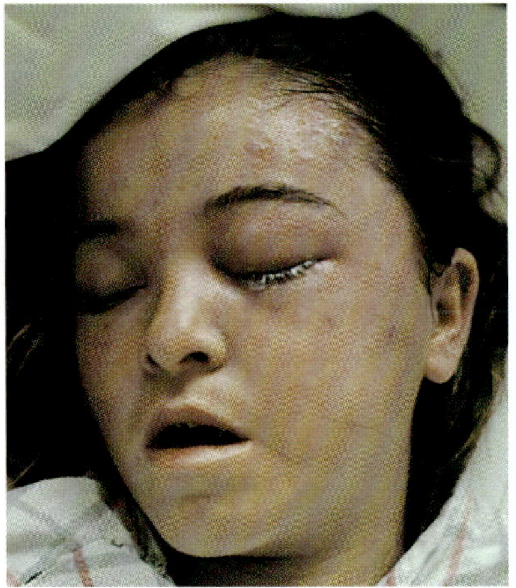

FIGURE 31-10. Romana sign (unilateral edema of the eyelid, unilateral conjunctivitis, and dacryoadenitis). This young woman's acute Chagas disease was complicated by meningoencephalitis.

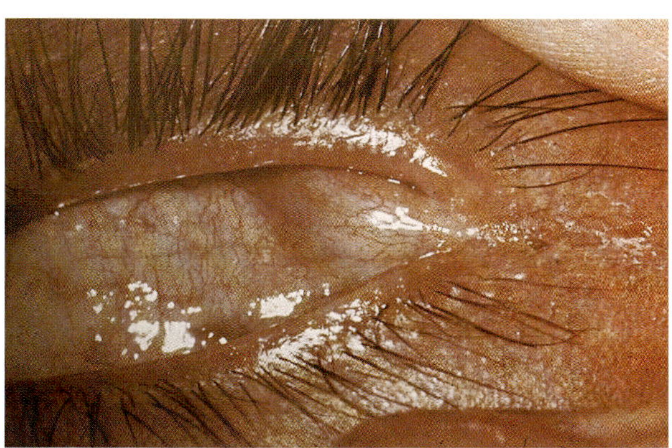

FIGURE 31-11. Enlarged lachrymal gland (part of Romana sign) in Chagas disease.

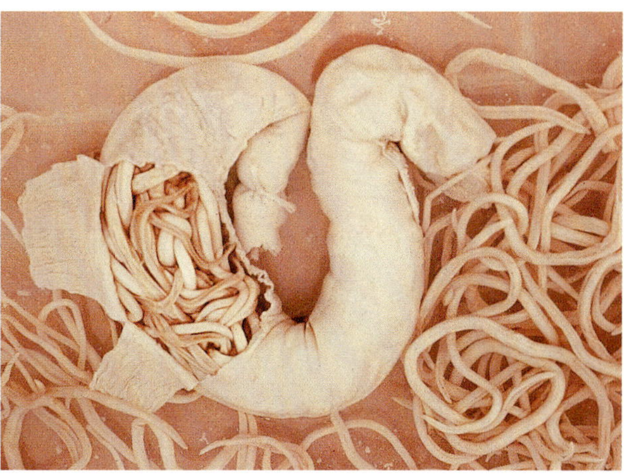

FIGURE 31-12. Massive numbers of ascaris in the intestines found at autopsy.

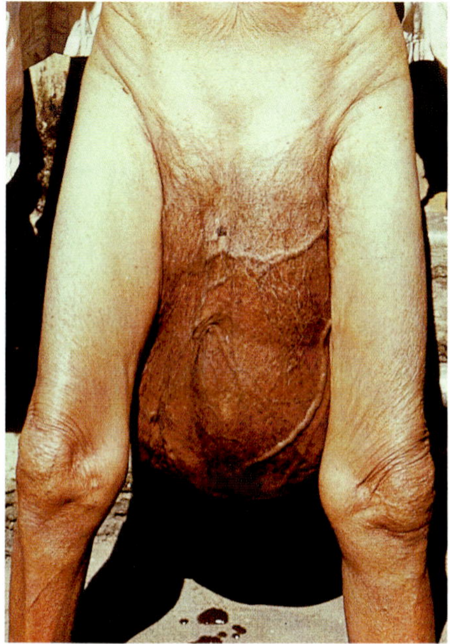

FIGURE 31-13. Filariasis in an old man with enormous scrotal edema. (Courtesy of Dr. William Hennessey.)

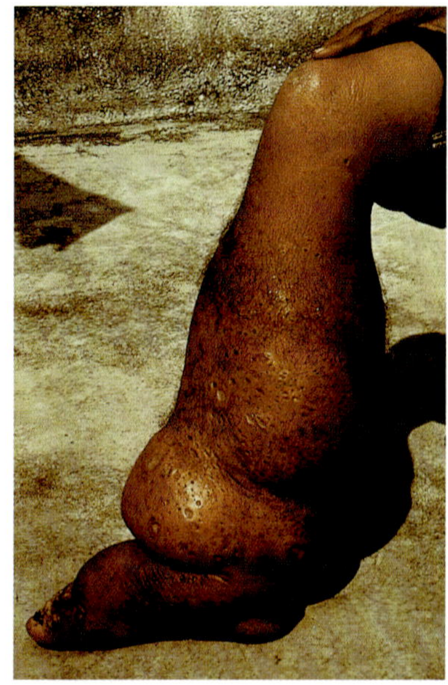

FIGURE 31-14. Filariasis with elephantiasis.

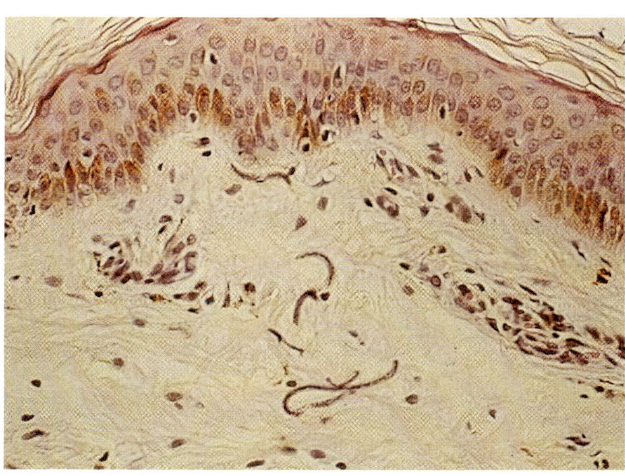

FIGURE 31-15. Microfilaria of *Onchocerca volvulus* in skin.

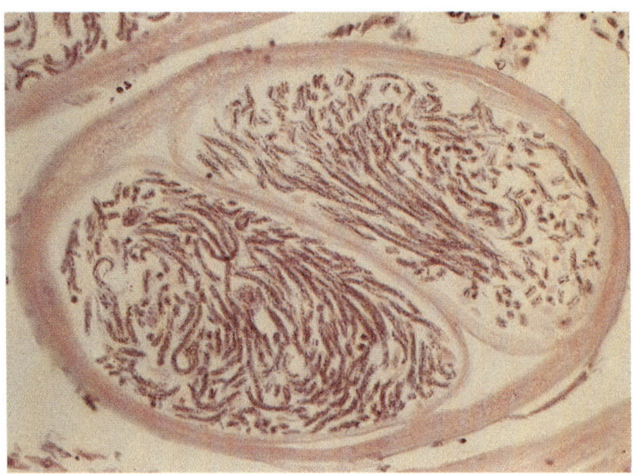

FIGURE 31-16. Cross sections of adult filaria in a fibrous capsule (onchocercoma).

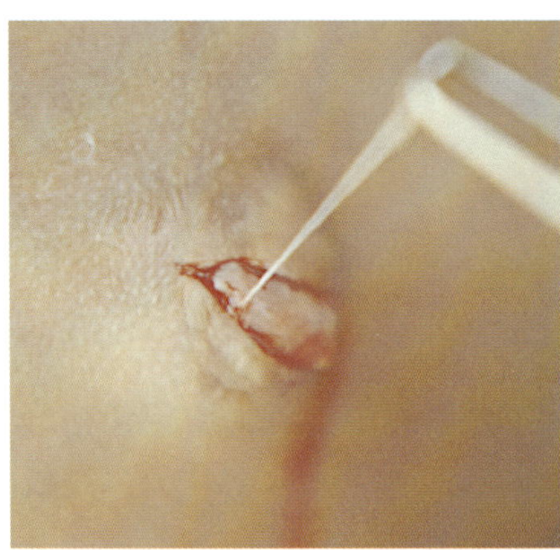

FIGURE 31-17. Adult filarial organism being extracted from an onchocercoma of the subcutaneous tissue, while performing an onchocercotomy on the young boy pictured in Fig. 31-19. The onchocercoma was inadvertently nicked, exposing the organism.

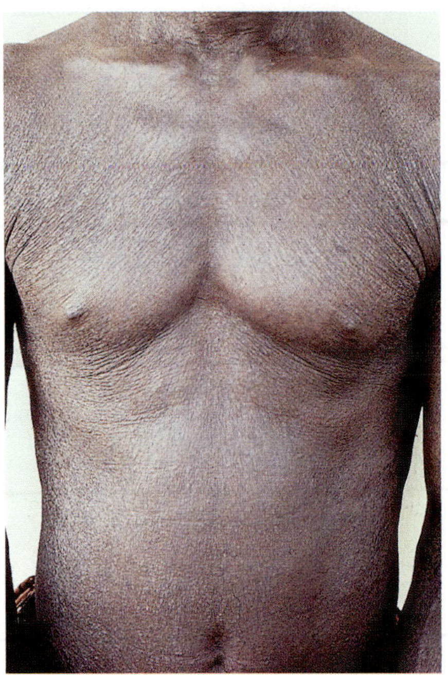

FIGURE 31-18. Chronic onchocerciasis showing dry, thickened skin.

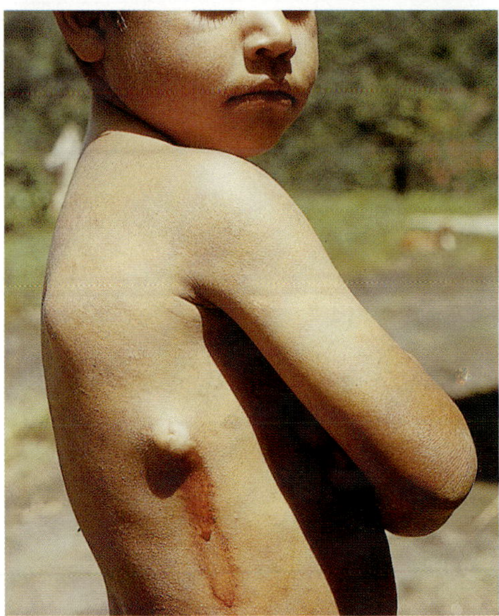

FIGURE 31-19. Onchocercoma in young Guatemalan boy. Bleeding is from injection of anesthesia before surgical removal. (Same patient as shown in close-up in Fig. 31-17.)

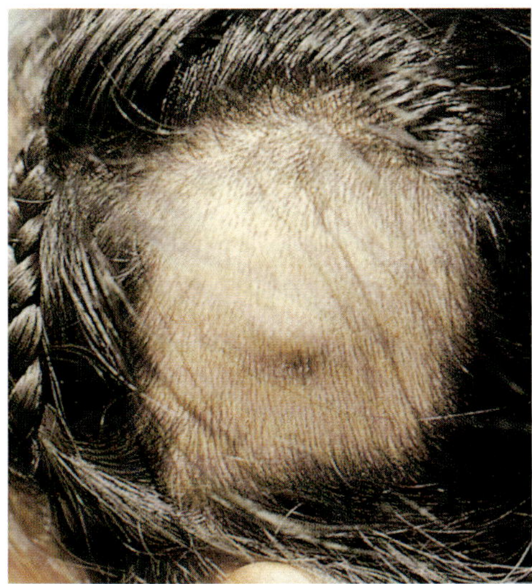

FIGURE 31-20. Onchocercoma of scalp in young Guatemalan girl shaved before surgery. Onchocercotomy reduces the number of microfilaria released by the adult worms in these nodules. It is the microfilaria that cause most of the pathology in this disease, especially of the eye.

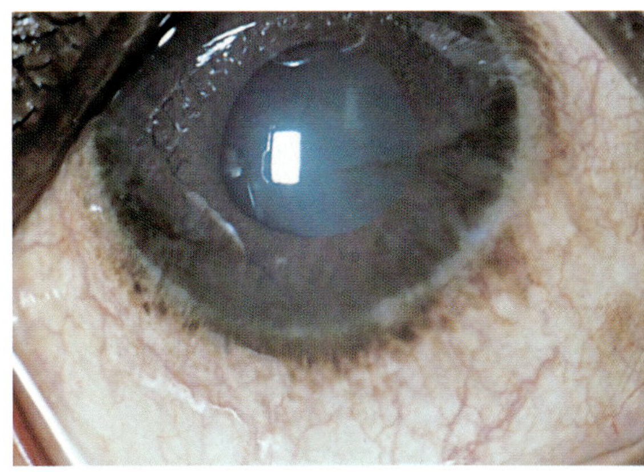

FIGURE 31-21. Onchocerciasis. Early sclerosing keratitis. (Courtesy of Dr. Mitchell Friedlaender.)

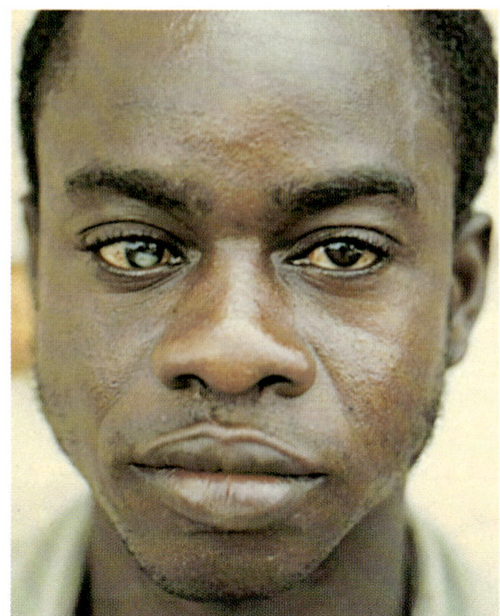

FIGURE 31-22. Onchocerciasis with sclerosing keratitis in a patient from Ghana. (Courtesy of Dr. John Reeves.)

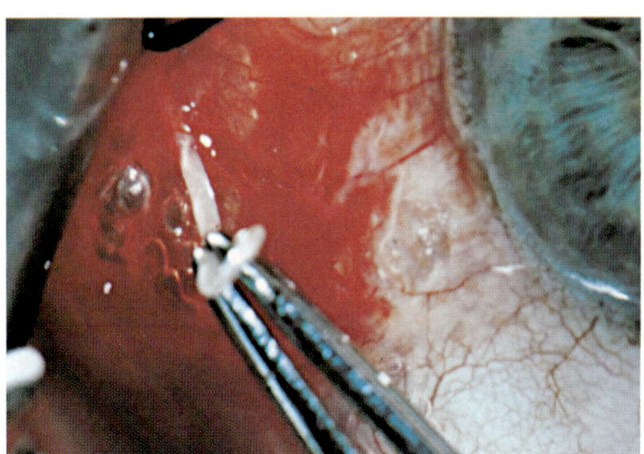

FIGURE 31-23. Loa loa under the conjunctiva.

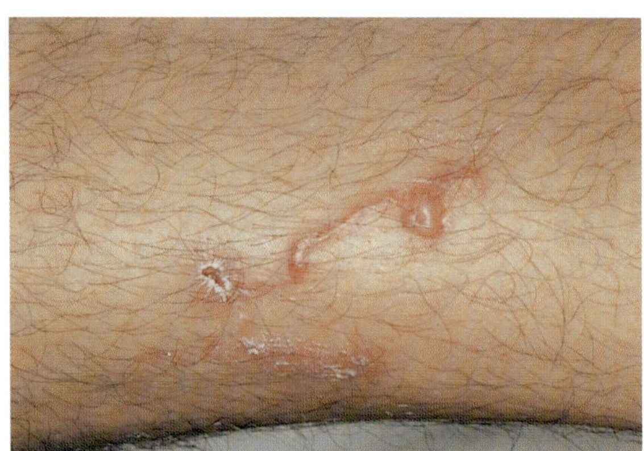

FIGURE 31-24. Cutaneous larva migrans (creeping eruption). The tortuous, erythematous lines are formed by the advancing larva.

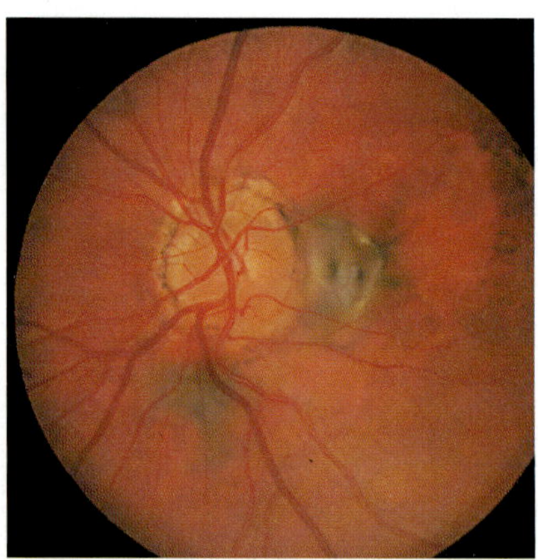

FIGURE 31-25. Toxocariasis of the uveal tract.

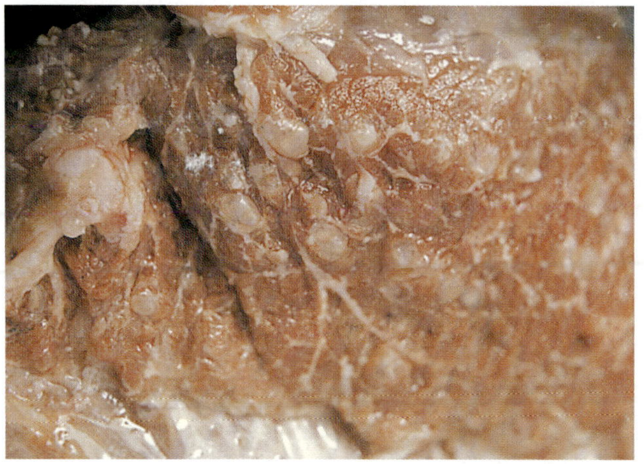

FIGURE 31-26. Cysticercosis (*Cysticercus cellulosae*) in pork. This photograph is of tainted meat available in the marketplace in a central American country. The customers were told to cook the meat well.

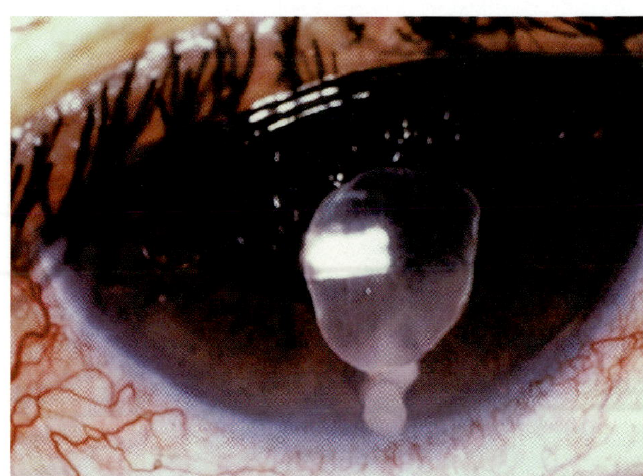

FIGURE 31-27. *Cysticercus* organism in the anterior chamber. (Courtesy of Dr. Phillips Thygeson.)

DISEASES CAUSED BY ARTHROPODS AND OTHER NOXIOUS AGENTS

Many arthropods cause skin and eye disease or serve as vectors for skin and eye disease. Each possesses a chitinous exoskeleton, segmental body, and jointed appendages.

LICE

Lice are blood ectoparasites and are the cause of pediculosis.

Pediculosis Pubis (*Pthirus pubis*)

The pubic louse (*Pthirus pubis*) usually infests the pubic hair, often extending to hairs on the abdomen, thighs, and axilla (Fig. 32-1). Occasionally, it also infests the eyebrows and eyelashes (Figs. 32-2 and 32-3). In prepubertal patients lacking pubic hair, it is sometimes found on the scalp and lashes. It is transmitted by close, most often sexual, body contact. Thus, when seeing *P. pubis,* always consider coexisting, other sexually transmitted diseases. This louse is somewhat broader than the head-and-body louse and is more capable of grasping the widely spaced hair (Fig. 32-4). The eggs are cemented to the hair near the skin surface (Fig. 32-4), where it is warmest, and are light brown, darker after a blood meal. An operculum through which the nymph emerges is evident at its free end.

Pediculus humanus var. *capitis* infests the scalp hair (Figs. 32-5 and 32-6); occasionally, the body hair; and, rarely, the lashes or brows. It is transmitted by the common use of combs, hats, and scarves or by direct head-to-head contact. Outbreaks occur frequently in schools. Factors favoring transmission include overcrowding, poor hygiene, and poverty. The nits are cemented to the hair shafts close to the surface of the scalp. They are flesh-colored until the nymph emerges through the operculum, when it becomes more white.

The body louse, *Pediculus humanus* var *P. corporis,* apparently does not affect the brow or lashes. It is prevalent in overcrowded and unhygienic conditions where individuals fail to remove their clothes (Fig. 32-7). It very closely resembles the head louse. The female cements her eggs to the seams of clothing (Fig. 32-8). It is important as a vector for epidemic typhus, trench fever, and louse-borne relapsing fever.

Skin Features

Persistent and intense itching is common to all forms of pediculosis. Redness and excoriation are usually found, and pyoderma may occur.

The adult *P. pubis* organisms and nits are readily seen close to the surface of the skin, especially if viewed with magnification (Fig. 32-1). Occasionally, they cause asymptomatic blue-gray skin macules (maculae caeruleae), believed to be due to altered blood pigments in the host.

P. capitis usually causes scalp itch. Pruritic papules occur on the nape of the neck (Fig. 32-6), and sometimes the hair becomes matted and crusted from secondary bacterial infection. Patients infested by *P. corporis* usually develop symptoms only if sensitized to the organism's salivary antigens, at which time there is itching and excoriation in the areas of infestations. Sometimes the skin becomes hyperpigmented during prolonged infestation.

Patients with *P. pubis* infestation usually complain of persistent, intense itching. In the eye, the involved area, such as the lid margin, is red and sometimes excoriated. Rust-colored speckles representing louse feces are often visible. Lid abscesses rarely occur from secondary infection. The adult organism and nits can usually be seen (Figs. 32-2 and 32-3).

DIPTERA (TWO-WINGED INSECTS)

Many flies, mosquitoes, gnats, and midges have ocular and dermatologic significance because of their ability to transmit disease, to bite man, and to cause myiasis.

Mosquitoes

Mosquitoes, apart from their ability to transmit disease by serving as vectors for malaria, filariasis, yellow fever, and dengue fever, through their venom and the immune reaction induced by antigens in their saliva, cause itching, erythema, a wheal at the site of the bite, and occasionally, chemosis that may be very severe. Rarely, bullae, cellulitis, and an eczematoid reaction are observed.

Flies

It is beyond the scope of this book to discuss the characteristics of the various flies; however, because the numbers of species and the diseases they transmit are extremely plentiful, we call attention to them and to the diseases they can transmit.

The housefly and the lesser housefly sometimes act as mechanical vectors for transmission of disease. The stable fly is similar in appearance and often causes painful bites.

Sandflies are tiny, hairy flies with long legs and sharp, pointed wings. They include the *Phlebotomus* species, vectors for Old World cutaneous and visceral leishmaniasis and sandfly fever, and the *Lutzomyia* species, vectors for New World cutaneous and visceral leishmaniasis and bartonellosis.

The black flies are small, humped-back flies with short, broad wings. They are found almost worldwide; besides causing severe misery by their tenacious persistence and biting, several species serve as vectors for the transmission of onchocerciasis. Bites usually occur on exposed parts of the body and are covered by a small crust of blood with surrounding ecchymosis; later, they become pruritic papules. Rarely, they induce severe edema, nodules, or an eczematoid reaction.

Gnats or biting midges cause misery worldwide through biting. They induce small papular lesions, nodules, and wheallike lesions or bullae.

Horse flies, deer flies, and clegs cause painful bites in man and serve as vectors for transmission of tularemia and loiasis. They have a large, stout body and short antennae. The snipe flies belong to the same family and are vicious biters and pests.

The eye gnats are small flies that are attracted to open sores and purulent material, such as that associated with conjunctivitis. The *Hippelates* and *Siphunculina* species belong to the same family and are mechanical vectors for the transmission of yaws and trachoma.

The housefly is often attracted to the conjunctiva and may feed on conjunctival secretions.

The flat flea, or ked, an ectoparasite of birds and animals, may cause persistent pruritic papules.

The tsetse fly serves as a vector for the transmission of trypanosomiasis.

Myiasis

Myiasis represents infestation of any body tissue by the larvae (maggots) of flies. Myiasis is divided into:

1. Cutaneous myiasis. Cutaneous myiasis represents infestation of the skin through deposition of larvae or ova into existing ulcers or wounds (traumatic or wound myiasis) (Fig. 32-9).
2. Furuncular myiasis (Figs. 32-10 to 32-15). Furuncular myiasis represents penetration and deposition of larvae or ova into apparently normal skin.
3. Nasopharyngeal myiasis (myiasis of the nose, sinus, and pharynx).
4. External ophthalmomyiasis (Fig. 32-16). External ophthalmomyiasis represents infestation of the ocular adnexa. In some instances, botfly larvae are found in the conjunctiva.
5. Internal ophthalmomyiasis (intraocular infestation).

Myiasis is more common in areas of squalor and filth.

Clinical Manifestations

The clinical and ocular features of myiasis are similar.

Furuncular myiasis often occurs in normal body orifices (e.g., ears, nasal passages, genital tract, and eye) as well as in wounds and sores. It often causes constitutional symptoms of malaise, regional lymphadenopathy, and lymphangitis. Recurrently painful (with movement of the larvae), boillike lesions with a central opening, often showing tiny telltale bubbles, develop several days following the infestation. The posterior end of the larvae may be seen in the opening, and serosanguineous fluid can be extruded through the opening. The lesion heals rapidly following expulsion of the larva. (*Hypoderma* species fail to mature in man and are therefore not expelled and thus induce migratory inflammatory nodules.) The *Gastrophilus* larvae produce a creeping eruption that appears under the skin as a tortuous, threadlike, red line with a vesicle at its end containing the larva.

Furuncular myiasis of the lid causes considerable edema; otherwise, the findings are similar to those seen in the skin.

Conjunctival myiasis causes moderate lid edema or, more frequently, considerable destruction of both lid and conjunctiva. The lids may be destroyed in the generalized destruction that occurs with orbital infection; in such instances, constitutional symptoms are usually severe.

Conjunctival infestation causes an acute catarrhal conjunctivitis associated with "small grains of sand," which represent very motile white larvae that move in an accordion fashion, attempting to avoid light. The larvae attach themselves firmly to the underlying conjunctiva when attempts are made to remove them. Occasionally, the larvae invade the conjunctiva, forming an inflammatory nodule, cyst, or subconjunctival swelling, or may be seen wriggling under the tissue.

Corneal involvement is uncommon and is manifested as a superficial epithelial keratitis or a marginal corneal ulceration. True corneal invasion or penetration is very rare.

The lacrimal system is usually involved in the destructive orbital or nasal myiasis. Infrequently, the lacrimal sac is involved and is characterized by a chronic dacryocystitis with discharge and sometimes a fistula.

Orbital destruction is found in the general scenario of destructive myiasis. In such instances, the orbit and its contents are converted into a crater filled with rotting flesh and maggots in less than 24 hours. Coma and death quickly supervene. Less frequently, only one or two larvae penetrate into the orbit and cause proptosis and chemosis, which later subsides as the parasites are expelled.

Intraocular myiasis usually develops only after an interlude of 6 to 8 months from the initial infection. It usually occurs in children from penetration of the sclera or, less commonly, the cornea. Anterior ophthalmomyiasis with the organism located in the anterior chamber is most common, causing a turbulent iridocyclitis with intense pain and sometimes lens subluxation. Occasionally, there is a gray-white mass that moves with the movement of the head.

Posterior ophthalmomyiasis often causes subretinal (linear, depigmented) tracks, retinal pigment epithelial changes, and subretinal and vitreous hemorrhages. Subretinal larvae cause an intense uveal reaction with retinal detachment. Intravitreal larvae cause a less intense reaction and may be self-limited.

Fleas

Fleas are bloodsucking ectoparasites that often affect man. They are wingless and measure 1 to 8 mm. Several fleas serve to transmit plague and murine typhus to man. Many others [e.g., human (Fig. 32-17), cat, dog, and bird fleas] cause a typical papular urticaria in sensitized patients. Sand fleas cause tungiasis.

Clinical Features—Dog, Cat, Bird, and Human Flea Bites

Clinically, the patient presents with pruritic, grouped or linear, pale erythematous papules with a tiny central punctum. Depending on the sensitivity of the host, one may also see evidence of hemorrhages (Fig. 32-18), urticaria (papular urticaria), and occasionally, small bullae.

Human and animal flea bites most commonly occur on the ankles, lower legs (Fig. 32-19), and waist. They are also found at sites of close contact, such as an arm or the chest, from holding or sleeping with a pet.

The eruption caused by the bite of bird fleas is similar but often more generalized and extensive, including the face, because the bites occur during sleep.

Clinical Features—Sand Fleas

The female sand flea burrows under the skin (especially the skin of the toes and soles) and sometimes under the skin of the eyelid to lay its eggs. The larvae hatch, causing intense irritation. At first, a black dot is visible at the site of the

organism and is later replaced by an inflammatory nodule or, in some cases, an abscess or ulceration with sloughing, especially if there is secondary infection.

STINGING ARTHROPODS (ANTS, BEES, WASPS, AND HORNETS)

The stinging arthropods have a narrow isthmus connecting the abdomen to the thorax. Humans are affected by venom released when a modified ovipositor is used to sting the unsuspecting individual. The clinical manifestations are dependent upon the type and amount of venom injected, the venom's allergenic nature, and the patient's allergic state to that particular venom. Multiple bites give more violent reactions than a single bite.

Honeybees have a barbed stinger that is left in the wound; thus they can only sting once. Bumblebees do not have a barbed stinger and can sting repeatedly, although they usually do so only when provoked. Bee, wasp, and hornet venom causes burning pain, edema, erythema, and rarely, gangrene. Patients who possess a local hypersensitivity reaction to the venom develop increasing edema for 30 minutes to several hours following the sting. Apart from anaphylaxis, constitutional reactions usually occur only following multiple stings. They include severe headache, vomiting, diarrhea, hypotension, generalized vasodilatation, and shock. Cutaneous anaphylaxis is manifested by pruritus, erythema, urticaria and angioedema, respiratory anaphylaxis by laryngeal edema and bronchospasm, and vascular anaphylaxis by tachycardia, hypotension, and shock. Late reactions to the venom include a reaction that resembles serum sickness—with urticaria, arthralgia, and joint swelling.

Wasps, social wasps, and solitary wasps have small or no barbs and thus can sting repeatedly, sometimes inflicting painful and troublesome stings.

Ants, especially the Australian jumper and bull ants and the red and black fire ants, may inflict much pain through bites and stings. The cutaneous reaction to fire ants is manifested by a cluster of two minute hemorrhagic points where the fire ant attaches its mandible to the skin. Initially, the hemorrhagic points are quickly surrounded by a wheal and then by a vesicle. The vesicle fluid becomes cloudy, and the lesion pustulates within 10 to 12 hours, followed after several days by crusting and healing with scarring.

Systemic hypersensitivity reactions to fire ants often increase in severity with subsequent bites. The reactions include generalized urticaria, angioedema, nausea, vomiting, wheezing, and hypotension. Ant bites cause severe lid edema.

Ocular Features—Bee, Wasp, and Hornet Stings

Bee, wasp, and hornet stings (Fig. 32-20) of the lid cause local pain, edema, erythema, and occasionally, gangrene.

The contiguous areas are usually indurated. In some instances, the stinger penetrates the lid, injuring the conjunctiva, sclera, or cornea.

HEMIPTERA (TRUE BUGS)

Hemiptera of dermatologic and ocular significance include bed bugs; bugs that parasitize bats or birds (martin and swallow bugs); Mexican chicken bugs; members of the family Anthocoridae that are usually found in granaries, haystacks, and clothing; and the Reduviidae, or kissing bugs.

Bedbugs cause linear and multiple bites on the skin and may affect the eyelid. Purpuric maculae develop at the site, and sensitized patients develop itching, wheals, or papules along with hemorrhagic dots in the center of the lesions. (Fig. 32-21).

Bites from the Mexican chicken bugs cause wheals, papules, vesicles, and pustules.

Bites from the assassin bug cause severe pain, whereas bites from the Triatominae cause minimal reaction unless the patient develops a hypersensitivity reaction, at which point pruritic papules, hemorrhagic nodules, and bullae may be observed.

The reduviid bugs are vectors for transmission of Chagas disease.

Beetles

Some beetles emit a blistering fluid while still alive (e.g., oil and blister beetles); others emit a vesicant only after being crushed (e.g., rove and *Paederus* beetles).

The vesicant causes a wheal that progresses to a blister. The lesions are usually linear. The *Paederus* beetles cause a vesicular narrow yellow line surrounded by edema that usually develops about 48 hours after the insect brushes the skin with its abdomen.

LEPIDOPTERA

Caterpillars

Caterpillars cause a toxic or foreign-body reaction by their hair (setae) (Fig. 32-22) coming in contact with the skin. The reaction, which may be delayed for several hours or days, is manifested by urticarial papules, wheals, and sometimes vesicles that last for several days. Pronounced lid edema may be associated.

The toxic pine caterpillar is a distinctive larvae of the Lepidoptera family that may cause severe blepharoconjunctivitis from the inorganic compounds, enzymes, and other toxic proteins in its setae. The toxin itself induces a short-lived violent inflammation. The barb and toxin together induce a longer-lasting and sometimes recurrent inflammation.

The flannel moth caterpillar induces immediate, intense burning pain along with spreading erythema at the puncture sites of the setae. It is usually associated with edema, lymphangitis, and regional lymphangitis.

Caterpillar hairs introduced into the conjunctiva or sclera may cause ophthalmia nodosa (Fig. 32-23), which is manifested by a granulomatous reaction surrounding the barb of the setae. The hairs of some caterpillars (*Isia isabella*, *Thaumetopoea wilkinsoni*) may even penetrate into the eye, causing violent inflammation and sometimes absolute glaucoma.

Moth Dermatitis

The hairs (setae) of various moths (Figs. 32-24 and 32-25) can cause severe pruritus and conjunctivitis on contact with the skin or eye. There is not only a mechanical irritation from the small, sharp spines, but also a chemical one from their urticating contents. Intense pruritus is soon followed by numerous papules (Figs. 32-26 and 32-27) and at times vesicles and urticaria. The tiny setae penetrate clothing so that even covered areas are affected. Eye lesions are similar to those resulting from contact with hair from certain caterpillars.

ARACHNIDS

Spider Bites

Spider bites may cause local or systemic symptoms of toxicity known as arachnidism. A bite from the black widow spider, the red-back spider, or the brown widow spider causes latrodectism with increasing pain and generalized symptoms within minutes. Colicky abdominal pain, profuse sweating, paresthesia, incoordination, and paralysis are common. In the young child or the very frail, death may ensue.

A bite from the violin or brown recluse spider family (Fig. 32-28) causes necrotic cutaneous loxoscelism or viscerocutaneous loxoscelism. Cutaneous loxoscelism begins with itching at the site of the bite, followed by severe pain, swelling, and ischemia; occasionally, the area becomes hemorrhagic. The area becomes necrotic 3 to 4 days later. An eschar develops, and sloughing occurs, leaving a slow-healing ulcer. Viscerocutaneous loxoscelism is associated with systemic symptoms of pyrexia, severe malaise, restlessness, headache, and vasomotor collapse. Ecchymosis, jaundice, hematuria, and hematoglobinuria may develop within 24 hours, leading to death from intravascular hemolysis.

Other spider bites may cause local pain, erythema, swelling, and sometimes small areas of necrosis.

Scorpions

Many scorpion stings cause severe pain, especially in infants and young children, although scorpions from the Middle

East, North Africa, the southern United States, and Mexico are the major species responsible for causing morbidity and mortality.

Most of the stings cause only local pain, although sometimes they cause severe burning pain, hyperesthesia, and edema. Constitutional effects include restlessness, difficulty with speech, muscle spasms, profuse sweating, increased salivation and tearing, tachycardia or bradycardia, and arrhythmias. Death is caused by cardiac or respiratory failure.

Ticks

Ticks are bloodsucking ectoparasites (Figs. 32-29 and 32-30). Ticks have important medical consequences, serving as vectors for tick-borne relapsing fever, tularemia, Lyme disease, ehrlichiosis, arbor virus, babesiosis, and a number of viral (several viral encephalitides) and rickettsial (Rocky Mountain spotted fever, Q fever, Siberian tick typhus, Colorado tick fever, and boutonneuse fever) infections. Ticks may also cause an ascending flaccid paralysis (tick paralysis) from the injection of a neurotoxin. The two major families of ticks having medical significance are hard-shell ticks and soft-shell ticks. Tick bite pyrexia, manifest by fever, chills, headache, abdominal pain, and vomiting, may occur while the tick is attached to the patient.

Depending on the species of tick, skin attachment may lead to intense local edema, especially if it attaches to the lid. Bullae and bruising may occur. Multiple ticks may cause a papular urticarial response and temporary alopecia if the scalp is involved, and eczematoid reactions from a tick granuloma if only part of the organism is removed. A blueish lid tumor has been observed to be caused by the larva of a tick.

Mites

Mites include the organisms causing scabies, chiggers, and *Demodex,* all of which have skin and eye significance.

Scabies

Scabies is characterized by intensely pruritic papulo-scaling lesions, often surmounted or accompanied by burrows. The itching is classically worse at night. Burrows (Fig. 32-31) are barely discernible, straight or tortuous, 1- to 3-mm, slightly elevated, grayish lines, often with a tiny dark or light dotlike papulovesicle at one end (representing the female scabies mite). The lesions are characteristically found at sites of thinner skin, such as finger webs, sides of the hands, volar wrist (Fig. 32-32), the axilla, umbilicus, areola, sacral area and buttocks, dorsal toe web areas, insteps (Fig. 32-33), and especially the penis and scrotum. In infants (Fig. 32-34) and in patients with reduced immunologic response, such as those with crusted (Norwegian) scabies

(Fig. 32-35), or AIDS, lesions may be widespread and include the face. The eruption may vary considerably from extensive lesions (chiefly eczematous sensitivity response) (Fig. 32-36) to very few in persons who wash frequently in whom the diagnosis may be difficult (scabies incognita).

To confirm the diagnosis, the examiner must first locate one or several burrows. Using a good magnifying light, place a drop of immersion oil on the slide and after dipping a #15 Bard-Parker blade in the oil, gently scrape the burrow or burrows at a right angle to the burrow's long axis, keeping the skin taut. Under the microscope at low magnification, one can usually find mites, eggs, and feces (Scybala) (Fig. 32-37). Since the mite feces are the most numerous, at times these may be all one can find as small, oval, pale golden-brown nuggets.

The ocular adnexa are not usually involved by scabies. However, in infants and following the use of topical glucocorticoids, the mite occasionally involves the eyelid, causing similar findings to those notes elsewhere.

The skin of the eyelid is also occasionally affected in crusted, or Norwegian, scabies (Fig. 32-35). Large crusted areas occur on the hands and feet, whereas erythema and scaling often exist on the face, neck, scalp, and trunk. Itching may be present and can be severe, although in many instances, the failure of the patient to scratch and thus destroy the mite's burrow allows for the enormous mite population that occurs in crusted scabies. In immunocompromised patients, such as persons with AIDS, itching may be minimal or nonexistent.

Chigger

The chigger or harvest mite prefers thin skin areas such as the ears, axillae, groin, and genitalia, although lesions may also occur around the feet, ankles, wrists, antecubital fossae, and areas constricted by clothing. The early lesions are severely pruritic, erythematous, hemorrhagic, punctate macules that later become papular (Fig. 32-38) or papulovesicular. Sometimes, ulcerated lesions covered by a black, necrotic crust occur on the skin of the eyelid. The surrounding area is indurated and erythematous.

Demodicidosis (Follicle Mite)

Follicle mites (*Demodex folliculorum*) are microscopic acarian parasites (Figs. 32-39 to 32-41). The organism has a cephalic, thoracic, and abdominal segment. The abdomen is striated, is vermiform, and ends in a conical point. There are four pairs of stubby legs. The organisms inhabit the meibomian glands, the hair follicles, and the sebaceous glands in all areas of the body, especially the forehead, lid margins, nose, cheek, and external auditory meatus.

Follicle mites of the lid are often asymptomatic but may cause itching, burning, and redness. Sleeves (small, 0.5- to 1.0-mm elongations of skin along the base of the eyelash suggesting the short sleeve of a coat) are almost pathognomonic. The lash is normal, and if the lash is removed, the sleeve is often removed along with it. Sleeves are often associated with redness of the lid margin; and occasionally, they involve the loss of lashes. The eyelid may also be involved in rosacea with Demodex infection.

Skin Features

Demodicidosis, pustular acne rosacea, various pigmentations of the skin, tuberculid rosacea of Lewandowsky, *Demodex* granuloma, and *Demodex* blepharitis have been attributed to *Demodex folliculorum.*

Pityriasis folliculorum (*Demodex*) occurs primarily in middle-aged and older women and is favored by use of makeup and of cleansing creams for makeup removal instead of soap and water. It is characterized by diffuse facial erythema, dryness, and a nutmeg grate or stippled appearance of the skin. White, frosty follicular scales are usually located about the facial lanugo hairs. Symptoms of itching and burning may occur.

The relationship of *Demodex* to acne rosacea is controversial. The findings are similar to pityriasis folliculorum (*Demodex*) with added superficial vesiculopustules and small papules or papulopustules. The skin is less oily, and the papules and pustules are smaller. Similar eruptions associated with *Demodex* may occur on the face or scalp of bald men.

The rosacea-like tuberculid (Lewandowsky) associated with *Demodex* is characterized by bluish or brownish red papules or papulopustules on the cheeks, forehead, and temples. The lesions appear to have a yellowish-brown color with diaphanoscopy. They vary in size from pinhead to hemp seed and are associated with hyperemia and variable telangiectasis.

Granulomas of the face, beginning as a progressive rash of the chin, upper lip, and other facial areas, have been found on biopsy to have *Demodex* deep within the epidermis. An intense inflammatory reaction surrounds the granuloma. A papulopustule and scaling also occurs, and the patient has symptoms of intermittent burning of the involved areas.

Skin pigmentation associated with *Demodex* varies from light-yellow wrinkled spots on the face and upper chest with a peculiar whitish substance (suggesting rice grains) around the follicular orifices, a cafe-au-lait hue with characteristic drying and scaling over the lips and chin, or a brownish zone surrounding a patch of atrophic lupus. In each instance, there are large numbers of *Demodex* on the skin surface.

Centipedes and Millipedes

Centipedes are elongated arthropods with many segments, each having one pair of legs. The first pair of legs is modified into claws that can grasp and inject venom into the skin. Centipedes cause local pain, erythema, edema, urticarial eruption, and wheals on the skin and eyelids; sometimes they cause only a foreign-body reaction. Small centipedes are of less importance because they are unable to penetrate skin.

Millipedes are elongated arthropods composed of many segments, each bearing two pairs of legs. Millipedes secrete substances that may cause a burning sensation followed by blisters within 24 hours and a yellowish-brown stain that gradually darkens to a mahogany or purple-brown color. The lesion desquamates after 10 to 14 days, but the pigmentation often remains or the area becomes hypopigmented.

If secreted in the conjunctival sac, the patient experiences severe irritative conjunctivitis.

Leeches

Lid edema may occur from the bite of a leech as it takes its blood meal. An urticarial or bullous reaction occurs if the patient is sensitized to the antigens introduced at the time of feeding of the leech.

NOXIOUS VERTEBRATES AND VERTEBRATE BITES

Spitting Snakes

The spitting cobra often ejects its venom toward the face of a trespasser when threatened. The venom causes severe blepharospasm, lid edema, and conjunctivitis, symptoms that persist for about a week to 10 days. Epithelial keratitis and corneal bullae may be found. The bite of the spitting cobra causes local swelling and skin necrosis along with hematologic abnormalities and depletion of complement.

Dog Bites

Dog bites (Fig. 32-42), apart from the physical trauma of the bite itself, may lead to secondary infection, especially with *Pasteurella multocida.*

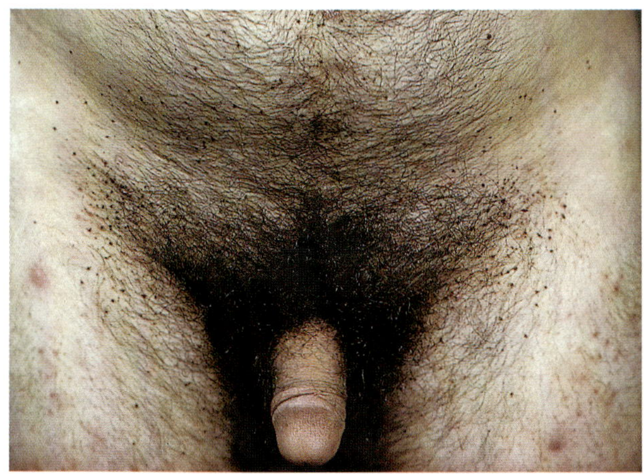

FIGURE 32-1. *Pediculosis pubis* showing heavy infestation extending to thighs and abdomen. The lice appear as small, dark specks (dark because they have had a blood meal). Note secondary folliculitis and small furuncles, a frequent complication.

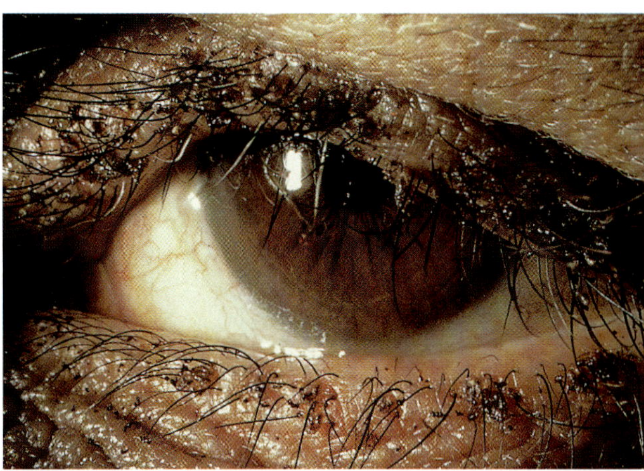

FIGURE 32-2. *Pediculosis palpebrarum* showing numerous pubic lice and nits along the eyelashes. The patient had complained of mild itching around the eyes.

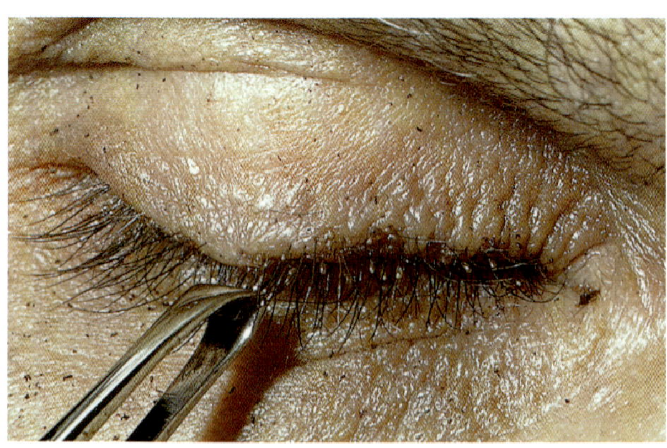

FIGURE 32-3. Completion of treatment is removing residual nits from lashes with serrated tweezers after smothering the lice by three-times-a-day application of an ophthalmic ointment for 1 week.

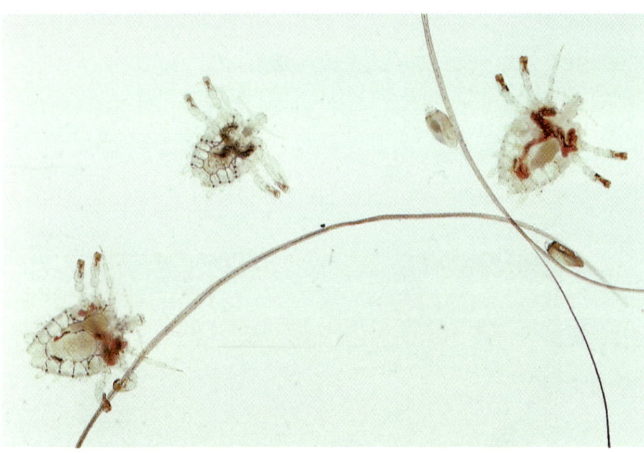

FIGURE 32-4. Pubic lice (*Phthirus pubis*) (40×) showing broader body than head and body lice. Note nits cemented to hairs.

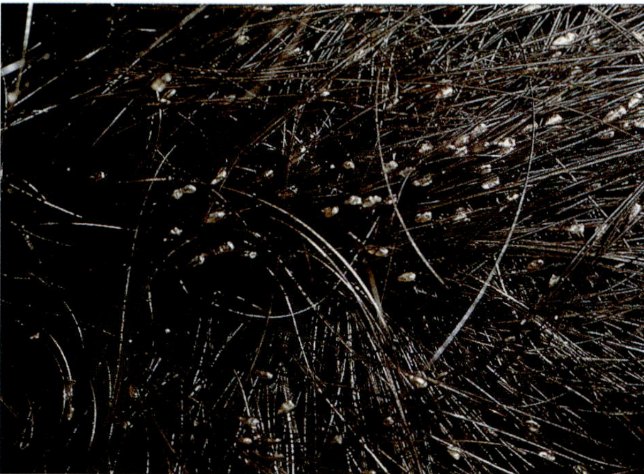

FIGURE 32-5. *Pediculosis capitis* showing numerous nits, which are usually easier to find than the lice.

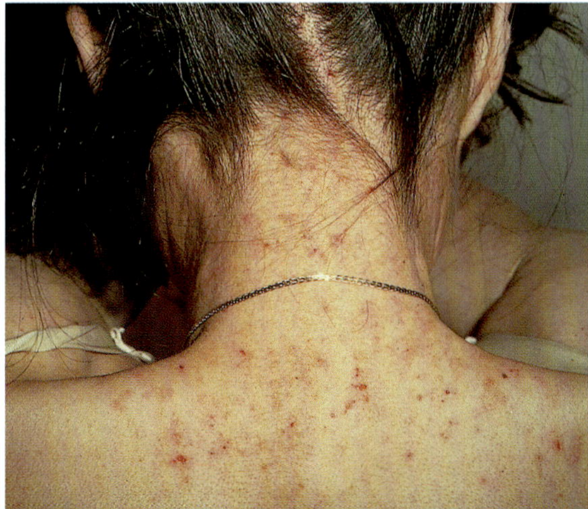

FIGURE 32-6. *Pediculosis capitis* with secondary folliculitis and impetiginization. Itching of the nape of the neck, especially with evidence of secondary bacterial infection, should always alert the examiner to possible *P. capitis*.

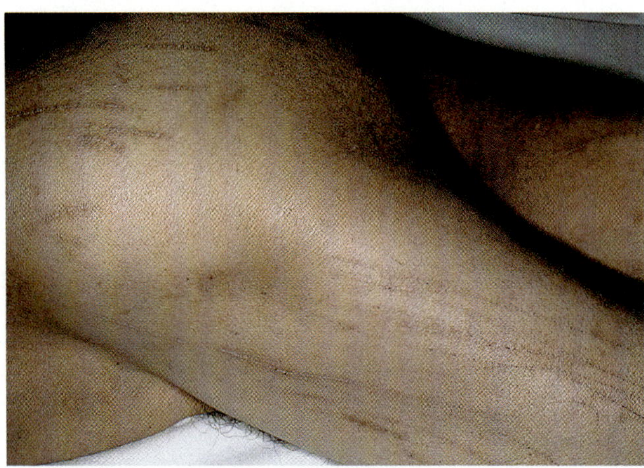

FIGURE 32-7. *Pediculosis corporis* showing typical long, linear excoriations.

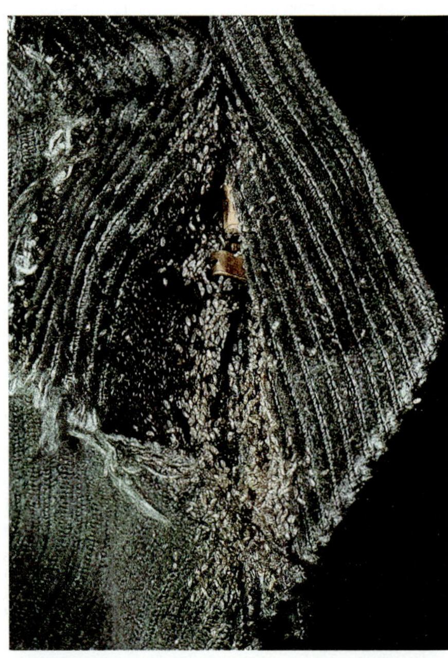

FIGURE 32-8. Multiple nits in zipper area of trousers. Lice and nits in *Pediculosis corporis* are most frequently located on the clothing (especially in seams) rather than on the skin. Thus, in suspected *P. corporis,* examine the clothing carefully. The frequent location in the seams especially in persons lacking in hygiene is the origin of the saying "the seamier side of life".

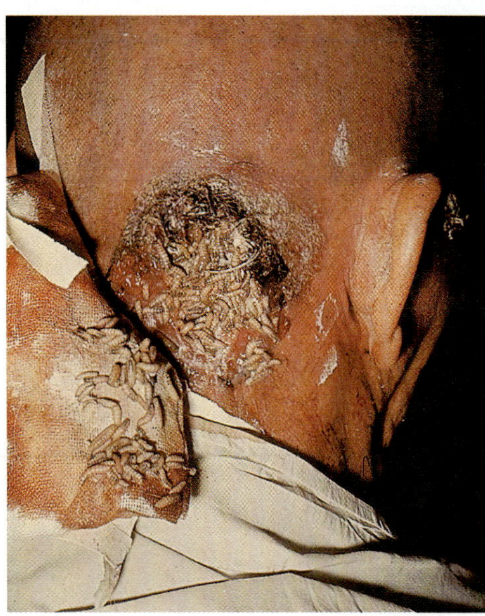

FIGURE 32-9. Wound myiasis. Fly maggots (nature's way of cleaning up wounds) are still available and occasionally used for debriding infected wounds.

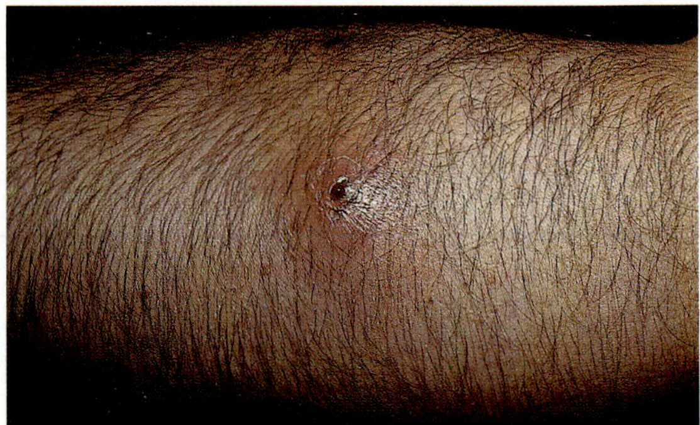

FIGURE 32-10. Furuncular myiasis caused by the human botfly (*Dermatobia hominis*) in a patient who had recently returned from Guatemala. Close inspection revealed intermittent, tiny air bubbles, a clue to the hidden larva.

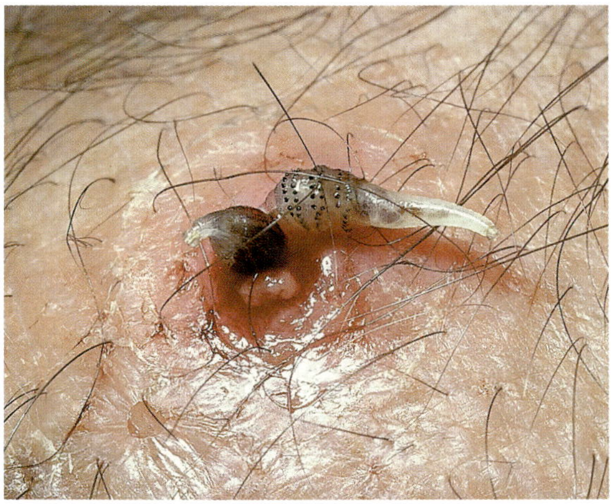

FIGURE 32-11. These two larvae were expressed after gently enlarging the opening with a probe. Myiasis is a significant problem in cattle as well as in humans.

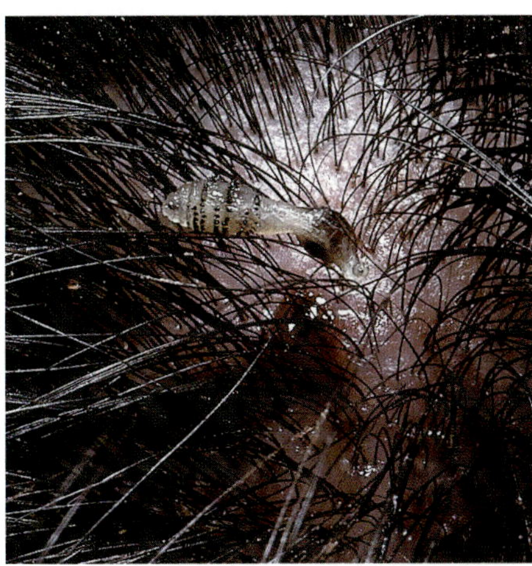

FIGURE 32-12. Furuncular myiasis of scalp showing extracted larva.

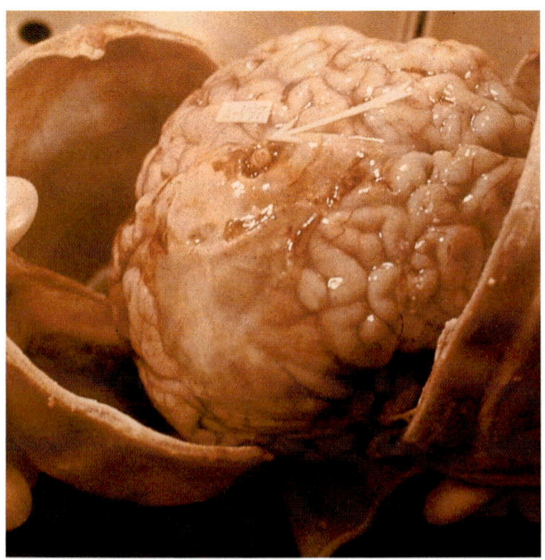

FIGURE 32-13. Myiasis with penetration of larvae into the brain, causing the death of the patient, a rare complication. (Courtesy of Department of Pathology, University of Guatemala Medical Center.)

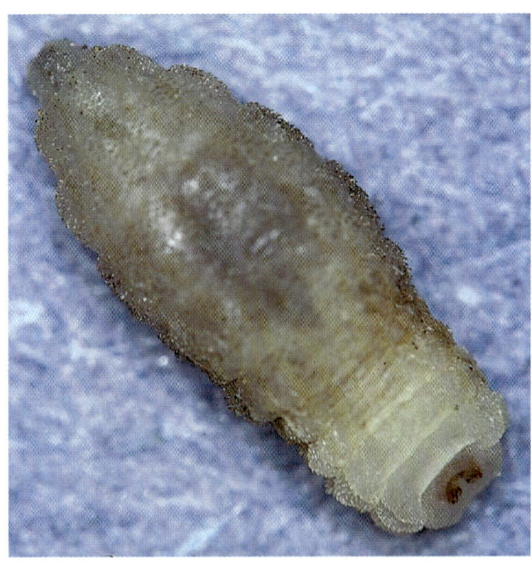

FIGURE 32-14. Larva of botfly (*Dermatobia hominis*), the most common cause of furuncular myiasis in Central America.

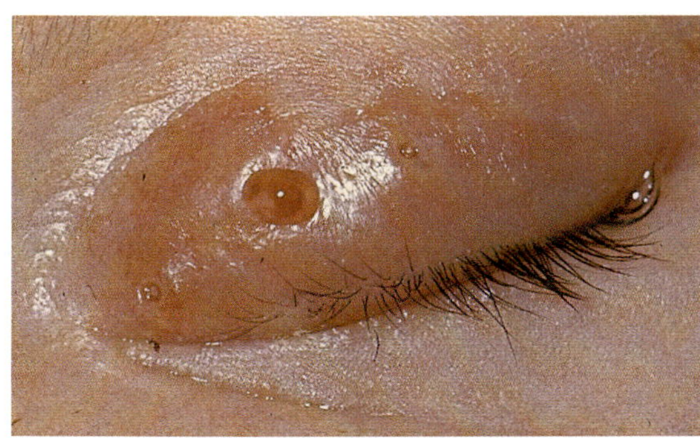

FIGURE 32-15. Furuncular myiasis with larva penetrating tarsal plate.

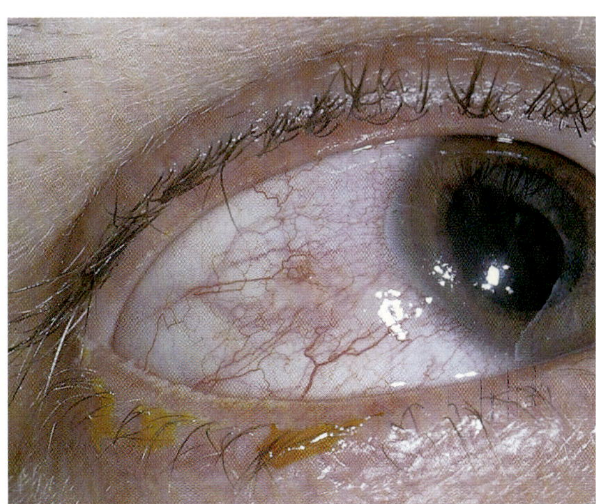

FIGURE 32-16. Larva of botfly has been removed from this conjunctiva (see Fig. 32-14). (Courtesy of Masao Okumoto.)

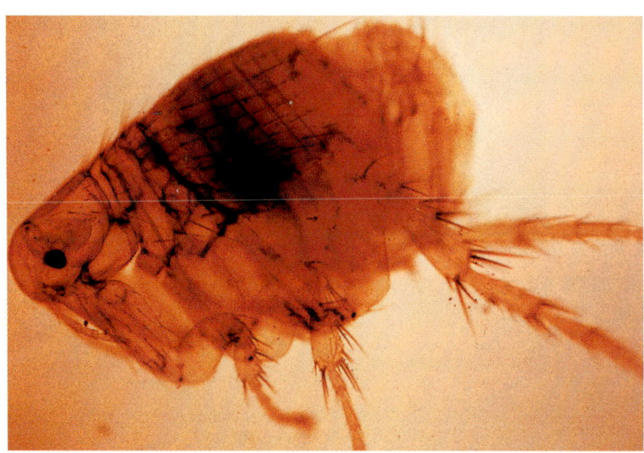

FIGURE 32-17. Human flea (*Pulex irritans*). Note strong legs for jumping.

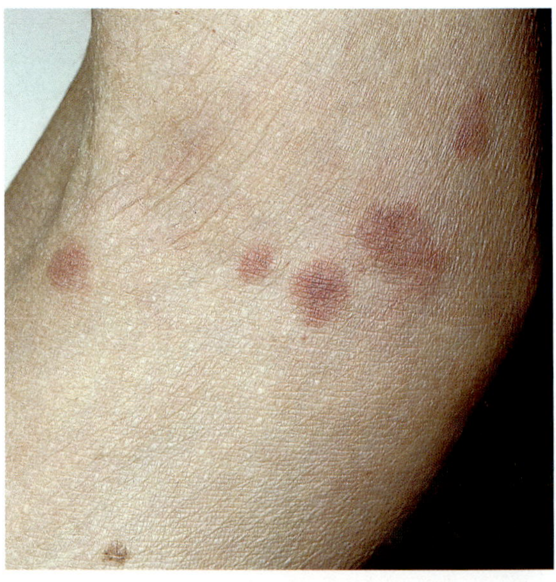

FIGURE 32-18. Flea bites showing grouped (so-called breakfast, lunch, and supper pattern) hemorrhagic punctae. The patient had held a stray kitten on her arm.

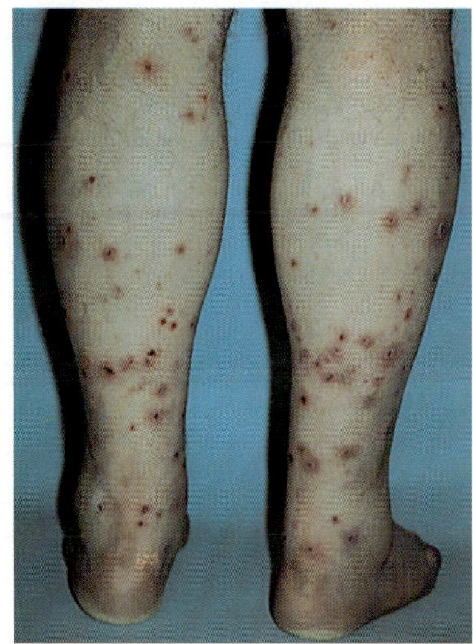

FIGURE 32-19. Multiple secondarily infected flea bites in a patient who was very sensitive to this organism. Self-treatment with over-the-counter antipruritic lotions was ineffective.

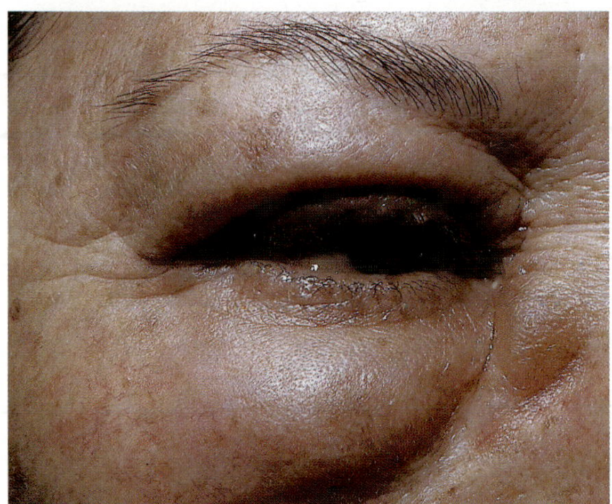

FIGURE 32-20. Periorbital edema and itching following a bee sting.

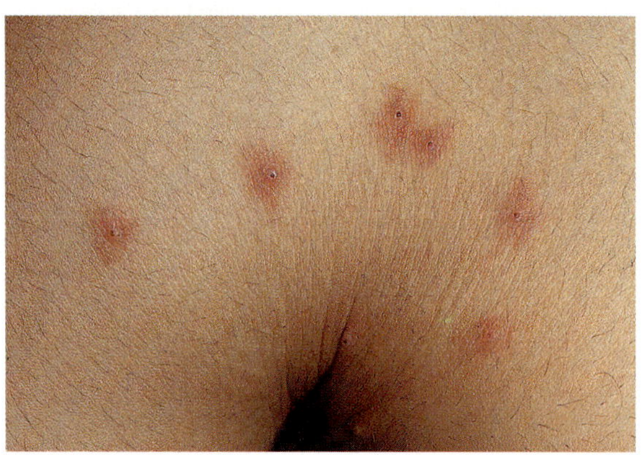

FIGURE 32-21. Bedbug bites. The bug hides in crevices during the day and feeds on human blood at night. The bite is initially asymptomatic, with itching, which is often severe, first noticed upon awakening. (Courtesy of Dr. John Reeves.)

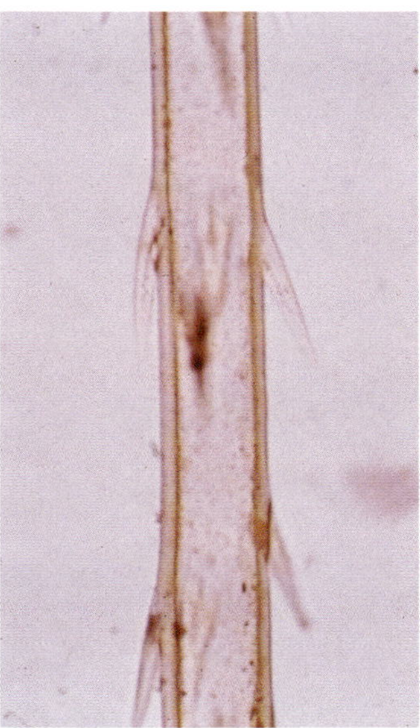

FIGURE 32-22. Caterpillar hair with spines. (Courtesy of Mr. Masao Okumoto.)

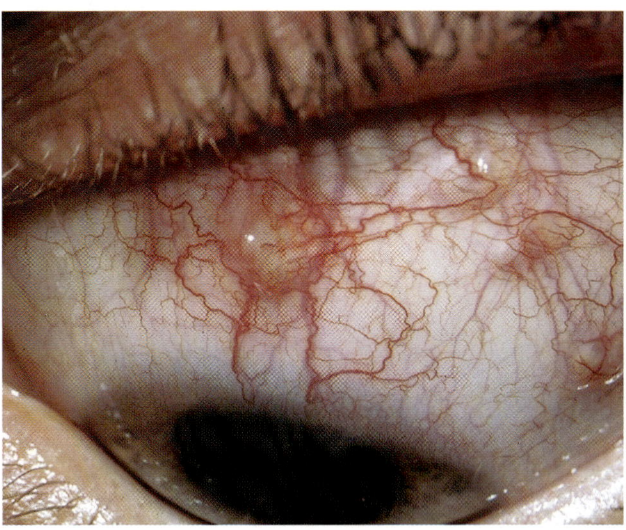

FIGURE 32-23. Ophthalmia nodosa, a granulomatous reaction to the caterpillar spine.

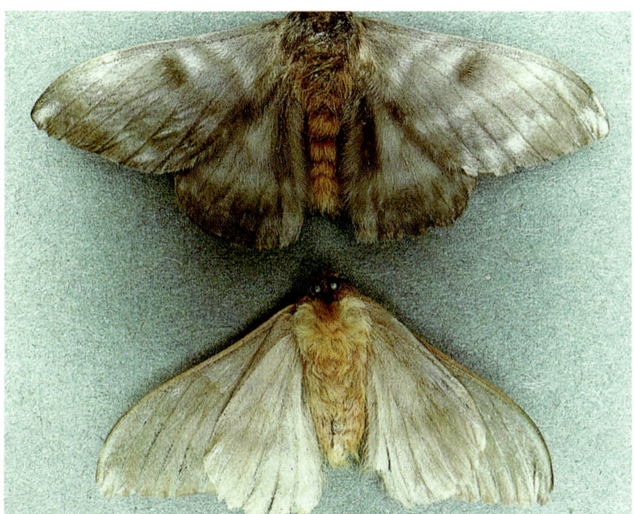

FIGURE 32-24. Moths of the genus *Hylesia,* the most frequent cause of moth dermatitis seen in Latin America.

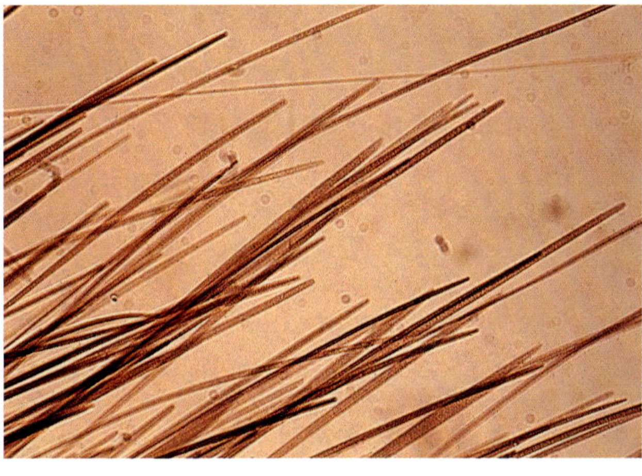

FIGURE 32-25. Close-up of the nettling hairs (setae) of moths in Fig. 32-24. These delicate spiny hairs contain an irritant that, when released on skin, causes intense itching with urticarial papules and vesicles. Eye contact causes a severe inflammatory and foreign-body reaction, as seen also with caterpillar hairs (Fig. 32-22).

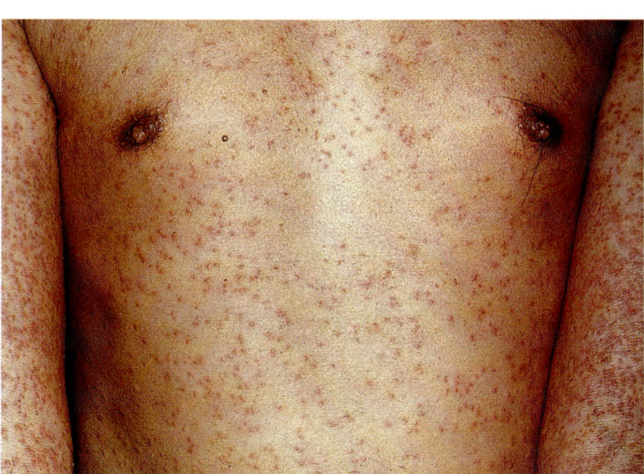

FIGURE 32-26. Moth dermatitis acquired while loading a tanker in the Venezuelan port of Caripito. Deforestation had reduced the habitat of these moths. Thus this once frequently seen problem (known among merchant seamen as "Caripito itch") is now rare.

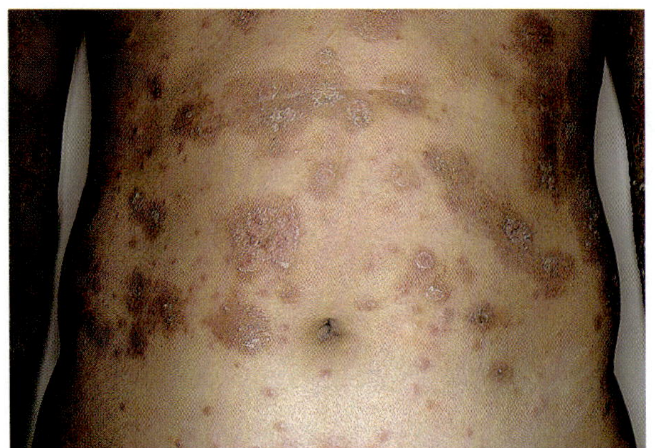

FIGURE 32-27. Moth dermatitis impetigenized.

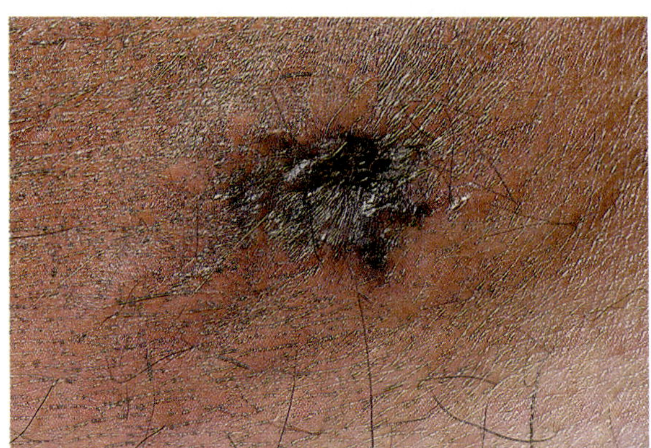

FIGURE 32-28. Bite from suspected brown recluse spider. Patient had experienced intensely painful bullous lesion for several days before developing the necrotic eschar.

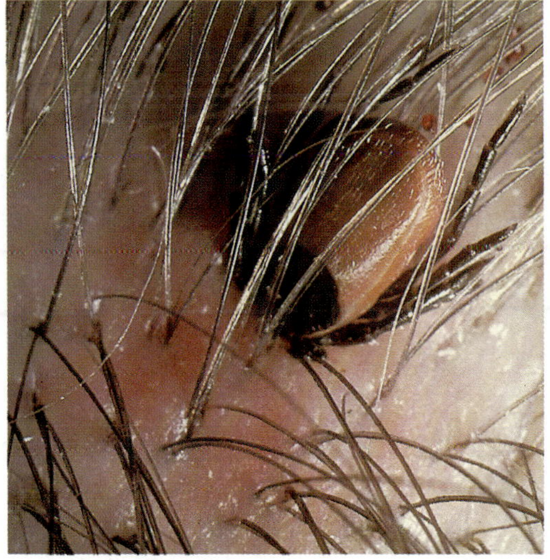

FIGURE 32-29. Tick feeding on scalp. An area that could easily be over looked.

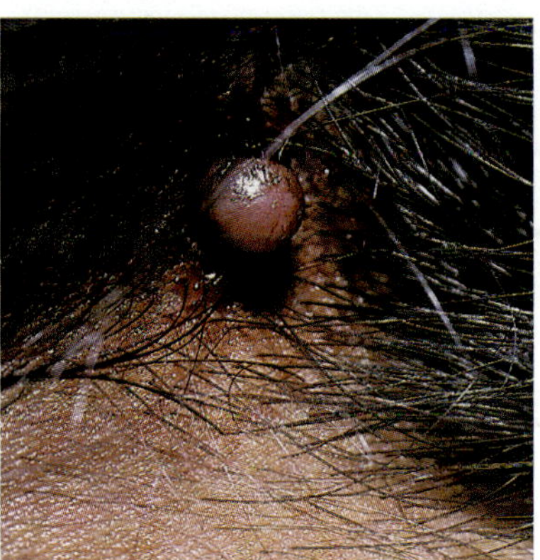

FIGURE 32-30. Blood-engorged tick on nape of neck. Ticks attached on head or neck can rarely result in tick paralysis. This engorged tick could be confused with a pyogenic granuloma.

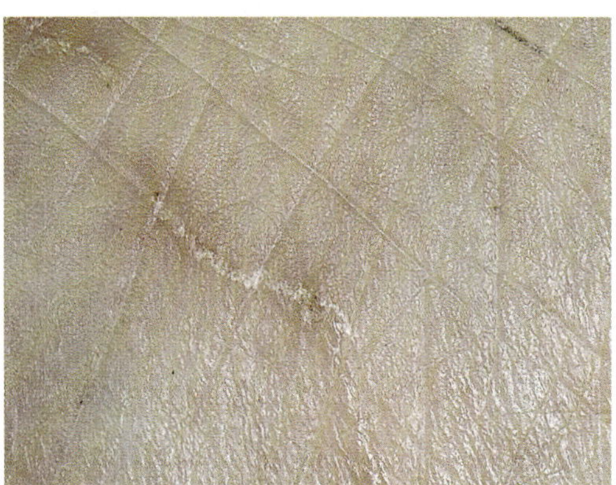

FIGURE 32-31. Scabies burrows on skin of ankle. Note long, thin, pale grayish-white, tortuous, slightly scaly lesion.

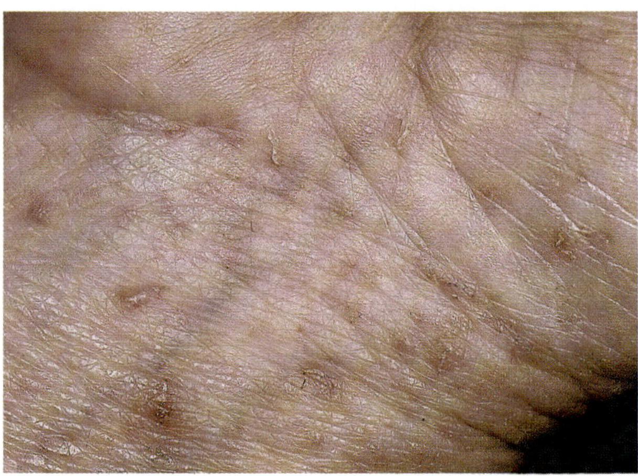

FIGURE 32-32. Multiple small scabies burrows on volar wrist, a frequent site.

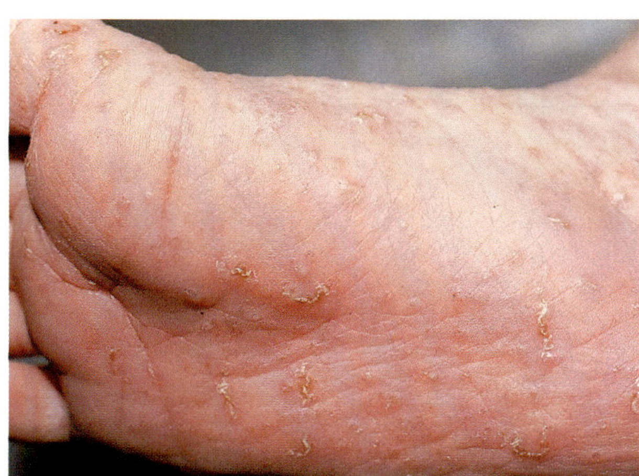

FIGURE 32-33. Multiple classic scabies burrows on the sole in a young infant. Burrows are frequently found intact in infants at this site, since they may not be able to scratch there.

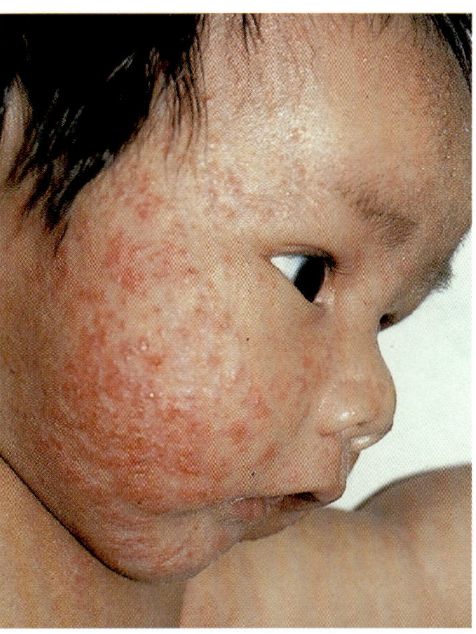

FIGURE 32-34. Eczematous lesions of scabies mimicking atopic eczema in an infant. (Courtesy of Dr. Richard Odom.)

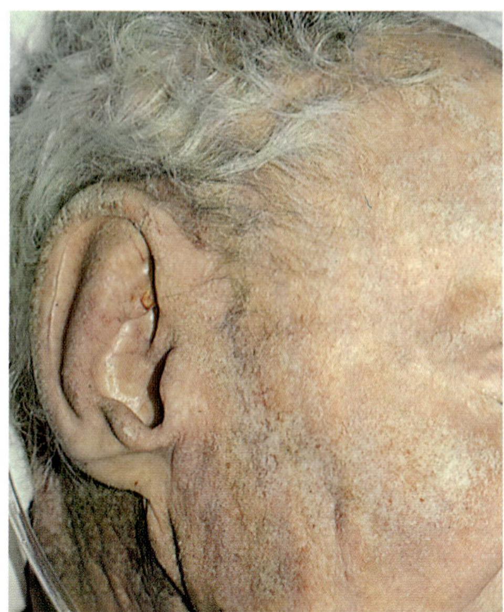

FIGURE 32-35. Crusted (Norwegian) scabies in an elderly terminally ill patient hopitalized in a large city convalescent hospital. Crusted patches on his face, palms, and chest revealed 54 mites under one microscopic coverslip. Thousands of scabies mites are shed in this rare type of scabies, causing repeated epidemics in hospitals and nursing homes (as was the problem at this institution) unless properly diagnosed and treated.

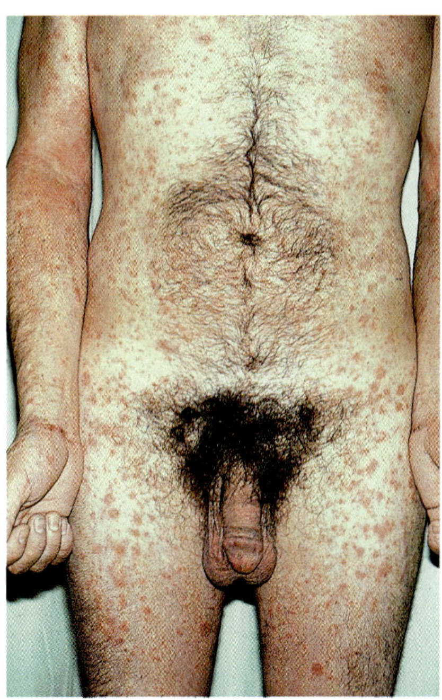

FIGURE 32-36. Extensive eczematoid reaction to scabies. Note typical scabetic papules on flexor wrist and penis. Scraping eczematous lesions for scabies mites is futile. Scrape only obvious burrows.

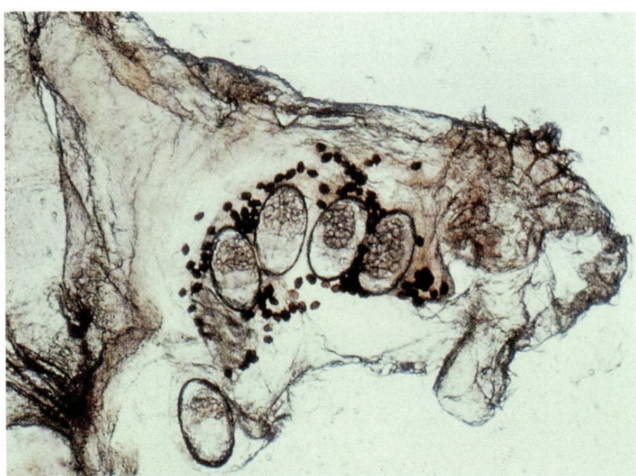

FIGURE 32-37. Low-power microscopic examination of scraped burrow, revealing multiple eggs, feces, and one mite. Once mastered, scabies preps are simple, rapid, and rewarding.

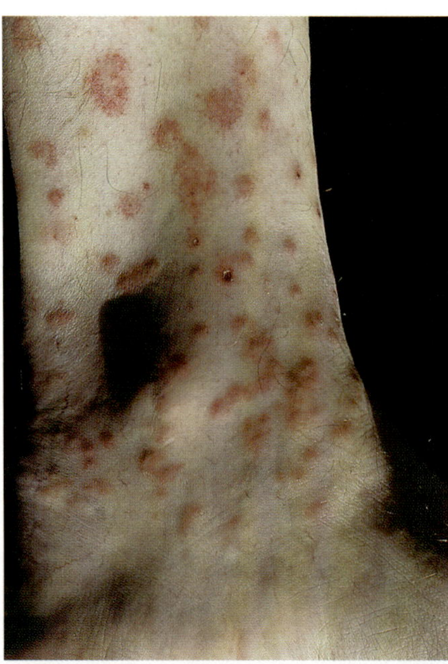

FIGURE 32-38. Chigger bites. Ankles are common sites, especially after hiking through mite-infested grasses or bushes.

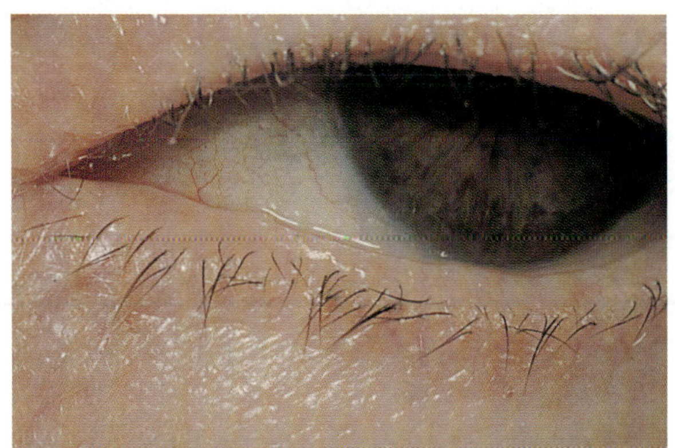

FIGURE 32-39. Lash sleeves associated with *Demodex.*

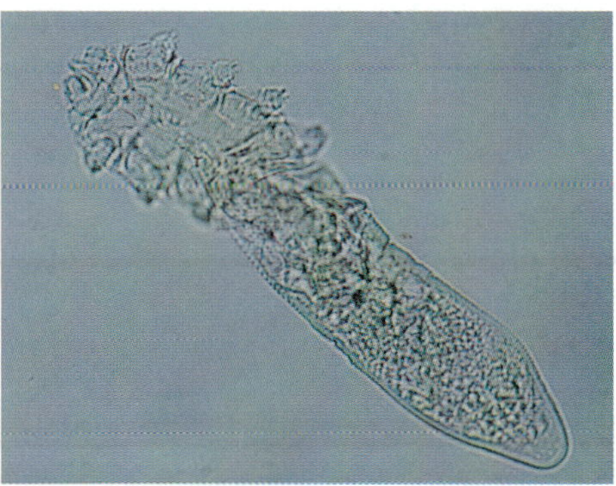

FIGURE 32-40. *Demodex folliculorum.* (Courtesy of Masao Okumoto.)

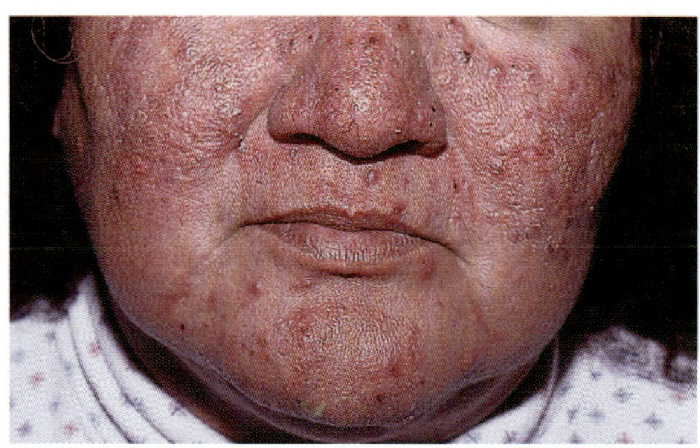

FIGURE 32-41. Demodicidosis in severe rosacea.

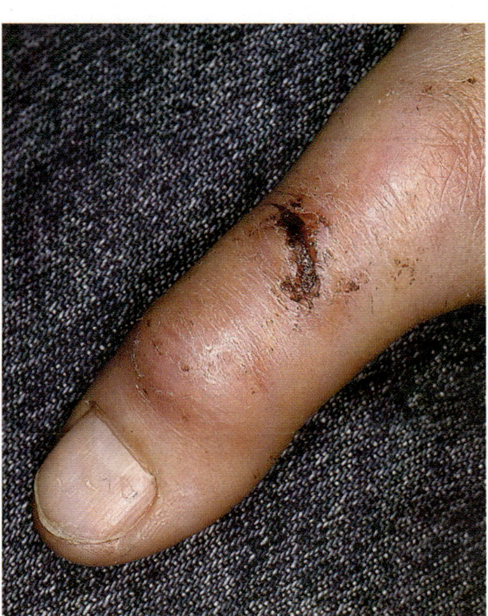

FIGURE 32-42. Dog bite. Secondary infection with *Pasteurella multocida* may occur. Cat bites are more contaminated with multiple organisms.

33

NUTRITIONAL DISORDERS

Nutritional disorders arise from inadequate food intake, malabsorption, intestinal parasites, inadequate transport mechanisms in the blood, vomiting, diarrhea, and intestinal fistulas. They are usually multifactorial. Rarely, intoxication syndromes can be seen with excessive intake of certain vitamins.

MALABSORPTION SYNDROMES

Malabsorption represents incomplete or impaired intestinal absorption of nutrients. It is usually associated with steatorrhea and often causes deficiencies of fat-soluble vitamins. Intestinal malabsorption may cause widespread desquamating eczema, which responds to systemic calcium.

Sprue and other malabsorption syndromes commonly cause scaly inflammatory plaques, followed by an addisonian pattern of hyperpigmentation or hyperpigmentation in well-defined patches on the face, neck, and occasionally, trunk. Dry skin, ichthyosis, brittle nails, and alopecia may also occur.

Steatorrhea is a major feature of Whipple disease. The disease has many of the features of sarcoidosis and is often associated with enlarged hilar lymph nodes, arthritis, myocarditis, and pericarditis. The skin manifestations include erythema, nodosum-like nodules on the legs, and diffuse skin hyperpigmentation. The ocular features include ptosis, keratitis, uveitis, retinal hemorrhages, and vasculitis, with vitreous opacities and hemorrhages, nystagmus, gaze palsy, ophthalmoplegia, and papilledema.

Cystic fibrosis of the pancreas (mucoviscidosis) has components of malabsorption. It is autosomal recessive and characterized by increased viscosity of mucous secretions that results in obstruction of the excretory ducts of the pancreas, the bile ducts of the liver, and the small bronchioles. The clinical manifestations can all be attributed to the increased viscosity of mucous secretions. Obstruction of the excretory pancreatic ducts and bile duct leads to malabsorption, retarded growth, and hepatic disease. Chronic pulmonary disease is often associated with clubbing of the fingers and periodic periods of dyspnea.

The skin changes are reminiscent of acrodermatitis enteropathica with a vesicobullous dermatitis of the hands, feet, and periorificial areas and alopecia of the scalp.

The ocular features include decreased tearing, retinal hemorrhages, and venous engorgement and tortuosity.

Nutritional Deficiency

Most nutritional deficiencies that affect the eye and skin are vitamin deficiencies with or without protein deficiency.

Vitamin A Deficiency

Vitamin A deficiency causes xerophthalmia (Figs. 33-1 to 33-3), follicular hyperkeratosis, and generalized xerosis. Vitamin A is found in yellow, orange, and green plants.

Follicular hyperkeratosis is characterized by horny follicular papules on the dorsal and lateral parts of the extremities. It is often associated with generalized pigmentation.

Bitot spots (Fig. 33-2) are common in xerophthalmia and often serve as a marker for vitamin A deficiency. They involve the interpalpebral area of the conjunctiva and are triangular in shape, with the base directed toward the limbus. The lesions are silvery-gray in color; their surface is foamy; often they appear like a lusterless, striated plaque. Conjunctival pigmentation also occurs and is especially striking in the lower fornix and bulbar conjunctiva. Xerophthalmia—a dry, lusterless, ocular surface—is usually associated with vitamin A deficiency. It is widespread in Africa, India, the Middle and Far East, and Central and South America. It is caused by vitamin A deficiency and frequently accompanies kwashiorkor. Rarely, zinc deficiency, which acts on the retinol-binding protein, leads to vitamin A deficiency.

Keratomalacia is not uncommon in xerophthalmia. The earliest changes consist of loss of corneal luster or development of a mild corneal haziness near the inferior limbus. The condition progresses rapidly to loss of luster of the entire corneal surface, giving a peau d'orange appearance. The most severe changes are found in a 2- to 3-mm zone adjacent to the inferior limbus. Later, there is a thick, heavy, xerotic plaque that covers the corneal surface in the interpalpebral zone. Corneal ulcers may occur (Fig. 33-4). A corneal ulcer with a smooth, regular margin usually develops in the inferior or nasal quadrant. As it increases in size, generalized corneal edema develops. Eventually, the entire cornea except for the peripheral rim is destroyed.

Occasionally, colliquative keratopathy occurs, characterized by dissolution of a small area of the cornea at 5:00 to 7:00 o'clock without other corneal signs. It leads to iris prolapse and then heals, resulting in an adherent leukoma. Sometimes the rest of the cornea becomes mildly vascularized.

Thiamine (Vitamin B₁) Deficiency

Thiamine is found in yeast, liver, meat, eggs, cereals, and vegetables. Deficiencies arise from use of polished rice as the main staple; from insufficient nutrition in the chronic alcoholic; from malabsorption as in ulcerative colitis, celiac disease, achlorhydria; and from vomiting and anorexia. Occasionally, it is associated with diabetes mellitus, pregnancy, or lactation.

Thiamine deficiency causes beriberi, which is characterized by anorexia, constipation, weakness, edema, muscle wasting, cardiac insufficiency, symmetric and progressive polyneuritis, and sometimes Wernicke encephalopathy or Korsakoff syndrome. The ocular features include optic atrophy, epithelial keratitis, ophthalmoplegia, and nystagmus.

Vitamin B₂ Deficiency

Riboflavin (vitamin B₂) is found in milk and in the same foods as thiamine. Deficiency of this vitamin is most often seen in alcoholic patients, persons suffering from malabsorption, chronic illness, and occasionally, hypothyroidism. It is often associated with pellagra and zinc deficiency. Vitamin B₂ deficiency leads to the classic triad of the oral-occulo-genital syndrome. The oral lesions consist of angular cheilitis, cheilosis, and atrophic magenta-colored tongue (Fig. 33-5). Ocular features include photophobia, angular blepharoconjunctivitis, and occasionally, peripheral corneal neovascularization. Genital dermatitis, which is worse in males, presents with a confluent dermatitis of the scrotum extending to the thighs.

Niacin (Nicotinic Acid) Deficiency (Pellagra)

Pellagra arises from a diet inadequate in niacin and tryptophan, the precursor amino acid. It is seen in chronic alcoholics; patients with carcinoid tumors (which direct tryptophan to serotonin); heavy infestations of intestinal parasites (especially hookworm); gastrointestinal disease; patients receiving isoniazid, azathioprine, and 5-fluorouracil, in Hartnup disease (impaired absorption of tryptophan); and patients with severe psychiatric disorders, including anorexia nervosa. Pellagra is manifested by the four Ds—dermatitis, diarrhea, dementia, and death. The skin findings include a photosensi-

tive dermatitis with redness and superficial scaling in areas exposed to sunlight (Fig. 33-6), heat, friction, or pressure. The redness is often followed by hyperpigmentation that may have an Addisonian pattern but is accentuated on the face and hands and in areas of friction or pressure; or it may occur as a sequel to the dermatitis. A distinct marginated, scaly, pigmented erythema may occur on the front of the neck (Casal necklace) (Fig. 33-7) and in a symmetric butterfly distribution over the cheeks.

Diarrhea, pain, and achlorhydria are common. Severe niacin-induced hepatotoxic reaction may cause a clotting-factor coagulopathy.

The dementia (Fig. 33-7) may be mild and manifested by slight depression or apathy, or patients may be frankly disorientated and restless. A peripheral neuritis and myelitis may also be found.

Pyridoxine (Vitamin B₆, Pyridoxal) Deficiency

Vitamin B₆ is found in various grains, yeast, eggs, and many other foods.

Pyridoxine deficiency can be seen in cirrhosis and uremia as well as following treatment with isoniazid, hydralazine, or penicillamine. It causes a seborrheic, dermatitis-like eruption, angular cheilitis, atrophic glossitis, intertrigo, and occasionally, a pellagroid eruption. Neurologic findings include somnolence, confusion, neuropathy, and acrodynia. Anemia may be present.

Ocular Features

Ocular features include an optic neuritis and angular blepharoconjunctivitis.

Vitamin B₁₂ (Cyanocobalamin) Deficiency

Vitamin B₁₂ deficiency usually occurs in patients with megaloblastic and pernicious anemia but may also be found in vegetarians. The deficiency causes a diffuse brown hyperpigmentation, which may be more pronounced in exposed areas such as the face and hands and also in the creases of the fingers and palms, resembling Addison disease. The nails are occasionally streaked with the same pigment. The hair is often prematurely gray. The tongue is characteristically bright red, sore, and atrophic (Fig. 33-8). A subacute combined degeneration of the spinal cord and brain results in weakness, paresthesias, numbness, and ataxia.

Ocular Features

Ocular changes are limited to optic neuritis with central or cecocentral scotomas.

Biotin Deficiency

Biotin deficiency is extremely rare. It may result from a diet containing many raw egg whites, the short bowel syndrome, loss of biotin through a gastrointestinal fistula, and biotinidase deficiency that is autosomal recessive. It causes a dermatitis similar to that seen in zinc deficiency with peri-orificial, patchy, red, erosive lesions around the eyes, nose, mouth, and groin.

Alopecia including the eyebrows and lashes may occur. Brain atrophy may be found. Neurologic manifestations are prominent and can include depression, lethargy, hallucinations, and paresthesias of the limbs. In infants, hypotonia, seizures, developmental delay, and death may occur.

Scurvy, Vitamin C (Ascorbic Acid) Deficiency

Scurvy is caused by deficiency of ascorbic acid, which is found in fresh fruits and vegetables, especially green, leafy varieties and potatoes. Scurvy has been recognized for centuries, especially among soldiers and sailors whose diets were often deficient in this vitamin. In the late eighteenth century, the British Navy required sailors to have a daily ration of limes to help prevent this common problem, a practice that gave rise to the slang term *limey*. Scurvy is still seen in the United States in persons with chronic alcohol problems; in depressed elderly people, especially those living alone; occasionally in food faddists; and in the very poor. Worldwide, it occurs as part of severe malnutrition as, for example, in World War II, during the 3-year siege of Leningrad by the Germans, when the starving population ate pine needles to try to treat scurvy.

Clinically, scurvy is characterized by the four Hs— hemorrhagic signs, hyperkeratosis of hair follicles, hematologic abnormalities, and hypochondriasis. Perifollicular petechiae and ecchymoses, especially of the lower extremities, are common (Figs. 33-9 and 33-10). Subungual bleeding can sometimes be seen (Fig. 33-11). Subcutaneous and intramuscular hemorrhage can produce tender nodules. Hemarthrosis and subperiosteal hemorrhage give rise to painful joints (Fig. 33-9) and extremities, and in children can lead to pseudoparalysis. Keratotic plugging of hair follicles, primarily on the forearms, anterior thighs, and abdomen, produces curling of hair shafts, resulting in "corkscrew hairs," a distinctive finding in scurvy (Fig. 33-10). Swelling and bleeding of the gums (scurvy buds) (Fig. 33-12), usually accompanied by loose teeth and fetor oris, is characteristic. If the patient is edentulous or practices exceptional dental hygiene, these may not be present. In patients with chronic scurvy, "woody" edema of the lower legs (Fig. 33-13), often accompanied by dry, scaly skin and pigmentation, may ensue.

Epistaxis and delayed wound healing are common. Signs and symptoms of other vitamin and mineral deficiencies may accompany those of scurvy. Anemia as a result of bleeding into the joints, periosteal areas, muscles and skin or through blood loss or deficiency of folate is common (Fig. 33-9). Depression may precede or accompany scurvy (Fig. 33-9). In patients with chronic, severe, untreated scurvy, death may result from cardiac tamponade.

Ocular Features

In patients with scurvy, one may see hemorrhages of the lid, conjunctiva, anterior chamber, and retina.

Protein-Calorie Deficiency

Kwashiorkor

Kwashiorkor represents a deficiency in protein. *Kwashiorkor* is an African term that means literally "the first child when the second child is born." At that time the first child is no longer breast-fed and nutritional problems begin. Kwashiorkor is common in developing countries, especially where the diet consists of corn, rice, or beans. It usually develops in children between the ages of 6 months to 5 years, and is characterized by retarded skeletal and mental development, depression, muscle wasting, and massive edema of the abdomen (Fig. 33-14) and spindly extremities.

The skin has a cracked or flaky lacquered appearance often accompanied by edema (Fig. 33-15). Patchy areas of hypopigmentation and hyperpigmentation often develop in the areas of inflammation (Fig. 33-16). The hair is dry, lusterless, light red-brown or reddish; sparse; fine; and brittle (Fig. 33-17). In some patients one sees alternating bands of dark and light hair referred to as the "flag wave sign". This is the result of alternating periods of poor and better nutrition (Fig 33-18).

Cheilosis, vulvovaginitis, scrotal eczema (Fig. 33-19), and xerophthalmia may also be seen. Children with kwashiorkor fail to smile and often appear apathetic or are irritable (Fig. 33-16).

In elderly patients, the skin over the shins and the lower abdomen has a cracked appearance. It is commonly associated with periorificial glazed erythema and hair loss similar to that seen in zinc deficiency.

Marasmus

Marasmus is caused by deficiency of protein and carbohydrates, and is common in developing countries where there are insufficient food supplies. It has many of the manifestations of vitamin A deficiency because of the lack of carrier protein for vitamin A and also because of zinc deficiency (Fig. 33-20). In marasmus, there is loss of skin elasticity, failure to develop body fat, muscle wastage, loss of muscle tone, mental dullness, and growth arrest. Skin ulcerations may occur. There is no peripheral edema. The hair is sparse and thin with a reddish tinge. The nails are fissured. In adults, there may be prominent follicular hyperkeratosis. Marasmus and kwashiorkor often coexist in patients.

HEAVY METAL DISORDERS

Zinc Deficiency and Acrodermatitis Enteropathica

Zinc (Zn) is found in shellfish, nuts, legumes, whole grains, and leafy vegetables. Zn deficiency may be acquired or inherited. Acquired deficiency occurs in severe malnutrition and may be seen when there is inadequate absorption of nutrients, as in significant inflammatory bowel disease, jejunoileal bypass, gastrointestinal malignancies, severe alcohol problems, and parenteral nutrition without adequate Zn supplementation. Occasionally, it may be seen in patients with anorexia nervosa and in patients with AIDS.

Zinc deficiency is more often found in premature than in full-term infants because, in the premature baby, there are inadequate stores of Zn, Zn requirements are high, and absorption may be suboptimal. Weaning classically precipitates Zn deficiency, both in premature infants and in babies with acrodermatitis enteropathica.

The dermatologic manifestations of Zn deficiency, with or without acrodermatitis enteropathica, are the same. There is an acral and periorificial patchy, erythematous, dry, scaling, exudative, and crusting eczematous picture (Figs. 33-21 and 33-22). Angular cheilitis, stomatitis, and periungual scaling and pustules are often present. Generalized alopecia is usually found.

Diarrhea is classically seen, as are growth retardation, poor wound healing, and central nervous system manifestations such as irritability. Patients with chronic Zn deficiency are mentally depressed and may show rashes seen in acrodermatitis enteropathica (Fig. 33-23). Ocular features include photophobia, angular blepharoconjunctivitis, and occasionally, peripheral corneal neovascularization.

Copper Abnormalities

Wilson Disease (Hepatolenticular Degeneration)

Wilson disease is autosomal recessive and is characterized by accumulation of toxic amounts of copper in the body. Symptoms usually begin by the age of 15.

At onset, the most prominent symptoms are usually related to the liver. The patient may have fatigue, jaundice, spider nevi, edema, ascites, hemorrhages, and hepatosplenomegaly.

Neurologic symptoms become manifest after some time and include tremors, slurring of speech, clumsiness, rigidity, gait disturbances, and personality changes. Other findings include a nephrotic syndrome seen in almost all patients, joint stiffness, and hypoparathyroidism.

Skin and Ocular Features

Hyperpigmentation of the skin is not uncommon in Wilson disease. A Kaiser–Fleischer ring (Figs. 33-24 and 33-25) and a sunflower cataract may also occur. The Kaiser–Fleischer ring is almost pathognomonic of Wilson disease. It appears as a golden brown or bronze deposition in Descemet membrane at the limbal area of the cornea.

Menkes (Kinky-Hair) Syndrome

Menkes (kinky-hair) syndrome is X-linked recessive and is characterized by sparse, kinky, coarse, brittle hair; growth retardation; developmental delay; seizures; and arterial disease. There is a defect in copper transport in the cells, and death frequently supervenes by age 3.

Ocular Features

The ocular features are limited to nystagmus.

NUTRITIONAL INTOXICATION

Hypervitaminosis A

Chronic vitamin A intoxication develops from prolonged ingestion of high doses of vitamin A. It causes anorexia, loss of weight, lethargy, and bone pain. The skin changes include pruritus; a rough, dry skin with desquamation; follicular keratosis; patchy erythema; purpura; and slowly progressive thinning of the hair. The lips become dry and cracked. Angular cheilitis is common (Fig. 33-26). In young children, painful swelling of the legs may occur from the bony changes. Pseudotumor cerebri may also be caused by excess intake of vitamin A; symptoms consist of headaches, increased intracranial pressure, papilledema, and the consequences of these signs and symptoms.

Carotenemia

Carotenemia occurs from eating large amounts of food rich in carotenoids, such as carrots. It may also occur during pregnancy or in patients with hyperlipidemia, such as diabetics, and in patients unable to convert ingested carotene into vitamin A. Unlike in patients with hypervitaminosis A, the liver is unaffected.

The stratum corneum, especially of the palms and soles, has an orange-yellow tinge similar to that seen in jaundice (Fig. 33-27). The sclera is not affected, however, as it would be in jaundice (Fig. 33-28).

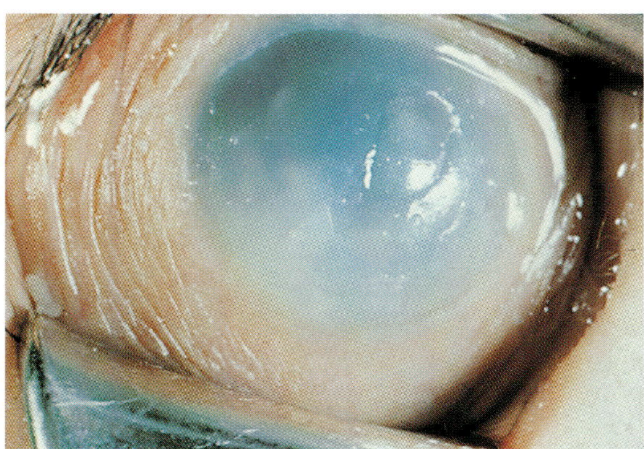

FIGURE 33-1. Xerophthalmia with pneumococcal corneal ulcer. There are severe, dry, lusterless conjunctiva and cornea with a central corneal infiltrate in this patient. (Courtesy of Dr. Mario Valenton.)

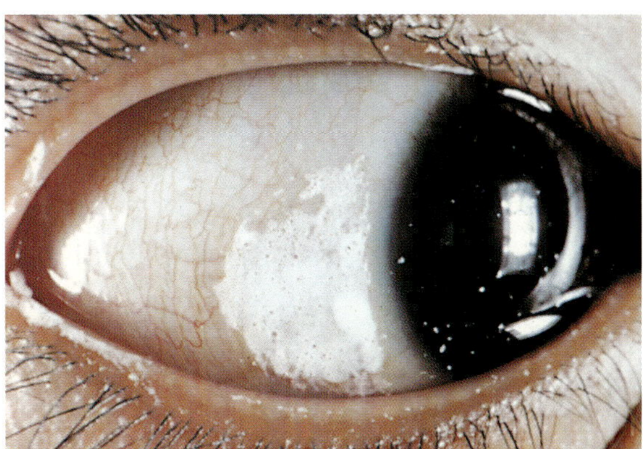

FIGURE 33-2. Bitot spot. (Courtesy of Dr. Mario Valenton.)

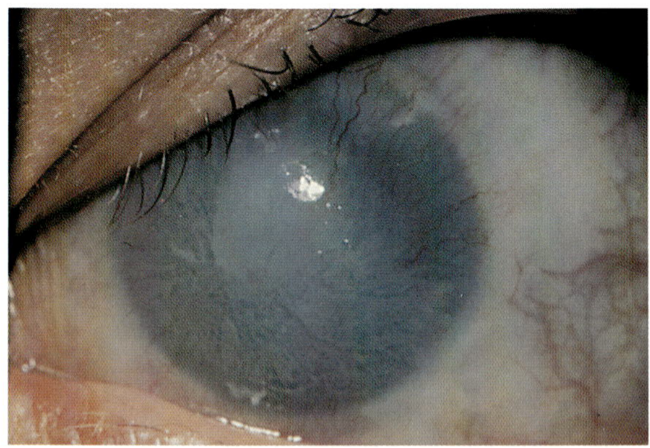

FIGURE 33-3. Dry, lusterless cornea in xerophthalmia.

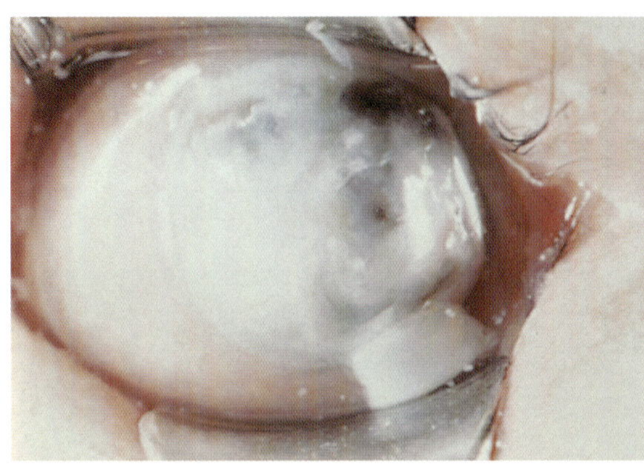

FIGURE 33-4. Corneal perforation in xerophthalmia. (Courtesy of Dr. Mario Valenton.)

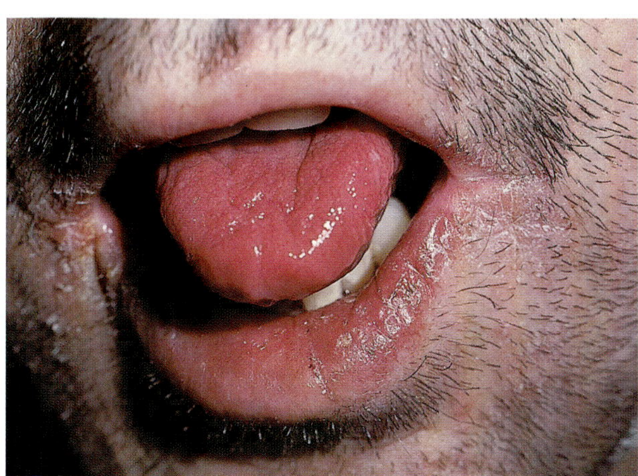

FIGURE 33-5. Vitamin B_2 deficiency showing angular cheilitis with atrophic magenta-colored tongue in an alcoholic patient.

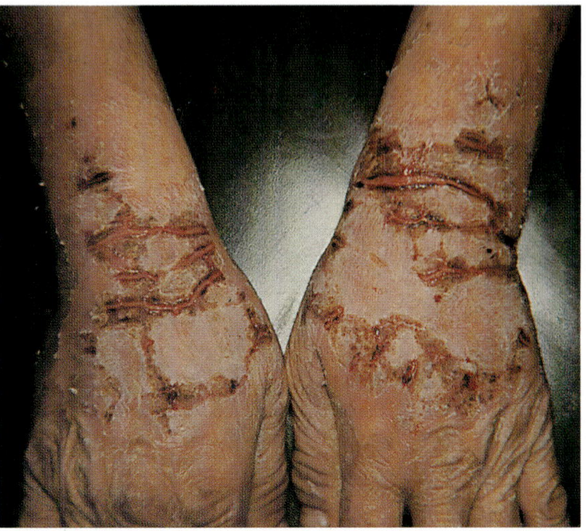

FIGURE 33-6. Sun-exposed sites of hands and wrists in an alcoholic patient with pellagra.

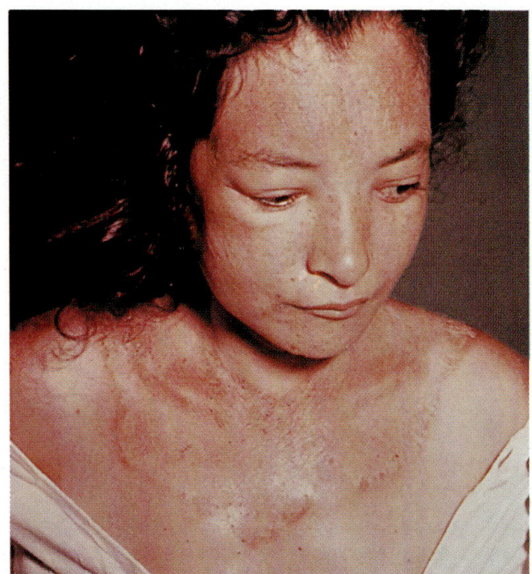

FIGURE 33-7. Hospitalized patient with advanced pellagra demonstrating the classic photo eruption of the upper chest known as Casal necklace. She also suffered with chronic diarrhea and dementia. (Courtesy of Dr. Bernard Gordon.)

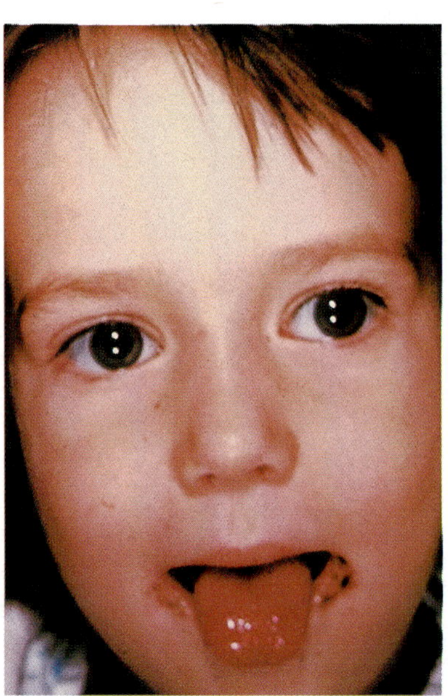

FIGURE 33-8. Pernicious anemia showing atrophic bright red tongue.

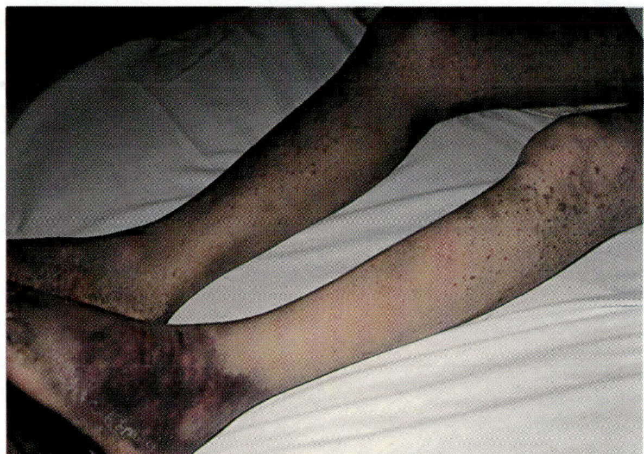

FIGURE 33-9. Scurvy in a 58-year-old man who, following the death of his parents, with whom he had been living, became severely depressed and lived for the preceding 4 months primarily on tea (without lemon) and crackers. The marked ecchymosis of his ankle was accompanied by hemarthrosis, as was his knee. His hematocrit was 18.

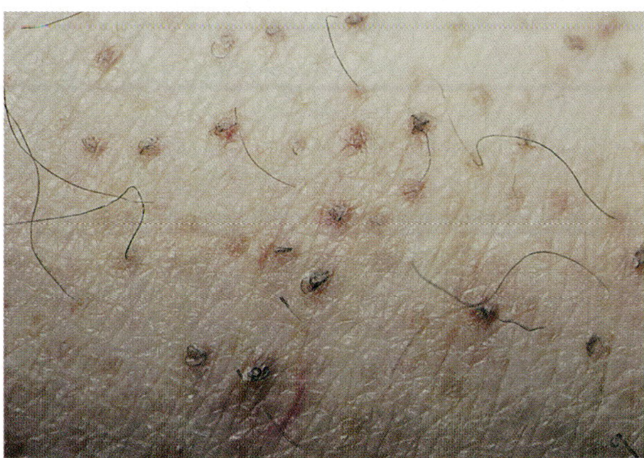

FIGURE 33-10. Perifollicular hemorrhages and "corkscrew" hairs on forearm in same patient as pictured in Fig. 33-9. When the patient was admitted to the hospital, he was lethargic and confused.

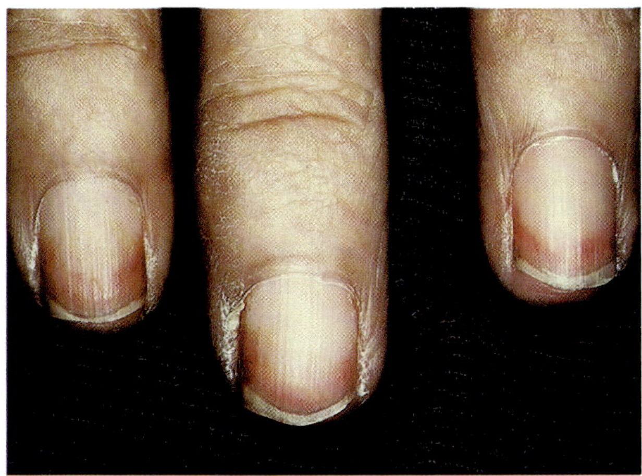

FIGURE 33-11. Subungual bleeding in scurvy.

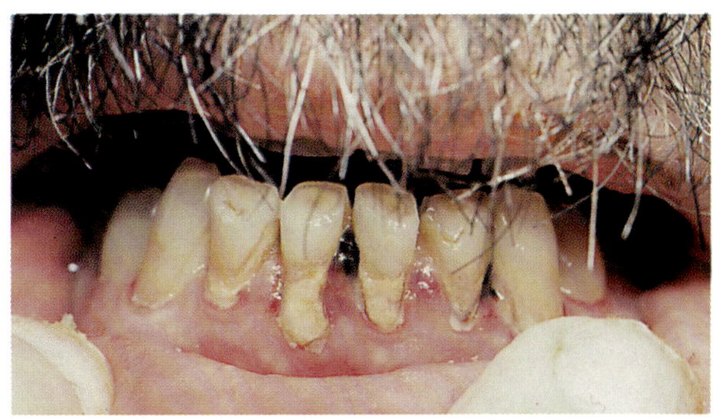

FIGURE 33-12. Gingivitis with swollen hemorrhagic gums (scurvy buds) in an elderly man with scurvy. His wife also had scurvy. Severe halitosis (fetor oris) was noticeable, as was depression.

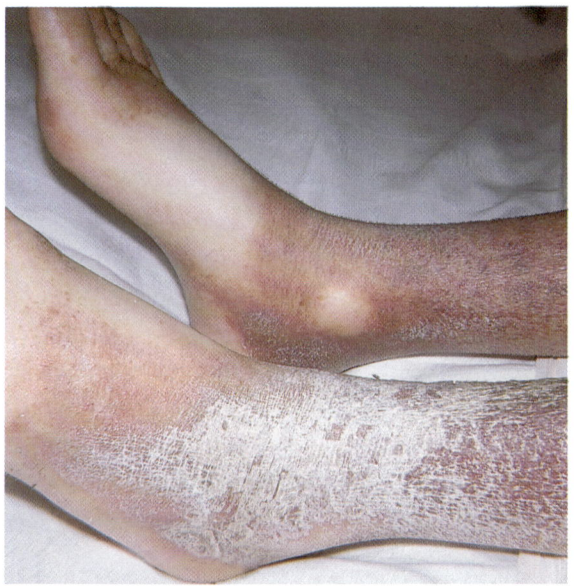

FIGURE 33-13. Chronic scurvy with "woody edema" of the lower leg and ankle.

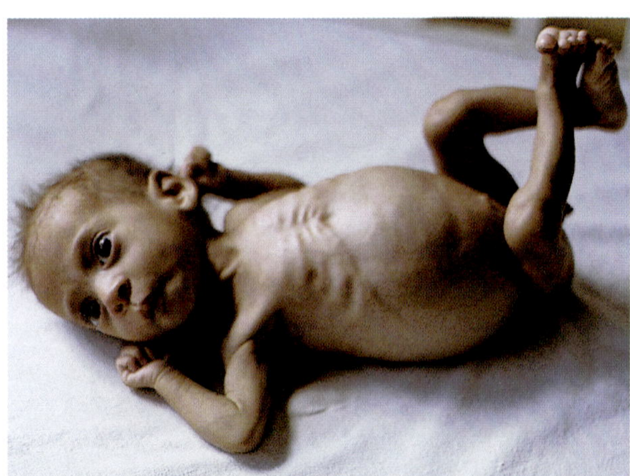

FIGURE 33-14. A young patient with a potbelly; spindly extremities; ribs showing; sparse, lackluster hair; and the apathetic expression so tragically characteristic of kwashiorkor and frequently associated marasmus.

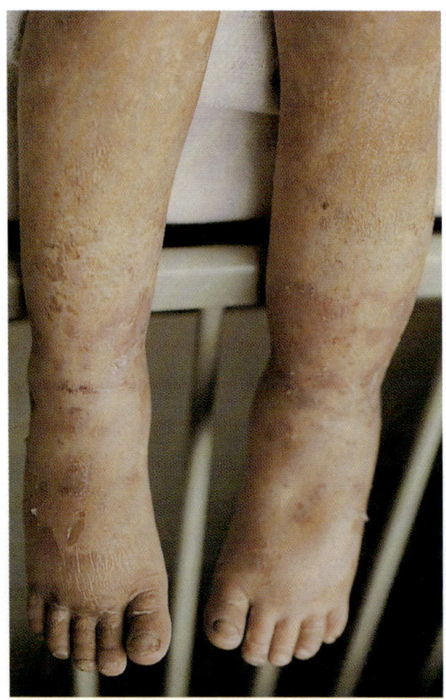

FIGURE 33-15. Edema and cracked desquamating skin sometimes referred to as "flaky enamel paint" or "crazy pavement pattern" in a 4-year-old boy with kwashiorkor.

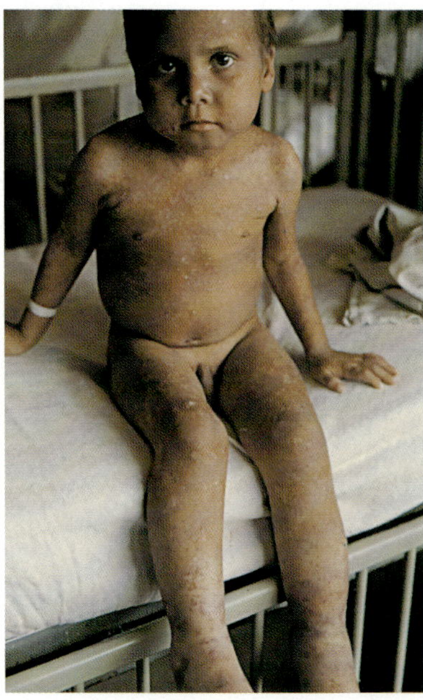

FIGURE 33-16. Kwashiorkor in a 4-year-old child with nine siblings. His diet consisted of rice, red kidney beans, molasses, and water. The liver was enlarged and the albumin/globulin ratio was 1.38/2.45. He had been in the hospital for 2 weeks when this photo was taken and still showed an apathetic expression. When seen 10 days later, he was able to smile. (Same patient as pictured in Fig. 33-15.)

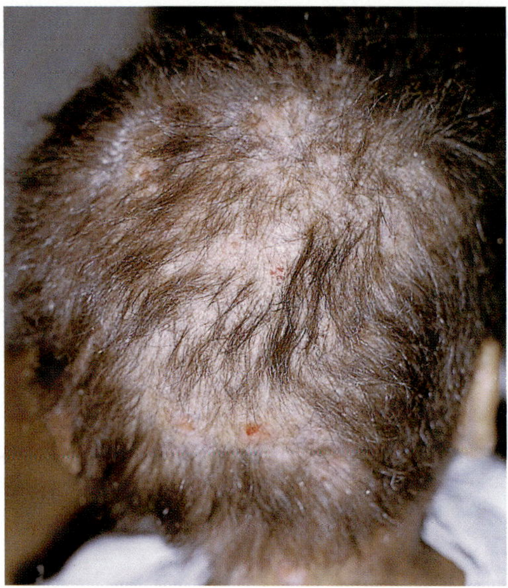

FIGURE 33-17. Hair in child with kwashiorkor showing sparse, lusterless appearance with scaling and inflammation of the scalp.

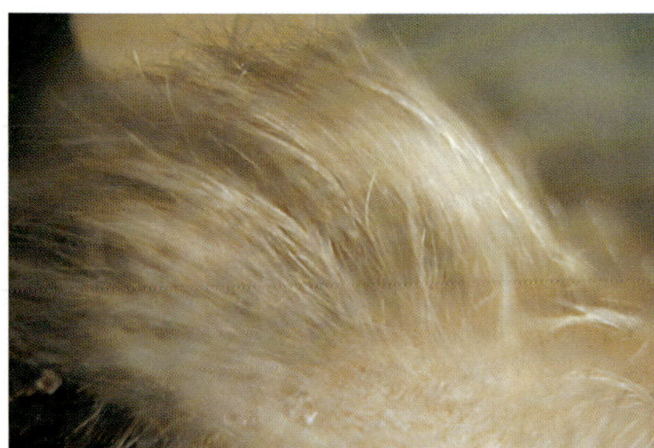

FIGURE 33-18. "Flag wave" sign, so called because of the alternating bands of light and dark hair, indicating periods of poor versus adequate nutrition.

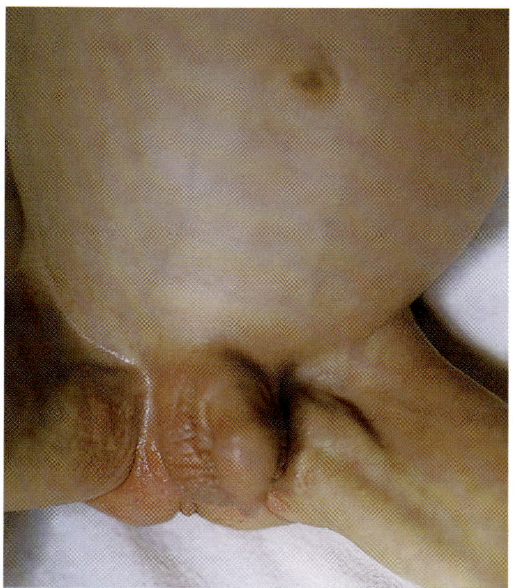

FIGURE 33-19. Scrotal and inguinal eczema commonly seen in kwashiorkor. Note the protuberant abdomen.

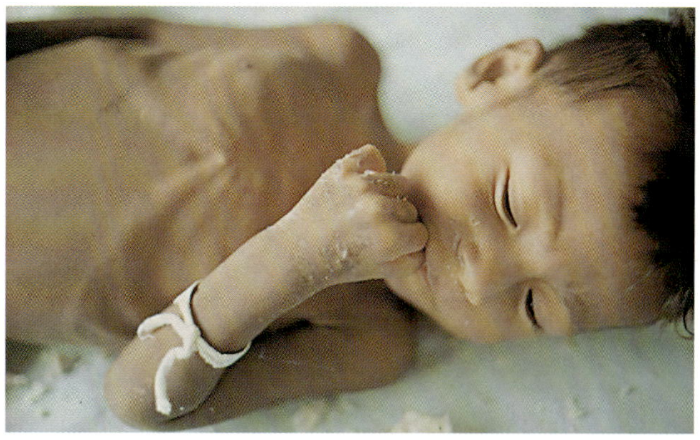

FIGURE 33-20. Marasmus and pellagra. This child had subsisted on sugar, milk diluted with water, and barley. With the onset of diarrhea (which may have been due, in part, to intestinal parasites as well as to the contaminated water), he was given milk further diluted. Note pellagroid scaling of dorsum of hand.

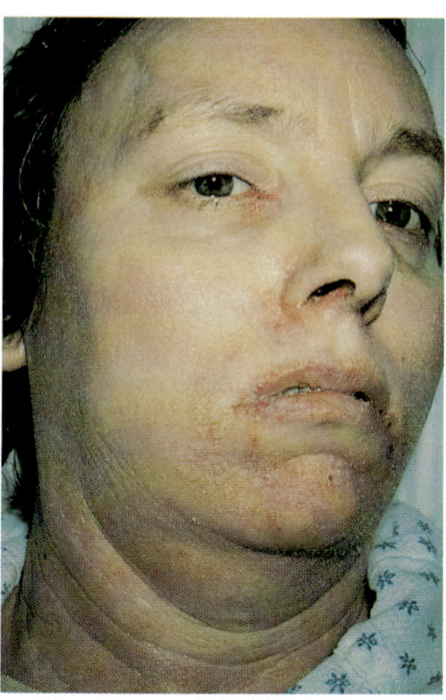

FIGURE 33-21. Zinc deficiency following jejunoileal bypass. The patient was receiving parenteral nutrition at a time when physicians were unaware that these products lacked adequate amounts of zinc. (Courtesy of Dr. John Reeves.)

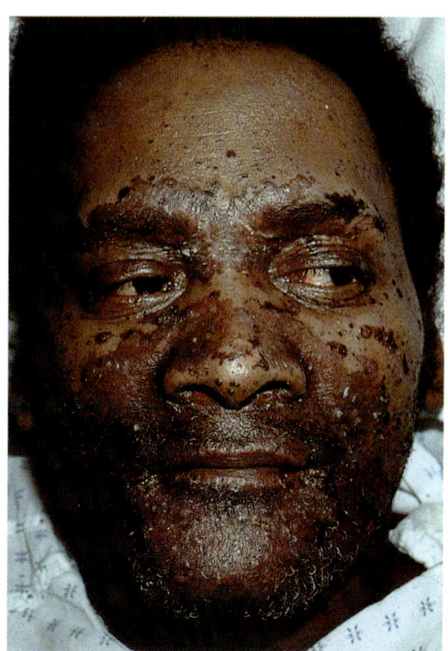

FIGURE 33-22. Zinc deficiency following gunshot wounds of abdomen requiring hyperalimentation before adequate zinc in this formula. (Courtesy of Dr. John Reeves.)

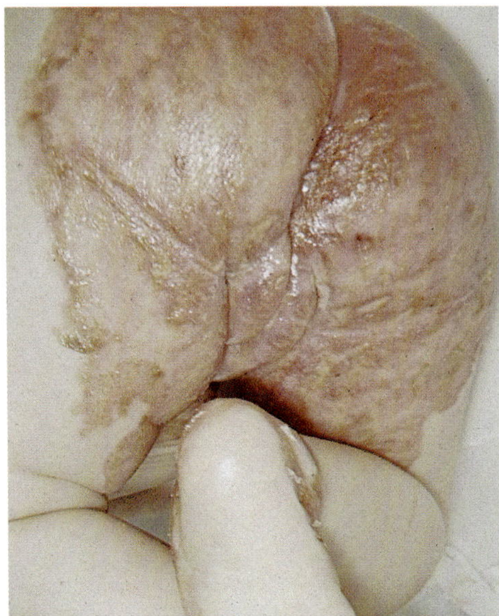

FIGURE 33-23. Acrodermatitis enteropathica showing extensive eczematous lesions in the anogenital and buttocks area. This baby also suffered from diarrhea, irritability, and alopecia.

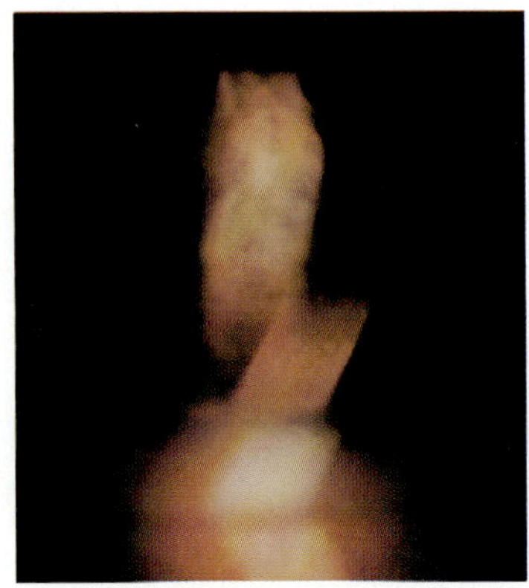

FIGURE 33-24. Kaiser–Fleischer ring in Wilson disease.

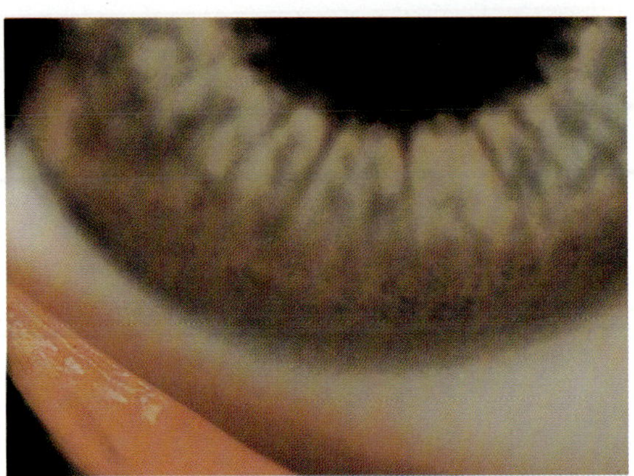

FIGURE 33-25. Kaiser–Fleischer ring in Wilson disease.

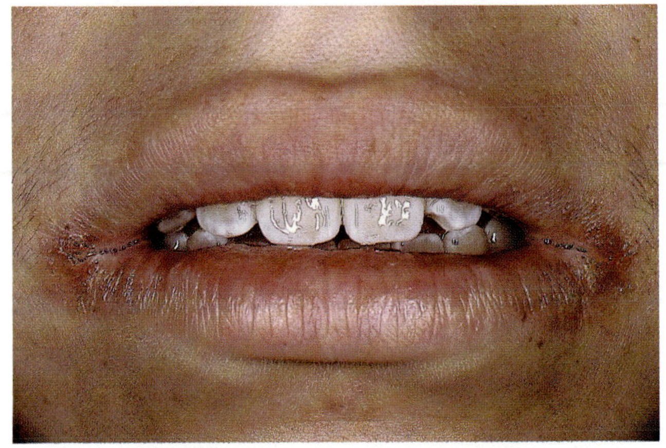

FIGURE 33-26. Angular cheilitis in patient with hypervitaminosis A due to treatment with Accutane.

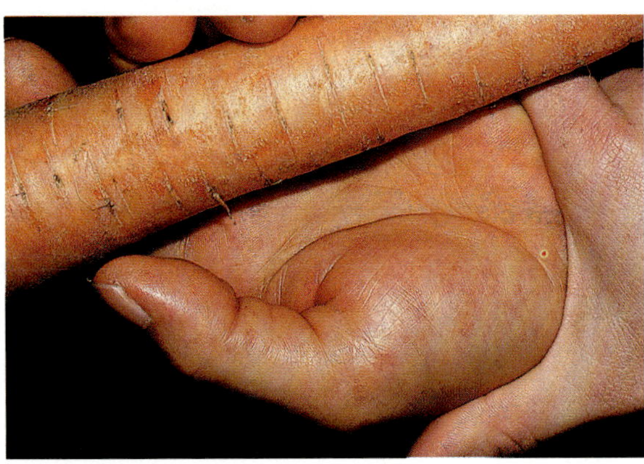

FIGURE 33-27. Carotenemia. This patient was drinking up to a quart of carrot juice per day in a futile attempt to treat carcinoma of the lung.

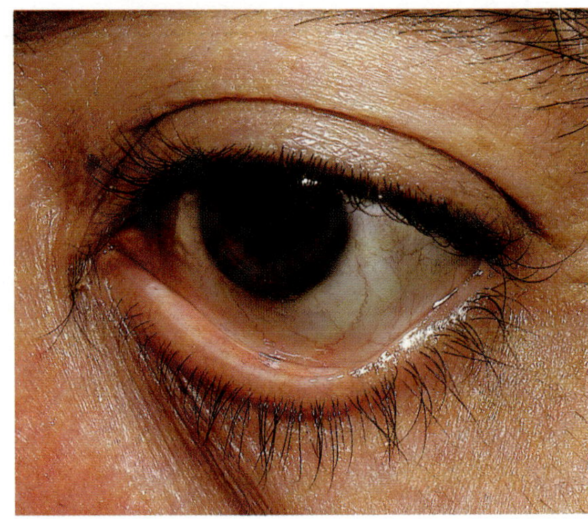

FIGURE 33-28. Carotenemia evident on the side of the nose. Note that the sclera is spared, a helpful finding to differentiate carotenemia from icterus. (Same patient as pictured in Fig. 33-26.)

Appendix

NOMENCLATURE AND GLOSSARY

A

Abscess   A focal collection of pus in a cavity produced by liquefactive necrosis of tissues.

Acantholysis (dermatology)   Separation of the prickle cells from each other.

Acrokeratosis (dermatology)   A hyperkeratotic skin lesion, usually of the extremities and occasionally of the nose or ear.

Allesthesia (ophthalmology)   A condition in which the sensation of a stimulus of one site is experienced at a point remote from that site.

Alopecia   Absence of hair (baldness) from an area that normally bears hair.

Anetoderma (dermatology)   Atrophy of the skin characterized by circumscribed translucent lesions that are wrinkled and baglike.

Aniridia (ophthalmology)   A congenital condition in which all of the iris except for its root is absent.

Ankyloblepharon (ophthalmology)   Complete fusion of the eyelids.

Ankyloblepharon filiform adnatum   Thin, finger-like adhesions of the eyelids.

Antihelix (dermatology)   An elevated ridge of cartilage anterior to the helix of the ear.

Antitragus (dermatology)   A projection of the cartilage posterior to the tragus.

Apocrine Gland   A coiled tubular gland that contributes part of its cytoplasm to the secretion.

Arrhinencephaly   A developmental defect of the brain.

Arthrogryposis   A congenital defect of the limb in which there are flexion and extension contractures.

Astichiasis (ophthalmology)   Lashes not arranged in rows.

Atrophoderma (dermatology)   Skin atrophy in circumscribed or widespread areas.

Atrophy   A loss of the epidermis, dermis, and/or subcutaneous tissue characterized by loss of the normal skin markings. In instances of sclerosis (see *sclerosis*), the epidermis may be atrophic, whereas the dermis and subcu-taneous tissue are thickened by a diffuse or localized induration.

B

Band-Shaped Keratopathy (ophthalmology)   Calcification of the superficial part of the cornea occurring in the shape of a band. The lesion usually occurs in the inter-palpebral fissure area.

Blaschko Lines (dermatology)   Anatomical markings that are indicative of embryologic cellular migration. They represent a nonrandom developmental pattern different from that of the dermatomes.

Blepharophimosis (ophthalmology)   Decrease in the aperture of the lid without evidence of fusion of the lids.

Blister   A fluid-filled vesicle in or under the epidermis.
   Intraepidermal Blister   A blister within the epidermis.
   Subcorneal Blister   A blister located under the horny layer of the epidermis.
   Subepidermal Blister   A blister located under the epidermis.

Bowman Layer (ophthalmology)   A thin, homogenous layer of the cornea located just beneath the epithelium.

Brachycephaly   A short skull.

Bromidrosis (dermatology)   Foul-smelling perspiration.

Brushfield Spots (ophthalmology)   Light areas in the outer one-third of the iris. They are seen in Down syndrome and in some normal individuals.

Bulla (pl. bullae)   A bulla is a large fluid containing blister (> 0.5 cm in diameter) that is located within or beneath the epidermis. Multiple bullae often develop during an intense inflammatory reaction (e.g., following burns or in an acute eczematous reaction to irritants), in drug reactions, and in pemphigus.

Bullar Shield (ophthalmology)   A type of plastic shield that can be applied over the orbit to help prevent drying of the eye through evaporation of the tears.

Buphthalmos (ophthalmology)   Enlargement of the eyeball during infancy resulting from glaucoma.

C

Camptodactyly A bent digit, especially a bent finger.

Canities (dermatology and ophthalmology) Grayness or whiteness of the hair.

Cellulitis (dermatology and ophthalmology) A diffuse acute inflammation of cellular tissue; it especially involves the deep dermis or subcutaneous tissue.

Central Serous Retinopathy (ophthalmology) Retinal or subretinal fluid in the area of the macula.

Chalazion (ophthalmology) A small granuloma of the meibomian gland.

Chilblain (perniosis) (dermatology) Dull erythema, itching, pain, and swelling, usually of the fingers, toes, or pinna resulting from a vascular response to low temperature and humidity.

Choanal Atresia Absence of the normal opening of the nose to the nasopharynx.

Chylothorax Accumulation of milky fluid in the thorax.

Clinodactyly Permanent deflection of one or more digits, especially the fingers.

Collarette (ophthalmology) This denotes a crust that is pierced by an eyelash, much like a piece of paper impaled on a stick. Collarettes are very suggestive of ulcerative blepharitis, such as is seen in staphylococcal lid infections.

Collarette of the Iris (ophthalmology) This denotes the iris frill that is present near the pupil.

Corps Rounds Cells showing premature partial keratinization histologically.

Coxa Valga (dermatology) Deformity of the upper end of the femur.

Crust (dermatology) Dried serum or secretion on the skin (a scab).

Cubitus Valgus Twisting in or bending in of the elbow.

Cyst (dermatology and ophthalmology) A normal or abnormal closed epithelial-, endothelial-, or membranous-lined sac containing fluid or a semisolid.

Cystic Hygroma A cystic swelling filled with serous fluid (usually located in the neck).

Cystoid Macular Edema (ophthalmology) Retinal fluid accumulated in cyst-like spaces in the area of the macula.

Cytoid Bodies (ophthalmology) Cotton-wool spots, which on histologic examination, resemble cells.

D

Dactylitis (dermatology) Inflammation of one or more digits, especially the fingers.

Deformation (dermatology and ophthalmology) A deformation represents a defect in form, shape, or position of an organ, part of an organ, or part of a body that arises from intrauterine mechanical forces. The body parts affected are usually musculoskeletal and arise from neuromuscular fetal problems.

Dermatoglyphics Fingerprints.

Deuteranopia (ophthalmology) Green color blindness.

Disruption A defect in form, shape, or position of an organ, part of an organ, or part of a body that arises from a destructive intrauterine influence, such as infection, circulatory compromise, or amniotic bands.

Distichiasis (ophthalmology) Two or more rows of lashes.

Dolichocephaly Elongation of the head.

Dystopia Canthorum (ophthalmology) Lateral displacement of the inner canthus. This condition is characteristic of Waardenberg type I syndrome.

E

Ecchymosis (dermatology and ophthalmology) A macular area of extravasated blood more than 2 cm in diameter.

Eccrine Gland A coiled tubular sweat gland other than an apocrine gland.

Elastosis Perforans (dermatology) A condition in which elastic tissue is expelled through the dermis.

Endophthalmitis (ophthalmology) Inflammation of the structures within the eye.

Ephelis (dermatology) A freckle.

Epicanthus (ophthalmology) A fold of skin running from the eyebrow to the root of the nose that overlaps the medial aspect of the interpalpebral fissure.

Epicanthus Inversus (ophthalmology) A fold of skin that runs from the medial aspect of the lower eyelid to the glabellar region.

Erosion (dermatology) Loss of the epidermis that heals without scarring.

Erosion (ophthalmology) Generally, a corneal erosion that is commonly recurrent; therefore it is called a recurrent erosion. The erosion represents loss of corneal epithelium and generally heals with minimal or no scarring.

Eventration Generally, protrusion of abdominal viscera through an open abdominal wall.

Excoriation (dermatology) A superficial loss of substance of the skin generally arising from scratching. It may be linear, sharply circumscribed, superficial, or deep. An excoriation is commonly found in prurigo and other causes of pruritus.

Exfoliation (dermatology) A desquamation or splitting off of the epidermal keratin layer in sheets or scales.

Exfoliation (ophthalmology) The appearance of a desquamation or splitting off of the anterior layer of the lens capsule. Generally, exfoliation of the lens capsule is called pseudoexfoliation and represents an abnormal deposit of material on the lens and sometimes on the iris.

Exomphalos Protrusion of the umbilicus.

F

Fibrosis (dermatology and ophthalmology) The formation of fibrous tissue or collagen, usually in the form of a scar.

Nodular Subepidermal Fibrosis The formation of fibrous tissue in the skin as a result of productive inflammation.

Proliferative Fibrosis The continued formation of fibrous tissue even after the initiating agent has ceased to exist.

Fissure (dermatology) A normal or abnormal cleft or groove in the skin surface.

Fistula (dermatology and ophthalmology) An abnormal sinus or passage leading from one structure to another or from a deep structure to the skin. Often it is lined with squamous epithelium.

Follicular Acuminate Papule (dermatology) A tapered or pointed papule in a follicle.

Follicular Atrophoderma Circumscribed skin atrophy surrounding the follicles in which the hair follicles remain open.

Freckle (dermatology) A light-brown pigmented macule probably resulting from the overactivity of melanocytes that are stimulated by ultraviolet irradiation.

G

Gangrene (dermatology and ophthalmology) Ischemic necrosis of tissue usually combined with invasion by bacteria.

Genodermatoses (dermatology) The genodermatoses comprise hereditary skin disorders that are determined by a single gene and are only minimally altered by environmental factors.

Gland of Moll Modified sweat glands found on the lid margin.

Gland of Zeis Sebaceous glands found on the lid margin and opening into the lash follicles.

Guttate (dermatology) In the shape of a drop.

H

Hamartoma (dermatology and ophthalmology) A benign (nonneoplastic) malformation composed of one or more tissues that are normal to the organ but are abnormally mixed and overgrown. Dermatologists also sometimes use the term to indicate absence of a particular tissue from the organ or to describe tissues that are normal anatomically but abnormal in function.

Hematoma (dermatology and ophthalmology) A localized tumor that is composed of effused blood.

Hemimelia A defect in the limbs.

Heterochromia (dermatology) The growth of hair of two distinct colors in the same patient.

Heterochromia (ophthalmology) Two distinct colors of the iris.

Holoprosencephaly (dermatology and ophthalmology) A developmental defect of the forebrain.

Hyaloid Artery (ophthalmology) Remnants of the fetal vessels that were present at the time of development of the eye.

Hypertelorism (ophthalmology) Wide-spaced eyes.

Hyphema (ophthalmology) Bleeding into the anterior chamber.

I

Iridodonesis (ophthalmology) Tremulousness of the iris that occurs from loss of support by the lens. It occurs when the lens is dislocated or has been removed. Separation of the anterior from the posterior layer of the iris.

J

Jaw-winking (ophthalmology) Drooping of the eyelid associated with lid movement during movement of the jaw. The condition arises from misdirection of motor fibers to the two areas.

K

Keratoconjunctivitis Sicca (ophthalmology) Literally, a dry eye.

Keratoconus (ophthalmology) A condition in which the central cornea becomes thin and ectatic, and forms a symmetric conical protrusion.

Keratoderma (dermatology) Hypertrophy or thickening of the horny layer of the epidermis.

Keratoglobus (ophthalmology) A diffuse corneal thinning most marked in the periphery.

Keratosis Pilaris Decalvans (dermatology) Loss of hair as a result of keratinization of the hair follicles.

Koebner Phenomenon (dermatology) Induction of a lesion in an area of physical trauma.

Reverse Koebner Phenomenon (dermatology) Clearing of a lesion in an area following physical trauma to that area.

Koilonychia (dermatology) Spoon-shaped nails with a concave surface, as seen in iron deficiency anemia.

L

Lagophthalmos (ophthalmology) Inability to completely close the eyelids.

Langerhans Cells Dendritic cells located in the epidermis that histologically have a rod or racket shape, a centrolinear density, and a clear cytoplasm.

Lentigo (dermatology) A small brown macule that histologically reveals melanocytic replacement of keratinocytes in the basal layer of the epidermis. (Note: A lentigo cannot be considered a junctional nevus because the dermis is not involved.)

Lester Iris (ophthalmology) Hyperpigmentation of the pupillary margin. It is seen in the nail–patella syndrome.

Leukonychia (dermatology) White spots in the nail.

Lichenification (dermatology) Lichenification represents a thickening of the epidermis that results in increased skin markings. It arises in response to prolonged or repeated rubbing.

Livido Reticularis (dermatology)   Purplish discoloration of the skin in a reticular pattern.

M

Macula, macule (pl. maculae, macules) (dermatology)   A macula is a flat, circumscribed patch or spot on the skin that possesses a color or texture different from the surrounding skin (e.g., a freckle). Maculae can be further classified as ephelides (multiple, irregular, circumscribed, smooth-pigmented spots); lentigines (irregular, circumscribed, smooth-pigmented spots that are darker and have a smoother margin than ephelides); and nevus spilus (a congenital speckled hyperpigmented macule of varied size).

The maculae that characterize many exanthemata consist only of localized patches of erythema arising from local vasodilation and mild inflammation. In purpura and hemosiderosis, maculae arise from deposition of blood pigments; in freckles, the maculae are due to excess melanin.

Macula (ophthalmology)   A corneal macula represents a faint gray or white scar, through which the details of the iris, although blurred, can still be distinguished.

Macula Retinae   Macula retinae represents a small spot, perceptively different from the rest of the retina, where the cones of the retina are highly concentrated. It is located about two disc diameters to the lateral side and slightly below the nerve head. Retinal blood vessels are not found in the macula; the fovea centralis is located in its center and gives a bright reflex.

Maculopapular (dermatology)   A maculopapular rash consists of both maculae and papules. It characterizes many of the exanthemata.

Madarosis   Loss of the lashes or eyebrows.

Malformation (dermatology and ophthalmology)   A primary abnormal development of a tissue or organ. Usually, it occurs as an isolated phenomenon and the affected child is otherwise healthy. Multiple malformations sometimes occur, however. When they occur in a recognizable pattern, they are thought of as a multiple malformation syndrome. Often they are associated with mental retardation.

Mamillations (dermatology)   Nipple-like projections.

Marcus Gunn Ptosis (ophthalmology)   Jaw winking.

Melanocyte (dermatology and ophthalmology)   A cell that bears or is capable of bearing pigment. The cell is capable of synthesizing melanosomes and contains the enzyme dihydroxyphenylalanine (DOPA).

Merkel Cell   A cell found in the epidermis, having a lobulated nucleus and characteristic membrane bound neurosecretory granules.

Milium (pl. milia) (dermatology)   A small, whitish nodule (cyst) on the skin containing lamellated keratin.

Mosaicism (ophthalmology and dermatology)   Composed of cells of more than one genotype.

Mutton-Fat Keratic Precipitate (ophthalmology)   A large precipitate on the posterior surface of the cornea resembling a glob of mutton-fat.

Myositis   Inflammation of the muscles.

N

Nevus (dermatology and ophthalmology)   A nevus represents a congenital localized skin or mucous membrane malformation in which there is an excess or deficiency of any one of the normal cutaneous structures.

Compound Nevus (dermatology and ophthalmology)   A melanocytic nevus having the histologic features of junctional activity along with the presence of nevus cells in the dermis. The nevi are usually pigmented.

Intradermal Nevus (dermatology and ophthalmology)   A nevus located only in the dermis (i.e., a collection of nevus cells in the dermis while the overlying epidermis shows no abnormality. These nevi are often nonpigmented clinically.

Junctional activity (dermatology and ophthalmology)   The presence of a group of melanocytes at the dermo-epidermal junction.

Junctional Nevus (dermatology and ophthalmology)   A melanocytic nevus in which large numbers of melanocytes are located at the dermoepidermal junction. Often a few nevus cells are also scattered in the underlying dermis.

Melanocytic Nevus   A hyperpigmented malformation of the skin arising from accumulation of melanocytes. A mole.

Nevus Spilus (dermatology)   A speckled mole with a smooth surface.

Nikolsky Sign (dermatology)   The ability to strip previously normal-appearing epidermis from the underlying dermis by tangential pressure on the skin.

Nodule (dermatology)   A solid lump measuring more than 0.5 cm in diameter. It is generally situated deep in the skin but can involve both the epidermis and dermis, the dermis and the subcutis, or the subcutis alone. The lump can usually be palpated or visualized. Nodules arise from neoplasia (epitheliomas), from aggregation of edema and inflammatory cells (erythema nodosum), or from granulomatous infiltration (lupus vulgaris).

Apple Jelly Nodules   Consisting of epithelioid tubercles, they are characteristic of lupus vulgaris and best seen by diascopy.

Busacca Nodules   These are small gelatinous nodules that are located on the surface of the iris in iridocyclitis.

Dalen–Fuchs Nodules   These are small nodules that are located in the choroid in sympathetic ophthalmia. The nodules are generally visible only histologically but occasionally can be seen with the ophthalmoscope.

Koeppe Nodules   These represent gelatinous nodules that occasionally develop at the pupillary border in iridocyclitis.

Rheumatic Nodule, Freol Node   These are cutaneous nodules in rheumatic disease that consist of noncaseating, palisading granulomata.

Sarcoid Granulomas   These are occasionally found in the conjunctival cul-de-sac. They appear as solid, often fleshy or yellow-colored nodules and are most commonly found in the inferior cul-de-sac attached to the bulbar conjunctiva.

Nodule (ophthalmology)   A nodule is a small solid lump of any size that can be visualized inside the eye.

O

Oculoglandular Syndrome of Parinaud (ophthalmology)   Granulomatous conjunctivitis associated with a grossly visible preauricular lymph node.

Oligophrenia   Defective mental development.

Onychia Striata (dermatology)   Linear streaks of the nail.

Onychogryphosis (dermatology)   Thickening, curvature, and increased length of the nail causing it to resemble a ram's horn.

Osteopoikilosis (dermatology)   Multiple small islands of dense bony tissue are found at the epiphyseal and metaphyseal ends of bones.

P

Pannus (ophthalmology)   A superficial fibrovascular membrane of the cornea.

Panophthalmitis (ophthalmology)   Purulent inflammation of all layers of the eyeball.

Papilla (pl. papillae) (dermatology)   Dermal papillae or papillae corii are small conical elevations that project from the dermis into the epidermis to interdigitate with the rete ridges of the epidermis.

Hair Papillae or Papillae Pili   These are the masses within the dermis upon which the hair bulbs rest.

Papilla (pl. papillae) (ophthalmology)   Conjunctival papillae are cone-shaped elevations that develop on the surface of the conjunctiva in response to inflammation. Each papilla contains a central core of vessels that branches over the surface of the papilla. Small conjunctival papillae when viewed with the naked eye give a velvety appearance to the conjunctiva. Giant conjunctival papillae give a cobblestone appearance to the conjunctiva and when viewed under magnification can often be found to contain several tufts of vessels that branch over the surface of the papilla. A conjunctivitis that is predominantly papillary in character is seen in the various types of bacterial conjunctivitis. Giant papillae are generally found in atopic keratoconjunctivitis, vernal keratoconjunctivitis, and giant papillary conjunctivitis arising from contact lens wear.

Bergmeister Papilla   This is a harmless remnant of the embryonic mesodermal tissue that commonly persists on the optic nerve head and can often be seen with the ophthalmoscope.

Lacrimal Papillae   These are cone-shaped elevations of the lid margin that contain the lacrimal puncta. They are located near the medial aspect of the lower and upper eyelid.

Papillary (ophthalmology)   Tiny, nipple-shaped elevations of the conjunctiva.

Papilloma (dermatology and ophthalmology)   An epithelial nipple-like mass in which the tumor projects from the surface of the skin or mucous membranes.

Papule (pl. papules) (dermatology)   A papule is a circumscribed, raised spot on the surface of the skin that is less than 0.5 cm in diameter.

Paronychia (dermatology)   Inflammation of the nail fold.

Pellucid Marginal Degeneration (ophthalmology)   A corneal degeneration in which the inferior cornea becomes thin and often ectatic.

Peridacryocystitis (ophthalmology)   Inflammation surrounding the lacrimal sac.

Perniosis (dermatology)   A cold injury (see *chilblain*).

Pes Equinus   A condition in which the patient walks on his toes.

Phthisis Bulbi (ophthalmology)   Degeneration and shrinkage of the eyeball.

Pili Torti (dermatology)   Twisted hair.

Pinguecula (ophthalmology)   A pinguecula is a small, yellow, triangular conjunctival elevation located in the medial and lateral aspect of the conjunctiva. The base of the triangle is located at the corneal side.

Plaque (dermatology)   A raised patch of skin measuring more than 2 cm in diameter. The lesion has a well-defined edge and a flat or rough surface.

Plaque (ophthalmology)   The term is limited to Hollenhorst plaques; these represent glistening cholesterol crystals (emboli from the carotid arteries) that are located within retinal arteries.

Poikiloderma (dermatology)   The variable association of skin atrophy, telangiectasia, and macular or reticulate pigmentation.

Poliosis (dermatology and ophthalmology)   Premature graying of the hair.

Polyhydramnios   Excess amniotic fluid.

Porencephaly   Presence of cavities in the cortex of the brain.

Porokeratosis (dermatology)   A keratotic lesions characterized by peripheral spread with a wall-like horny border and an atrophic center.

Posterior Subcapsular Cataract (ophthalmology)   A lens opacity that is located immediately anterior to the posterior lens capsule.

Protanopia (ophthalmology)   A form of color blindness that is characterized by retention of the sensory mechanism for two hues in the blue and yellow ranges, but not in the red and green ranges. Also described as red–green color blindness, it affects about 1% of adult males.

Pseudogerontoxon   An arcus of senilis-like opacity arising from prolonged hyperemia of the limbus.

Pterygium (dermatology)   An abnormal skin web or fold.

Pterygium (ophthalmology)   A weblike vascular conjunctival tissue that encroaches from either side on the superficial cornea in the interpalpebral space.

Pterygium Unguis   This represents a fusion of the dorsal nail fold to the nail bed, causing partial destruction of the nail.

Ptosis (ophthalmology)   Drooping of the eyelid.

Pustule (pl. pustules) (dermatology)   A skin bleb that is filled with pus. Pustules occur in or beneath the epidermis and are usually associated with the pilosebaceous unit or a sweat duct. Occasionally, they are seen on the glabrous skin. They are commonly found in staphylococcal infections, occasionally in other bacterial or in candidal infections, and infrequently in psoriasis.

Pyoderma (dermatology)   A pyogenic skin disease.

R

Raynaud Phenomenon (dermatology)   Episodic tricolor changes of the skin of the digits (blanching with numbness and pain followed by cyanosis, then redness with burning sensation).

Rete Ridge   The undulating shape of the dermoepidermal border caused by downward thickening of the epidermis between the dermal papillae.

Rubeosis (dermatology)   A peculiar, rosy reddening of the face and, occasionally, of the hands and feet. It is usually found in long-standing diabetes mellitus.

S

Scale (dermatology)   A thin flake of horny epithelium (stratum corneum) such as may be seen in psoriasis or in many other inflammatory disorders.

Collarette Scale   This represents a centrally detached but peripherally attached scale of the epithelium as classically seen in pityriasis rosea.

Furfuraceous Scale   A scale such as is seen in fine, loose dandruff.

Ichthyotic Scales   These are polygonal in shape and often quite large.

Scale (ophthalmology)   The term *scale* is generally not used in ophthalmology, whereas *scurf*, which properly means "a branny scale arising from the epidermis in dandruff," is commonly but often improperly used to denote the oily substance that is seen clinging to the eyelashes in seborrhea.

Collarette in Ophthalmology   See *collarette*

Collarette of the Iris   See *collarette*

Scaphocephalic   A long, narrow skull.

Scar (cicatrix) (dermatology and ophthalmology)   A mark that develops during the healing process of a wound or other injury. It is composed of fibrous tissue.

Atrophic Scar   A mark that is thin and wrinkled.

Hypertrophic Scar   A mark in which the fibrous tissue is elevated and excessive.

Sclerodactyly (dermatology)   A term used to describe the tapering and cutaneous sclerosis or atrophy that occurs distal to the proximal interphalangeal joint of the digits. It is seen in Raynaud phenomenon, mixed connective-tissue diseases, lupus erythematosus, dermatomyositis, scleroderma, pangeria, and various chemical poisonings.

Scleroderma (dermatology)   This constitutes a localized or generalized hardening of the skin. It may be seen in systemic sclerosis, localized and generalized morphea, lupus erythematosus, and dermatomyositis.

Sclerokeratitis (ophthalmology)   Inflammation of the sclera that extends to involve the adjacent cornea.

Sclerosis (dermatology)   This represents a diffuse or circumscribed induration of the dermis or subcutaneous tissues. When the dermis is involved, the epidermis is often atrophic.

Sclerosis (ophthalmology)   Nuclear sclerosis represents an aging form of cataract in which the nucleus of the lens becomes hardened and opaque due to compression of the lens fibers as the lens matures.

Staphyloma (ophthalmology)   A bulging of the choroid and sclera.

Sugiura Sign (ophthalmology)   Perilimbal depigmentation that serves as an early sign of onset of vitiligo in some patients.

Symblepharon (ophthalmology)   Adhesion of the eyelid to the eyeball.

Syndactyly   Webbing or fusion of the soft parts of the digits.

Synophrys (ophthalmology)   A continuity of the eyebrows at the midline.

Syringoma   A benign tumor of the sweat glands.

T

Taurodontia   Enlarged pulp cavity.

Thèque (dermatology)   An aggregate of four or more melanin-containing nevus cells in contact with the epidermal basal layer. The cells usually bud downward into the dermis.

Trichilemmoma (dermatology)   A benign tumor arising from the outer root-sheath of a hair follicle.

Trichorrhexis Invaginata (dermatology)   A condition in which the hair readily breaks within its sheath.

Tumor (ophthalmology)   A swelling or enlargement of tissue arising from any cause such as inflammation or proliferation of cells. The lesion may represent a benign or malignant lesion.

Tylosis (dermatology)   Diffuse keratoderma. Often indicates involvement of the palms and soles.

Tylosis (ophthalmology)   Hypertrophy, thickening, and deformity of the lid border, especially the posterior border. The lid border is red, thickened, and rounded. Loss of lashes usually accompanies the tylosis.

U

Ulcer (dermatology)　An ulcer is characterized by total loss of epithelium of the skin or mucous membrane. In many instances, some of the dermis is also involved; occasionally, there is loss of the underlying tissue. Ulcers generally develop from slough of necrotic tissue.

Ulcer (ophthalmology)　In ophthalmology, the term *ulcer* generally refers to the loss of the epithelium and often of Bowman layer and some of the corneal stroma. In such instances, the term *corneal ulcer* is used, which is then frequently modified by stating the location, other characteristics, or type of agent. Thus a corneal ulcer that seems to migrate toward the center of the cornea and away from the vascularized limbus is often called a *central corneal ulcer*, whereas an ulcer that remains confined to the peripheral cornea and appears to favor the area near the vascularized limbus is often called a *marginal* or *peripheral corneal ulcer*. In many instances, central corneal ulcers are associated with an intense anterior chamber reaction and the presence of pus (a hypopyon) in the anterior chamber, as manifested by a layer of cells in the inferior part of the anterior chamber; such ulcers are also called *hypopyon ulcers*. Infectious agents that can cause corneal ulcers include bacteria, fungi, viruses, and parasites.

Conjunctival Ulcers　These are uncommon and often are mistaken for a pseudomembrane because of the overlying mucous. Scleral ulcers are very uncommon and when they occur often are accompanied by loss of the overlying epithelium.

Dendritic Ulcer　A corneal dendritic ulcer is most frequently caused by herpes simplex infections. The ulcer generally involves the epithelium only, is linear, branches, and has bulbous ends.

Ulerythema (dermatology)　This term is derived from the Greek words *ul,* meaning "scarring," and *erythema,* meaning "redness." Generally, it connotes an erythematous follicular reaction that leads to cicatricial alopecia without pustulation having occurred.

Ulerythema Ophryogenes　Keratosis pilaris atrophicans faciei.

V

Vegetation (dermatology)　A luxuriant growth of pathologic tissue, often having a fungoid appearance.

Vesicle (pl. vesicles) (dermatology)　A small blister or sac (<0.5 cm in diameter) that contains fluid. Vesicles are usually grouped and are characteristically seen in herpes simplex infections. In eczema, the lesions are associated with papules.

W

Wernicke Pupil (ophthalmology)　A bilateral hemianopic pupil that may be caused by chiasmatic and optic track compression.

Wheal (dermatology)　A transient, white, or pinkish elevation of the skin arising in urticaria or from strokes to the skin. The lesion is often surrounded by a red area, and the two combined represent the axon-mediated wheal and flare.

Wickham Striae (dermatology)　Fine, white striae that are often found on the surface of papules in lichen planus.

Y

Y-sutures (ophthalmology)　The normal lines in the lens formed by junction of the lens fibers.

SUGGESTED READINGS

OPHTHALMOLOGY

Albert DM, Jakobiec FA. *Principles and practice of ophthalmology,* 2nd ed. Philadelphia: WB Saunders, 2000.

Bohigian G, Valluri S. *Handbook of ocular infections, inflammation and external diseases,* 4th ed. Thorofare, NJ: Slack, Inc., 2000.

Fraunfelder FT, Roy FH, eds. *Current ocular therapy,* 5th ed. Philadelphia: WB Saunders, 2000.

Gold DH, Weingeist TA, eds. *Color atlas of the eye in systemic disease.* Philadelphia: Lippincott Williams & Wilkins, 2001.

Hoeprich, PD, Jordan MC, Ronald AR. *Infectious diseases: a treatise of infectious processes.* 5th ed. Philadelphia: JB Lippincott, 1994.

Mackie IA. *External eye diseases: a systemic approach.* Woburn, MA: Butterworth–Heinemann, 2004.

Mannis MJ, Macsai MS, Huntley AC, eds. *Eye and skin disease.* Philadelphia: Lippincott-Raven, 1996.

Michelson JB, Friedlaender MH, *Color atlas of the eye in clinical medicine.* St. Louis: CV Mosby, 1996.

Ostler HB, Ostler MW. *Diseases of the external eye and adnexa. a text and atlas.* Baltimore: Williams & Wilkins, 1993.

Spencer WH, ed. *Ophthalmic pathology: an atlas and textbook,* 4th ed. Philadelphia: WB Saunders, 1996.

Tasman W, Jaeger EA. *Duane's ophthalmology on CD-ROM,* vol. 23. Philadelphia: Lippincott Williams & Wilkins, 2003.

Tierney LM Jr, McPhee SJ, Papadakis MA, eds. *Current medical diagnosis and treatment.* 41st ed. New York McGraw-Hill, 2002.

Zierhut M, Thiel HJ, eds. *Immunology of the skin and the eye.* Buren, The Netherlands : Aeolus Press, 1998.

DERMATOLOGY

Aly R, Maibach HI. *Atlas of infections of the skin.* New York: Churchill Livingston, 1999.

Arndt KA, LeBoit PE, Robinson JK, et al., eds. *Cutaneous medicine and surgery.* Philadelphia: WB Saunders, 1996.

Bolognia JL, Jorizzo JL, Rapini RP. *Dermatology.* St. Louis: Mosby, 2003.

Callen JP, Greer KE, Paller AS, et al. *Color atlas of dermatology.* 2nd ed. Philadelphia: WB Saunders, 2000.

Callen JP, Jorizzo JL. *Dermatologic signs of internal disease,* 3rd ed. Philadelphia: WB Saunders, 2000.

Champion RH, Burton JL, Elbling, FJG, eds. *Rook/Wilkinson/Elbling textbook of dermatology,* 5th ed. Oxford: Blackwell Scientific Publications, 1992.

Epstein E. *Common skin disorders,* 5th ed. Philadelphia: WB Saunders, 2002.

Fitzpatrick TB, Johnson RA, Wolff K, et al. *Color atlas and synopsis of clinical dermatology,* 4th ed. New York: McGraw-Hill, 2000.

Freedberg IM, Eisen AZ, Wolff K, et al., eds. *Fitzpatrick's dermatology in general medicine,* 6th ed. New York: McGraw-Hill, 2003.

Habif TP. *Clinical dermatology,* 3rd ed. St. Louis: CV Mosby, 1996.

Harper J, Pembrey ME, eds. *Inherited skin disorders: the genodermatoses.* Oxford: Butterworth-Heinemann, 1997.

Larsen WB, Adams RM, Maibach HI. *Color text of contact dermatology.* Philadelphia: WB Saunders, 1992.

Litt JZ. *Drug eruption reference manual,* 8th ed. New York: Parthenon Publishing Group, 2002.

Lynch PJ, Edwards L. *Genital dermatology.* New York: Churchill-Livingston, 1994.

Maibach HI, Bashir SJ, McKibbon A. *Evidence-based dermatology.* London: B.C. Decker, Inc., 2002.

Moshella SL, Hurley HJ, eds. *Dermatology,* 3rd ed. Philadelphia: WB Saunders, 1992.

Odom RB, James WD, Berger TG. *Andrews' diseases of the skin,* 9th ed. Philadelphia: WB Saunders, 2000.

Reeves J, Maibach H. *Clinical dermatology illustrated: a regional approach,* 3rd ed. Philadelphia: FA Davis, 1998.

Tyring SK, ed. *Mucocutaneous manifestations of viral diseases.* New York: Marcel Dekker, Inc., 2002.

SUBJECT INDEX

Page numbers followed by f refer to figures; page numbers followed by t refer to tables.